CONTRIBUTORS

Lori R. Arent, MS
Rehabilitation Coordinator, The Raptor Center
University of Minnesota, St. Paul, Minnesota

Robert L. Bill, DVM
Associate Professor, Veterinary Physiology and Pharmacology
School of Veterinary Medicine
Purdue University, West Lafayette, Indiana

Joann Colville, DVM
Fargo, North Dakota

Keith Nelson Strickland, DVM, Dipl ACVIM (Cardiology)
Assistant Professor of Cardiology
Department of Veterinary Clinical Sciences
School of Veterinary Medicine
Louisiana State University, Baton Rouge, Louisiana

To Joann, Jeff, and Carolyn—my wife, son, and sister,
and my three best friends.
TC

To Ed, Edward, and William—the scientists I cherish.
And to the memory of my father,
Dr. David E. Bassert,
who first introduced me to
anatomy and physiology when I was eight.
JMB

Clinical Anatomy & Physiology for Veterinary Technicians

1

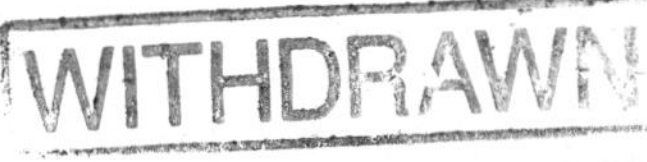

Clinical Anatomy & Physiology for Veterinary Technicians

Thomas Colville, DVM, MSc
Program Director, Veterinary Technology Program
North Dakota State University
Fargo, North Dakota

Joanna M. Bassert, VMD
Professor and Director, Program of Veterinary Technology
Manor College
Jenkintown, Pennsylvania

with 372 illustrations

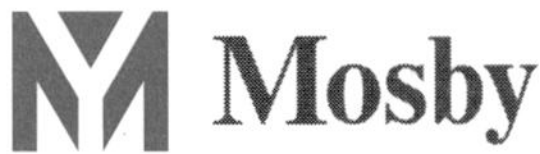

A Harcourt Health Sciences Company
St. Louis London Philadelphia Sydney Toronto

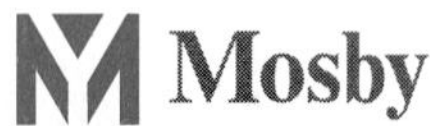

A Harcourt Health Sciences Company

Publishing Director: John A. Schrefer
Editorial Manager: Linda L. Duncan
Senior Developmental Editor: Teri Merchant
Project Manager: John Rogers
Designer: Kathi Gosche
Cover Art: Kathi Gosche

Notice

Pharmacology is an ever-changing field. Standard safety precautions must be followed, but as new research and clinical experience broaden our knowledge, changes in treatment and drug therapy may become necessary or appropriate. Readers are advised to check the most current product information provided by the manufacturer of each drug to be administered to verify the recommended dose, the method and duration of administration, and contraindications. It is the responsibility of the licensed prescriber, relying on experience and knowledge of the patient, to determine dosages and the best treatment for each individual patient. Neither the publisher nor the editor assumes any liability for any injury and/or damage to persons or property arising from this publication.

Mosby, Inc.
A Harcourt Health Sciences Company
11830 Westline Industrial Drive
St. Louis, Missouri 63146

Printed in the United States of America

Library of Congress Cataloging in Publication Data

Colville, Thomas P.
Clinical anatomy and physiology for veterinary technicians / Thomas Colville, Joanna M. Bassert.
p. ; cm.
Includes bibliographical references and index.
ISBN 0-323-00819-4
1. Veterinary anatomy. 2. Veterinary physiology. I. Bassert, Joanna M. II. Title.
[DNLM: 1. Animals, Domestic—anatomy & histology. 2. Animal Technicians. 3. Animals, Domestic—physiology. SF 761 C727c 2002]
SF761 .C65 2002
636.089'1—dc21 2001032643

01 02 03 04 05 GW/RRD 9 8 7 6 5 4 3 2 1

Preface

Animals represent a fascinating array of forms. They may be vertebrates or invertebrates; large or small; feathered, scaled, or furred. They are beautiful, diverse products of our planet, carved by the evolutionary forces of a changing world. Even among mammals, which constitute a minute portion of the total number of animals on earth, there are remarkable differences in their sizes, behavior, diet, and abilities. But there are countless similarities among them as well. It would be impossible to write a single text that addresses all species of animals or even all species of mammals. This book, therefore, concentrates on the anatomy and physiology of those domestic species that are most often encountered by the veterinary technician in practice, such as cats, dogs, horses, and cattle. A separate chapter at the end of the book is devoted to birds. This is one of the first anatomy and physiology texts written specifically for the veterinary technician.

The text is lavishly illustrated with more than 370 drawings that clarify and enliven the chapter discussions. "Test Yourself" boxes are integrated throughout the chapters to emphasize important study points and reinforce learning. Key terms are highlighted in the text and included in an extensive end-of-book glossary.

For many veterinary technician students, the anatomy and physiology course offers a first-time glimpse into the inner workings of animals. It is an opportunity to leave the human-centered world and examine, at the systemic and cellular levels, the diverse ways in which the bodies of animals function. The digestive, reproductive, and musculoskeletal systems, for example, and the diseases that afflict them may be similar among various mammalian species but, at the same time, distinctly different from one another. The ability to understand and appreciate these similarities and differences is a critical part of veterinary science. It is what differentiates veterinary from human medicine.

As veterinarians, we have had the pleasure of examining, studying, and treating many animals. They have inspired us, humbled us, and taught us in countless ways. We, therefore, have incorporated clinically relevant material into each chapter, in the form of "Clinical Application" boxes, to share our experiences and enable the reader to connect the study of anatomy and physiology with the treatment of animals. Thus we hope this textbook not only will provide an introduction to anatomy and physiology of domestic mammals but also will inspire our readers to think independently and to consider the animal world as a whole. For in the face of such broad diversity among animals, the veterinarian and veterinary technician cannot rely exclusively on the information taught in school. There is simply too much to know. However, we are proud to offer you, within the contents of this text, a starting point and the building blocks for greater understanding. Use it well.

Thomas Colville
Joanna M. Bassert

ACKNOWLEDGMENTS

The development of a new book has many similarities to pregnancy. A lot of exciting commotion accompanies the start of the process. Then things seem to settle down, but there's a lot of activity going on that is not apparent to outside observers. The whole process concludes with the delivery of the finished newborn book. The gestation of this book involved a lot of work, humor, discipline, and creativity on the part of the team of people who helped us turn ideas and concepts into the educational resource you have in your hands. We would like to acknowledge the contributions of some of the key members of that team.

Dr. Robert "Pete" Bill helped originate the concept for this book and get the project off the ground. He also contributed two chapters. Dr. Joann Colville, Dr. Keith Strickland, and Ms. Lori Arent also took time out of their busy schedules to write chapters for the book. Our editors at Harcourt Health Sciences, Linda Duncan and Teri Merchant, were encouraging and helpful through all the ups and downs of the book's creation. Artist Don O'Connor transformed our many ideas and scribbles of illustrations into the finished images that comprise such an important part of this book. Ms. Nancy Lewis painstakingly compiled material for the book's glossary. To each of these people, and others who played roles in the book's development, we would like to express our sincere gratitude and admiration for a job well done.

Finally, we would like to thank the many English teachers who struggled to teach us to compose and organize complete sentences in an interesting and informative manner. This book is evidence that their efforts were not in vain.

Thomas Colville
Joanna M. Bassert

CONTENTS

CHAPTER 1

Introduction to Anatomy and Physiology

Thomas Colville

The animal body is an amazing machine. We usually don't think of it in these terms, but the study of anatomy and physiology is really the study of the animal machine, its parts, and how the whole thing works. The language of anatomy and physiology uses terms like *cells, tissues, organs,* and *systems,* but we're really talking about the remarkable parts of this extraordinary machine. "Parts is parts," but when we're discussing a *living* machine, the "parts" are really intricate and their functions extremely interrelated. As veterinary health care professionals, we must understand how animals are put together and how their bodies work. Fortunately, the animal body is fascinating to study in and of itself, but even more so when we consider how important normal anatomy and physiology are to animal health.

The various parts of the body must work together in near-perfect harmony to maintain the life and well-being of an animal. The interesting part of this truth is that the apparently simple and automatic states of life and health are not what they seem. Life is not simple and health is not automatic. Life is extraordinarily complicated, and health is the result of numerous things going just right. At first glance it seems like health is the normal state of affairs and disease and death result from some awful *outside* influences attacking the body. However, outside influences alone usually play smaller roles than we might think. Disease and death often result from the *absence of normal body structure and functioning.* Normal anatomy and physiology are critical to an animal's health and survival, and our knowledge of them is critical to our ability to *influence* the animal's health and survival in case of disease or injury.

ANATOMY AND PHYSIOLOGY

Anatomy and physiology describe two complementary but different ways to look at the animal body. **Anatomy** deals with the *form and structure* of the body and its parts—what things look like and where they are located. **Physiology** deals with the *functions* of the body and its parts—how things work and what they do. They are often studied as separate subjects, but such an approach makes it difficult to obtain a complete picture of how the amazing animal machine works. This book examines anatomy *and* physiology as we go along.

Table 1-1 Main Body Systems

System	Main Components
Skeletal	Bones and joints
Integumentary	Skin, hair, nails or hooves
Nervous	Central nervous system and peripheral nerves
Cardiovascular	Heart and blood vessels
Respiratory	Lungs and air passageways
Digestive	Gastrointestinal tube and accessory digestive organs
Muscular	Skeletal, cardiac, and smooth muscle
Sensory	Organs of general and special sense
Endocrine	Endocrine glands and hormones
Urinary	Kidneys, ureters, urinary bladder, and urethra
Reproductive	Male and female reproductive structures

We can approach the study of anatomy in different ways, for example, **microscopic anatomy** vs. **macroscopic anatomy.** Microscopic anatomy deals with structures so small we need a microscope to see them clearly, such as cells and tissues. Macroscopic anatomy, also called "gross" anatomy, deals with body parts large enough to be seen with the unaided eye, such as organs, muscles, and bones. Both aspects are presented in this book as we examine the animal body in detail. We also delve into the submicroscopic level occasionally to explain things occurring at the microscopic and macroscopic levels. Discussions at the submicroscopic level include the components that make up cells and the chemical molecules and ions that serve important roles in the body.

Another way to approach anatomy is to study individual *regions* of the body **(regional anatomy)** vs. individual *systems* of the body **(systematic anatomy).** In the regional approach, all the components of each region of the body are examined; for example, the anatomy of the neck (cervical) region would include all the cells, tissues, blood vessels, nerves, muscles, organs, and bones present in the neck. The problem is that the body is not always easy to subdivide this way and there is often overlap between adjacent regions; that is, where does the neck region end and the shoulder region begin? It's not always clear.

The systematic approach to anatomy, on the other hand, deals with the systems of the body, such as the nervous system and the skeletal system, as separate topics. The many interrelationships between the body systems can be described as the systems are examined. This approach lets us look at the whole body by breaking it down into clear, logical components. The main systems of the body are listed in Table 1-1. We will take a systematic approach to anatomy and physiology in this book, and in addition to these systems, we examine cells, epithelial and connective tissues, and blood, lymph, and immunity.

TEST YOURSELF

1. How does the anatomy of a muscle or bone differ from its physiology? Which describes appearance and location and which describes function?
2. How might abnormalities in an animal's anatomy or physiology have a negative impact on its health and well-being?

TERMINOLOGY

To be clear and accurate with descriptions of body parts, we have to use terms that leave no doubt as to their meaning. Terms such as *up, down, above, below,* and *beside* are not very useful because they depend on the orientation of the animal (upright, on its side, on its back, etc.). If an animal is lying on its left side, is its right lung *above* its left lung or *beside* it? If the animal stands up, what is the relationship between the lungs then? Even the position of the observer can make a difference in terms such as *left* and *right.* If a structure in an animal is located "to the right" of another structure, does the meaning change if the observer is facing the animal head-on or facing the same direction as the animal? Anatomical terms must have the same meaning regardless of the orientation of the animal or the position of the observer. Basic anatomical terminology is based on imaginary slices, called *planes,* through the animal body that can be used as points or areas of reference and on sets of directional terms that have opposite meanings from each other.

ANATOMICAL PLANES OF REFERENCE

There are four anatomical **planes of reference,** two of which are variations of each other. Each plane is an imaginary "slice" through the body that is oriented at right angles to the other two. The four reference planes (Figure 1-1) are as follows:

- **Sagittal plane:** A plane that runs the length of the body and divides it into left and right parts that are not necessarily equal halves.
- **Median plane:** A special kind of sagittal plane that runs down the center of the body lengthwise and divides it into *equal* left and right halves. It is also known as a midsagittal plane.
- **Transverse plane:** A plane across the body that divides it into cranial (head-end) and caudal (tail-end) parts that are not necessarily equal.
- **Dorsal plane:** A plane at right angles to the sagittal and transverse planes. It divides the body into dorsal (toward the back) and ventral (toward the belly) parts that are not necessarily equal. If an animal stands in water with its body partially submerged, the surface of the water describes a dorsal plane.

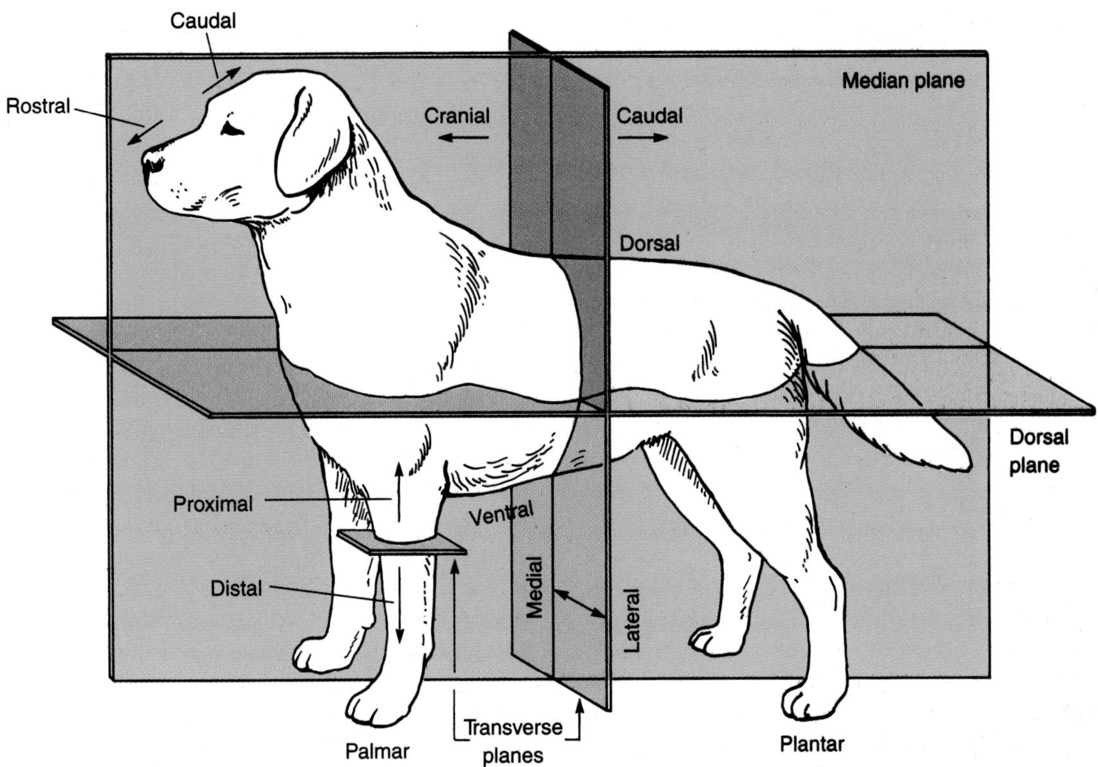

FIGURE **1-1** **Anatomical Planes of Reference and Directional Terms.** (From McBride DF: *Learning veterinary terminology,* ed 2, St Louis, 2002, Mosby.)

DIRECTIONAL TERMS

Directional terms in anatomy provide a common language for accurately and clearly describing body structures regardless of the position of the animal's body. These terms generally occur in pairs that have opposite meanings and are used chiefly to describe relative positions of body parts (Table 1-2).

Table 1-2 Directional Terms	
Term	**Definition**
Left	The animal's left
Right	The animal's right
Cranial	Toward the head
Rostral	Toward the tip of the nose (head only)
Caudal	Toward the tail
Dorsal	Toward the back
Ventral	Toward the belly
Medial	Toward the median plane
Lateral	Away from the median plane
Deep (internal)	Toward the center (whole body or part)
Superficial (external)	Toward the surface (whole body or part)
Proximal	Toward the body (extremity)
Distal	Away from the body (extremity)

- *Left* and *right* always refer to the *animal's* left and right sides. The spleen, an organ with several important functions, is located on the left side of a cow's abdomen. The duodenum, the first short portion of the small intestine, exits the stomach on the right side of a dog's abdomen.
- *Cranial* and *caudal* refer to the ends of the animal as it stands on four legs. **Cranial** means toward the head (cranium), and **caudal** means toward the tail (cauda). A horse's shoulder is located cranial to its hip. The caudal end of the sternum (breastbone) is called the *xiphoid process.*
- *Rostral* is a special term used only to describe positions or directions on the head. The term *cranial* loses its meaning on the head because the cranium is part of the head. *Caudal* retains its normal meaning on the head because it still means toward the tail end of the animal. **Rostral** means toward the tip of the nose (rostrum). An animal's eyes are located rostral to its ears.
- *Dorsal* and *ventral* refer to "up and down" directions or positions with the animal in a standing position. **Dorsal** means toward the back (top surface) of a standing animal, and **ventral** means toward the belly (bottom) of a standing animal. Dorsal and ventral are easiest to visualize in a standing animal, but they retain their meanings regardless of the animal's position. When preparing to ride a horse, the saddle is placed on the

animal's dorsal surface, and the cinch goes around the horse's ventral surface.

- *Medial* and *lateral* refer to positions relative to the median plane. **Medial** means toward the median plane (toward the center line of the body), and **lateral** means away from the median plane. The medial surface of an animal's leg is the one closest to its body. The lateral surface of the leg is the outer surface.
- *Deep (internal)* and *superficial (external)* refer to the position of something relative to the center or surface of the body or a body part. **Deep** means toward the center of the body or a body part. (**Internal** is sometimes used in place of deep.) **Superficial** means toward the surface of the body or a body part. (**External** is sometimes used in place of superficial.) The deep digital flexor muscle is located closer to the center of the leg than the superficial digital flexor muscle, which is located nearer to the surface of the leg.
- *Proximal* and *distal* are used to describe positions only on extremities, such as legs, ears, and tails, relative to the body. **Proximal** means toward the body, and **distal** means away from the body. The proximal end of the tail attaches it to the body. The toes are located on the distal end of the leg.

TEST YOURSELF

1. How does each of the anatomical planes of reference (sagittal, median, transverse, and dorsal) divide a cow's body?
2. If you are facing a cat head-on, is its left ear on your left or right side?
3. Why must the term *rostral* be used instead of *cranial* to describe structures on a hedgehog's head, but the term *caudal* works just fine?
4. If your left hand is on a goat's belly and your right hand is on its back, which hand is on the animal's dorsal surface and which is on its ventral surface?
5. The next time you see a dog, differentiate between the medial and lateral surfaces of one of its elbows and the proximal and distal ends of one of its legs.
6. If you insert a hypodermic needle into a horse's muscle to give it an injection, which end of the needle (tip or hub) is located deep in the muscle and which end is located superficially?

GENERAL PLAN OF THE ANIMAL BODY

Before studying the individual parts of the animal body, let's take a look at the overall arrangement of the body. Our focus is on the principle of bilateral symmetry, the two main cavities (spaces) in the body, and the levels of organization that make up the body.

BILATERAL SYMMETRY

Bilateral symmetry means that the left and right halves of an animal's body are essentially mirror images of each other. Although not absolute, the principle of bilateral symmetry accurately reflects the basic inner and outer structure of the body. Paired structures, such as the kidneys, lungs, and legs, are approximately mirror images. For example, in looking at your hands, you see that they are not identical (the thumb of one of your hands is where the little finger is on the other hand), but they are mirror images of each other. Paired internal organs are similar.

Single structures in the body are generally found near the center of the body—near the median plane. This is true of structures such as the brain, the heart, and the gastrointestinal (GI) tract. At first glance the GI tract does not seem to obey this rule. After all, it is extensively folded and more or less fills the abdominal cavity. Actually the GI tract *is* located near the median plane, but it is so long that it has to be intricately folded so it fits in the abdomen. If we were to stretch it out, it would form one long tube. Even with all its twists, turns, and convolutions, the GI tract does not wander far from the median plane.

BODY CAVITIES

The animal body has two main cavities (spaces)—a small dorsal cavity and a much larger ventral cavity (Figure 1-2).

Dorsal Body Cavity

The **dorsal body cavity** contains the brain and spinal cord, that is, the central nervous system. It consists of two parts—a somewhat spherical cranial cavity in the skull and a long, narrow spinal cavity running down the spine. The cranial cavity is also known as the **cranium.** It is formed from several bones of the skull, and it houses and protects the brain. The spinal cavity is also known as the **spinal canal.** It is formed from the vertebrae of the spine, and it houses and protects the spinal cord.

Ventral Body Cavity

The **ventral body cavity** is much larger than the dorsal one. It contains most of the soft organs (**viscera**) of the body. It is divided by the thin diaphragm muscle into the cranial thoracic cavity, also known as the *thorax* or *chest,* and the caudal abdominal cavity, also known as the *abdomen.*

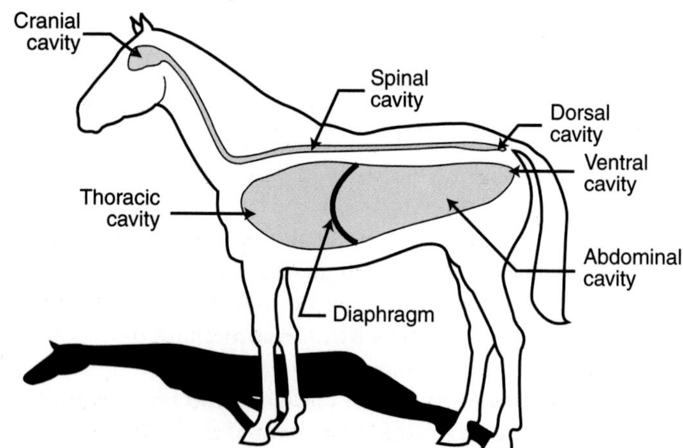

FIGURE 1-2 **Body Cavities.**

Major structures in the thoracic cavity include the heart, lungs, esophagus, and many major blood vessels coming to and going from the heart. All of the organs in the thoracic cavity are covered by a thin membrane called the **pleura.** Even the cavity itself is lined by pleura. The layer that covers the organs is called the **visceral layer** of pleura because it lies right on the **viscera** (the organs). The layer that lines the whole thoracic cavity is called the **parietal layer** of pleura. A potential space between the two layers is filled with a small amount of lubricating fluid. The smooth pleural surfaces lubricated by the pleural fluid ensure that the two surfaces slide over each other easily during breathing. If the pleural surfaces become thickened and roughened by inflammation, a condition called *pleuritis* or *pleurisy,* the surfaces scrape over each other with each breath, making breathing very painful.

The abdomen contains the digestive, urinary, and reproductive organs. It is lined by a thin membrane called the **peritoneum,** which also covers its contents. The visceral layer of peritoneum covers the abdominal organs, and the parietal layer lines the abdominal cavity. As in the thorax, a potential space filled with peritoneal fluid separates the two layers. Inflammation of the peritoneum (peritonitis) is very painful and most commonly results either from a wound that penetrates into the abdomen from the outside or from a rupture or perforation of the GI tract. When performing surgery on the digestive tract, we must take care to securely suture it closed to prevent leakage, which could lead to peritonitis.

TEST YOURSELF ✓

1. According to the principle of bilateral symmetry, single structures in the body are located on or near which anatomical plane of reference?
2. Where is the pleura found? The peritoneum?
3. What is the difference between the visceral and parietal layers of pleura and peritoneum?

LEVELS OF ORGANIZATION

Cells

Cells are the basic functional units of animal life—the smallest subdivisions of the body that are capable of life. A simple, single-celled animal like an amoeba has to carry out all the life functions necessary to support itself within its one cell. It must do things such as grow; respond to positive and negative stimuli; seek out, engulf ,and absorb food; eliminate wastes; and reproduce. It has no ability to influence its environment and has to take things as they come. If environmental conditions are favorable, the amoeba survives. If not, it dies.

In the complex animals we discuss in this book, the body's cells must divide the work. The sheer size of a dog or horse results in most of the animal's cells being far removed from the outside environment. The animal's body must create and support an internal environment that allows all of its cells to live and function. To accomplish this, cells must specialize in some functions and eliminate others. For example, some cells specialize in absorbing nutrients (intestinal lining cells), others in carrying oxygen (red blood cells), and still others in organizing and controlling body functions (nerve cells). A particular cell in the body depends on the rest of the body's cells all doing their jobs to ensure its survival. At the same time, all the other cells in the body rely on that cell doing its job to contribute to their survival.

Tissues

When specialized cells group together, they form **tissues.** The entire animal body is made up of only four basic tissues—epithelial tissue, connective tissue, muscle tissue, and nervous tissue.

Epithelial tissue is composed entirely of cells, and its main job is to cover body surfaces. The surface of the skin is covered by epithelium, as are the linings of the mouth, intestine, and urinary bladder. Epithelial tissue also forms glands, which are structures that secrete useful substances and excrete wastes. The secreting units of sweat glands, salivary glands, and mammary glands are all composed of specialized epithelial tissues.

Connective tissue holds the body together (connects its cells) and gives it support. Cells are very soft and cannot support themselves without outside help. Connective tissues range from very soft, such as adipose tissue (commonly called fat), to very firm, such as cartilage and bone. Connective tissues are composed of cells and a variety of nonliving intercellular substances, such as fibers, that add strength.

Muscle tissue moves the body inside and out. It exists as three types—skeletal muscle, cardiac muscle, and smooth muscle. Skeletal muscle moves the bones of the skeleton and is under conscious nervous system control. Cardiac muscle makes up the heart and works "automatically" (no conscious effort is required). Smooth muscle is found in internal organs such as the digestive tract and urinary bladder. It also works pretty much automatically.

Nervous tissue transmits information around the body and controls body functions. It transmits sensory information from the body to the brain, processes the information, and sends instructions out to tell the body how to react to changing conditions.

Epithelial and connective tissues are discussed in more detail in Chapter 4. Muscle and nervous tissues are more complicated, so each has its own chapter.

Organs

The next level up from tissues in complexity is **organs.** Organs are made up of groups of tissues that work together for common purposes. For example, the kidney is an organ composed of various tissues that function together to eliminate wastes from the body. Some organs, such as the eyes, lungs, and kidneys, occur in pairs. Others, such as the brain, heart, and uterus, are single structures.

Systems

Systems are the most complex level of body organization. Systems are groups of organs that are involved in a common set of activities. For example, the digestive system is concerned with obtaining, digesting, and absorbing nutrients to fuel the rest of the body. It is composed of the organs that make up the digestive tube, such as the esophagus, stomach, and intestine, as well as accessory digestive organs, such as the salivary glands, pancreas, and liver. Table 1-1 lists all the major systems of the body.

TEST YOURSELF

1. What is the difference between a cell, a tissue, an organ, and a system in an animal's body?
2. What are the four basic tissues that make up an animal's body?

HEALTH

The term **health** has a lot of meanings. Probably the simplest way to think of health is a state of normal anatomy and physiology. When the structures or functions of the body become abnormal, disease results. Maintaining health is a complicated process. In terms of the levels of organization of the body, the health of the body as a whole depends on the health and proper functioning of each of its systems, organs, tissues, and cells. On the other hand, each of the body's cells depends on the health and proper functioning of all the tissues, organs, systems, and the body as a whole. All structures and functions in the body are interrelated; nothing takes place in isolation. We can represent these interrelationships with the following diagram:

Body health ⇆ System health ⇆ Organ health ⇆ Tissue health ⇆ Cell health

HOMEOSTASIS

Imagine that you are driving a car. To reach your destination, you cannot just put the car in gear and then sit back, relax, and expect it to automatically take you there. You have to be actively involved in the process. You must accelerate to the proper speed, monitor and avoid other traffic, steer as the road twists and turns, accelerate up hills, brake while going down hills, stop when necessary, and generally oversee conditions and make adjustments throughout the journey. This description is an analogy for homeostasis in the body. The road is life, the car is the animal's body, and homeostasis is all the little inputs and corrections necessary to keep the body (car) alive (on the road).

Homeostasis is the maintenance of a dynamic equilibrium in the body. The word *dynamic* implies activity, energy, and work, and *equilibrium* refers to balance. Together they summarize all the physiological processes that actively maintain balance in the various structures, functions, and properties of the body. Consider this: An animal's body temperature cannot vary more than a few degrees from either side of the normal range without starting to interfere with other body functions. Or consider how acid-base balance, fluid balance, hormone levels, nutrient levels, and oxygen levels cannot vary by much if the body is to operate normally; they must be kept within fairly narrow operational ranges. The processes that monitor and adjust all the various essential parameters of the body are summarized by the term *homeostasis*.

Is some particular part of the body responsible for homeostasis? The answer is no. The *whole body* is responsible for homeostasis. All the body systems are involved in the many mechanisms of homeostasis, which require a lot of energy and work. Like all the little inputs and corrections that keep a car safely traveling down the road, the various homeostatic mechanisms in the body keep it functioning amid the twists and turns of life. To put it more mechanistically, the processes of homeostasis help maintain a fairly constant internal environment in the body as conditions inside and outside the animal change. Along with normal functioning of the body's cells, tissues, organs, and systems, the processes of homeostasis make life possible.

TEST YOURSELF

1. How does the normal anatomy and physiology of cells in an animal's body impact the health of the animal as a whole? How does the normal anatomy and physiology of the animal's body as a whole impact the health of its cells?
2. How do homeostatic mechanisms influence the health of an animal?

If you are beginning to view the concepts of life and health as a little less ordinary and more unique, you are starting to appreciate the amazing complexity of the animal body. Only by understanding what is normal in the body can we hope to help sick or injured animals. With this in mind, we can proceed with our examination of the fascinating machine that is the animal body.

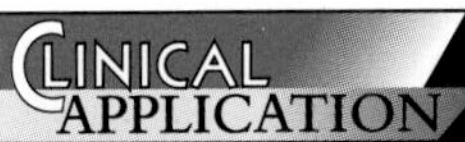

Homeostasis and Congestive Heart Failure

The processes in the body that try to maintain the functioning of a failing heart offer some excellent illustrations of how important homeostasis is as it attempts to maintain the health and life of an animal. *Congestive heart failure* is a clinical term used to describe a heart that is not pumping adequate amounts of blood. This results in blood "backing up" in the body, which produces congestion (abnormal fluid accumulation) upstream from the failing heart. There are many causes and forms of congestive heart failure, but the overall homeostatic mechanisms that attempt to maintain normal blood circulation in the body are basically the same.

The first indication that the heart is starting to fail is a drop in the cardiac output, that is, the amount of blood the heart pumps out per minute. The decreased blood flow and blood pressure are picked up by receptors in the vascular system and relayed to the central nervous system. Signals then go out to activate the sympathetic portion of the nervous system. This system, also called the "fight or flight" system, helps prepare the body for intense physical activity. Its effect on the cardiovascular system is to increase blood flow and blood pressure by stimulating the heart to beat harder and faster and constricting blood vessels. In the short term, these mechanisms help bring blood flow and blood pressure back up to normal levels.

Unfortunately, these compensatory mechanisms are causing a weak heart to work harder, which is kind of like whipping an exhausted horse to get it to move faster or pull harder. The result is a further weakening of the heart and further decreases in cardiac output. This causes more sympathetic nervous system stimulation. The cycle continues to repeat until either the heart gives up completely or we intervene with medical therapy. Homeostatic mechanisms cannot change the basic defects that are causing the heart to fail, but they help the damaged heart maintain vital blood flow to the rest of the body for as long as possible. By adding good medical care to the body's natural homeostatic mechanisms, we can often extend the length, and significantly increase the quality, of life.

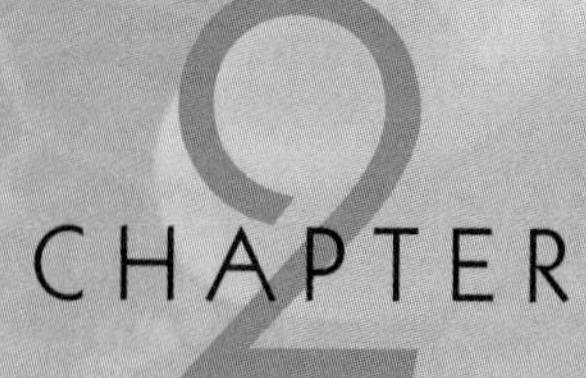

CHAPTER 2

THE AMAZING CELL

Joanna M. Bassert

The **cell** is the remarkable basic unit of living things. It can exist alone as a single, free, living plant or animal, or it can combine with other cells to form elaborate complex **organisms,** such as trees, horses, and people. The cell is dynamic and carries all of the functions by which life is defined. It can grow, develop, reproduce, adapt, become influenced by outside stimuli, maintain a stable internal environment, and convert food into usable energy. Each cell carries vital **genetic material** that governs its own **development, metabolism,** and **specialization.** A great diversity is seen in the appearance of cells. They can be small, biconcave red blood cells; long, thin **myofibrils;** or octopus-like **osteocytes.** Each form reflects its own specialized function (Figure 2-1). In a **multicellular** organism, such as a dog, cells have differentiated and become grouped into specialized tissues that work collaboratively to sustain life for the animal as a whole. These tissues, as well as the systems they form, are the focus of anatomy and physiology, but it is important to remember that their functional unit is the cell. It is *in* the cell that molecular messages are transmitted and received, electrical impulses generated, oxygen absorbed, and energy manufactured. Thus we must first learn about the *cell* before we can understand the anatomy and physiology of the tissues and systems they compose.

EVOLUTION OF CELLS

When our solar system was born about 4.5 billion years ago, the earth was fortunately placed at a distance from the sun that supported fairly stable and moderate temperatures that allowed molecular interaction. It was also of a size and density that afforded the formation of a protective atmosphere. Hydrogen, oxygen, carbon, and nitrogen—four elements that make up 95% of living tissue—were present on earth in the form of methane gas (CH_4), water (H_2O), and ammonia (NH_3). Energy from lightning storms and the sun may have caused these molecules to break apart and reform into organic molecules such as amino acids, the building blocks of **proteins.** Later, it is thought, the organic molecules were washed from the atmosphere by driving rains and aggregated into droplets in the warm, shallow seas below. When life actually began on earth is unclear, but these droplets are believed to have developed into the first cells nearly 3 billion years ago.

These primitive cells resembled present-day bacteria and contained a single strand of **deoxyribonucleic acid (DNA),** which floated freely in a gelatinous **protoplasm.** The cells did not possess a **nucleus** and were therefore called **prokaryotes,** which means "before nucleus." For 1.5 billion years prokaryotes were the only forms of life on this planet. **Eukaryotes** (meaning "true nucleus") developed later and are found in all multicellular organisms today. Eukaryotic cells are characterized by having a distinct nucleus in which the DNA has combined with protein to form chromosomes. These, in turn, are surrounded by a protective **nuclear envelope,** which, like a guard station, monitors the flow of molecules in and out of the nucleus.

THE CELL THEORY

In 1665 **Robert Hooke,** having made his own microscope, examined the structure of cork. He noticed that the cork was

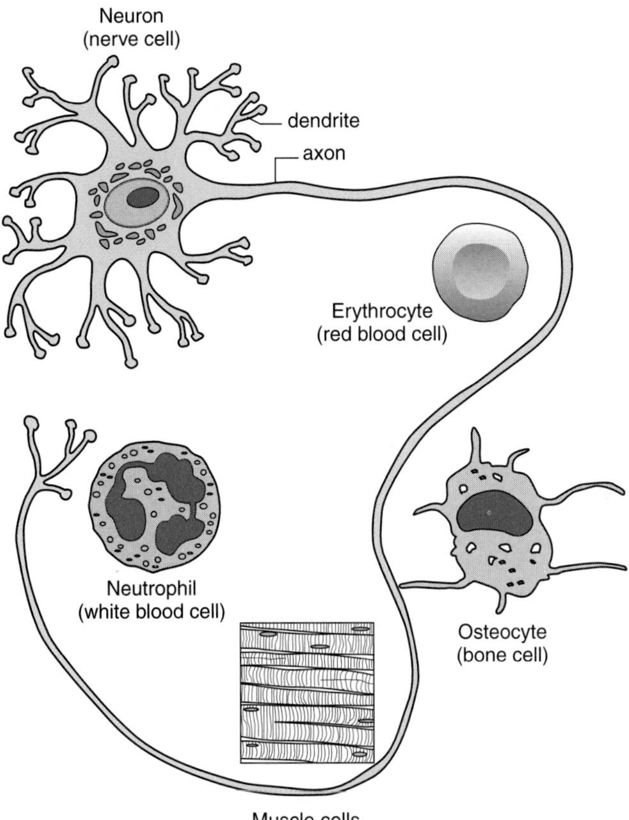

FIGURE **2-1** **Examples of Cell Types.** Differentiation and specialization of cells in the multicellular organism has led to a diverse array of cell types. Shape and size of the cell are related to its function.

composed of thousands of small rooms, and he called these rooms "cells" based on the Latin *cella* meaning "little chamber." He did not know at the time that the actual "cell," as we know it, had died and that he was actually examining the honeycomb-like structure of the remaining cell walls. Not until much later, in 1772, was the gelatinous inner protoplasm in living cells first observed; however, scientists did not understand the full ramifications of what they were seeing microscopically.

In the early nineteenth century, a definitive cell theory was born. **Mathias Schleiden,** who worked with plants, and **Theodor Schwann,** who worked with animal tissue, developed the theory that all living organisms are composed of cells. This seemingly simple theory had important and widespread ramifications for scientific research because, like the theory of evolution, it presented a unifying concept for the basis of life. Today we know that, with the exception of viruses, all living things are composed of one or more of these fundamentally similar units known as *cells.*

In 1858 a noted pathologist, Rudolf Virchow, expanded the cell theory by stating that modern cells can arise only from preexisting cells. This important concept challenged the widely accepted theory of spontaneous generation, which proposed that living organisms could spontaneously arise from fetid meat, garbage, or soil. Today, with the aid of electron microscopy, scientists have been able to learn even more about cells and how they work. For example, we now know that cells contain hereditary information, which is passed from mother to daughter cell, and that the chemical reactions of living organisms occur within the cell itself.

SIZE LIMITATIONS

The size of most animal cells is restricted to a range of 10 to 30 μm in diameter because of the relationship between the surface area and the volume of a cell. Small cells have smaller nutritional requirements than large cells but have a proportionately larger surface through which they can absorb the substances they need. Thus a small cell with a proportionately larger surface area will be able to complete its metabolic functions more rapidly and efficiently than a large cell with a relatively small surface area. In other words, if cells were the size of basketballs, they would not be able to take in nutrients fast enough to feed themselves and would die. A second limiting factor in cell size is related to the governing capability of the nucleus. A single nucleus can control the metabolic activity of a small cell better than a large one. Also, the more active a cell is, the greater are its metabolic needs. Therefore it is not surprising that some very large cells or cells that are very active, such as cardiac and skeletal muscle cells, have two or more nuclei. Also, these cells are long and thin, thereby creating a larger surface area through which nutrients can be absorbed. The combination of increased nuclei and expanded surface area enables muscle cells to function at a very high metabolic rate.

TEST YOURSELF ✓

1. What are the basic cellular functions that define life?
2. Describe the series of events that scientists believe led to the formation of the first cells on earth.
3. What is the difference between a prokaryote and a eukaryote?
4. Why are cells called "cells"?
5. Why aren't cells the size of watermelons?

MAMMALIAN CELL ANATOMY

Since their first appearance over 3 billion years ago, cells have evolved into diverse shapes and have taken on a wide range of specialized functions within multicellular organisms. Despite these changes and the **morphological** diversity that evolved among them, certain essential structures can be found in all mammalian cells. These structures are the **cell membrane,** the cytoplasm, and the nucleus (Figure 2-2).

All cells are separated from their environment by a cell membrane, which is also known as a plasma membrane or **plasmalemma** (plaz-ma-LEM-a; *lema* meaning "husk"). Everything inside the cell membrane other than the nucleus and genetic material is known as the **cytoplasm.** Cytoplasm is a

Clinical Application: Viruses and Prions: What Are They? Are They Alive?

There are many microorganisms called pathogens that cause diseases in animals. Many of us are familiar with bacteria and fungi, for example. We know that they are cellular and are found just about everywhere, such as on our skin, in soil, in air, on furniture, and even in the kitchen sink. Most bacteria and fungi therefore do not cause disease in healthy animals. Those bacteria and fungi that are pathogenic, however, cause diseases that often can be treated effectively with antibacterial and antifungal medications. But what about viruses and prions? What are they?

Viruses

Viruses are much smaller than cells and, unlike bacteria or fungal spores, are not visible with **light microscopy.** They are composed of a protein-covered capsule and contain either one strand of DNA or one strand of **ribonucleic acid (RNA),** but not both. Viruses are parasitic because they cannot live independently. They lack the biochemical mechanisms to reproduce by themselves and must rely on cells for the nutritional, structural, and molecular assistance needed to multiply. After attaching to a cell's surface, a virus injects its genetic material into the cytoplasm, where it interferes with the cell's normal metabolic processes, and in this way "reprograms" the cell to manufacture viruses—lots of them. Ultimately, the viruses rupture and kill the host cell, releasing hundreds of newly formed viruses into the extracellular environment, where they travel to other cells to continue the reproductive process.

Many diseases in animals are caused by viruses, including feline leukemia, canine parvoviral enteritis, rabies, western equine and eastern equine encephalitis, and bovine papular stomatitis. Many of the diseases caused by viruses can be prevented with immunization, but far more cannot be prevented. Viruses therefore continue to be a clinical challenge for many veterinarians. Although some antiviral medications are available, most animals infected with viral diseases are treated symptomatically.

Viruses, like bacteria and fungi, are considered to be alive. They are able to reproduce, grow, develop, adapt, respond to stimuli, and maintain a stable internal environment using energy resources from their environment. Prions, however, are pathogens that are not considered to be alive.

Prions

Prions are believed to be proteins or proteinaceous infectious particles. Although they lack DNA and RNA, they can cause both inherited and transmissible disease. This fact is surprising because it contradicts the long-held belief that transmissible diseases must possess nucleic acid (either DNA or RNA). All of the known prion diseases are fatal and cause a progressive neurodegenerative disorder that leaves grossly visible holes in the brain. Affected brains are said to resemble sponges; therefore the condition that they incur is called spongiform encephalopathy. **Scrapie,** which occurs in sheep and goats, is the most common prion-causing disease in animals. Afflicted animals lose coordination and become recumbent. They also become irritable, may develop tremors, and become highly itchy (pruritic), particularly over the rump. Often they scratch themselves until their coat is scraped off (hence the term *scrapie*).

Researchers, such as **Stanley Prusiner,** who won the Nobel Prize in 1997 for his work on prions, believe that prion proteins exist normally in all mammals. It is thought that normal prion proteins can be converted into deadly killers simply by changing their shape. In addition, the abnormal proteins can influence other proteins to change their shapes and become pathogenic as well. Many believe that the conversion of prions occurs inside neurons, specifically in enzyme-containing units called **lysosomes.** The lysosomes are filled with **enzymes** that normally break down nutrient molecules. However, the prions cause the lysosome to rupture, and the enzymatic contents spill into the cell. The cell subsequently digests itself and dies. The abnormal prions are then free to attack other cells. If enough cells are killed, prions can generate grossly visible holes in brain tissue.

Research studies indicate that animals may become infected with abnormal prions either by inheriting them from their dam or by ingesting the flesh, particularly the brain and spinal cord, of infected animals. The latter was presumed to have occurred in 1986 when a disease called mad cow disease, or **bovine spongiform encephalopathy (BSE),** first appeared in cows in Great Britain that were fed meat and bone meal from dead sheep. Humans can contract a fatal spongiform encephalopathy called **Creutzfeldt-Jakob disease (CJD).** Although the incidence of CJD in Great Britain has not increased, a new manifestation of the disease occurred among a cluster of British dairy farmers, which has raised questions about a possible link between CJD in humans and mad cow disease. Other prion-based diseases in animals include feline spongiform encephalopathy, chronic wasting disease in deer and elk, and transmissible mink encephalopathy.

colloidal, jamlike protoplasm that is highly structured and composed of proteins, electrolytes, **metabolites,** a flexible cytoskeleton, and complex structures called **organelles.** Organelles, like the organs in our own bodies, work collaboratively to carry out necessary metabolic functions (Table 2-1). As already mentioned, all mammalian cells are eukaryotic and therefore possess a nucleus, which contains vital genetic material in the form of chromosomes.

Cell Membrane

The cell membrane acts as a flexible, elastic barrier between the inner cytoplasm and the outside environment (Figure 2-3). It includes many infoldings and outpouchings that provide extra surface area and is continually removing and recycling different segments of itself, updating surface receptors, and renewing its sticky outer coating. Like our own skin, the cell membrane is capable of self-repair, but if damaged to the extent that intracellular contents are released, the cell quickly dies. The cell membrane governs the movement of atoms and molecules in and out of the cell. Although the actual consistency and complexity of the cell membrane are based largely on the function of the cell as a whole, cell membranes usually consist primarily of protein (55%) and **phospholipids** (25%) but also include quantities of **cholesterol** (13%), miscellaneous **lipids** (4%), and **carbohydrates** (3%).

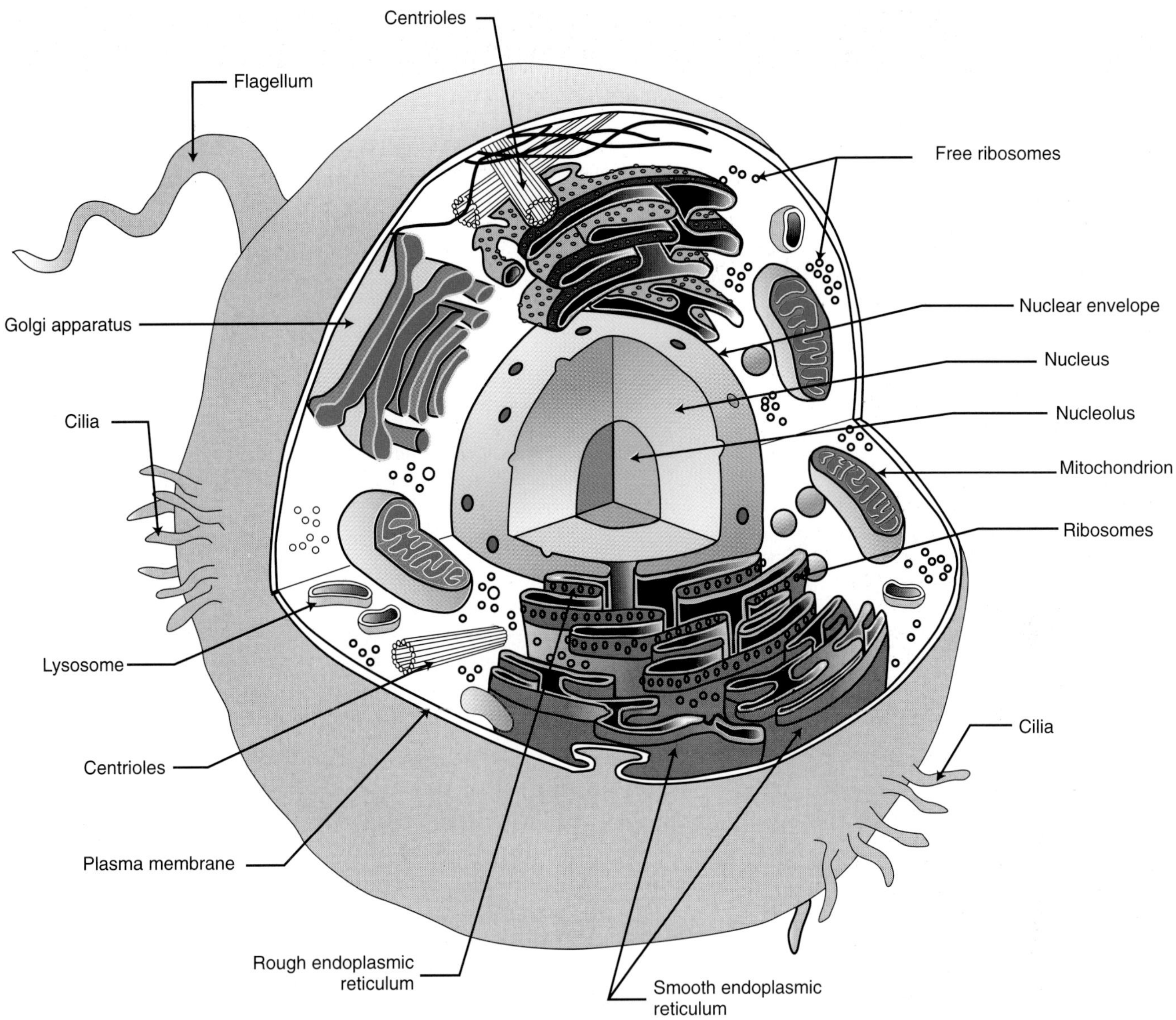

FIGURE **2-2** **Example of a Mammalian Cell.**

Membrane Structure

Because of its surprising thinness (about 60 to 100 angstroms), the cell membrane is not visible using light microscopy. Under the **electron microscope,** however, the cell membrane appears as two thin, dark layers with a seemingly empty space between them. At the molecular level, the cell membrane is composed of two layers of phospholipid molecules arranged so that the **hydrophilic** (soluble in water) "heads" are on the outside and the **hydrophobic** (not soluble in water) fatty acid "tails" are on the inside. This is called a **lipid bilayer.** Proteins that are suspended in the bilayer can move easily throughout the membrane to create a constantly changing mosaic pattern known as the **fluid mosaic.** Most lipid-soluble materials, such as oxygen and carbon dioxide molecules, pass through the membrane with ease, whereas ionized and water-soluble molecules, such as amino acids, sugars, and proteins (which are not lipid soluble), do not readily pass through.

The membrane also contains cholesterol molecules that wedge themselves between phospholipids and help to stabilize the membrane. In this way, cholesterol not only prevents the lipids from aggregating and therefore helps to keep the membrane fluid but also adds to the oily nature of the internal layer, which increases the membrane's impermeability to water-soluble molecules.

The cell membrane is composed of a wide variety of important structural and **globular proteins,** which are responsible for the membrane's special functions. Compact globular proteins may occur either on the cell surface or inside the lipid bilayer. Those that occur within the bilayer are called **integral proteins.** These molecules span the entire width of the mem-

Table 2-1 Anatomical Parts of the Cell

Morphology	Part	Description	Function
Cell Membrane			
	Cell membrane	Phospholipid bilayer with integral and peripheral proteins	Boundary between extracellular and intracellular compartments; controls passage of substances into and out of cell, maintains receptors for ligands
	Cilia	Fine hairlike structures on surface of cells; composed of nine pairs of microtubules arranged to encircle a central pair	Rhythmic beating propels mucus and debris across luminal surface of cell
Nucleus			
	Nucleus	Important "information bank" or "CEO of operations" for cell	Contains and processes genetic information; controls cell metabolism and protein synthesis
	Nuclear envelope	Double membrane–bound structure with pores; Outer membrane is continuous with endoplasmic reticulum	Separates nucleus from surrounding cytoplasm; controls movement of molecules in and out of nucleus
	Chromatin	Deoxyribonucleic acid (DNA) and proteins normally arranged in loose strands condense to form chromosomes during cell division	Regulates protein synthesis and other molecular interactions
	Nucleolus	Dense body containing ribosomal ribonucleic acid (RNA) and protein; nucleoli are not membrane bound	Location where ribosomal subunits are synthesized
Cytoplasm			
	Cytosol	Fluid containing dissolved electrolytes, nutrients, and protein	Media for transport of intracellular substances; contains enzymes needed for metabolic reactions

Table 2-1 Anatomical Parts of the Cell—cont'd

Morphology	Part	Description	Function
Cytoplasm—cont'd			
	Inclusions	Vesicles, vacuoles, and lipid droplets	Storage and transport of substances containing manufactured or absorbed substances
	Cytoskeleton	Protein arranged into microtubules and microfilaments	Strength, structure, and support; maintains cell shape, aids movement of organelles and intracellular materials
Organelles			
	Mitochondria	Double-membrane bound, internal cristae for expanded surface area	Site of adenosine triphosphate production from respiration
Nucleus	Endoplasmic reticulum (ER)	System of collapsed sacs extending throughout cytoplasm; rough ER has ribosomes on outer surface; smooth ER has no ribosomes	Transport and storage of materials in cell; synthesis of lipids, carbohydrates, and secretory proteins
	Ribosomes	RNA in combination with special proteins form large and small subunits; fixed ribosomes are found on rough ER; free ribosomes are scattered throughout cytoplasm	Site of protein synthesis
	Golgi apparatus	Network of connected flattened tubes or sacs stacked on top of one another	Packaging and alterations of substances for secretion or internal use; lysosome formation
	Lysosome	Vesicle filled with hydrolytic enzymes; pinches off Golgi apparatus	Digestion of absorbed material; autolysis
	Peroxisomes	Membrane-bound vesicle containing enzymes; produced by pinching in half	Detoxify various molecules such as alcohol and formaldehyde; remove free radicals

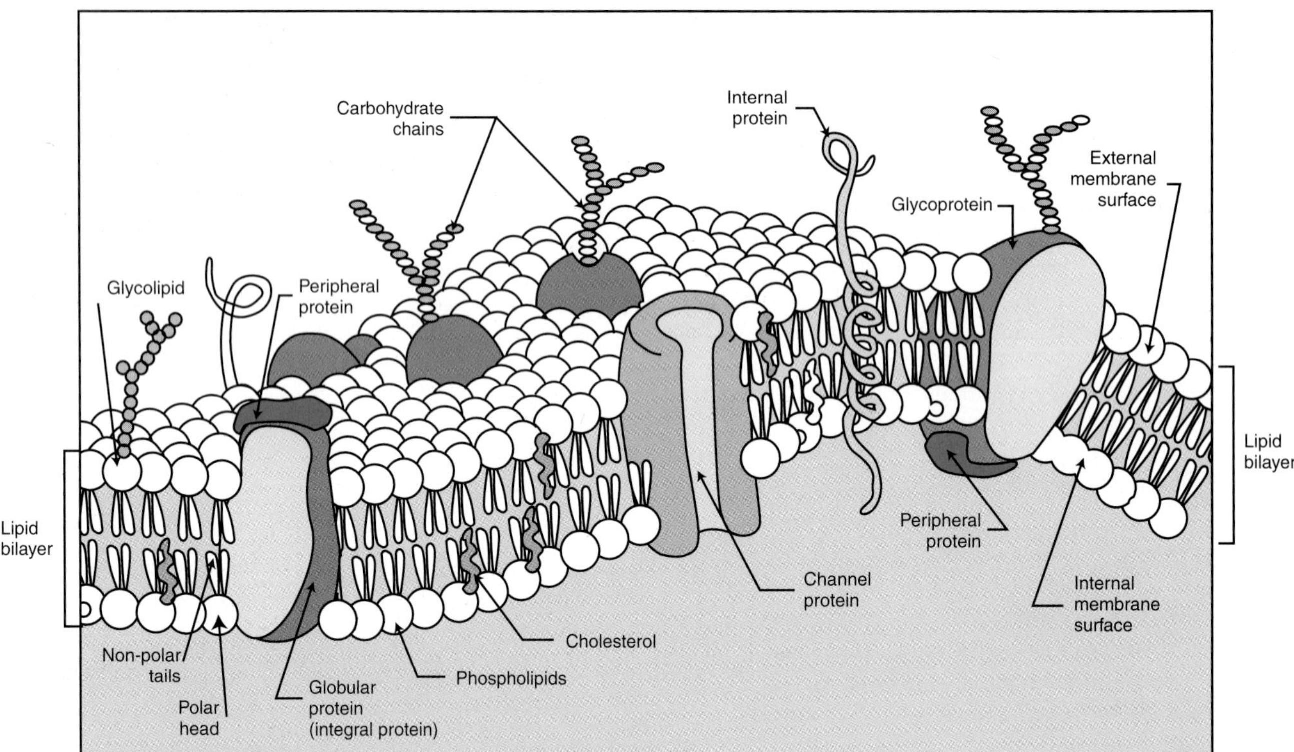

FIGURE **2-3** **Cell Membrane.** Cell membrane is composed of a lipid bilayer. Proteins help govern the movement of atoms and molecules in and out of the cell.

brane and may create channels through which other molecules can cross. Some integral proteins form selective passageways that permit only particular substances to enter or exit the cell, whereas others create **pores** (tunnels within the protein molecule) that allow substances such as water to pass through with no resistance. Pores are scattered over the surface of the cell and make up approximately 0.2% of the cell's surface area. Other globular proteins form **peripheral proteins,** which are bound to the inside and outside surfaces of the cell membrane. The inside peripheral proteins are more restricted in their movement than integral proteins because they are often attached to portions of the internal cytoskeleton or to the exposed parts of some integral proteins. Peripheral proteins sometimes act as enzymes to catalyze specific chemical reactions and may be involved in the mechanics of changing the cell's shape, an event which is quite dramatically seen, for example, during the contraction of a muscle cell.

The inner and outer layers of the cell membrane are different from one another. Proteins that reside on the inner surface of the membrane may be bound to components of the cytoskeleton, **keratin fibers,** or peripheral proteins. Phospholipids and the externally protruding ends of proteins on the outer layer, however, are attached to various sugar groups. These **glycoprotein** (sugar and protein) and **glycolipid** (sugar and phospholipid) molecules are the principal components of the "sugar coating" that covers the surface of some cells. This coating is called the **glycocalyx.** Like the stripes on zebras or the fingerprints on human hands, the glycocalyx is unique. It provides improved cell-to-cell adhesion and represents an important biological marker for intercellular recognition and for the interactions between the cell and antibodies and the cell and viruses. The interaction between the glycocalyx and extracellular molecules may incur changes in the membrane and possibly in the activity of the cell as a whole.

The glycocalyx is composed of two families of molecules: **cell adhesion molecules (CAMs)** and membrane receptors. CAMs are sticky glycoproteins that cover the surfaces of almost all of the cells in mammals and allow them to bond to extracellular molecules and to each other. These molecules are also important in helping cells move past one another and in signaling circulating cells, such as white blood cells, to areas of inflammation or infection.

Membrane receptors are integral proteins and glycoproteins that act as binding sites on the cell surface. Some of them play a vital role in cell-to-cell recognition, a process called **contact signaling.** This is particularly important during **cell-mediated immune responses** and assists bacteria and viruses in finding preferred "target" cells. Membrane receptors are also involved in a process called **chemical signaling.** Hormones, neurotransmitters, and other chemical messengers called **ligands** bind to specific binding sites on cell surfaces. Once bound to the cell membrane, ligands can bring about a change in the cell's activity. Some ligands act as enzymes to activate or inactivate a particular cellular activity.

Flagella and Cilia

Flagella and cilia are extensions of the plasma membrane that extend into the extracellular space. They are energetic, motile "hairs" that are structurally identical but function differently from one another. Cilia and flagella are composed of nine pairs of microtubules that encircle a central pair of microtubules. Both cilia and flagella originate from a pair of **centrioles,** called *basal bodies*, which are located at the periphery of the cell, just under the plasma membrane. During their formation, cilia and flagella grow outward from the basal bodies and exert pressure on the plasma membrane.

Cilia occur in large numbers on the exposed surface of some cells (Figure 2-4). They are shorter than flagella and measure only about 10 μm long. They move synchronously, one after the other, creating waves of motion that propel fluid, mucus, and debris across the cellular surface. Cilia are best known for their important functions (1) in the upper respiratory tract, where they propel bacteria and mucus away from the lungs, and (2) in the oviduct, where their beating motion pulls the ovulated egg away from the ovary and into the opening of the oviduct.

Flagella generally occur singly and are significantly longer than cilia. They are typically attached to individual cells and propel the cell forward by undulating. Flagella move cells through fluid, whereas cilia move fluid across cell surfaces. The tail of a sperm cell is an example of a **flagellum.** It is the only mammalian cell that is propelled by a single flagellum although many disease-causing organisms are propelled in this manner.

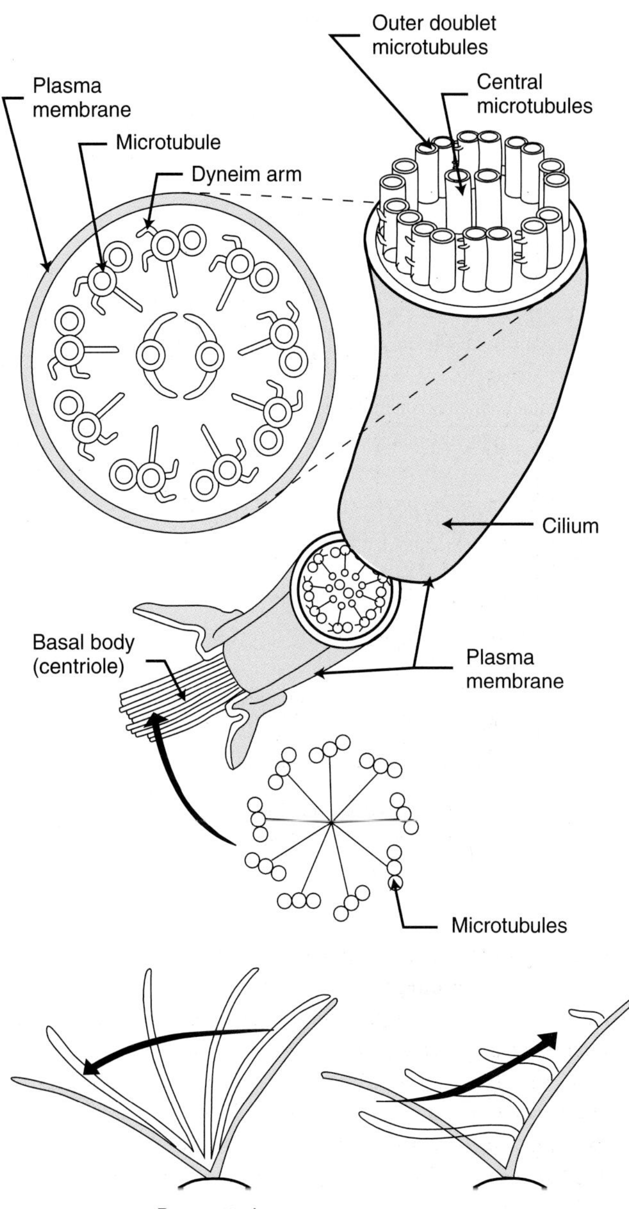

FIGURE **2-4** **Cilia and Flagella.** Cilia and flagella are composed of nine pairs of microtubules that surround a central pair. Cilia have a fast, powerful stroke in one direction. In the trachea, this helps to propel particles away from the lungs toward the mouth where they can be coughed up and swallowed.

TEST YOURSELF

1. Name three structures that all mammalian cells possess?
2. Draw a picture of the lipid bilayer. Which part is hydrophobic and which part is hydrophilic?
3. What types of protein are found in the cell membrane?
4. Where are the proteins located and what are their functions? Add them to your drawing.
5. What is the glycocalyx?
6. What are CAMs and what do they do?
7. What are membrane receptors and what do they do?
8. How are cilia and flagella different?
9. Which are found more commonly in mammalian cells: cilia or flagella?

Cytoplasm

The cytoplasm is the inner substance of the cell, excluding the nucleus. Initially seen under light microscopy, it appears as a nondescript bag of gel with a few opaque speckles. Now, with the increased use of electron microscopy, **cytologists** (*cyto,* "cell"; *ologist,* "one who studies") have the ability to visualize minute internal structures that define the complex internal workings of the cell. The principal components of cytoplasm are the cytosol, cytoskeleton, organelles, and inclusions.

Cytosol

The fluid of the cell is called **cytosol.** It is a viscous, semitransparent liquid composed of dissolved electrolytes, amino acids, and simple sugars. Proteins are also suspended in the cytosol and give it its thick, jellylike consistency. These proteins are mostly enzymes that are important in the metabolic activities of the cell.

Cytoskeleton

Like the skeleton in our bodies, the **cytoskeleton** is a three-dimensional frame for the cell; but unlike our bones, it is neither rigid nor permanent (Figure 2-5, *A*). It is a flexible, fibrous structure that changes in accordance with the activities of the cell. It gives support and shape to the cell, enables it to move, provides direction for metabolic activity, and anchors the organelles. Three different types of fibers comprise the cytoskeleton, all of which are made of protein. They are microtubules, intermediate fibers, and microfilaments (Figure 2-5, *B*). These fibers are not enclosed in a membrane.

The thickest fibers are the **microtubules,** which are long, hollow tubes that grow out from the cell center near the nucleus. They form secure "cables" to which mitochondria, lysosomes, and **secretory granules** attach. Proteins that act as "motors" move the attached organelles along the microtubule from one location in the cell to another. Because microtubules act as the "railroad tracks" for organelle travel, they can be easily disassembled and then reassembled to form new paths or to take on new direction. They appear, for example, in greater numbers during cell division to assist in the separation of chromosomes and organelles. Microtubules are composed of a pair of spherical molecules called **tubulins,** which are linked together into a spiraled chain. The spiral shape provides strength and flexibility to cilia and flagella, as well as to the cell as a whole.

Intermediate fibers are woven, ropelike fibers that possess high tensile strength and are able to resist pulling forces on the cell by acting as internal guy wires. These fibers are the toughest and most permanent element of the cytoskeleton. They are composed of different proteins depending on the

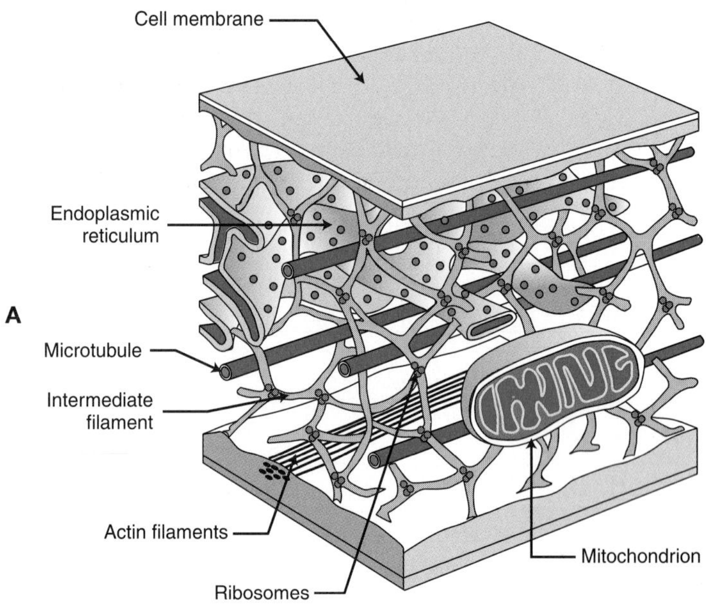

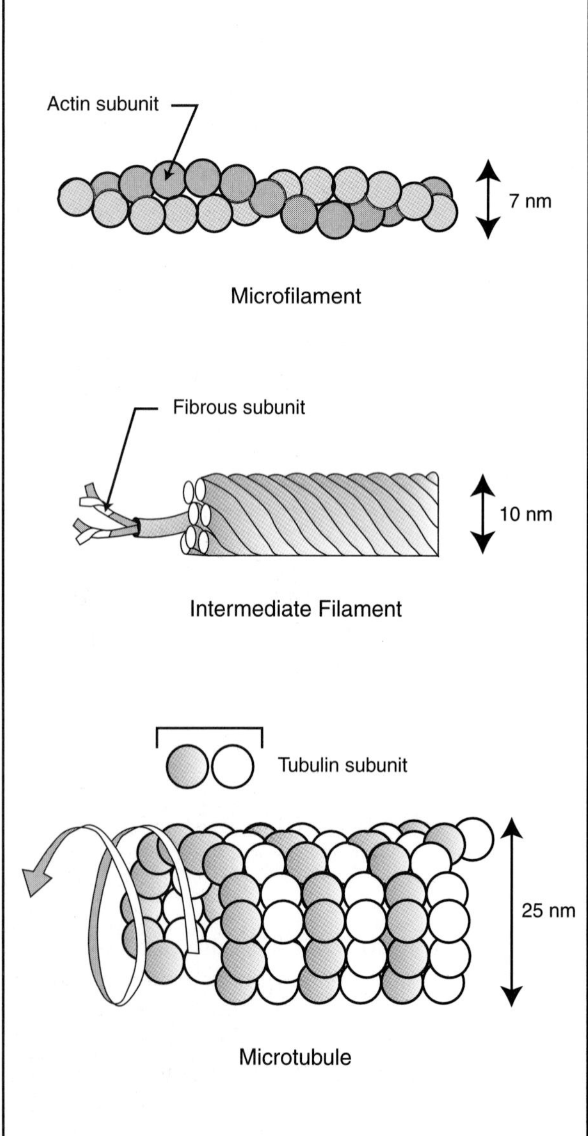

FIGURE **2-5** **Cytoskeleton. A,** Cytoskeleton is an important structural frame for the cell. It is strong, but flexible, and can be dismantled in some regions and rearranged as needed. **B,** Cytoskeleton is composed of three different types of fibers: microtubules, intermediate fibers, and microfilaments.

function of the cell and often take on different names depending on the type of cell in which they are found. In epithelial cells, for example, they are composed primarily of keratin and are known as *tonofilaments* or *keratin filaments,* whereas in nerve cells they are known as *neurofilaments.*

Microfilaments are located near the cell surface on the cytoplasmic side of the plasma membrane and are arranged in bundles and meshworks. They are composed of the contractile protein **actin** and, together with the motor protein **myosin,** play a key role in the cell's ability to change shape, break apart during cell division, and form outpouchings and involutions. In most cells, microfilaments are assembled where and when needed. Their position and quantity within the cell vary depending on the cell's activity. In muscle cells, however, the microfilaments are permanent, highly developed myofibrils, which shorten to cause muscle contraction.

Some cytologists believe that minute **microtrabeculae** exist as a fourth component of the cytoskeleton. These fibers are thought to form a lattice that interconnects larger cytoskeletal elements, suspends free ribosomes, and gives cytosol its jamlike consistency.

Organelles

Organelles, or "little organs," are membrane-bound structures within the cytoplasm that possess specialized cellular functions. The membranes of the organelles are similar in composition to those in the plasma membrane but do not have glycocalyx coatings. In this way, each organelle is separated from the surrounding cytosol and is able to maintain its own internal environment. This compartmentalization is crucial for effective metabolic processes because it enables the cell to separate and control various molecular interactions, which are the basis for food absorption, energy production, and excretion.

Mitochondria. Among the largest of the organelles is the mitochondrion (*plural,* mitochondria). This is known as the "powerhouse" of the cell because it produces 95% of the energy that fuels the cell. In the **mitochondria,** large nutrient molecules, such as glucose, are processed and broken down into smaller ones such as that can be used intracellularly to fuel most metabolic processes (Figure 2-6). It is also where respiration takes place: oxygen is consumed, and carbon dioxide is excreted. Numerous biochemical reactions, such as amino acid and fatty acid catabolism, respiratory electron transport, oxidative phosphorylation, and the oxidative reactions of the citric acid cycle, all occur in the mitochondria. (See Chapter 3 for more detailed descriptions of these metabolic processes.) Active cells, which have high-energy demands, have greater numbers of mitochondria within their cytoplasm than inactive cells. Heart cells, for example, have far more mitochondria than relatively inactive endothelial cells.

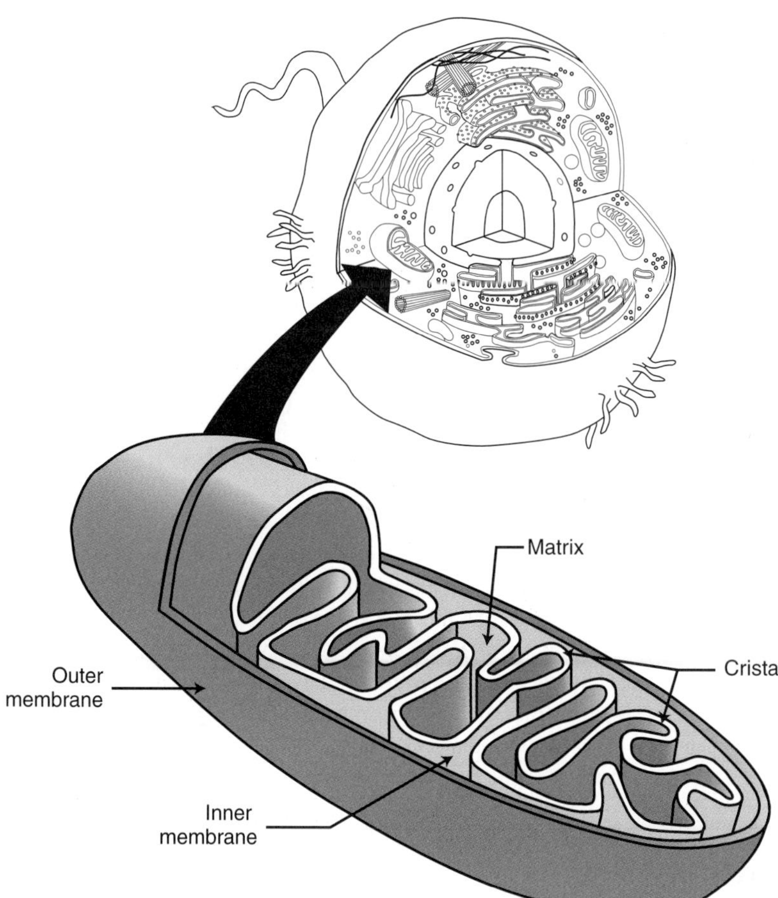

FIGURE **2-6** **Mitochondrion.** Mitochondrion is the powerhouse of the cell. Using oxygen, it produces 95% of the energy that fuels the cell.

When cellular requirements for energy increase, the mitochondrion divides by pinching itself in half and then grows to normal size, a process called **fission.** In addition, mitochondria tend to congregate in areas of the cell where greater amounts of energy are required, such as at the base of a flagellum.

Mitochondria contain the DNA, RNA, and enzymes necessary to make protein, but they provide themselves with only 13 of the proteins required for their metabolic functions; the nucleus provides the remaining 50. Thus most of the protein needed by the mitochondria is produced elsewhere in the cell and is later taken up by the mitochondria.

Mitochondria may take on a variety of shapes but tend to be elliptical or round. They can move throughout the cell and can elongate or change shape with ease. Mitochondria are enclosed by two membranes; the outer one is smooth and featureless, and the inner one involutes dramatically, forming shelflike folds called **cristae.** These folds increase the internal working area and allow greater contact between the cristae and the enzyme-rich liquid, called the **matrix,** which fills the spaces between the cristae. In addition to containing vital enzymes, the matrix is composed of calcium ions and the substrates required for metabolic reactions. Additional enzymes are available in the form of small particles that are found attached to some of the cristae. Because the cristae are the site of ATP production, it is not surprising that active mitochondria possess more cristae than inactive ones.

The DNA and RNA found in mitochondria are similar to those found in bacteria but are quite different from those found in the nucleus and cytoplasm. Mitochondria are thought to have originated as independent, bacteria-like organisms billions of years ago that later moved into the bodies of unicellular plants and animals, developing a symbiotic relationship with them.

Ribosomes. The most common organelle in the cell is the small, dark-staining **ribosome** (Figure 2-7). It is composed of two globular subunits, which fit together like cupped hands. These subunits contain protein and a specific type of RNA, known as **ribosomal RNA.** Although only 25 nm in diameter, the ribosome is an important site for protein synthesis. Soluble protein intended for intracellular use is manufactured on ribosomes that are evenly distributed freely throughout the cytoskeleton. Protein intended for use in the plasma membrane or meant for cellular export, on the other hand, is synthesized on ribosomes attached to the endoplasmic reticulum. Ribosomes are flexible in their abilities to attach and detach from membranes and to move freely within the cell. Thus they can move back and forth between the cytoskeleton and endoplasmic reticulum, depending on the type of protein they are making. When manufacturing protein, the ribosomes assemble the amino acids into long chains using specific instructions that are determined by the cell's genetic material. In this way, a wide range of proteins, such as cellular enzymes, hormones, collagen, and mucus, may be created based on the needs of the cell and of the organism as a whole.

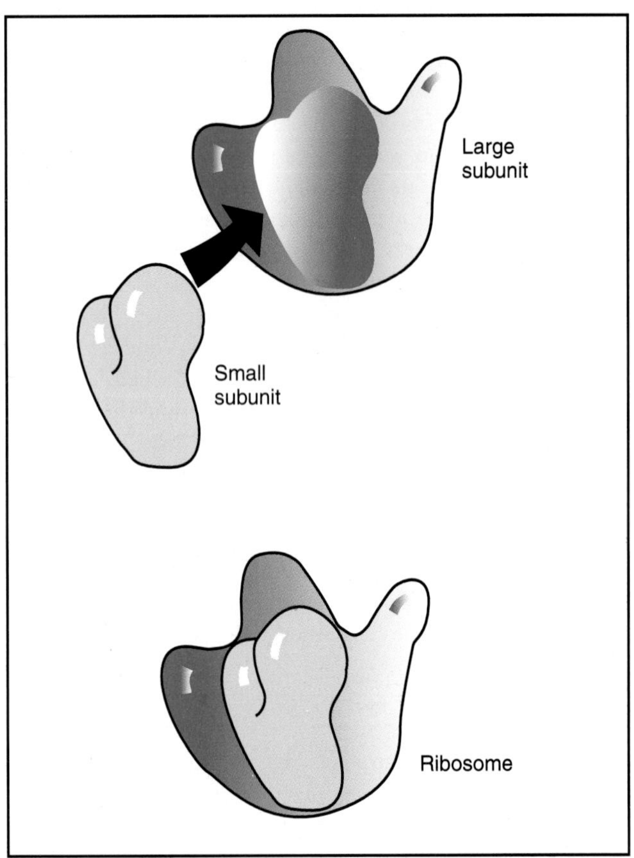

FIGURE **2-7** **Ribosome.** Each ribosome is composed of one large and one small subunit. When joined together, these two subunits form one ribosome.

Endoplasmic Reticulum. The **endoplasmic reticulum (ER)** is a series of flattened tubes stacked on one another and bent into a crescent shape. Its surface area is enormous and may be 30 times larger than that of the plasma membrane. The walls of the ER are composed of a single lipid bilayer and are continuous with the membranes of the nucleus and Golgi apparatus.

The two types of ER are rough, which has ribosomes on its surface, and smooth, which does not have ribosomes on its surface. **Rough ER** is involved in the production of protein, which is assembled by the ribosomes. These newly manufactured molecules are moved internally into passageways known as **cisternae** (sis-TUR-ne; a reservoir of water). Here the proteins are modified before being moved on to the Golgi apparatus for further modification and packaging. **Smooth ER,** which is connected to rough ER, is active in the synthesis and storage of lipids, particularly phospholipids and steroids, and is therefore seen in large quantities in gland cells. In liver cells, it may also function to eliminate drugs and break down glycogen into glucose. The proportion of smooth to rough ER varies depending on the synthetic activities of the cell.

Golgi Apparatus. The **Golgi apparatus** is often found near the nucleus and, like the ER, is composed of

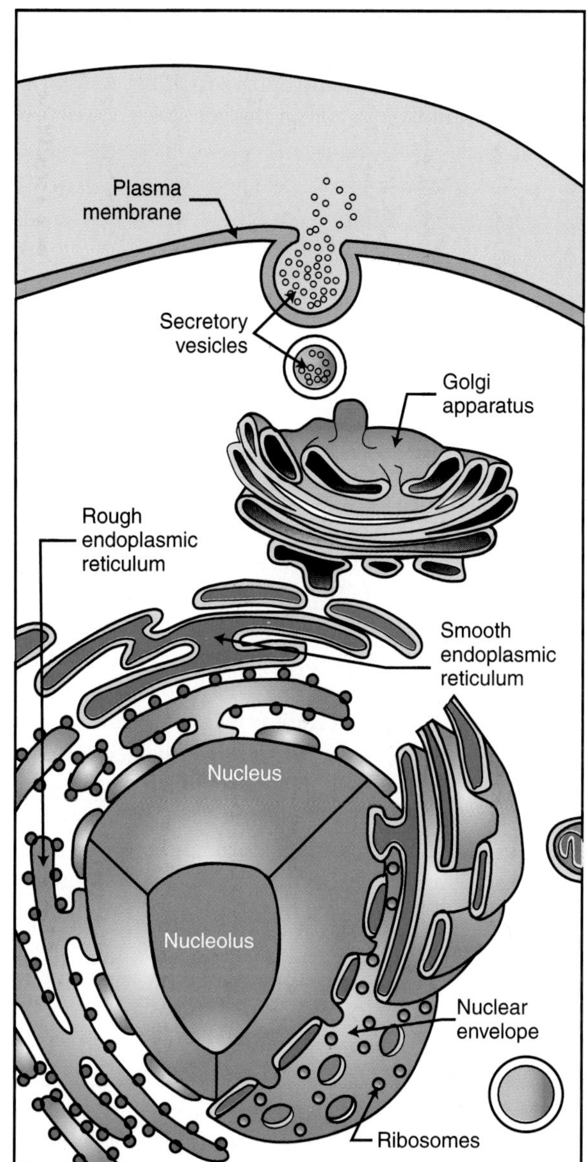

FIGURE **2-8** **Golgi Apparatus and Endoplasmic Reticulum.** Endoplasmic reticulum (ER) is continuous with the nuclear envelope and is divided into two types. Rough ER, which is covered by ribosomes, and smooth ER, which does not have ribosomes. Molecules produced by ER are transported to the Golgi apparatus, where they are modified and packaged into vesicles. Vesicles transport molecules to other regions of the cell.

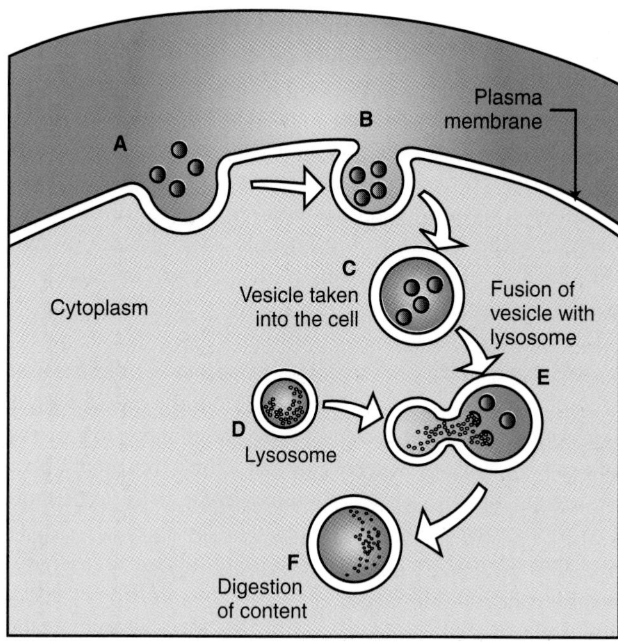

FIGURE **2-9** **Lysosomal Action.** *A,* Material from outside the cell is drawn into a forming vesicle. *B,* The plasma membrane surrounds the material and pinches off to form a vesicle. *C,* Vesicle transports material to internal regions of the cell. *D,* A lysosome approaches the vesicle. *E,* The lysosome fuses with the vesicle and dumps digestive enzymes into it, which break down the material. *F,* Contents of vesicle are digested and transported to other regions of the cell.

stacks of flattened, crescent-shaped tubes called cisternae (Figure 2-8). Small, spherical transfer sacs from the ER containing newly manufactured proteins are received by the Golgi apparatus. These sacs fuse with the membrane at the ends of the Golgi apparatus and dislodge their contents into the Golgi cisternae. The protein molecules are then moved from stack to stack through the Golgi body where they are modified. Sugar groups, that the Golgi apparatus manufactures, for example, may be added to the proteins to form glycoproteins. When the modified proteins reach the outermost layer of the Golgi's flattened tubes, they are packaged into small spherical **vesicles.** The vesicles are formed as they pull away from the cisternae and venture out into the cytosol, destined for other parts of the cell, particularly the cell membrane. Thus the Golgi body acts as a modification, packaging, and distribution center for molecules destined either for secretion or for intracellular use. It also functions in polysaccharide synthesis and in the coupling of polysaccharides to proteins (glycoproteins) that are found on the cell surface.

Lysosomes. The lysosome is a specialized vesicle formed by the Golgi apparatus (Figure 2-9). It contains powerful hydrolytic enzymes enclosed in a single protective membrane that fuses with vacuoles containing engulfed bacteria or foodstuffs and digests them. In this way, the lysosome is considered the "stomach" of the cell. Its principal responsibility is the breakdown of nutrient molecules into usable smaller units and the digestion of intracellular debris.

When cells die, the lysosomes within them are triggered to burst open and release their caustic enzymes into the cytosol, which immediately begin to dismantle and digest the various organelles and nuclear components of the cell. The process of self-digestion is called **autolysis.** The organism as a whole recycles the used parts of the dead cell to create new cells or to help maintain existing ones. As cells age, the number of lysosomes within them increases.

Lysosomes may also release their enzymes outside of the cell to assist with the breakdown of extracellular material. During the process of bone remodeling, for example, osteocytes use lysosomes to help break down and remove unnecessary bone. This process is seen radiographically (in an x-ray film) as bone resorption and a decrease in opacity of the affected area. In addition, lysosomal digestion is responsible for decreasing the size of body tissues, for example, after parturition with shrinkage of the uterus and in the atrophy of muscles in paralyzed animals.

Peroxisomes. Like lysosomes, **peroxisomes** are membranous sacs containing enzymes found throughout the cell. But unlike lysosomes, which are formed in the Golgi apparatus, peroxisomes reproduce by pinching in half. They commonly occur in liver and kidney cells and are important in the detoxification of various molecules. Peroxisomes contain enzymes that use oxygen to detoxify a number of harmful substances, including alcohol and formaldehyde. They also assist in the removal of **free radicals,** which are normal products of cellular metabolism but can be harmful to the cell in large quantities because they interfere with the structure of proteins, lipids, and nucleic acids. Peroxisomes carry two major types of enzymes: **peroxidases,** which assist in the conversion of free radicals to hydrogen peroxide, and **catalases,** which reduce hydrogen peroxide to water.

TEST YOURSELF

1. What are the four principal components of cytoplasm?
2. What is cytosol and what kind of molecules are found in it?
3. What is the cytoskeleton and what is its function?
4. How many types of fibers make up the cytoskeleton? Can you name them? How do they function differently?
5. Draw a picture of each of the six organelles described earlier.
6. How do each of these organelles function within the cell?

Inclusions

Inclusions are packaged units of metabolic products or substances that the cell has engulfed. They may be delineated by a surrounding single-layer membrane, as seen in secretory granules, vacuoles, and vesicles, or they may be non–membrane-bound inclusions, such as lipid droplets and fat globules. Vacuoles are larger than vesicles but are otherwise identical in structure. They are often filled with water and solutes that are transported to and from the cell surface. Some vesicles act simply as storage units, holding substances within the cell until its contents can be used.

Centrioles

Centrioles are small hollow cylinders composed of microtubules (Figure 2-10). They are found in pairs with their long axis perpendicular to one another and are visible during cell division near the nuclear envelope in a region of the cell known as the cell center, or **centrosome.** Centrioles help to organize the **spindle fibers** during cell division by taking a central position in the **spindle apparatus.** They also form the bases of cilia and flagella and in this role are known as **basal bodies.**

Nucleus

The nucleus is the largest organelle in the cell and is considered the "control center," the central processing unit, the CEO of operations, or the "brain" of the cell. It is a dominating, dark-staining, spherical or multisegmented body. The primary functions of the nucleus are to maintain the hereditary information of the species and to control cellular activities through protein synthesis. Thus the nucleus contains the hereditary information that enables the cell to divide and produce an identical daughter cell and, on a larger scale, determines whether an animal will develop into a dog, cat, or horse. It also contains all of the instructions, blueprints, and information required to make over 2000 proteins that are needed for normal cell activity.

Although most cells have at least one nucleus, extremely large cells, such as muscle cells, may have many nuclei and are therefore called **multinucleated.** Mature mammalian red blood cells, on the other hand, have no nuclei because the nuclei are removed from the cells during their development in the bone marrow. These cells are therefore called **anucleated.** Without a nucleus, they cannot divide, make protein or enzymes, or repair themselves as they start to age. For this reason, the supply of vital molecules in mammalian red blood cells allows them to survive in circulation for only 3 or 4 months. The red blood cells found in birds and reptiles, on the other

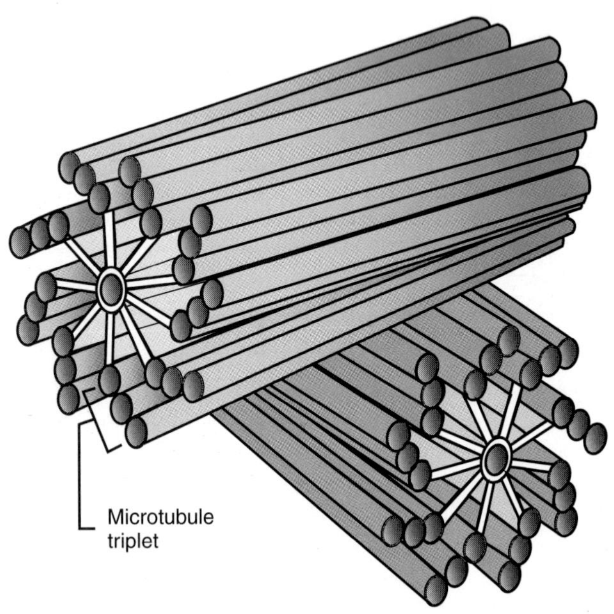

FIGURE **2-10** **Centriole.** Each centriole is composed of nine triplets of microtubules arranged around a central axis, much like a pinwheel.

hand, are nucleated and therefore are able to produce the proteins and other molecules needed by the cells to survive for longer periods.

The anatomy of the nucleus is divided into the following four parts:

1. Nuclear envelope or membrane
2. Nucleoplasm
3. Chromatin
4. Nucleoli

Nuclear Envelope and Nucleoplasm

The nucleus is separated from the cytosol by a nuclear envelope or membrane composed of two lipid bilayers (unlike the cell membrane, which is composed of one bilayer). The outer layer is continuous with the ER and is studded with ribosomes. Over 10% of the nuclear surface consists of **nuclear pores**—places where the two layers of the nuclear envelope have fused to form a channel that spans its entire thickness (Figure 2-11). Although similar in structure and composition to the plasma membrane, passage of molecules into the nucleus is less selective because the nuclear pores are relatively large (0.1 μm in diameter). Typically, protein molecules are moved into the nucleus from the cytoplasm, and RNA molecules are exported. The nuclear pores represent the principal channels of communication between the cytoplasm and the nucleus. Between the bilayers of the nuclear envelope is a space called the **perinuclear cisterna.** The nucleus is filled with a gel-like substance called **nucleoplasm** that resembles cytosol.

Chromatin

Genetic material (DNA) is connected to globular proteins called **histones,** and together they form **chromatin.** Chromatin is composed of units of eight histone proteins connected by a single strand of DNA. The DNA winds around the histones, which helps keep it organized and untangled. As the histones change shape, they expose different **genes,** or sections of the DNA. This determines what proteins will be made. In this way, histones play an important role in gene regulation. The DNA contains all of the important instructions required for synthesis of the various proteins and macromolecules that govern cellular activity. When the cell is not actively dividing, the chromosomes are arranged in loose fibers that appear as dark-staining granules throughout the nucleoplasm. These granules are called chromatin. During cell division the chromatin reorganizes and condenses into thick bodies called **chromosomes.**

Nucleoli

Nuclei usually contain one or more small, dark-staining spherical patches known as **nucleoli.** The nucleoli are

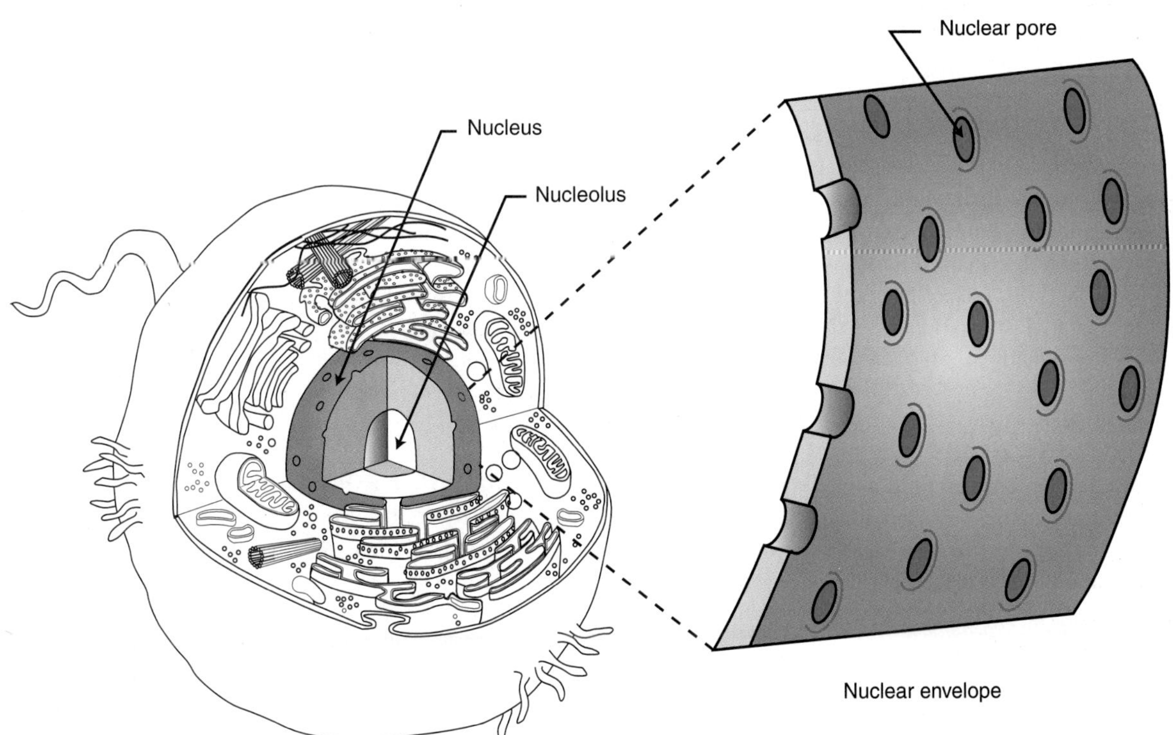

FIGURE **2-11** **Nucleus.** The nucleus contains a central nucleolus surrounded by clumps of chromatin. The entire nucleus is surrounded by a nuclear envelope, which contains hundreds of pores. Pores permit substances to pass between the nucleus and cytoplasm.

not membrane bound and are the places in the nucleus where ribosomal subunits are made. These subunits are exported separately from the nucleus and are assembled in the cytoplasm to form functional ribosomes. In addition, nucleoli contain the DNA that governs the synthesis of ribosomal RNA (rRNA). (See Chapter 3 for further discussion of rRNA.)

TEST YOURSELF

1. Why do inclusions vary in appearance? What function do they perform?
2. What role does the centriole play in the formation of cilia and flagella?
3. How are centrioles structurally similar to cilia and flagella?
4. Why is the nucleus considered the "CEO of operations"?
5. Can a cell that does not contain a nucleus live as long as a cell that does contain one? Why or why not?
6. Describe the nuclear envelope. How is it different from the cell membrane?
7. How do histones play a role in gene regulation?
8. What is the significance of the nucleolus? What happens in that region of the nucleus?

CELL PHYSIOLOGY

THE CELLULAR ENVIRONMENT

Body Fluids

Mammals are composed primarily of water. Water is in blood, saliva, urine, sweat, and all other bodily secretions. It is found in the tissues of organs and in the cells that make up the tissues. Put simply, animals are primarily composed of water and cannot live without it. Surprisingly, most of the water in animals is found inside the cell and is called **intracellular fluid.** Fluid outside the cell is called **extracellular fluid.** Extracellular fluid specifically found in tissues, rather than in lymphatic or blood vessels, is called **interstitial fluid.** Intracellular and extracellular environments are separated and defined by the plasma membrane, which regulates the flow of fluid and nutrients into and out of the cell.

Ions, Electrolytes, and pH

Extracellular and intracellular fluid is filled with many different kinds of charged particles, called **ions,** that may be either positively or negatively charged. Salt is a good example of an ionic compound because it is composed of oppositely charged ions that separate from one another when mixed in water. The salt sodium sulfate ($Na_2SO_4^{2-}$), for example, separates into two sodium ions (Na^+) and one sulfate ion (SO_4^{2-}). Positively charged ions, such as Na^+, are called **cations** (pronounced "cat-ions"), and negatively charged ions, such as SO_4^{2-}, are called **anions** (unfortunately, they are not called "dog-ions," which would seem logical in the veterinary world). A salt, by definition, is made up of anions other than the hydroxyl ion (OH^-) and of cations other than the hydrogen ion (H^+). Because anions and cations are capable of conducting an electrical current in solution, they are called **electrolytes.** All ions are electrolytes.

Acids and bases are also electrolytes because they dissociate in water and can conduct an electrical impulse. However, unlike salt, acids release hydrogen ions (H^+) and bases release hydroxyl ions (OH^-) when in solution. Because the nucleus of a hydrogen atom contains one proton, a hydrogen ion is therefore simply a proton. For this reason, acids are molecules that release protons and are called "proton donors." Conversely, bases are "proton receivers" because they release hydroxyl ions, which readily bind to free hydrogen ions (protons). When a hydroxyl anion and a hydrogen cation unite, two things happen: water is formed, and the acidity of the solution is reduced.

The more free protons or hydrogen ions (H^+) in a solution, the greater is its acidity. In contrast, the greater the concentration of hydroxyl ions, the more basic or **alkaline** the solution becomes. Body fluids are rich with hydrogen and hydroxyl ions, and their relative proportion to one another determines the acidity or alkalinity of the fluid. The concentration of hydrogen ions in fluid is measured *inversely* by pH units on a scale from 0 to 14. Pure water, for example, has a neutral pH of 7. Gastric juices, on the other hand, are acidic, which means a lot of H^+ ions are present in them. Therefore they have a pH *below* 7. In contrast, an alkaline substance, such as bleach, has a pH *above* 7 because it contains a low concentration of hydrogen ions and a high concentration of hydroxyl ions, as shown below:

0 (Acidic)	7 (Neutral)	14 (Alkaline)
Lots of H^+ ions	Equal concentration	Few H^+ ions
Few OH^- ions	of H^+ and OH^- ions	Lots of OH^- ions

In sick or injured animals, the electrolyte concentrations and pH of intracellular and extracellular fluid can become abnormally high or low. Normal body functions, such as the transmission of nervous impulses, muscle contraction, and respiration, can be adversely affected by changes in electrolyte concentration and pH. For this reason, additives such as bicarbonate or potassium chloride may be placed in intravenous fluids to help adjust the ionic imbalances of animal patients.

MEMBRANE PROCESSES: EXCRETION AND ABSORPTION

In addition to containing electrolytes, tissue fluids are loaded with fatty acids, vitamins, amino acids, regulatory hormones, and dissolved gases. For the cell to maintain homeostasis, the cell must select what it needs from the extracellular fluid and bring it into the intracellular environment. Similarly, it must excrete waste products or transport resources, needed in other parts of the body, to the extracellular compartment.

The function of the plasma membrane is complex, and therefore it may work differently at various times and locations

Table 2-2 Summary of Membrane Processes

Type of Process	Description	Substances Transported	Example
Passive Processes (Does Not Require Adenosine Triphosphate [ATP])			
1. Diffusion	Kinetic movement of molecules from higher to lower concentration	1. Small molecules diffuse through membrane 2. Lipid-soluble gases pass through lipid bilayer 3. Charged ions move through specialized channel proteins	1. Water 2. Oxygen and carbon dioxide 3. Chloride and urea
2. Facilitated diffusion	Selective carrier proteins assist in movement of molecules from higher to lower concentration; speed of diffusion is limited by saturation of carrier molecules	Some large molecules and nonlipid-soluble molecules	Movement of glucose into muscle and fat cells
3. Osmosis	Passive movement of water through a semipermeable membrane from dilute solution to more concentrated one	Water	Water moves from stomach into bloodstream
4. Filtration	Hydrostatic pressure (caused by the beating heart) forces liquid through a membrane.	Water and small molecular solutes	Filtration of blood in kidney enables all solutes and liquid to pass through it except blood cells and proteins
Active Processes (Uses ATP)			
1. Active transport	Active movement of molecules by specific carrier protein; molecules may move against concentration gradient	Molecules too large to pass through channels or unable to penetrate lipid bilayer because of polarity; may be on wrong side of concentration gradient	Ions such as K^+, Na^+, and Ca^{2+}
2. Endocytosis			
a. Phagocytosis	Cell engulfs solid substances	Microinvaders and foreign debris	White blood cell or macrophage engulfs bacteria
b. Pinocytosis	Cell engulfs liquid substances	Water and other solutes	Absorptive cells in small intestine take in water into intracellular vesicles
c. Receptor mediated	Specialized protein receptors bind to ligands specific to receptors	Hormones, iron, and cholesterol	Insulin produced by pancreas only binds to cells with insulin receptors
3. Exocytosis	Excretion of waste products and secretion of manufactured substances; these substances are packaged in secretory vesicles, which fuse with cell membrane; contents are ejected to the extracellular space	Waste products, secretory proteins, hormones, and lipids	Digestive enzymes produced in pancreas and released into ducts connected to small intestine

on the cell surface (Table 2-2). For example, the absorption of nutrients or excretion of waste may occur with or without the expenditure of energy (ATP) from the cell. Absorptive or excretory processes that require energy are considered active, whereas those that do not require energy (ATP) are passive. In addition, the cell membrane may be **impermeable** to some substances and **freely permeable** to others. Thus the cell membrane is generally considered to be **selectively permeable** because it allows some molecules to pass through, but not others.

Passive Membrane Processes

Diffusion. Whether in liquid or in gas, molecules are constantly moving, gyrating, and, at times, bouncing into one another. This activity, called kinetic energy, can be increased in warmer temperatures and slowed in cool temperatures. Concentrated molecules gyrate away from one another until they are evenly distributed within the space that confines them. The spectrum between the most concentrated region and the area that is least filled with molecules is called the **concentration gradient.** As the molecules move from an area of high concentration to a region of low concentration, they are said to be moving down the concentration gradient; therefore **diffusion** can be defined as the process of moving down the concentration gradient. Examples of diffusion are everywhere. When you place a drop of lemon in your tea, the drop slowly spreads out until it is uniformly mixed within the liquid (Figure 2-12). The rate of diffusion depends on the temperature of the tea in that it occurs faster in hot tea than in iced tea. When a dog expresses its anal sacs in the waiting room of a veterinary office because it is nervous, this may not be noticeable at first to the people waiting on the other side of the room; however, with time, diffusion of anal sac molecules released into the air will make everyone aware of a foul odor.

The plasma membrane forms an obstacle to the diffusion of some molecules into or out of the cell. Molecules, such as water, oxygen, and carbon dioxide, pass through the membrane easily, whereas others, such as sodium, may not. The following three principal factors determine whether a molecule may pass through the cell membrane by passive diffusion:

1. *Molecular size:* Very small molecules, such as water (H_2O), may pass through cellular membrane pores (approximately 0.8 nm in diameter), but larger molecules, such as glucose, cannot pass through.
2. *Lipid solubility:* Lipid-soluble molecules, such as alcohol and steroids, and dissolved gases, such as oxygen (O_2) and carbon dioxide (CO_2), can pass through the lipid bilayer with ease, whereas other molecules may not.
3. *Molecular charge:* Ions are small in size, but their charge prevents easy passage through the membrane pores. Specialized pores called channels selectively allow certain ions to pass through, but not others. For example, chloride channels permit only chloride ions through, and urea channels permit only urea to pass through.

Facilitated Diffusion. Some large molecules and nonlipid-soluble molecules can pass through the cell membrane with the assistance of an integral protein or carrier protein that is located in the bilayer. The molecule outside the cell binds to a particular binding site on the carrier protein. This causes the carrier protein to change its shape in such a way that the molecule is able to pass through the membrane and enter the cell. Once exposed to the cytoplasm, the molecule is released intracellularly. This process is known as *facilitated diffusion* and requires no energy (ATP) from the cell.

An example of facilitated diffusion in animals is the movement of glucose into the cell (Figure 2-13). Glucose is normally of a higher concentration outside the cell, but it is too large to fit through the tiny membrane pores and therefore cannot rely on **simple diffusion** to enter the cell. However, glucose is able to pass with the assistance of a carrier protein. Each carrier protein in the cell membrane is selective about the molecules that it transports. As the level of glucose rises in the bloodstream, more carrier molecules specific for glucose are employed. Eventually, if the blood sugar level becomes high

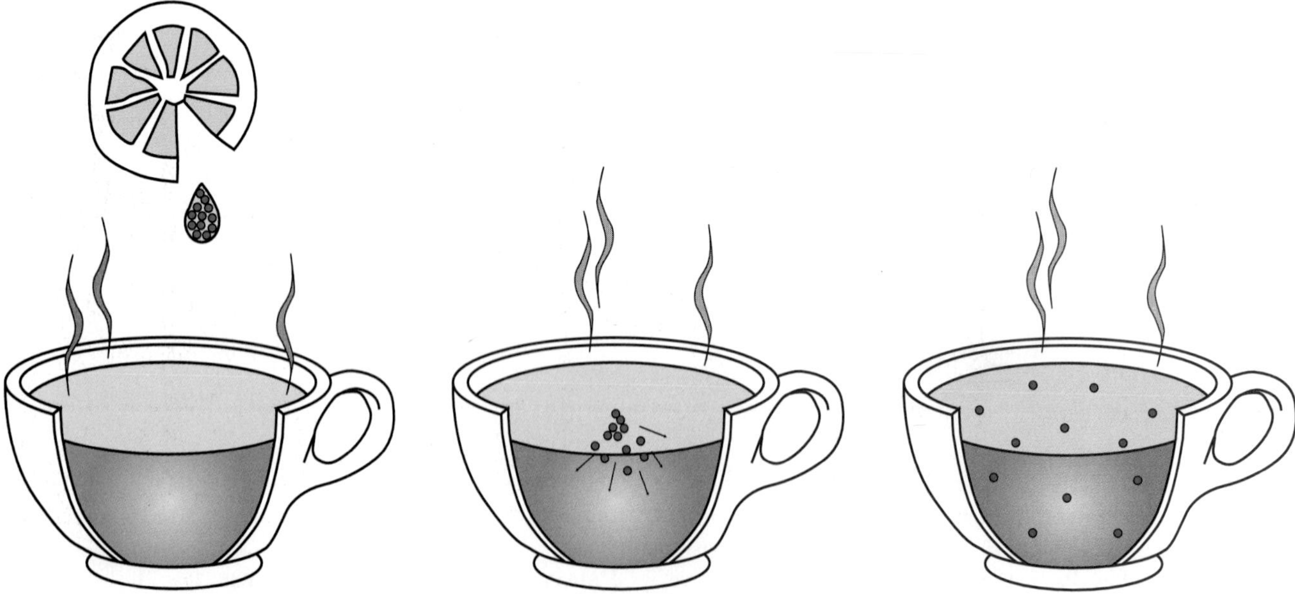

FIGURE **2-12** **Diffusion.** Molecules in solution are active and collide into one another. The hotter the solution, the more active the collisions. With time, molecules become evenly distributed throughout the liquid, having moved from the highest concentration to the lowest. This process, called diffusion, occurs more rapidly in hot liquids than in cold ones.

enough, all of the carrier molecules become engaged and glucose is unable to enter the cell at a faster rate. Thus facilitated diffusion is different from ordinary diffusion in that the process is limited by the number of available **carrier proteins.** Increasing the amount of glucose given to an animal under these circumstances is not going to increase the rate at which glucose is taken into the cell. Hormones such as insulin, however, play an important role in controlling the activity of the glucose-specific carrier proteins and can act on them to speed up their rate of transport.

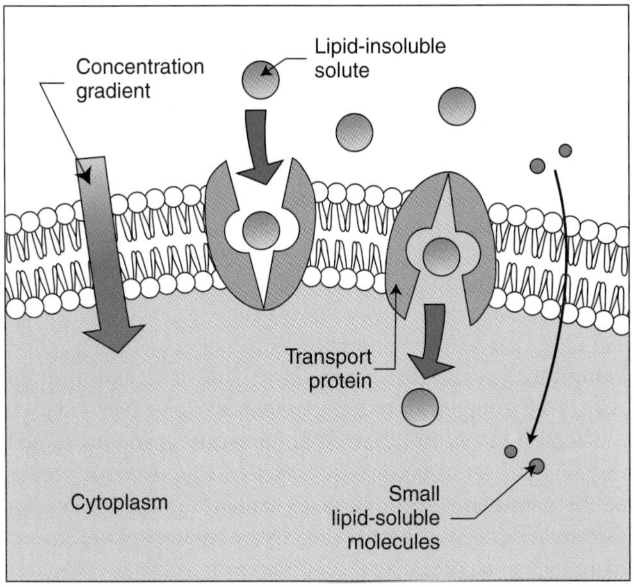

FIGURE **2-13** **Simple and Facilitated Diffusion.** Large, lipid-soluble molecules, such as glucose, are transported into the cell by binding to a transmembrane carrier protein. Small, lipid-soluble molecules, on the other hand, can pass through the cell membrane via simple diffusion.

Osmosis. **Osmosis** is the passive movement of water through a semipermeable membrane into a solution where the water concentration is lower. In other words, when two solutions of different concentrations are separated by a semipermeable membrane, water molecules move from the dilute solution, across the membrane, to the concentrated solution (Figure 2-14). In osmosis the movement of water occurs to achieve the same concentration of solution on both sides of a semipermeable membrane. This state is called a concentration balance or **equilibrium.** The greater the difference in solute concentration, the greater the osmotic flow. The force of water moving from one side of the membrane to the other is called the **osmotic pressure.** Note that osmosis occurs in the opposite direction of diffusion and that in osmosis the water, not solutes, is moving. In addition, osmosis requires a selective membrane, whereas diffusion does not.

Water can move rapidly into and out of cells through the pores in integral proteins, but large molecules and lipophobic substances cannot pass through. Normally the extracellular fluid has the same concentration of dissolved substances as the intracellular fluid and is therefore called **isotonic.** In isotonic environments, the cell does not change size and water moves freely in and out of the cell. If the extracellular fluid is **hypotonic,** however, the inside of the cell is more concentrated then the outside. In this scenario, water flows into the

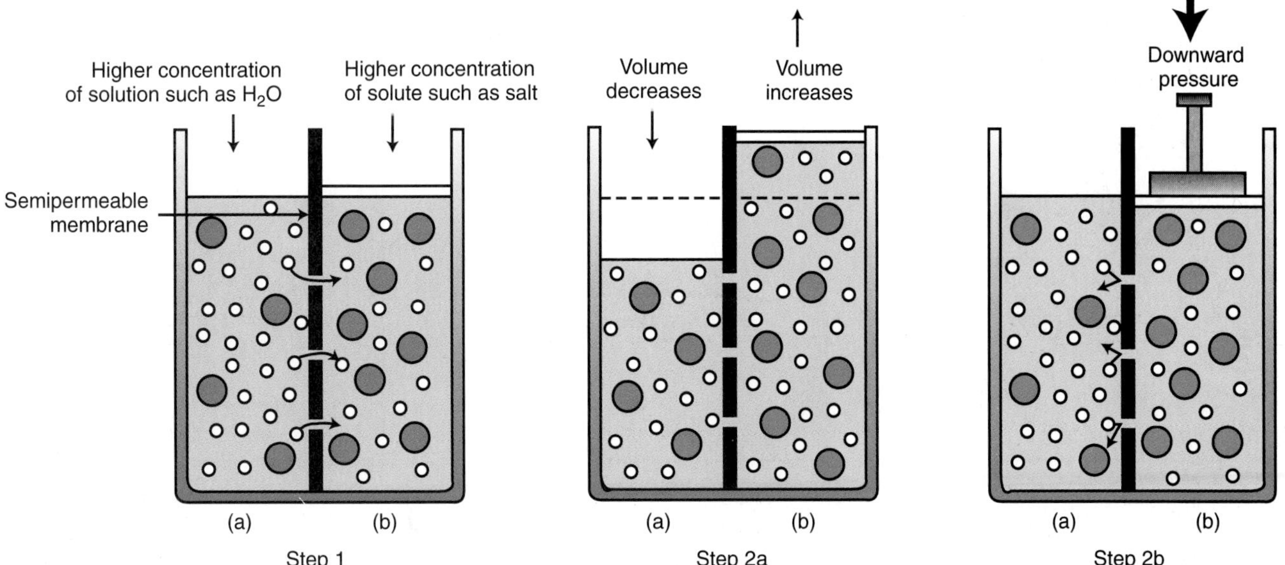

FIGURE **2-14** **Osmosis.** *Step 1:* Semipermeable membrane prevents larger solute molecule in side *(b)* from passing into side *(a)*. However, smaller solution molecules can pass readily from side *(a)* to side *(b)*. *Step 2a:* As solution moves from side *(a)* to side *(b)*, volume of side *(b)* increases until the concentration of solute is the same on both sides. *Step 2b:* Osmosis can be reversed via filtration when hydraulic pressure is placed on side *(b)*. This forces solution back through the semipermeable membrane to side *(a)*.

cell and causes it to swell and possibly burst. If the extracellular fluid is **hypertonic** and more concentrated than the cytoplasm, water is excreted into the extracellular space, causing the cell to shrink and become shriveled (Figure 2-15).

Osmosis is an important aspect of passive membrane physiology. It illustrates the importance of the extracellular environment and the necessity for stable concentration gradients. In regions of the body where isotonic environments cannot always be maintained, such as the kidney, the body has developed protective mechanisms. The endothelial cells, for example, that line the ducts of the urinary system are coated with thick mucus to separate them from urine, which would otherwise be caustic to the cells. Urine can be hypertonic, isotonic, and hypotonic at various times. These large swings in concentration would be fatal to unprotected cells.

The difference between the osmotic pressure of blood and the osmotic pressure of interstitial fluid or lymph is called the **oncotic pressure.** This is an important force in maintaining fluid balance between the blood and lymph in vessels and the fluid in surrounding tissues. In some disorders the balance of fluid between these two spaces is disrupted, particularly if there is a decrease in the number of protein molecules in blood plasma. Starvation, liver failure, and intestinal disorders, for example, can cause the levels of plasma proteins to decrease. If the levels become low enough, fluid can move via osmosis across the vessel wall into surrounding tissue or into open body cavities. When fluid leaks into the tissue under the skin, it is called subcutaneous edema. When it leaks into the abdomen, it is called ascites.

Filtration. Unlike the processes of diffusion and osmosis, which rely on concentration gradients to drive the activity of molecules, **filtration** is based on a **pressure gradient.** Liquids may be pushed through a membrane if the pressure on one side of the membrane is greater than that on the other side. The force that pushes a liquid is called **hydrostatic pressure.** In animals, hydrostatic pressure is blood pressure and is generated by the pumping heart. Blood, as it circulates in the body, is forced through vessels and minute capillaries. Small molecules and cells may be pushed through, but large cells may not. One of the best examples of filtration in animals is evident in the kidney, where blood is filtered through specialized capillaries in the process of making urine.

CLINICAL APPLICATION — Dialysis

In dogs with kidney failure, dialysis of their blood can be performed in some veterinary hospitals to remove toxic materials such as urea, uric acid, and creatinine. At abnormally high levels, these substances make animals feel nauseated, so they stop eating, lose weight, and become lethargic. Clinically, dogs tend to lick their lips excessively and cats tend to drool when they feel nauseated. To remove these toxic substances, the blood of the animal is diffused across a semipermeable membrane. Because the toxins possess different diffusion rates than other blood constituents, they are separated from the rest of the blood. This process involves the diffusion of particles from a higher to a lower concentration and the simultaneous movement of water (via osmosis) from a lower to a higher concentration. The "clean" blood is returned to the animal after the toxins have been diffused away.

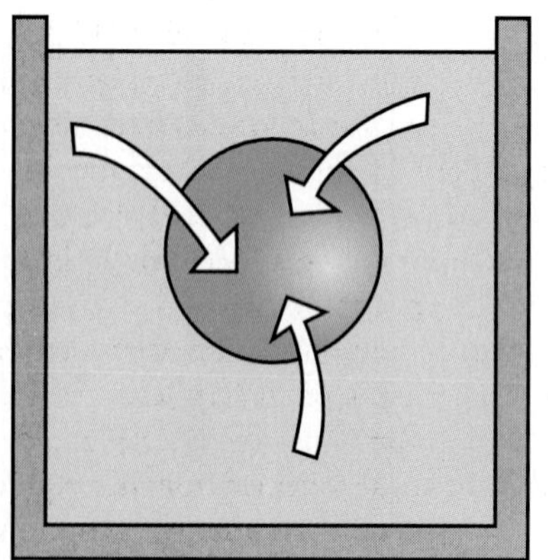

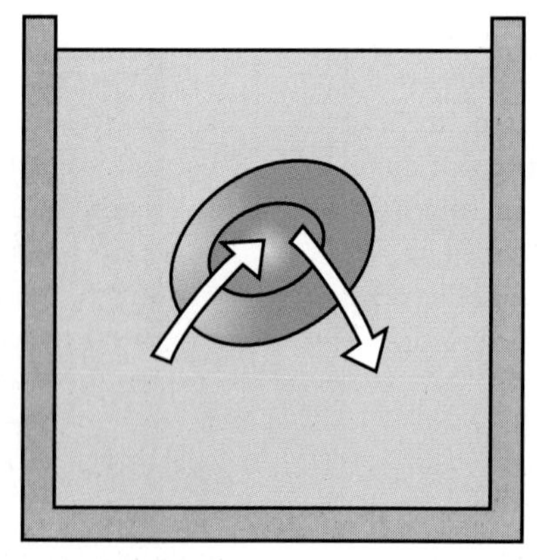

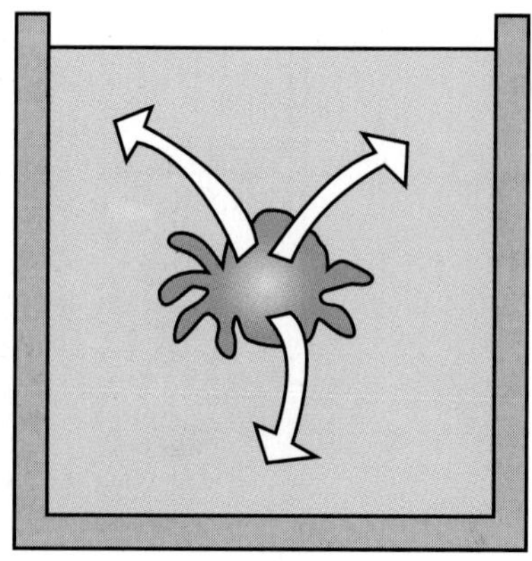

FIGURE 2-15 **Effects of Osmosis on Cells. A,** In hypotonic solutions, red blood cells swell and can burst as a result of movement of water into the cell. **B,** In isotonic solutions, cells maintain the same size and internal pressure because movement of water into the cell is equal to movement of water out of the cell. **C,** In hypertonic solutions, the cell loses fluid and deflates. Projections from the cytoskeleton become visible and look like "spikes" on the cell's surface.

TEST YOURSELF

1. Where is most of the water in animals found?
2. What is diffusion? Is it an active or a passive membrane process?
3. What molecules are more likely to diffuse into a cell? What three principles are involved?
4. How is facilitated diffusion different from simple diffusion? What is the limiting factor in the rate of facilitated diffusion?
5. What effect does a hypotonic solution have on a cell? What passive membrane process causes this effect?
6. What is the relationship between hydrostatic pressure and filtration?
7. What is another name for hydrostatic pressure in the body?

Active Membrane Processes

The movement of molecules and substances across the cell membrane is considered active when the cell is required to use energy (ATP). Some molecules are unable to enter the cell via the passive routes, perhaps (1) because they are not lipid soluble and therefore cannot penetrate the lipid bilayer, (2) because they are too large to pass through a membrane pore, or (3) because they are on the wrong side of the concentration gradient.

Regardless of the reason, these substances must rely on an active cellular process to enter the cell. Substances can be actively moved into or out of the cell by two processes: active transport and cytosis.

Active Transport. Some amino acids and ions must enter and exit cells without the assistance of a concentration gradient. They cannot move through the plasma membrane passively and must rely on energy, in the form of ATP, to assist in their transport across the cell membrane. Like facilitated diffusion, the **active transport** of a substance relies on a carrier protein with a specific binding site, but unlike facilitated diffusion, it does not require a concentration gradient. All cells demonstrate the active transport of electrolytes, specifically sodium (Na^+), potassium (K^+), calcium (Ca^{2+}), and magnesium (Mg^{2+}). In addition, specialized cells can transport iodide (I^-), chloride (Cl^-), and iron (Fe^{2+}). Many active transport systems move more than one substance at a time. If all of the substances are moved in the same direction, the system is called a **symport system.** However, if some substances are moved in one direction and others moved in the opposite direction, the system is called an **antiport system.**

One of the best understood examples of active transport is the antiport sodium-potassium pump. Na^+ and K^+ are the most common cations in the cell, and active transport sites for them can be found speckled throughout the plasma membrane. Normally, the concentration of potassium in the cell is 10 to 20 times higher than it is outside the cell. Conversely, sodium is 10 to 20 times higher outside the cell than it is inside. Because of this concentration gradient, potassium tends to diffuse out of the cell and sodium diffuses in. To maintain appropriate levels of intracellular potassium and extracellular sodium, the cell must pump potassium into the cell and move out sodium. Because diffusion is ongoing, the active transport system must work continuously. The rate of transport depends on the concentration of sodium ions in the cell.

When an ion is transported, it binds to a specific carrier protein in the cell membrane that triggers the release and use of cellular energy (ATP). This response, in turn, causes the orientation of the carrier protein to be altered, the ion to become lipid soluble, and the carrier protein to be able to move the ion through the cell membrane. ATP is provided by cellular respiration and, with the assistance of the enzyme ATPase, is broken down on the inner surface of the cell membrane for energy. The pump can cycle several times using one molecule of ATP, so that for every molecule of ATP, two K^+ ions are moved intracellularly and three Na^+ ions are moved extracellularly (Figure 2-16).

Differences in ionic concentrations are critical for maintaining proper fluid balances in all cells and tissue types. In addition, differences in ionic concentrations are of particular importance in the normal functioning of so-called irritable cells such as myofibrils and neurons, where up to 40% of the energy produced from cellular respiration is used to fuel active transport.

Cytosis. Cytosis is another mechanism for bringing nutrients into the cell and ejecting waste. Like active transport, cytosis requires ATP and is therefore considered an active process. The two types of cytosis are **endocytosis,** which means "going into the cell," and **exocytosis,** which means "going out of the cell."

Endocytosis. Endocytosis enables large particles, liquid substances, and even entire cells to be taken into the cell by engulfing them (Figure 2-17). In this case, the plasma membrane involutes, engulfs the particle or liquid, and forms a vesicle by closing the cell membrane around it. If the cell engulfs solid material, the process is called **phagocytosis,** which means "cell eating." The vesicle formed from phagocytosis is called a **phagosome.** If the cell engulfs liquid, the process is called **pinocytosis,** which means "cell drinking."

In mammals the **macrophage,** a giant cell found in many tissues throughout the body, is notorious for its ability to gobble up debris, dead cells, and outside invaders with ease. The phagosomes of macrophages often fuse with lysosomes that empty their digestive enzymes into the vesicles and digest their contents. The small molecules formed from this digestion can diffuse through the phagosome's membrane into the surrounding cytoplasm. Some white blood cells also can phagocytize material. They police tissues and keep them free of foreign invaders, such as bacteria and viruses. Many macrophages and white blood cells have very dynamic and motile cell membranes that allow them to move via **amoeboid motion.** Their steaming cytoplasm can branch out into armlike

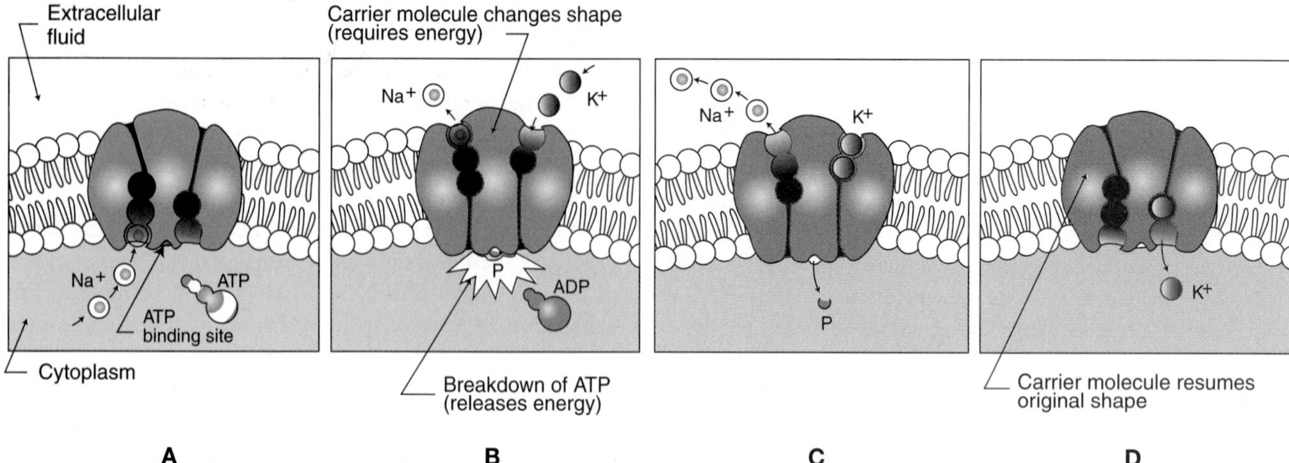

FIGURE **2-16 Sodium-Potassium Pump (an Antiport System).** Sodium and potassium ions are transported in and out of cells against their concentration gradients; therefore the pump is called an antiport system. **A,** A carrier molecule located in the plasma membrane accommodates three Na^+ ions. **B,** Energy in the form of adenosine triphosphate (ATP) binds to the carrier molecule and releases energy by breaking off one phosphate; adenosine diphosphate (ADP) remains. **C,** For each molecule of ATP, one carrier protein can transport three Na^+ ions and two K^+ ions. **D,** The carrier protein returns to its original shape when transportation of molecules is complete. It is once again prepared to accept Na^+ ions.

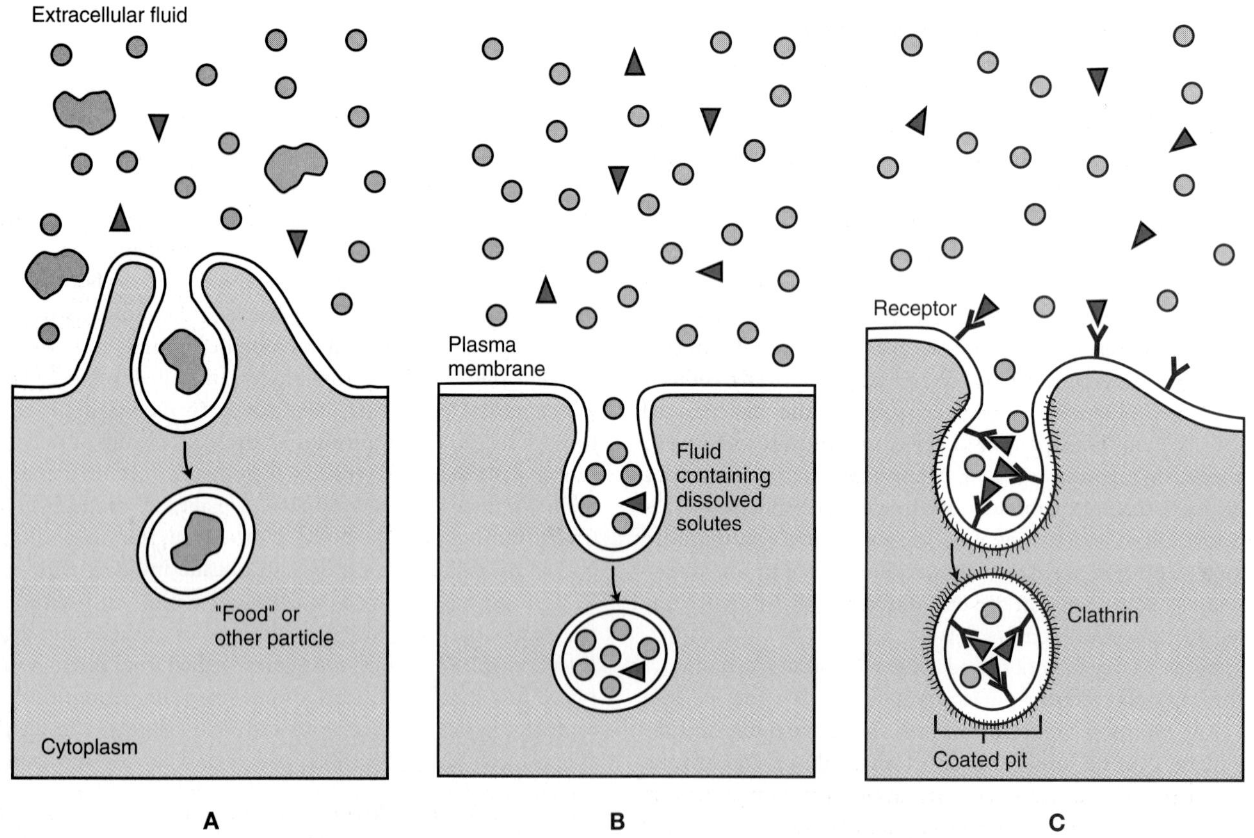

FIGURE **2-17 Three Types of Endocytosis. A,** Phagocytosis ("cell eating"): cell consumes solids, such as invading bacteria, viruses, or sick or damaged cells. **B,** Pinocytosis ("cell drinking"): cell consumes liquid substances, such as plasma. **C,** Receptor-mediated endocytosis involves selective consumption of substances.

projections called **pseudopods** (false feet), which enable these cells to move throughout tissue.

Unlike phagocytosis, pinocytosis involves only a minute infolding of the plasma membrane. Tiny droplets of liquid and the particles dissolved in them are taken into pinocytic vesicles, which pinch off from the plasma membrane. Eventually the membrane surrounding the vesicle breaks down, and the liquid contents spill into the surrounding cytoplasm. Pinocytosis is particularly important in cells that have absorptive responsibilities, such as the cells lining the small intestine and the cells that line the renal tubules in kidneys.

Unlike the processes of phagocytosis and endocytosis, which are primarily nonspecific ingestion processes, **receptor-mediated endocytosis** is very specific, occurring in cells that have specific proteins in their plasma membrane. These proteins act as specialized receptor sites for ligands such as hormones, iron, and cholesterol, which are found in the extracellular fluid. Insulin, for example, is a ligand that, once secreted from the pancreas, will only bind to those cells in the body that display the specialized protein receptor for insulin.

When a ligand successfully binds to a cell, it is taken into the cell with a small amount of involuted cell membrane and forms a vesicle called a **coated pit.** Like other endocytic vesicles, receptor-mediated coated pits fuse with lysosomes so that the ligands they contain can be broken down into smaller units and used by the cell.

Exocytosis. Cells may export substances from the intracellular environment into the extracellular space by exocytosis. Exocytosis of waste products is called **excretion,** and the exocytosis of manufactured molecules is known as **secretion.** Substances to be exported are packaged in vesicles by the ER and Golgi body. They move through the cytoplasm to the cell surface, fuse with the plasma membrane, and release their contents into the extracellular fluid. A neuron, for example, stores packages of acetylcholine (a neurotransmitter) in the synaptic region of the axon. When the proper electrical stimulus is initiated, these packages are released into the extracellular space where they quickly affect the postsynaptic neuron. Other examples of exocytosis are seen in the secretion of mucus by the endothelial cells lining the trachea and in the secretion of hormones by the adrenal and pituitary glands. One of the most dramatic examples of exocytosis, however, is evident during an allergic reaction in which thousands of granules containing histamine are released from mast cells. (Some of us are all too aware of the clinical signs of histamine secretion during ragweed season.)

Resting Membrane Potential

Charged particles (ions) exist within the intracellular and extracellular environments of all tissues. The amount, type, and distribution of these ions are important in maintaining cellular homeostasis. The plasma membrane, as you now know, is more permeable to some of these molecules than others. This difference in permeability leads to changes in the distribution of the charged particles on either side of the cell membrane, which, in turn, forms a **membrane potential** or **voltage** (Figure 2-18). A voltage is potential electrical energy created by the separation of opposite charges. All cells possess and maintain a membrane potential, which can range from -20 to -200 millivolts (mV), depending on the type of cell. The minus sign indicates that the cell is negative along the inner layer of the cell membrane relative to the outer cell surface. Cytoplasm and extracellular fluid generally have no net charge although they are both rich with ions.

How does the cell control the distribution and flow of ions that create the membrane potential? Although many ions are contained within the intracellular and extracellular fluids, the principal ions involved in maintaining membrane potential are K^+ and Na^+. As mentioned earlier, there are normally more potassium ions inside the cell than outside, and therefore potassium moves out of the cell via diffusion. Sodium, on the other hand, is more concentrated outside the cell than inside, but unlike potassium, it cannot enter the cell easily. The influx of sodium is lower than the outflow of potassium. In addition, for every cycle of active transport, three sodium molecules exit the cell for every two potassium molecules that are retrieved. Thus both active and passive membrane processes help to place more positively charged ions on the outside of the cell than on the inside. Cytoplasmic proteins, which are too large to leave the cell, tend to be negatively charged and further add to the voltage potential.

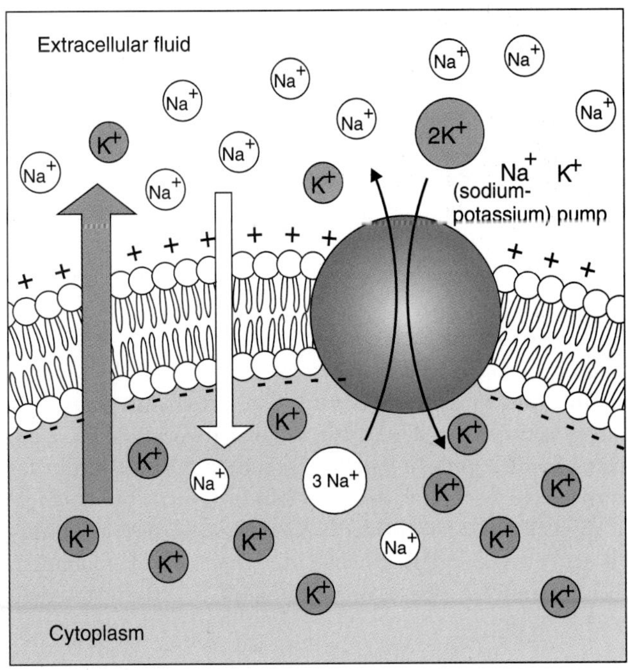

FIGURE **2-18** **Membrane Potentials.** Membrane potential is voltage or electrical potential caused by the separation of oppositely charged particles. Typically, the outside of the cell is slightly more positive than the inside of the cell as a result of the Na^+-K^+ pump and because Na^+ diffuses into the cell more slowly than K^+ diffuses out.

Cells are acutely aware of changes in the membrane potential. Changes in environmental tonicity, osmotic pressures, temperature, and contact with neighboring cells may alter **resting membrane potentials,** which, in turn, alter the flow of metabolites and the behavior of some structural and enzymatic proteins. Some specialized cells, such as muscle cells, owe their ability to contract to changes in membrane potential. Subsequent chapters (Chapters 7, 8, and 12) further address the role of membrane potential in the normal functioning of neuronal tissue, heart, and muscle, respectively.

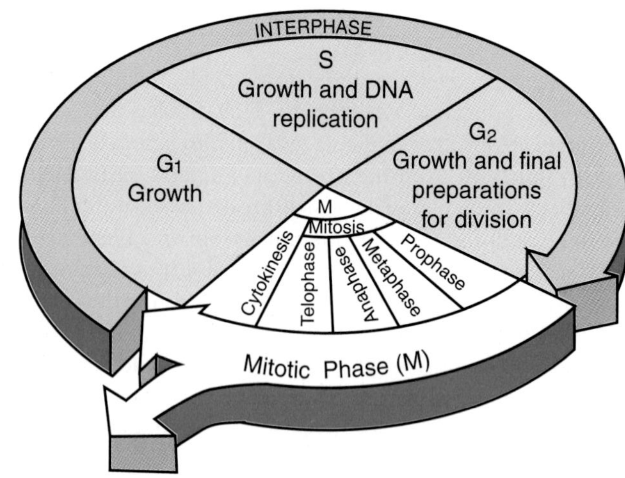

FIGURE **2-19** **Somatic Cell Cycle.**

TEST YOURSELF

1. When is a membrane process considered "active"?
2. How do electrolytes enter the cell?
3. What is the difference between a symport and an antiport system?
4. Describe how sodium and potassium enter and exit the cell.
5. Describe the three types of endocytosis.
6. What is the difference between excretion and secretion? These are both examples of what?
7. What are the principal ions involved in maintaining a cell's resting membrane potential?
8. Is there normally a higher concentration of sodium inside or outside of the cell? Where is there a higher concentration of potassium?

LIFE CYCLE OF THE CELL

In multicellular animals, cells are divided into two broad categories based on the way in which they divide. **Reproductive cells,** which are found in the ovary and testicle and give rise to eggs and sperm, respectively, divide via a process known as **meiosis.** (Meiosis is discussed later in Chapter 16, The Reproductive System.) **Somatic cells,** on the other hand, constitute all of the cells in the body except the reproductive cells. These cells divide via **mitosis.**

Mitosis

An animal's ability to grow and repair tissue is based on the division of somatic cells. In mitosis a cell divides by separating into two roughly equal parts. The cytoplasm, organelles, and genetic material separate to form two daughter cells, each of which grow and perform countless biochemical reactions before becoming ready to divide again. The life cycle of the cell has been divided into two major periods: **interphase,** when the cell is growing, maturing, and differentiating, and the **mitotic phase,** when the cell is actively dividing (Figure 2-19).

Interphase. Interphase is the period between cell divisions. Early cytologists were not aware of the complex metabolic activities of the cell and therefore erroneously considered interphase to be the "resting" phase. However, the cell is carrying out its normal life-sustaining activities during this time and therefore might be more accurately called the "metabolic" phase. During this time, the nucleus and nucleoli are visible and the chromatin is arranged loosely throughout the nucleus. In addition, the centrioles can be seen in various stages of replication. Interphase has been divided into three subphases (growth 1, synthetic, and growth 2), and cell growth occurs throughout all of them.

The first part of interphase is called the **growth 1 (G1) phase**. This stage can last for variable periods, from a few minutes in rapidly dividing cells to several weeks or even years in slowly dividing cells. The G1 phase is defined by intensive metabolic activity and cellular growth. During this time, the cell doubles in size and the number of organelles also doubles. In addition, centrioles begin to replicate in preparation for cell division.

The last two phases of interphase progress more rapidly. The **synthetic (S) phase** is marked by DNA synthesis and replication. New histones are formed and are assembled into chromatin, forming new identical replicas of the genetic material. The **growth 2 (G2) phase** is very brief and includes the synthesis of enzymes and proteins necessary for cell division and continued growth of the cell. The centrioles complete their replication by the end of the G2 phase. Although interphase is divided into distinct stages, these phases flow as a smooth, continuous process.

Mitotic Phase. The mitotic (M) phase is the time when the cell is actively dividing. From a single cell, two daughter cells are produced—each with the identical genetic material of the mother cell and each with the potential to divide and, once again, to pass on an identical copy of its DNA. Mitosis is separated into four stages—prophase, metaphase, anaphase, and telophase—and concludes with the division of the cytoplasm, which is called **cytokinesis** (Fig-

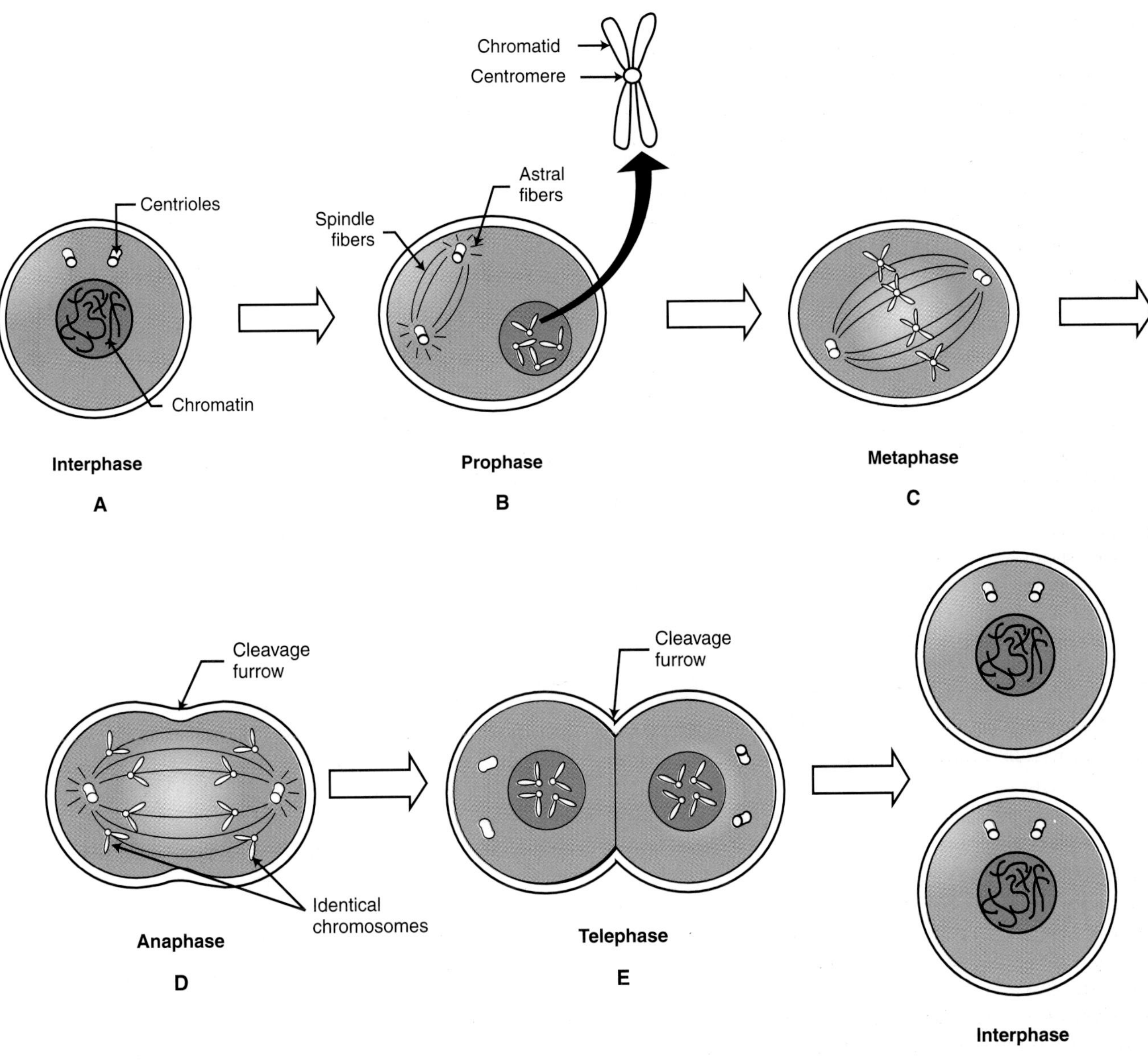

FIGURE **2-20** **Stages of Mitosis. A,** *Interphase:* Before a cell can divide, it must first make a copy of its DNA and another pair of centromeres. **B,** *Prophase:* Chromatin strands coil and condense to form chromosomes, which are linked at a central kinetochore. A spindle apparatus takes form while the nuclear envelope disintegrates. **C,** *Metaphase:* Chromosomes line up in the center of the spindle. The centromere of each chromosome is attached to a spindle fiber. **D,** *Anaphase:* Chromatids are pulled apart by spindle fibers to form a duplicate set of chromosomes. The cytoplasm constricts at the metaphyseal plate. **E,** *Telophase:* Chromatin begins to unravel at the poles of the cell, and a nuclear envelope appears. Cytokinesis marks the end of telophase. **F,** *Interphase:* Cycle of growth is repeated.

ure 2-20). A clue that a cell is about to divide is evident in the nucleus, where the chromatin starts to condense, coil, and form discrete chromosomes. The formation of chromosomes is important in enabling the cell to equitably divide its genetic material without tangling or breaking the long molecular chains.

In early **prophase,** chromatin coils and condenses to form barlike chromosomes that are visible with light microscopy. These chromosomes are composed of two identical **chromatids** that are linked together at a constriction in their middle, known as the **centromere** or **kinetochore.** The cytoplasm becomes more viscous as microtubules from the cytoskeleton are disassembled and the cell becomes round. Two pairs of centrioles form anchors on which new microtubules are constructed, and as the microtubules lengthen, they push the centrioles farther and farther apart. In this way a mitotic spindle is formed that provides the structure and machinery necessary to separate the chromosomes. Because transcription and protein synthesis cannot occur while the DNA is tightly coiled, the appearance of chromosomes marks the cessation of normal synthetic processes. Prophase is thought to conclude with the disintegration of the nuclear envelope.

Metaphase is distinguished by the lining up of chromosomes in the exact center of the spindle, known as the **equator.** The chromosomes are evenly spread apart and form what is called the **metaphase plate** midway between the poles of the cell. The centromere of each chromosome is attached to a single spindle fiber.

In **anaphase,** the centromeres of the chromosomes split apart and each chromatid becomes its own chromosome. The spindle fiber separates, each spindle segment shortens, and the twin chromosomes are pulled away from each another. The chromosomes take on a V shape as they are dragged at their midpoint toward the centrioles at opposite ends of the cell. The cell becomes elongated, and the cytoplasm begins to constrict along the plane of the metaphase plate. Although anaphase is the shortest phase of mitosis and usually lasts only a few minutes, its importance is clear in light of the devastating consequences if an error were to occur in chromosome separation. In anaphase the advantages of separating compact bodies of chromosomes, rather than long thin threads of chromatin, is particularly obvious.

Telophase is the final stage of mitosis and is said to begin when chromosomal movement stops. The chromosomes, having reached the poles, begin to unravel, elongate, and return to a diffuse threadlike form (chromatin). A nuclear envelope appears around each new set of chromosomes, and nucleoli appear in each nucleus. The microtubules that made up the spindle in the earlier phases of mitosis disassemble, and a ring of peripheral microfilaments begins to squeeze the cell into two parts. Ultimately, the cell pinches itself in half, dividing the cytoplasm and forming two completely separate daughter cells. The process of cytoplasmic division is called cytokinesis and marks the end of telophase. After cytokinesis, the daughter cells enter interphase, and the cycle of growth and reproduction is repeated once more.

Control of Cell Division. Cell division is important in the growth of an animal, but once adult size is reached, cell division becomes primarily a function of tissue repair and cellular replacement. Some cells, such as skin cells, must divide continuously to replace outer layers that have sloughed off. Nerve cells and fat cells, on the other hand, do not divide readily and are held in check. Why do some cell types divide rapidly whereas others, not at all? The control of cell division is poorly understood, but some important observations have been made. First, normal cells stop dividing when they come into contact with surrounding cells. This phenomenon is called **contact inhibition.** Second, growth-inhibiting substances may be released from cells when their numbers reach a certain point. Third, a number of checkpoints are reached during cell division when the cell reassesses the division process. These checkpoints occur during the G1 and G2 phases of interphase. For example, when the proper level of maturation promoting factor (MPF) is acquired at the end of the G2 phase, the cell is given the "go-ahead" to begin the mitotic phase of the cell cycle.

Cell Differentiation and Development. The development of a complex multicellular animal from a single fertilized egg is a miraculously choreographed event. It incorporates that which we understand biologically with that which is incomprehensible, for all living, breathing, thinking animals begin life as a single cell: the fertilized egg. The egg divides to form two cells, and they in turn divide, forming four cells, then eight, sixteen, and so on. Each generation of new cells gives rise to greater specialization. Ultimately the cells assume the diverse shapes and functions of the various tissues with which we are familiar: heart, lung, kidney, liver, and so on. However, because all of the cells in an individual contain the same genetic material, how can they take on diverse forms, shapes, and functions if they are all given the same set of instructions?

The answer lies in the position of genes in chromosomes. Some genes may be located on a region of the chromosome that is available for transcription, whereas other genes may be located inside the molecule and cannot be reached by transcription molecules. We say that one gene is "turned on" while the other gene is "turned off." Genes can be turned off permanently or temporarily. Chromosomes are dynamic in their ability to twist so that a gene that was once inaccessible on the inside can be moved to the outside of the molecule for use.

Some genes, like the ones that code for protein synthesis, are active in all cells, but the genes that govern the production of hormones and neurotransmitters are only turned on in some cells and not in others. The DNA in a muscle cell that codes for the production of acetylcholine, for example, is turned off because it is not needed, but the same gene in a nerve cell is turned on. Thus **differentiation** involves the temporary or permanent inhibition of genes that may be active in other cells.

Differentiation is important because no one cell can contain all of the metabolic and structural machinery needed to perform the secretion, absorption, contraction, conduction, storage, and elimination processes that are required for homeostasis in the body. The genetic material therefore "tells" the cell what types of protein to make and, consequently, what functions to perform. The proteins may be enzymes or catalysts for specific metabolic reactions. Thus the types of proteins that a cell makes are key to its specialization.

The specialization of cells also leads to a morphological or structural variation and influences the types and quantities of organelles contained within the various cell types. Some cells, such as striated muscle cells, are long and thin because the contractile proteins that they contain are long and thin. On the other hand, other cells, such as lymphocytes, are small and spherical, enabling them to pass through tiny blood vessels. In addition, cells such as macrophages, which are important phagocytic cells, are rich with lysosomes, whereas red blood cells contain no lysosomes because they do not need them to perform their job of carrying blood gases.

How does the cell know which genes to express and which to repress? As cells multiply, they become sensitive to chemicals released by neighboring cells that alter the expression of genes. Also, differences in oxygen and carbon dioxide concentrations between superficial and deeper cell layers may affect gene expression early in the developmental process. Regardless of these findings, there is still much to be learned about gene expression, about cell differentiation, and about the mysterious link between the life of an individual cell and that of an entire multicellular organism.

TEST YOURSELF

1. What are the two major periods that compose the life cycle of the cell?
2. Is interphase a time when the cell is resting? Why or why not?
3. What are the four stages of the mitotic phase?
4. What happens in each of these stages?
5. Why is it important for chromatin to coil and form discrete chromosomes before cell division?
6. What three factors play a role in the control of cell division?
7. What is the genetic basis of cellular differentiation?

CLINICAL APPLICATION Cancer

The word **cancer** is frightening to many of us. It is mysterious in its ability to affect some animals and people and not others. Sharks, for example, are not known to develop cancer, whereas certain breeds of dogs such as boxers are considered "tumor factories" by many veterinarians. Why is it that some of us have had or will have cancer, but others of us will not?

The causes of cancer are complex. Many factors influence the development of a normal cell and transform it into a killer. Environmental pollutants, certain food additives, radiation, some kinds of viruses, and certain chemicals have all been known to be **carcinogenic** (cancer causing). Also, certain genes have been linked to cancer in humans, and we see indications of this in animals as well. Rats, for example, carry a high risk for developing mammary carcinoma, and large dogs are far more likely to develop osteosarcoma, a tumor of bone, than small dogs.

Cancer develops when cells lose their normal control over cell division. Any cell can become cancerous and can divide unchecked in any tissue anywhere in the body. When cells proliferate excessively, they form abnormal masses called **neoplasms,** which are classified as either **benign** (kind) or **malignant** (*mal-*, meaning bad). Benign neoplasms are well circumscribed and may be encapsulated. Because they do not spread to other parts of the body and tend to grow slowly, they are rarely of danger to the patient as long as they are not affecting vital organs. Some benign neoplasms, such as lipomas, are common in older animals and are often found in the subcutaneous fat layer.

Malignant neoplasms, on the other hand, are invasive, are aggressive, and can spread to other parts of the body and form secondary tumors. Malignant cells are less sticky than normal cells and therefore tend to break away from the primary tumor. These cells are carried through blood and lymph to other parts of the body, where they may establish secondary tumors. This process is called **metastasis,** and the secondary tumors are called **metastatic masses.** In animals, primary lung cancer is extremely rare because animals do not smoke. Thus, when an animal is found to have lung cancer, every effort is made to find another tumor (the primary tumor) somewhere else in the body. Malignant cells form disorganized clumps rather then the neatly arranged rows of cells seen in normal tissue. Because they have lost their sense of contact inhibition, malignant cells invade the surrounding normal tissue by "walking" over the normal cells. In contrast, benign cancer cells tend to push the normal cells away. The invasive nature and ability to metastasize make complete surgical removal of malignant cancer difficult. Cancer cells also tend to be immature in nature. They tend to be larger and less well differentiated than their normal adult counterparts.

So how do the carcinogenic chemicals, viruses, and genes actually cause cancer? The answer is deceivingly simple; they cause mutations in the DNA, which alter the expression of certain genes. Genes that were permanently turned off may be turned on, and genes that should be turned on may be turned off. The cell is unable to perform normally because the programming has been altered. A **proto-oncogene** is a gene with fragile parts that are easily broken off or damaged by carcinogens. When the gene is damaged, it becomes known as an **oncogene** and provides incorrect instruction to the cell. Not all cancers are attributed to the formation of oncogenes, but their discovery has offered greater insight into the important relationship between carcinogens and genetics in the development of cancer.

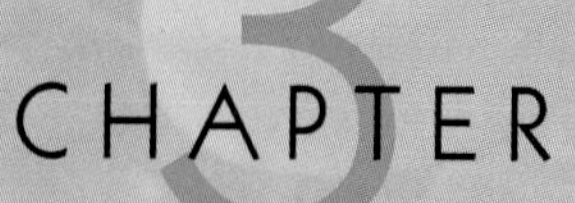

CHAPTER 3

CELL METABOLISM

Joanna M. Bassert

The cell is a dynamic, living powerhouse. It undergoes hundreds of metabolic reactions in its lifetime: building molecules and breaking down nutrients, manufacturing, packaging, and excreting. All of these biochemical events are part of the cell's metabolism. **Cell metabolism** is divided into two categories: **catabolism,** reactions that *break down* nutrients and *produce* energy, and **anabolism,** reactions that *build* large molecules from smaller ones and, in the process, *consume* energy. Catabolic and anabolic reactions occur simultaneously, and each must be in exquisite balance with the other so that adequate levels of energy are maintained (Figures 3-1 and 3-2).

CATABOLIC METABOLISM

The breakdown of large molecules into small ones is the basis of catabolism. As you know, the digestion of food occurs in the digestive tract, where stomach acids break down bits of food into molecular units that can be absorbed in the intestine and distributed throughout the body via blood or lymph. Potatoes, for example, may be broken down into molecules of carbohydrates, and a steak may be broken down into protein and fat molecules. Carbohydrates, proteins, and fat are further broken down before being absorbed through the wall of the intestine and placed in the bloodstream of the gastrointestinal tract (Figure 3-3). This part of the catabolic process is called **hydrolysis** (*hydro-,* "water"; *lysis,* "to break down") because at least one molecule of water is used up each time a nutrient molecule is broken down. Hydrolysis is the first stage of catabolism. A large sugar molecule such as a disaccharide can be broken down (hydrolyzed) into two smaller sugar molecules called **monosaccharides** as follows:

$$\text{1 Disaccharide + Water} \rightarrow \text{1 Monosaccharide + 1 Monosaccharide}$$

(*di-,* "two")(*mono-,* "one")

Through the process of hydrolysis, protein is broken down into **amino acids;** carbohydrates, into monosaccharides; **nucleic acids,** into nucleotides; and fat (lipids), into fatty acids and glycerol. Once hydrolysis is complete, the smaller nutrient molecules are taken up by absorptive cells that line the small intestine and are transported to various parts of the body via the circulatory and lymphatic systems.

The second and third stages of catabolism occur in the intracellular environment. Amino acids, glucose, glycerol, and fatty acids enter the cell and are further catabolized in the cytoplasm through a process called **anaerobic respiration.** Because *an-* means "not" and *aerobic* means "using oxygen," anaerobic respiration therefore is simply a metabolic process that does not use oxygen. An important molecular product of anaerobic respiration is acetyl-CoA. Acetyl-CoA is a molecule that is subsequently transported to the mitochondria, where it is used in **aerobic respiration,** the third and final stage of catabolism. As its name implies, aerobic respiration requires oxygen and involves the attachment of an inorganic phosphate group (PO_4) to a molecule of **adenosine diphosphate (ADP).** The result is the formation of **adenosine triphosphate (ATP): the**

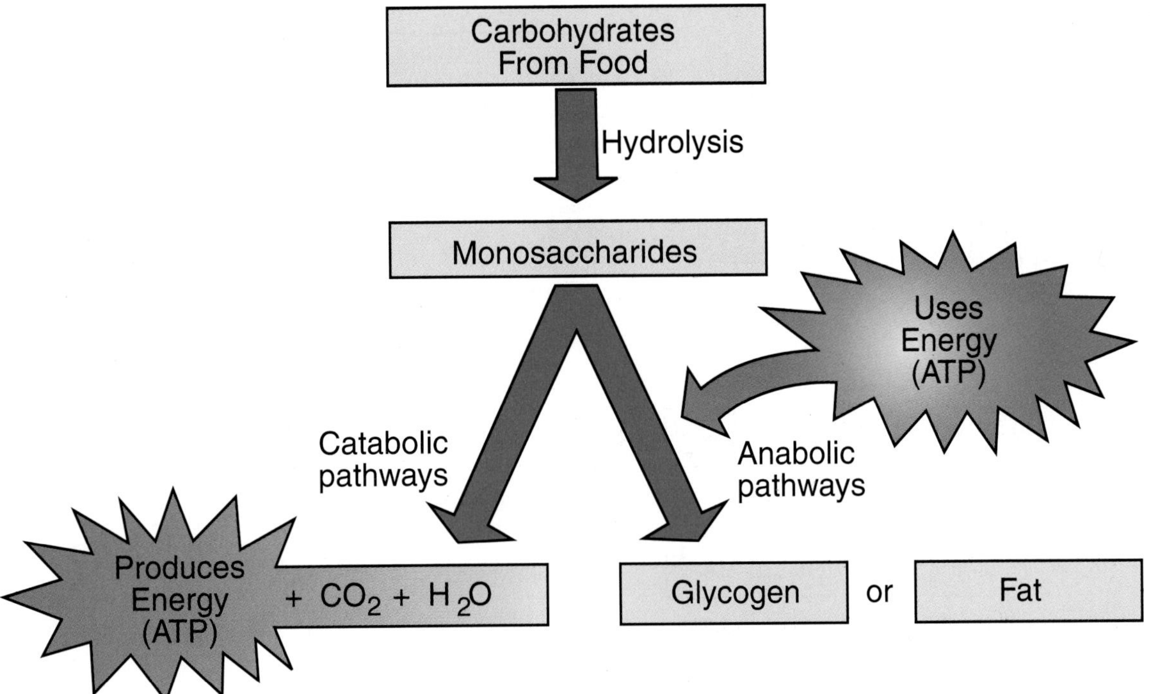

FIGURE 3-1 **Hydrolysis of Carbohydrates Leads to the Formation of Simple Sugars (Monosaccharides).** These, in turn, may be further catabolized to produce energy or may be used to build new molecules (anabolized) and stored as glycogen or fat.

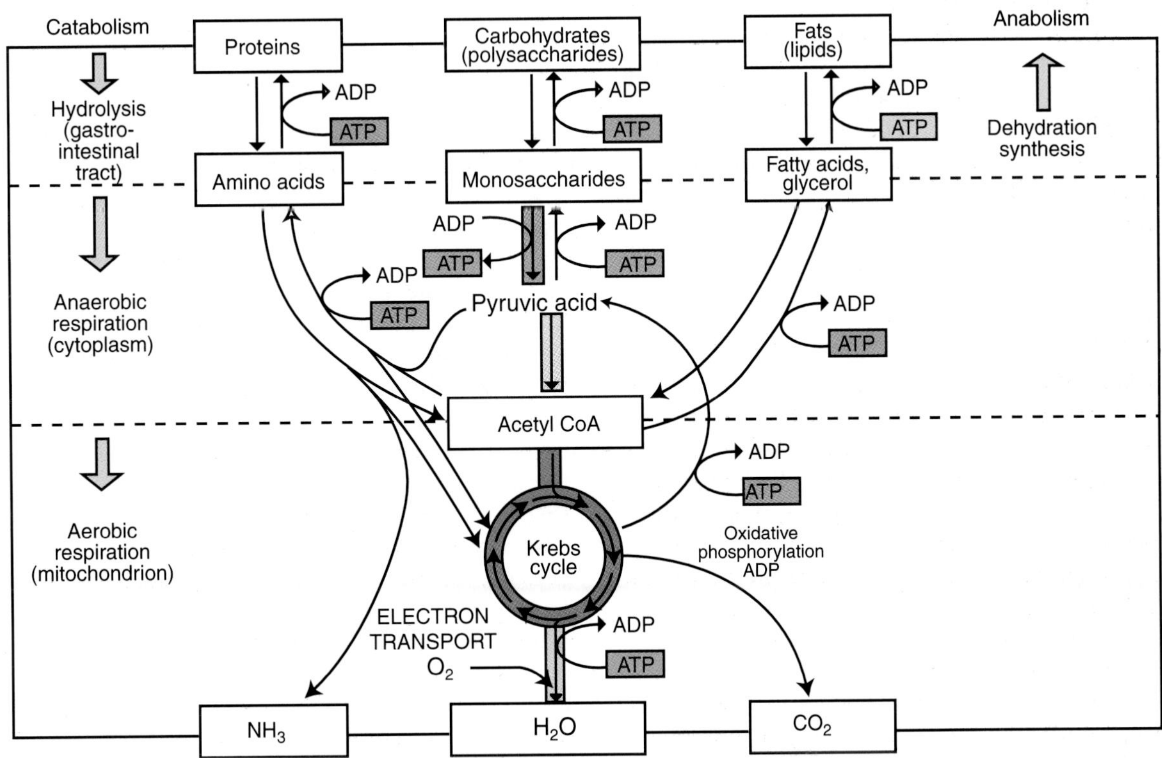

FIGURE 3-2 **Summary of Catabolism and Anabolism in the Cell.**

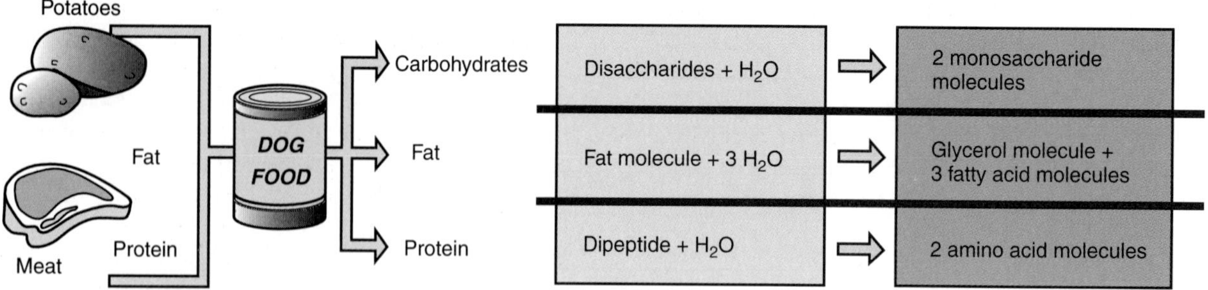

FIGURE **3-3** **Catabolism of Carbohydrates, Fats, and Proteins.**

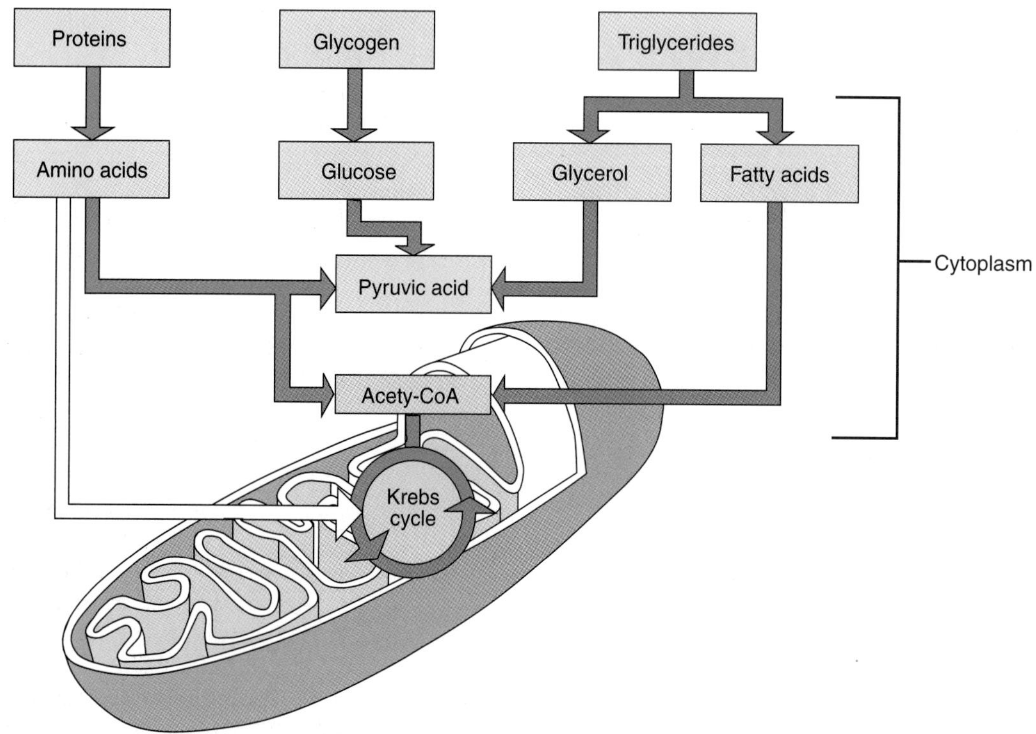

FIGURE **3-4** **Mitochondrion Is the Energy-Producing Factory for the Cell.** Energy is stored in molecules of ATP and is later used by the cell to maintain and repair itself and, ultimately, to divide. Therefore new proteins and enzymes are constantly being manufactured.

energy unit used in the cell to drive its **biosynthetic** processes. In this way, the mitochondrion can be viewed as an energy-producing factory in which the energy made is stored in the bonds of the ATP molecule (Figure 3-4). The catabolic pathways of protein, carbohydrate, and fat are vital to the survival of the cell, as well as the organism as a whole, because they generate energy for the cell in the form of ATP.

ANABOLIC METABOLISM

The cell uses energy in the form of ATP to manufacture a wide range of substances and to perform many vital functions. These *constructive* duties define anabolism, and the ATP that powers them is supplied by catabolism. Anabolic events are also called *biosynthetic processes* because a biochemical substance is manufactured. Examples of anabolism are evident in many aspects of cellular life. When cells grow, for example, additional proteins are needed for the expanded cell membrane. The cytoskeleton and additional organelles are manufactured. Cell locomotion, the production and secretion of hormones, the movement of materials from one place to another inside the cell, active membrane processes, and preparation for cell division are all examples of cellular activities that require the production of biochemical substances via anabolism. With the exception of deoxyribonucleic acid (DNA), molecular substances routinely break down, and replacement molecules are manufactured continuously. This process is called **metabolic turnover** and represents the largest demand for protein and enzymes in the cell.

An important part of anabolism is **dehydration synthesis,** the effect of which is the opposite of hydrolysis. **Simple sugars,** called *monosaccharides*, for example, are assembled (not broken down) to form chains called *polysaccharides*. A disaccharide (a chain of two monosaccharides) can be constructed as follows:

Monosaccharide + Monosaccharide → Disaccharide + Water

Glycerol and fatty acid molecules are connected to form fat molecules, and proteins are created from chains of amino acids. All of these anabolic processes begin with dehydration synthesis.

TEST YOURSELF

1. What is cellular metabolism? Can you think of routine cellular processes that represent specific examples of cell metabolism?
2. Cellular metabolism is divided into two categories. What are they?
3. What is the first stage of cellular catabolism called? Is energy produced or consumed?
4. Is energy produced or consumed during an anabolic process? What is an example of anabolism?
5. What cellular process represents the largest demand for protein and enzymes?

CONTROL OF METABOLIC REACTIONS

Living cells are composed of and contain thousands of molecules. How is it possible for all of these molecules to interact in a structured and orderly fashion that maintains life for the cell? As discussed in the last chapter, compartments are created within or on the surface of organelles, such as the mitochondria, endoplasmic reticulum, or ribosome. These "work areas" help to isolate molecules and allow chemical reactions to take place without interference. The organelles not only create separate environments for the different metabolic pathways but also assist in storing the enzymes and cofactors required for various biochemical processes. However, grouping molecules together does not guarantee that they will react with one another. Molecules must collide with sufficient force to initiate a reaction. The moderate temperatures of the intracellular environment and the relative stability of intracellular organic molecules preclude forceful collisions. How then are molecular reactions initiated and controlled? The answer is simple: through the formation and use of specialized proteins called **enzymes.**

Enzymes

Each enzyme reacts with a particular molecule called a **substrate** to produce a new molecule called a **product.** Because one enzyme reacts only with one substrate or combination of substrates, enzymatic reactions are considered highly specific. Hundreds of different biochemical reactions take place within the cell, so there must be hundreds of different enzymes available, each with the ability to locate and bond to its own special substrate. The DNA contained within the nucleus of the cell carries instructions for manufacturing all of the enzymes needed to drive these vital metabolic pathways. Metabolism therefore is a multienzyme sequence of events in which the product of one step is the substrate of the next. Some metabolic pathways include as many as 20 enzyme-driven steps. Although many of these pathways are linear, some are circular, and all have branches leading into or out of them (Figure 3-5).

Most chemical reactions require an input of energy to get started. The energy needed to initiate a biochemical reaction is called the **energy of activation.** In the laboratory the energy of activation is often supplied by heat. Heat causes molecules to become more active and to bang into one another. When molecules collide, existing bonds can be broken and new bonds can be formed. In this way, new substances are created. However, increased temperatures would be destructive to organelles and other structures within the cell. In addition, temperature changes would affect *all* of the chemical reactions at once and would not be selective for a particular type of reaction. The cell therefore relies on enzymes to initiate and control metabolic reactions.

An enzyme's ability to locate and bond to a particular substrate depends on the molecular *shape* of the enzyme. Enzymes are globular proteins that consist of one or more flexible polypeptide chains. These chains twist and coil to form a unique three-dimensional shape that fits the special shape of the substrate molecule(s). When the enzyme and substrate bind together, they form a temporary enzyme-substrate complex. The region of the enzyme molecule that binds to the substrate is called the **active site.** Like other portions of the enzyme, the active site is flexible and can exert pressure on the substrate that, in turn, weakens the bonds that keep the substrate molecule intact. In this way, one or more **product molecules** are formed, which subsequently separate from the enzyme. In biosynthetic reactions, enzymes unite smaller molecules to form one large one. These enzymes therefore require more than one active site, as shown in Figure 3-6. The enzyme is not altered by the reactions that it initiates and is able to move on to other substrate molecules and to complete more of the same kind of reaction.

Because enzymes bring reactant substrate molecules into proximity of one another and form temporary associations with them, they are able to speed up the rate of molecular reactions. For this reason, enzymes are also called **catalysts,** which are substances that speed up reactions by lowering the activation energy. Heat and various elements, ions, and chemicals can also act as catalysts. In the cell, enzymes speed up molecular reactions by a factor of a million or more. The rate at which a catalyzed reaction occurs is related to the amount of substrate and enzyme present. In general, an increase in the

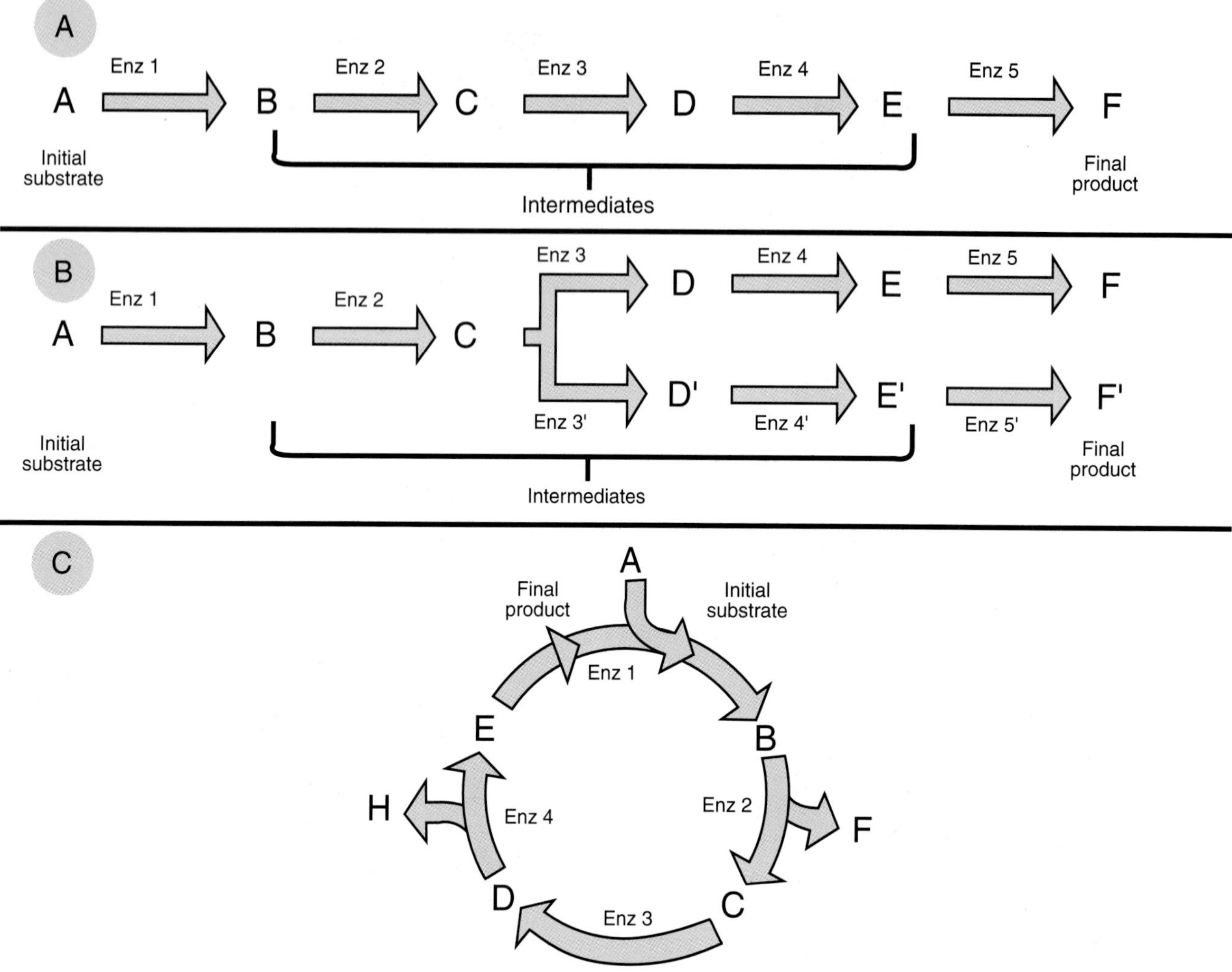

FIGURE **3-5** **Multienzyme Reactions.** Enzymes are specialized proteins that react with a particular molecule, a *substrate,* to produce a new molecule, a *product.* The enzyme is not altered in the process and can be used again and again to repeat the same reaction. **A,** Linear pathways are formed when the product of one reaction becomes the substrate of the next. Notice that the final product may be completely different from the initial substrate. **B,** Branched pathways occur when more than one product is formed from the initial substrate. **C,** Circular pathways terminate with a product that is identical to the initial substrate.

amount of an enzyme or a substrate causes an increase in the rate of the reaction. In addition, different enzymes have varying innate rates, that is, one type of enzyme might perform fewer reactions per second than another type of enzyme. As mentioned earlier, each enzyme is specific for a particular reaction; for example, hexokinase is an enzyme that converts glucose to glucose-6-phosphate (G6P), and this is the *only* reaction that hexokinase initiates and controls. It binds with glucose and ATP to create G6P and ADP, and it repeats this reaction over and over again. The amount of enzymes needed by the cell to carry out thousands of reactions is therefore relatively small because the enzymes are not used up during the reactions but are used multiple times to complete more reactions.

When studying cell metabolism, you can easily pick out the enzyme because its name ends with the suffix *-ase.* In addition, the enzyme is usually named for the substrate on which it acts. For example, proteinases are enzymes that break down protein, lipase breaks down lipid, lactase breaks down lactose, and so on. The name of the enzyme may also indicate the kind of reaction that the enzyme initiates. For example, synthetases are enzymes that synthesize or make new substances, and transferases are enzymes that move one part of a molecule to another molecule. Phosphotransferase, for example, is an en-

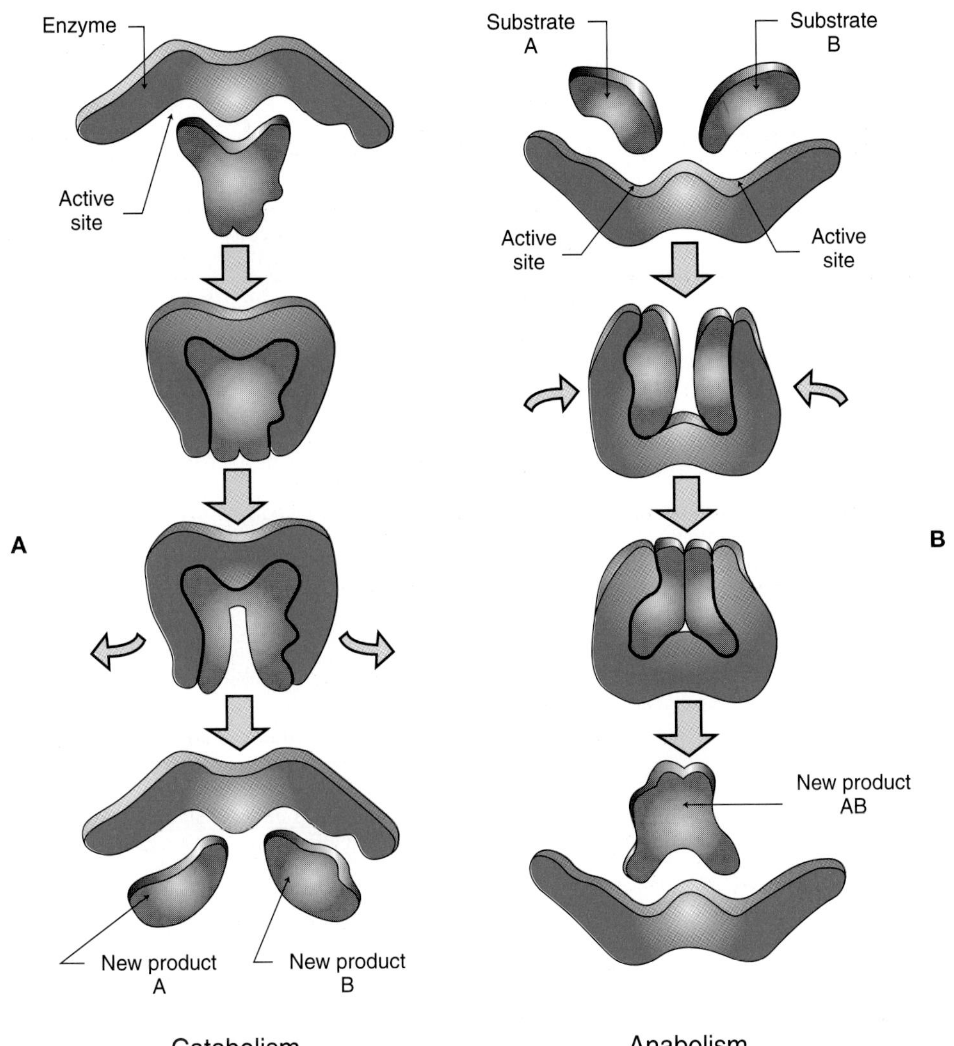

FIGURE **3-6** **Enzyme Activity.** Enzymes are flexible molecules with dynamic active binding sites. As shown in **A,** they are able to bond to one substrate to produce two product molecules via catabolism, or, as in **B,** can bind to two substrates to form a single product molecule via anabolism.

zyme that transfers a phosphate group from one molecule to another molecule. For these reasons, enzymes may have long names, such as glucose-1-phosphate uridylyltransferase and phosphoglucomutase. Although they may be a linguistic challenge at times, the names of enzymes are very useful and may indicate the biochemical reactions that are taking place.

Coenzymes and Cofactors

Some enzymes are not able to complete a reaction without the assistance of another substance. Elements such as iron, zinc, or copper, for instance, are needed to complete the shape of a binding site. These nonprotein substances are called **cofactors.** Certain ions, such as magnesium, are cofactors in reactions that involve the transfer of a phosphate group and are therefore found in virtually all cells. The negative charges on the phosphate group are attracted to the positive charges on the magnesium cation. The attraction of these opposite charges helps to stabilize the enzyme-substrate complex. K^+ and Ca^{2+} play a similar role in other molecular reactions.

Nonprotein organic substances may also act as cofactors. These substances are called **coenzymes** and are often derived from vitamins. They may be bound temporarily or permanently to the enzyme and are usually located near the active site (Figure 3-7). **Nicotinamide adenine dinucleotide (NAD),** for example, is a commonly encountered coenzyme in the cell and is critical in powering important cellular functions.

Clinical Application: Thermolabile Enzymes

Because enzymes are protein molecules with complicated three-dimensional structures, they are able to bend and move to accommodate bonding activities. Their shape is critical in enabling the enzyme to bond with the correct substrate. However, the shape of the binding site in some enzymes is affected by changes in the surrounding temperature. These enzymes are called **thermolabile enzymes** because changes in temperature bring about changes in the structure and shape of the enzyme molecule. For example, in the Siamese cat a thermolabile enzyme that affects coat color functions well in cooler temperatures but is rendered nonfunctional in higher temperatures; therefore a dark brown or black pigment is produced in the cooler regions of the body, such as the tips of the ears and tail, face, and paws, but not in warmer areas, such as the torso, neck, and thighs. Himalayan rabbits also carry thermolabile enzymes that affect coat color. For example, Himalayan rabbits raised in temperatures of around 5° C are entirely black; those raised in moderate temperatures are white with black ears, tail, and paws; and those raised in temperatures above 35° C are completely white.

An Easy Diagnosis

It is not uncommon for cats or dogs to develop Horner's syndrome, a condition caused by damage to a chain of nerves that extend from the chest, up the neck, and into the head and face. Ear infections (particularly those caused secondarily to ear mites), trauma to the neck (often from misuse of choker chains), tumors in the chest, and trauma to the nerves in the "armpit" region are all possible causes of Horner's syndrome. Usually only one side of the face is affected, and the most pronounced clinical signs include abnormal changes to the affected eye. Horner's syndrome also causes profound dilation of blood vessels in the muscles and skin of the face, an abnormality that is obvious in horses because they sweat profusely on the affected side. However, in domestic dogs and cats that do not sweat, this change is usually not clinically apparent. In Siamese cats the increased blood flow and temperature in their faces change the shape of thermolabile enzymes, making them unable to function normally. The production of pigment in the hair is halted, and in cases of long-term Horner's syndrome, the characteristic dark brown or black color of the Siamese face fades to a light tan or buff. Keep in mind that the appearance can look comical because this condition usually affects only one side of the face. Fortunately, for most cats, Horner's syndrome is a short-term disorder.

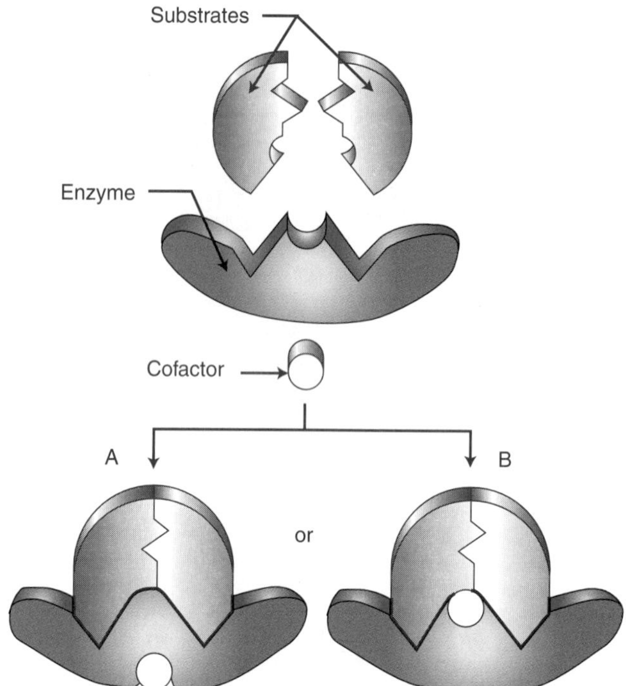

FIGURE **3-7 Cofactors and Coenzymes Assist in Activity of Enzymes in One of Two Ways. A,** Cofactor is added to structure of molecule in such a way that it indirectly changes the shape of the active site to enable a better fit between substrate and enzyme. **B,** Cofactor is part of active site and plays a direct role in creating the correct shape of the active site.

Energy for Metabolic Reactions

Energy is required for the survival of all living cells. In mammals, energy is supplied to cells by the breakdown of nutrients and is transferred to various "energy-holding" molecules, such as ATP, NADH, and $FADH_2$. In these convenient molecular packages, energy can be stored for extended periods and easily transported to regions of the cell where energy is in demand. Energy is captured and stored in the formation of atomic bonds but is released when these bonds are broken. ATP, for example, stores energy in the terminal phosphate bond. When the phosphate group is broken off, energy is released and the molecule is transformed into ADP (Figure 3-8). The released energy is used during subsequent biochemical reactions. The molecules that make up animal cells are adept at transforming themselves, from nutrient molecules to molecular energy stores and from substrate to product, cleaving off portions here and adding extensions there. Thus it is the *molecule* that stores, transforms, and uses energy in the cell through the formation and breakage of its molecular bonds.

Test Yourself

1. Why are enzymatic reactions considered highly specific?
2. What is a substrate? What is a product?
3. Why is the total number of enzymes present in the body relatively low when compared with the number of metabolic reactions?
4. What is the energy of activation in a biochemical reaction?
5. Why are enzymes catalysts? What is a catalyst?
6. How can you tell that a molecule is an enzyme? List three characteristics of enzymes.
7. What are some specific examples of cofactors?
8. How might vitamins play a role in enzyme-driven reactions?
9. How is energy stored in molecules? When is it released?
10. Can you give three examples of energy-holding molecules?

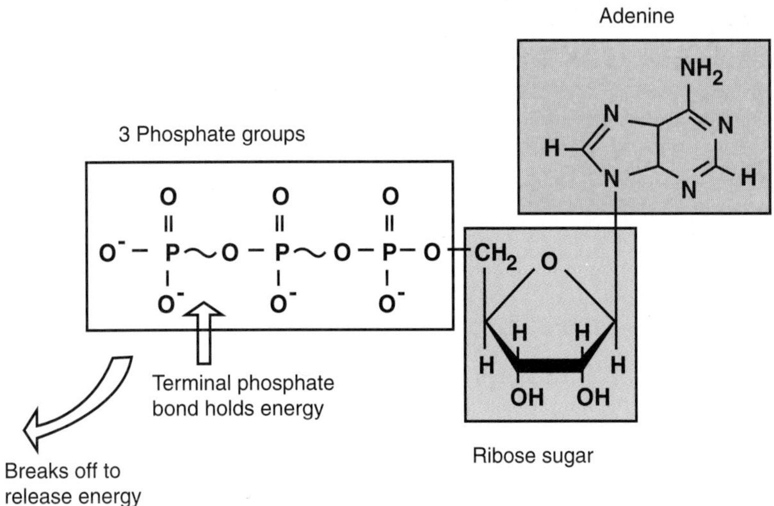

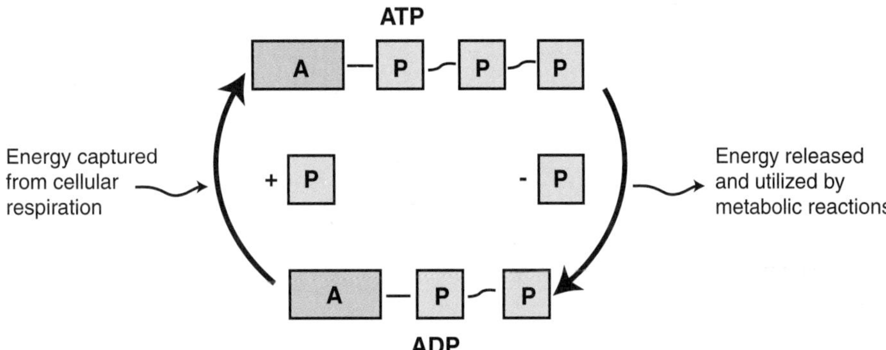

FIGURE **3-8** **ATP Conversion to ADP.** When the terminal phosphate bond in an ATP molecule is broken, it releases stored energy that can be used by the cell to make other molecules. The remaining molecule, ADP, has two remaining phosphate groups.

METABOLIC PATHWAYS

The breakdown of nutrients such as carbohydrates, proteins, and fats each follows a different metabolic pathway. Parts of these pathways occur in the cytoplasm and do not require oxygen (anaerobic), whereas other parts occur in the mitochondria and do require oxygen (aerobic). These pathways represent a complex series of biochemical steps that must occur in a particular sequence, and each step involves an enzyme specific for that particular step.

CARBOHYDRATE METABOLISM

Carbohydrate metabolism occurs in virtually all living cells and includes all of the catabolic and anabolic processes involving carbohydrates. In mammals, carbohydrates may be supplied either through the diet or from the breakdown of glycogen, glycerol, or, in the case of ruminants, propionate stored in the liver (Figure 3-9). In most mammals, carbohydrates provide well over half the energy required to fuel metabolic functions, such as absorption, secretion, excretion, mechanical work, growth, and repair.

Most dietary carbohydrates are in the form of polysaccharides, such as starch, **cellulose,** and glycogen. (A polysaccharide is a molecule composed of many saccharide molecules linked together.) Other dietary sources include disaccharides (two saccharide molecules linked), such as sucrose, maltose, and lactose, and monosaccharides (one saccharide molecule; also called *simple sugars*), such as glucose and fructose. The digestion of carbohydrates in nonruminants begins in the mouth with the activity of salivary amylase and is completed in the small intestine, where enzymes break down disaccharides into monosaccharides through hydrolysis. The resulting monosaccharides are absorbed by villi in the intestine and are transported via blood to the liver. Once in the cell, monosaccharides may either enter catabolic pathways and be used to make energy in the form of ATP or they may follow anabolic pathways and be converted to glycogen or fat. In **herbivores** the cellulose found in grass, hay, and other leafy plants is converted to short-chain or **volatile fatty acids (VFAs)** by microbial **fermentation** in the **alimentary canal.** These VFAs, such as butyrate, acetate, and propionate, provide a major portion of the energy needed by ruminants. *Dietary* sources of monosaccharides, however, play a less important role in herbivores.

Glucose is the primary carbohydrate found in blood. It is absorbed from the extracellular fluid by all cells and is used to

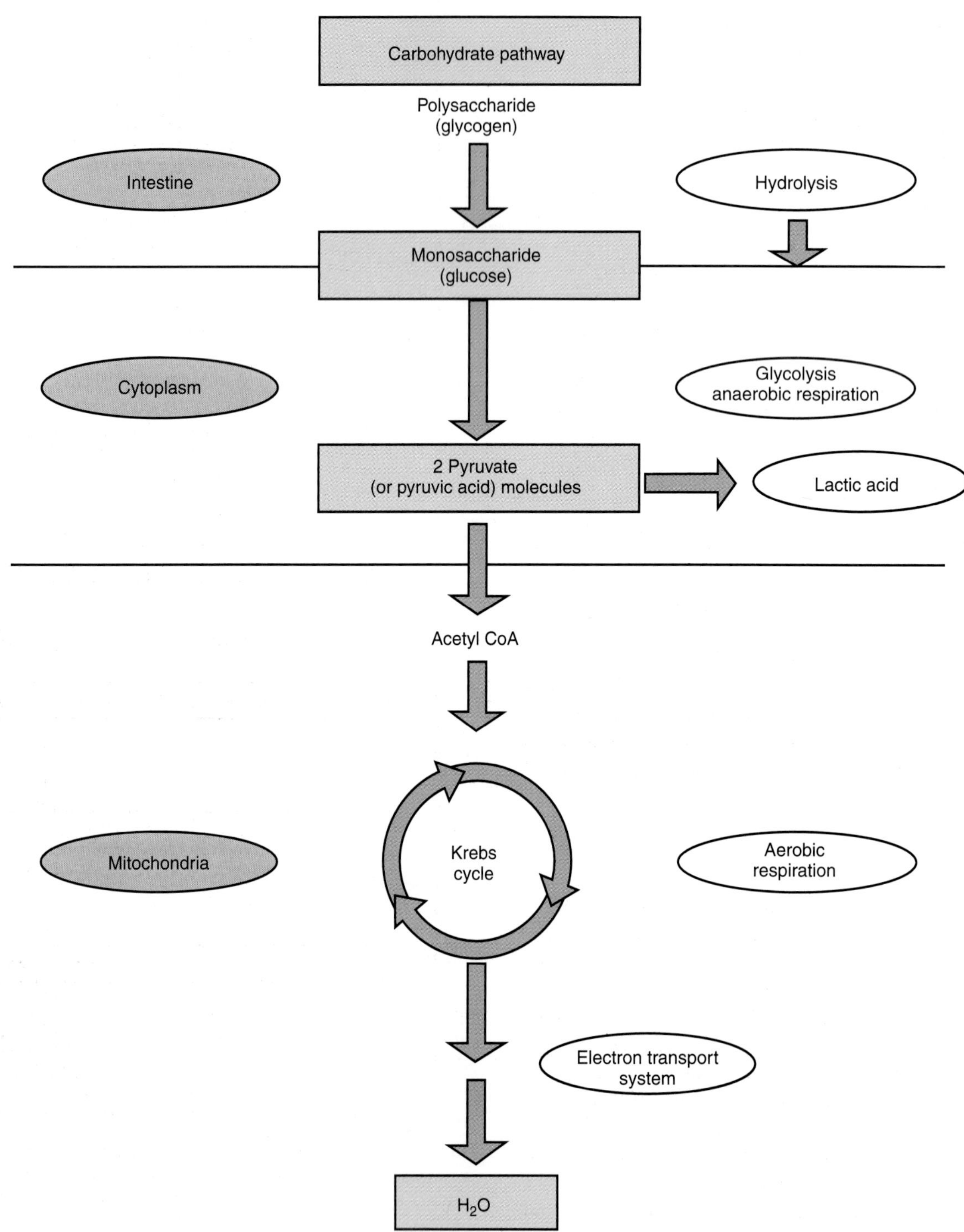

FIGURE **3-9** **Overview of Carbohydrate Metabolism.**

produce energy in the form of ATP. Certain types of cells, such as red blood cells and brain cells, are exquisitely sensitive to fluctuations in blood glucose levels because they cannot derive energy from other sources. Other cells, however, such as skeletal muscle cells, can derive energy from ketones and fatty acids and therefore are not as affected by falls in blood glucose supplies. Nevertheless, when glucose is urgently needed and in short supply, the body is able to provide it quickly by mobilizing stores of glycogenic molecules in the liver.

Glucose may enter a cell either by facilitated diffusion or via active transport. Once inside the cell, it is converted to G6P and is then further broken down to form pyruvate (or pyruvic acid). This process is called **glycolysis** (*glyco-*, "glucose"; *lysis,* "break apart") and occurs in the cytosol. Because glycolysis does not require oxygen, it is referred to, in some texts, as anaerobic glycolysis.

After pyruvate is formed from glycolysis, one of several pathways may follow. Most of the time, cells are fed with good quantities of oxygen via circulating red blood cells. In an oxygen-rich environment, pyruvate is transported from the cytosol to the mitochondria, where it undergoes further degradation as part of **cellular respiration.** However, some cells, such as skeletal muscle cells, may take a different pathway if the oxygen supplied to them has been depleted. During vigorous exercise, for example, skeletal muscle cells rapidly consume oxygen. Once the oxygen is depleted, the cells take a different metabolic pathway and convert pyruvate to **lactic acid.** We have all experienced the effects of lactic acid production in our own muscles at one time or another, particularly after performing strenuous work that we do not normally do. Lactic acid builds up in muscles during and after exercise and causes a "stiff" feeling the next day. In horses, this stiffness can be severe and can cause a condition called *tying up.* It is not uncommon for horses ridden for pleasure to "tie up" on Mondays because many owners only ride them on weekends. For this reason, "tying up" is sometimes called *Monday morning syndrome.*

The biochemical pathways of glycolysis and cellular respiration have been studied extensively by biochemists and therefore are discussed in detail. However, keep in mind that the biochemical principles involved in their function and regulation are common to all pathways of cell metabolism.

Glycolysis

Glycolysis occurs in all animals and includes nine biochemical steps, each of which relies on a specific enzyme found in the cytosol. It does not require oxygen and is therefore considered an anaerobic process. For every molecule of glucose metabolized, the cell must use two molecules of ATP and two molecules of NAD to initiate the process. Two molecules of pyruvic acid, four molecules of ATP, and two molecules of NADH are produced. Thus the net energy yield from glycolysis is two molecules of NADH and two molecules of ATP.

The chemical reactions of glycolysis are outlined in Figure 3-10. In the initial stage, one molecule of ATP is used to supply the energy needed to add one phosphate group to the sixth carbon in glucose. This process is called **phosphorylation** and results in the formation of G6P. Although this process costs the cell one molecule of ATP, it is important in preventing the glucose molecule from leaving the cell because phosphorylated glucose cannot cross the cell membrane. It also prepares the glucose molecule for further manipulations either in a catabolic or anabolic pathway. In glycolysis, G6P is rearranged to form fructose-6-phosphate. From here, phosphorylation occurs again using one more ATP molecule to form fructose-1-6-diphosphate. This molecule is then cleaved into two molecules of glyceraldehyde 3-phosphate. Each of these molecules is transformed into pyruvic acid via a five-step process that also gives rise to four molecules of ATP.

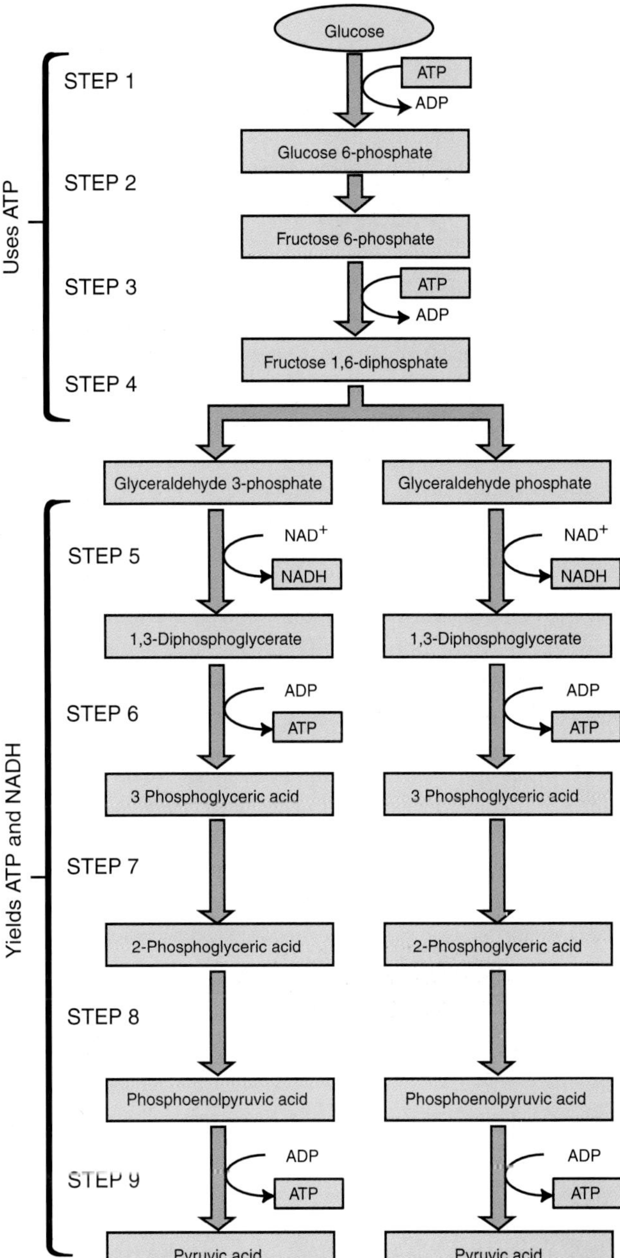

FIGURE **3-10** **Glycolysis.** In glycolysis, a six-carbon glucose molecule is catabolized into two molecules of pyruvic acid (pyruvate), each with three carbons. This process includes nine steps and produces six energy-holding molecules: two molecules of NAD and four molecules of ATP.

Although its contribution of energy to animal cells is important, glycolysis is *not* the cell's primary source of ATP. A great deal of potential energy from the original glucose molecule still remains in pyruvic acid. This molecule can be further broken down in the mitochondria to form larger quantities of energy for the cell through an aerobic sequence of biochemical events known as **cellular respiration,** or **oxidation.**

Cellular Respiration (Oxidation)

When we breathe in air, we are performing a vital function. If we do not breathe, we die. We can only survive for a short time without oxygen before the cells in our body start to die because oxygen is required for the production of energy (ATP) by the cell. Many cell types cannot live without ATP for very long. As you know, the process of breathing is called *respiration*, so the cellular process of taking in oxygen molecules and producing ATP molecules is called *cellular respiration*. Blood carries oxygen to cells throughout our bodies. After blood releases oxygen molecules to the cells, it picks up carbon dioxide molecules that have been discharged by the cell. These molecules are then circulated back to our lungs, where they are exhaled. We exhale carbon dioxide because our cells give off carbon and oxygen atoms in the process of making ATP. They are subsequently made into molecules of carbon dioxide before being exhaled from the body.

Cellular respiration occurs in the mitochondria in two stages: the **Krebs cycle** (also known as the **citric acid cycle**) and the **electron transport system.** The smooth outer membrane of the mitochondria is permeable to most small molecules, but the undulating inner membrane is more selective and permits the passage of only certain molecules, such as pyruvic acid and ATP. The folds of the inner membrane are called *cristae* and contain within their walls some of the enzymes and cofactors needed in the Krebs cycle and electron transport system. Other enzymes are found in the **matrix,** which is the thick solution that bathes the cristae within the mitochondria. Enzymes in the mitochondria that are responsible for aerobic respiration have positioned themselves on the cristae in the order in which they are needed for oxidation. This "assembly line" approach is an efficient way to carry out molecular alterations and, at the same time, minimizes the potential for errors (Figure 3-11).

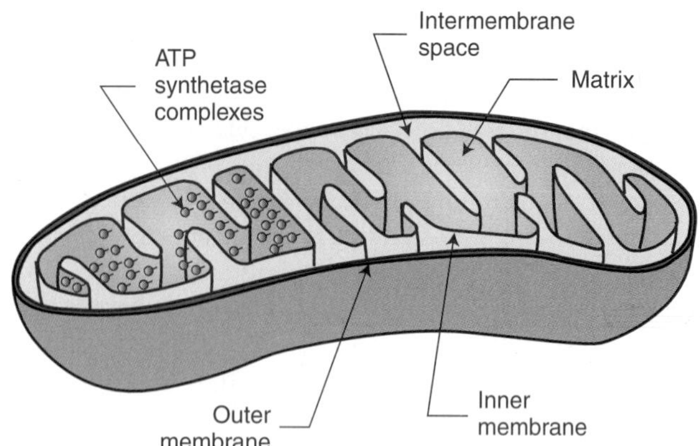

FIGURE **3-11** **Mitochondrion: Cellular Powerhouse.** The mitochondrion is uniquely designed to support cellular respiration and ATP production. The inner membrane of the mitochondrion, for example, has infoldings and outpouchings, called *cristae*, which form separate "work spaces" for the Krebs cycle and the electron transport system. Many of the enzymes involved in ATP production, such as ATP synthetase, are built into the wall of the inner membrane. These molecules form an "assembly line," which improves efficiency and helps to prevent errors. The matrix that fills internal spaces of cristae is rich with electron carriers, phosphates, coenzymes, and other solutes necessary for ATP production.

Krebs Cycle. Pyruvic acid enters the mitochondria from the cytosol by passing through both the outer and inner membranes. Before it enters the Krebs cycle, it is transformed from a three-carbon molecule of pyruvic acid into a two-carbon acetyl group; this, in turn, binds to a compound known as coenzyme A to form acetyl-CoA—a molecule that represents the link between glycolysis and the Krebs cycle. During this process, one molecule of carbon dioxide and one of NADH are also generated for every molecule of pyruvic acid.

Acetyl-CoA enters the Krebs cycle and reacts with oxaloacetic acid to form citric acid; therefore the Krebs cycle is also known as the citric acid cycle (Figure 3-12). As citric acid is produced, coenzyme A is released and is used repeatedly to make acetyl-CoA. After seven additional steps, citric acid is converted back to oxaloacetic acid and the entire process is repeated. Each turn of the Krebs cycle generates energy in the form of one ATP, one FADH2, and three NADH molecules. For every molecule of glucose, the Krebs cycle can run twice and in doing so produces two molecules of ATP, two of FADH2, and six of NADH. Carbon dioxide, which is formed as a byproduct of respiration, diffuses out of the cell and into the bloodstream as waste, is carried to the lungs, and is exhaled.

Electron Transport System. The final stage of cellular respiration, which produces the majority of ATP for the cell, occurs in the inner wall of the mitochondrion and is known as the electron transport system. NAD and FAD molecules released from the Krebs cycle, glycolysis, and the conversion of pyruvic acid to acetyl-CoA bind to hydrogen atoms to form NADH and FADH2. The electrons in NADH and FADH2 are at a very high energy level because they hold most of the energy once held by the original glucose molecule. In a sense, they are at the top of an energy hill and, from here, are carried down a chain of electron carrier molecules collectively known as the **cytochromes** (Figure 3-13). Each cytochrome molecule contains a central core of iron that accepts electrons and then releases them at a lower energy level. At each step, large amounts of free energy are released and used to pump protons from the mitochondrial matrix through the inner membrane to the intramembranous space (the space between the inner and outer membranes of the mitochondria). This establishes a difference in electrical charge because more positive hydrogen ions are pumped to the outside than remain on the inside of the inner mitochondrial membrane. Thus the outside has a positive charge relative to the matrix side of the membrane. The result is the formation of potential energy that is available when the protons flow back to the matrix side of the inner mitochondrial membrane (Figure 3-14). The energy released during this downhill pathway is captured in the formation of ATP from ADP. At the end of the electron transport chain, oxygen accepts the low-energy electrons, joins with hydrogen

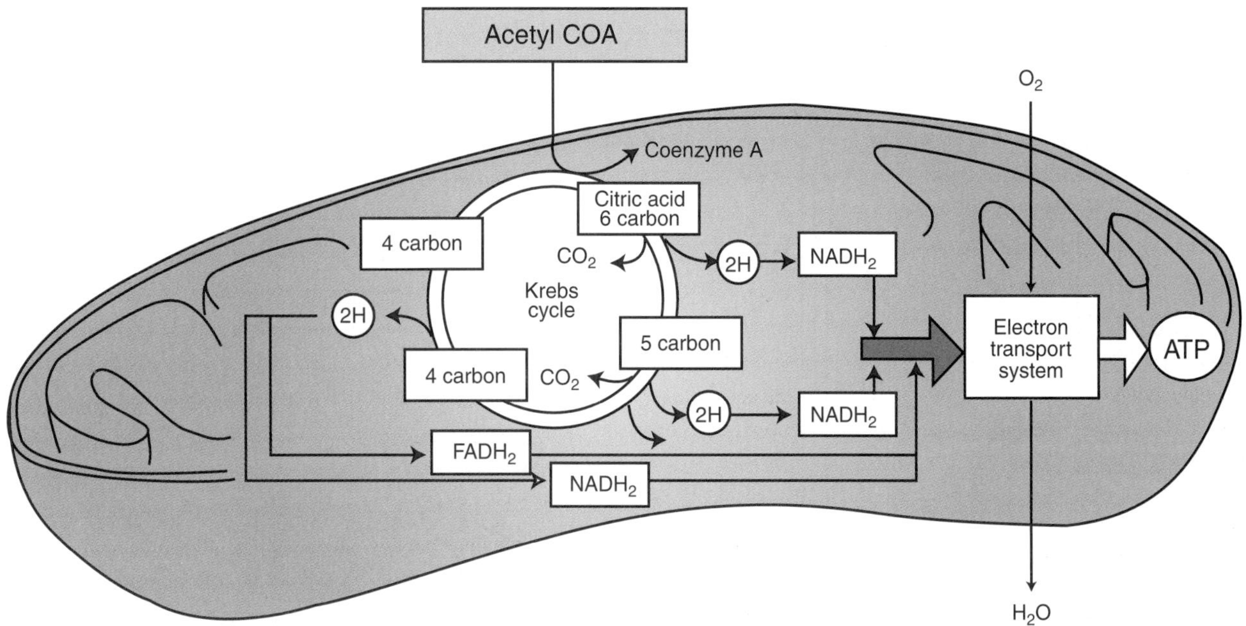

FIGURE **3-12** **Krebs Cycle.** Pyruvic acid is converted to acetyl-CoA, which in turn enters the Krebs cycle in the mitochondrion. The Krebs cycle produces hydrogen atoms that are funneled into the electron transport system to produce ATP. Carbon and oxygen are released from the cycle as waste and are ultimately exhaled by the animal in the form of carbon dioxide.

ions, and forms water (H_2O). Thus oxygen is the final acceptor of the electrons.

Summary of ATP Synthesis

The biochemistry of glucose catabolism is complicated, so let's take a step back and look at the overall picture of what the cell is doing.

Through the breakdown of glucose, the cell produces units of usable energy called *ATP*. For every molecule of glucose metabolized by an animal, a maximum of 38 ATP molecules is formed, although in some cells only 36 ATP molecules are formed. Two ATP molecules are made in the cytoplasm, and the rest are made in the mitochondria.

In the cytoplasm, glycolysis gives rise to two molecules of ATP directly and two molecules of NADH. The NADH molecules are shuttled to the electron transport system in the mitochondria, where they produce six ATP molecules (three for every molecule of NADH). Thus the total gain from glycolysis is eight ATP molecules. However, in certain cells, such as brain and skeletal muscle cells, there is energy cost for transporting NADH into the mitochondria. In these cells, each NADH molecule produces only two ATP rather than three. Thus, in some cells, glycolysis produces only six ATP, not eight.

Inside the mitochondria, pyruvic acid is converted to acetyl-CoA before it enters the Krebs cycle. During this process, two molecules of NADH are formed, one from each of the two molecules of pyruvic acid. Each of these NADH molecules forms three molecules of ATP so that a total of six ATP molecules are derived from the conversion of pyruvic acid to acetyl-CoA.

Also in the mitochondria, the Krebs cycle yields two molecules of ATP, two of FADH2, and six of NADH. The electron transport system converts the NADH and FADH2 molecules into 22 ATP. Thus the Krebs cycle produces a total of 24 ATP.

Table 3-1 provides a summary of ATP production in the cell. Notice that all but 2 of the 38 ATP molecules are produced in the mitochondria and that all but 4 ATP result from the passage down the electron transport chain of electrons carried by NADH and FADH2. Once formed, the energy-carrying ATP molecules are exported across the mitochondrial membrane, and a molecule of ADP is brought into the mitochondria for each ATP exported.

LIPID METABOLISM

Lipids are molecules composed of carbon, hydrogen, and oxygen, which are insoluble in water but dissolve easily in other lipids or organic solvents. Two common types of lipids are **triglycerides** and **phospholipids.**

Triglycerides are commonly known as neutral fats or just plain fat. As humans, we are acutely aware of the risks associated with a diet that is too rich in fat. We know that diets high in fat are associated with heart disease, hypertension, obesity, and, perhaps, some kinds of cancer. However, few people realize that fats play an important role in the health of both humans and animals. Fat forms protective pads around vital organs such as the kidneys and orbits of the eye. It insulates the body and prevents heat loss and is an important structural element of cell membranes. Fat-soluble vitamins such as A, D, E, and K play important roles in night vision, calcium uptake, wound healing, and blood clotting, respectively.

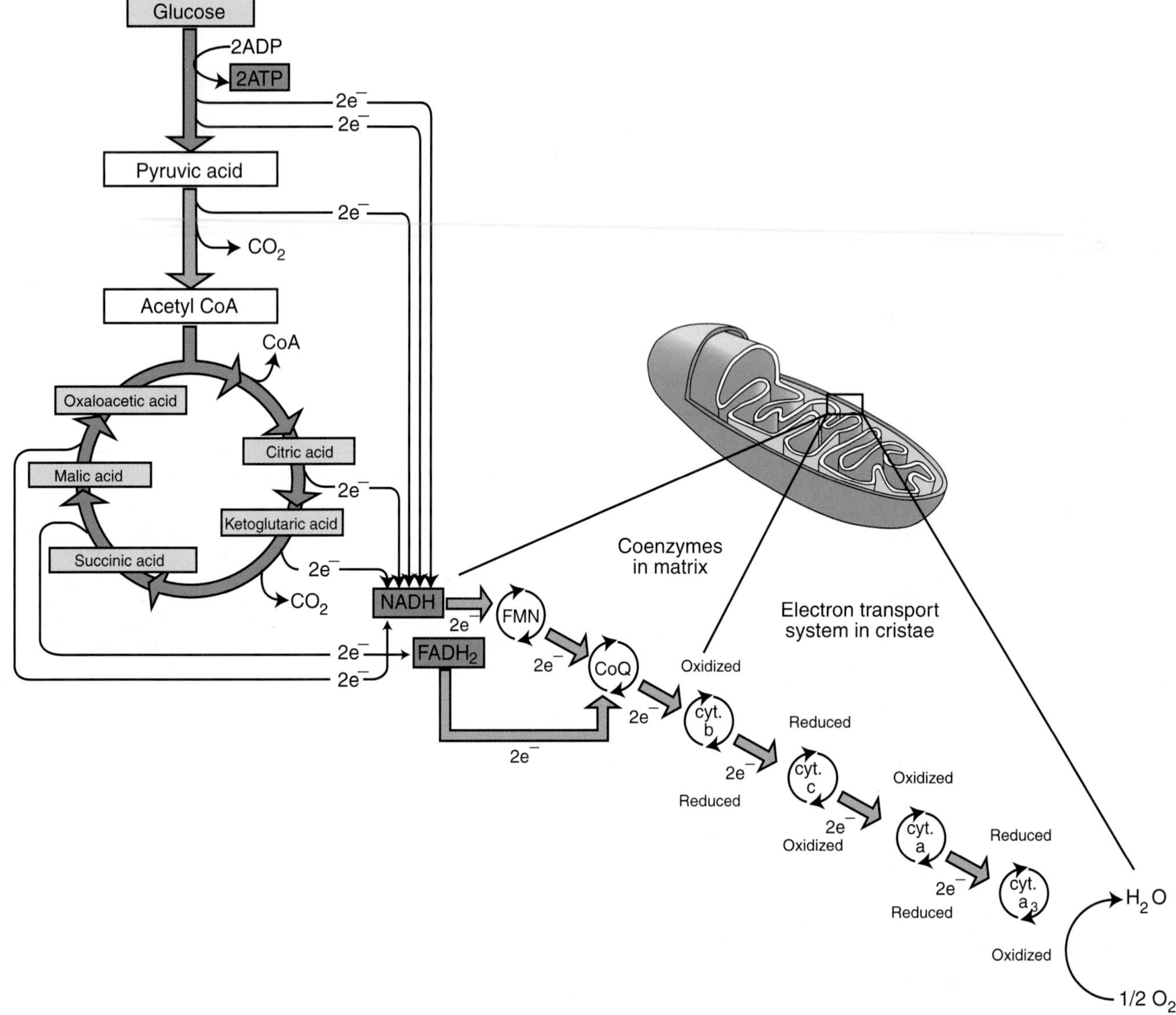

FIGURE **3-13** **Summary of Glycolysis and Cellular Respiration.** Glycolysis: *a,* in the cytoplasm of the cell, glucose is broken down to form two molecules of pyruvic acid; *b,* subsequently, pyruvic acid is transported to the mitochondria, where it is converted to acetyl-CoA. Cellular respiration: *c,* acetyl-CoA is then altered in inner folds of the mitochondria by a circular multienzyme reaction known as the Krebs cycle; *d,* the Krebs cycle transforms electron carrier molecules NAD^+ and FAD^+ into NADH and FADH by giving them electrons; *e,* these molecules then pass their electrons on to a series of cytochrome molecules in the electron transport system; *f,* electrons are passed from one cytochrome molecule to another down a long chain. Each time electrons are transferred from one cytochrome to another, energy is released. Energy is used to transport protons across the inner mitochondrial membrane to the intramembranous space and, in this way, establishes a proton gradient. *g,* Energy stored in the gradient is later released when protons rush back across the inner membrane. This energy ultimately transforms ADP into ATP.

Triglycerides contain a higher number of carbon-hydrogen bonds than other nutrient molecules and therefore contain more chemical energy than either carbohydrates or protein (remember that energy is stored in the bonds between atoms). Gram for gram, fat contains over *twice* as much chemical energy as carbohydrates and stores *six* times as much energy as glycogen. This fact is important, particularly in birds, because it illustrates that fat concentrates energy in a form that is relatively lightweight; an essential requirement for flight. Herbivores do not consume the large amount of fat that is prevalent in the diet of meat eaters. For them, the formation of fat is derived primarily from the conversion of carbohydrates that is in excess of what can be stored as glycogen.

Triglyceride molecules are neutral, hydrophobic structures composed of one central **glycerol** molecule and three chains of **fatty acids** (Figure 3-15, *A*). There are about 70 different fatty acids. They vary in their lengths and in the number and position of double bonds present. Fatty acids that have no double bonds, for example, such as those found in animal fat and butter, are said to be **saturated** because all of the possible

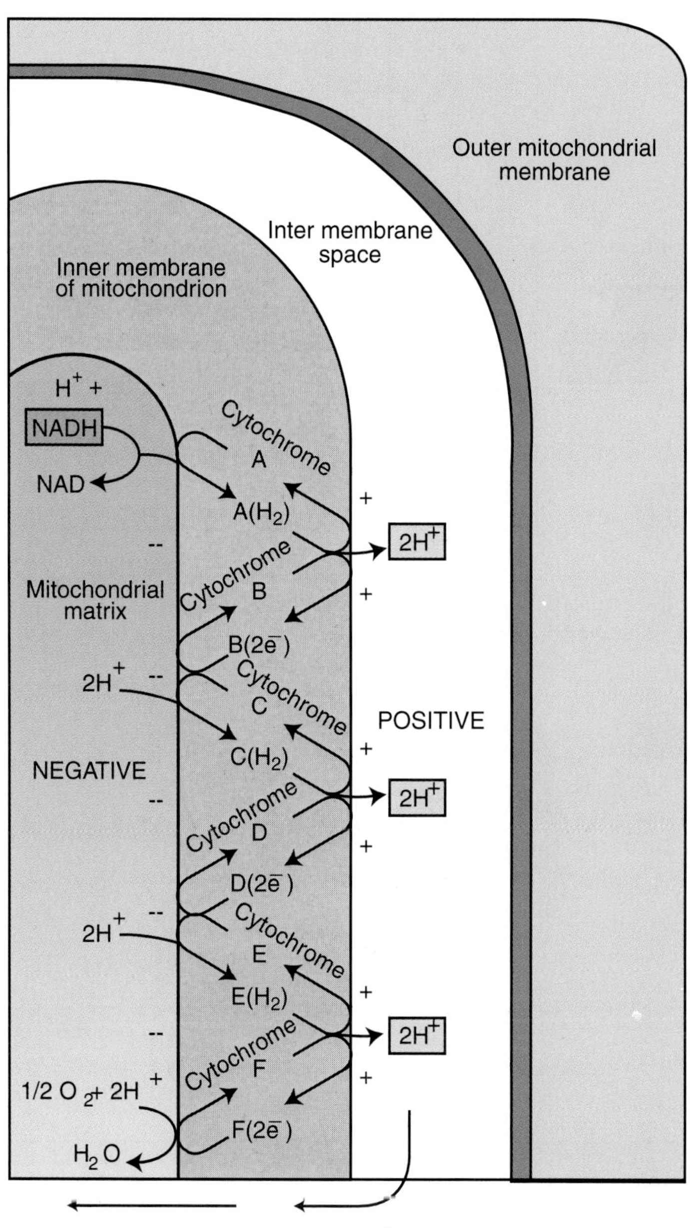

FIGURE **3-14** **Formation of Proton Gradient in Mitochondrion.** As electrons are passed from one cytochrome molecule to another, energy is released that is used to transport protons from the mitochondrial matrix across the inner membrane to the intermembrane space of the mitochondrion. Because protons are positive, this establishes a positive charge on the outside of the inner membrane relative to the matrix side. The electrical gradient that is established is a form of stored (potential) energy. Energy is released when protons rush back into mitochondrial matrix. This release of energy is the ultimate power source that converts ADP into ATP.

Table 3-1 Summary of Energy Production From One Glucose Molecule

Cytoplasm			
Glycolysis	2 ATP	2ATP	2 ATP
Mitochondria			
From glycolysis	2 NADH—(electron transport)—6 ATP		6 ATP
From cellular respiration			
Pyruvic acid—acetyl-CoA	2 NADH—(electron transport)—6 ATP		6 ATP
Krebs cycle	2 ATP	2 ATP	
	6 NADH—(electron transport)—18 ATP		
	2 FADH2—(electron transport)—4 ATP		24 ATP
		TOTAL	38 ATP

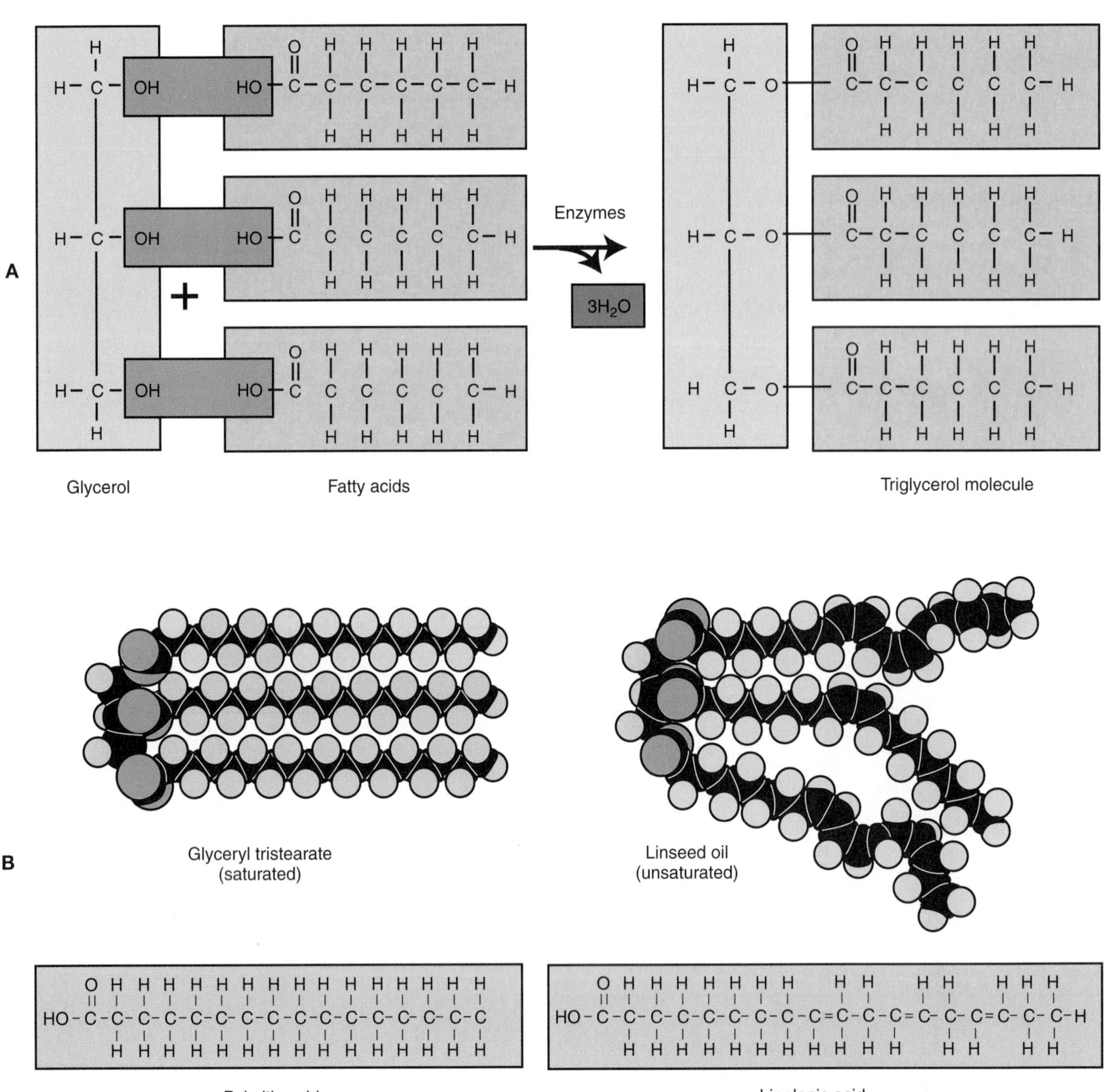

FIGURE **3-15 Formation of Triglycerides From Glycerol and Fatty Acids. A,** Triglyceride is composed of a central core of glycerol with three chains of fatty acids attached to it. **B,** There are two types of fatty acid chains—saturated and unsaturated. Saturated fatty acids are found in foods that are known to cause plaque formation in blood vessels. They are called *saturated* because all of the possible bonding sites on the molecule are used up. Unsaturated fatty acids, on the other hand, are found in oils that are liquid at room temperature. These fats are thought to be better for heart health than saturated fats because they do not tend to clog blood vessels. They are called *unsaturated* because they contain double bonds, which later can be broken to accommodate additional atoms.

bonding sites are occupied. On the other hand, fatty acids that *do* contain double bonds, such as those found in plant oils, are said to be **unsaturated** because the carbon atoms have the potential to bond to other atoms (see Figure 3-15, *B*).

Phospholipids are modified triglycerides with a phosphorous head and two, rather than three, chains of fatty acids (Figure 3-16). The phosphate-containing portion of the molecule is polar and attracts other polar molecules, such as water; therefore it is said to be **hydrophilic** (*hydro-*, "water"; *-philic,* "love"). The fatty acid chains, on the other hand, are insoluble in water but dissolve readily in other lipids. This region is therefore called **hydrophobic** (*phobic,* "fear of"). The hydro-

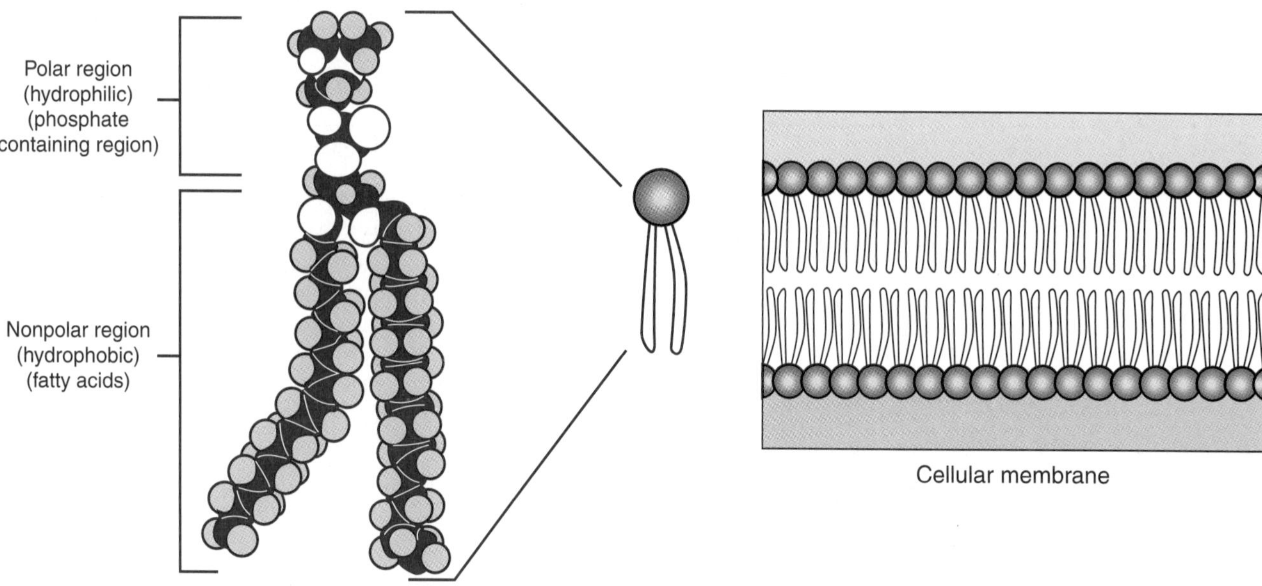

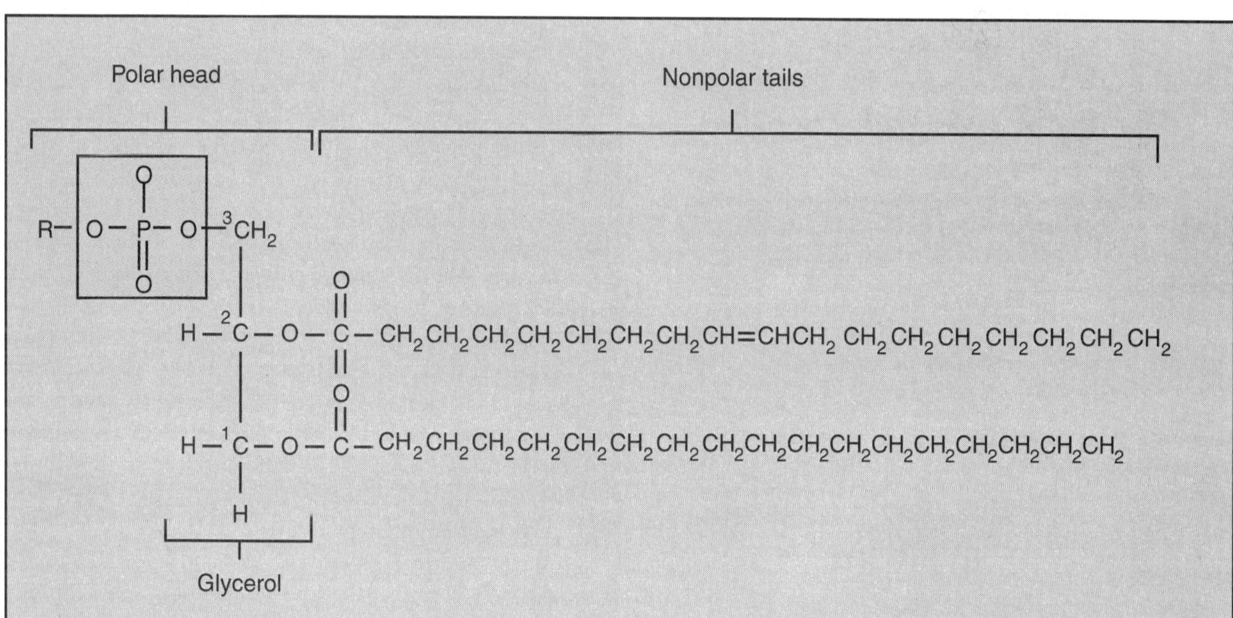

FIGURE **3-16** **Anatomy of a Phospholipid.** Example of hydrophilic and hydrophobic regions of phospholipid molecule.

philic "heads" and hydrophobic fatty acid "tails" are characteristic of phospholipids, which, as mentioned in the previous chapter, play a vital role in the composition of cell membranes.

The liver is the primary controller of lipid metabolism. Triglycerides and phospholipids can be removed from circulating blood by the liver and structurally altered. For example, lipids may be broken into smaller fragments that enable them to enter the glycolytic pathway to form pyruvic acid or may be fed directly into the Krebs cycle. This process is called **lipolysis.**

Triglycerides, specifically, are hydrolyzed into one molecule of glycerol and three fatty acid chains. The glycerol "head" is further catabolized in the cytoplasm to acetyl-CoA and subsequently enters the Krebs cycle, or it may be used to synthesize glucose. The fatty acid tails, on the other hand, are long chains of 18 carbon atoms or more and are handled by enzymes found in the mitochondria. Through a process known as **beta-oxidation,** each fatty acid chain is broken into multiple two-carbon fragments. Some of these fragments are converted to acetyl-CoA, whereas others are converted into

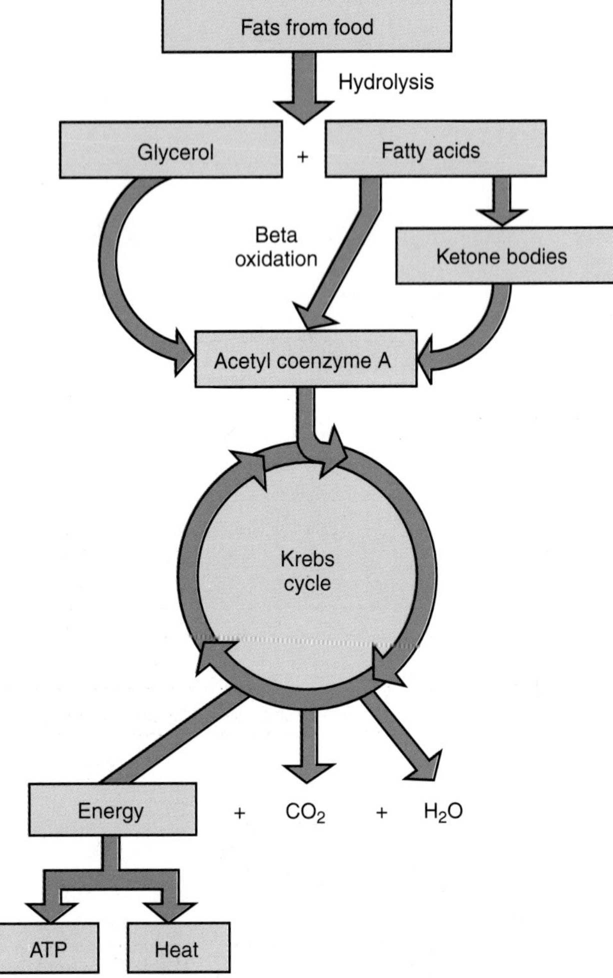

FIGURE **3-17 Trigylceride Metabolism.** Triglycerides from food are digested into glycerol and fatty acids. These can be further broken down to form acetyl-Co-A, which enters the Krebs cycle to form ATP. Excess nutritional triglycerides not immediately catabolized for energy are stored in tissue as fat.

compounds called **ketone bodies.** Later, the ketones can be converted to acetyl-CoA, which can be further catabolized in the Krebs cycle to form ATP (Figure 3-17). The energy gains from the complete oxidation of an 18-carbon fatty acid chain is substantial—about 148 ATP, which is about four times more energy than that generated from the catabolism of one molecule of glucose. Because fat, for the most part, is not soluble in water and is therefore difficult to mobilize, it serves primarily as a reserve energy source rather than a supply to meet immediate energy demands.

Glycerol and fatty acid chains, if not immediately used to produce energy, may be reconstructed into lipids and stored in fatty tissue. This is nature's way of protecting the health of animals and humans when food supplies become low.

Although most fatty acids can be synthesized by the cell, certain fatty acids cannot be and must be provided in the diet. These are called the **essential fatty acids,** and they vary from species to species. Linoleic acid and arachidonic acid are examples of two essential fatty acids in humans.

TEST YOURSELF

1. What is the most common carbohydrate found in blood?
2. Where does carbohydrate metabolism begin in nonruminant animals?
3. What part of carbohydrate metabolism occurs in the cytoplasm?
4. Under what conditions is lactic acid formed in muscle cells?
5. How many biochemical steps are involved in glycolysis? Does glycolysis require oxygen?
6. Cellular respiration is composed of what two parts?
7. How does the membrane structure of the mitochondrion assist in the process of cellular respiration?
8. What role does oxygen play in the electron transport system?
9. What is oxidative phosphorylation?
10. What is the maximum number of ATP molecules that are formed from the catabolism of one molecule of glucose?

PROTEIN METABOLISM

Proteins are found in great abundance in animals. The body of a cow, for instance, may contain several thousand different proteins, each with a unique function and a unique structure to fit its function. Proteins include **structural proteins,** such as hair, microtubules, and collagen; **regulatory proteins,** such as insulin and other hormones; **contractile proteins,** such as actin and myosin in muscle tissue; **transport proteins,** such as hemoglobin and myoglobin; **storage proteins,** such as those found in egg whites; **protective proteins,** such as antibodies; **membrane proteins,** such cell receptors and membrane transport molecules; and **osmoregulators,** such as albumin and enzymes. Clearly the diversity of proteins and the functions they perform are extensive.

Amino Acids: Building Blocks of Proteins

Structurally, proteins are remarkably similar because they are all composed of chains of amino acids, strung together like beads in a necklace. Their differences lie in the types, number, and sequence of the amino acids that they comprise. There are 20 different kinds of amino acids used to make proteins, and each protein may contain several hundred amino acids, so you can see that the number of possible combinations is very large.

Every amino acid has the same basic structure consisting of a central carbon atom bonded to a hydrogen atom (H), to a carboxyl group (—COOH), and to an amino group (—NH_2). In addition, every amino acid has a group attached that is unique for that kind of amino acid (called the *"R" group* for simplicity). R groups can be simple, as seen in alanine, or they can be elaborate, as in tryptophan. See Figure 3-18 for the structural makeup of each type of amino acid.

Most amino acids are derived from the breakdown of tissue proteins that must be continually replenished in the body. Smaller percentages come from dietary sources such as meat and soy. Proteins from food are broken down in the lumen and mucosal cells of the gastrointestinal tract, where enzymes, collectively known as **proteases** and **peptidases,** hydrolyze the

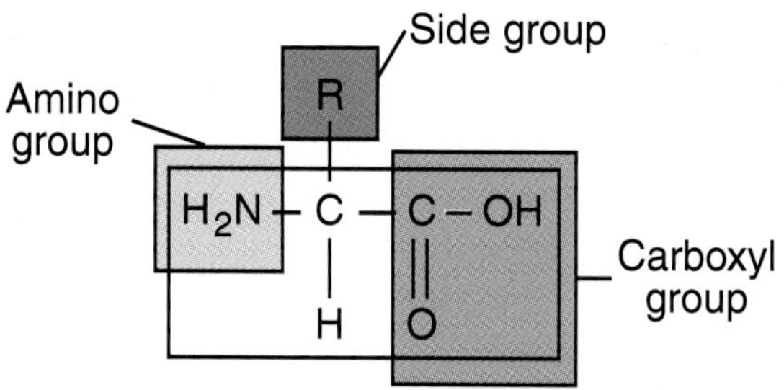

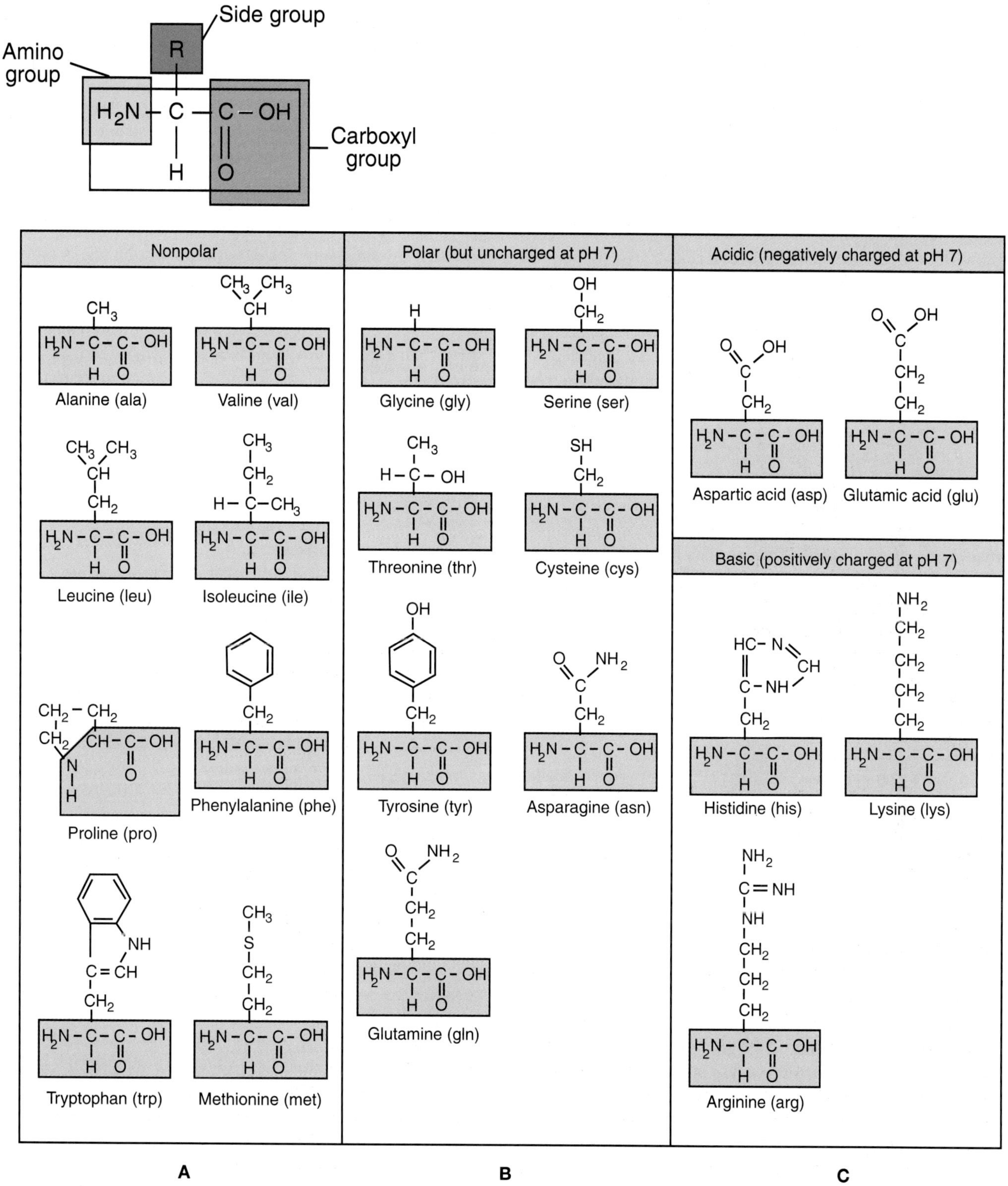

Nonpolar		Polar (but uncharged at pH 7)		Acidic (negatively charged at pH 7)	
Alanine (ala)	Valine (val)	Glycine (gly)	Serine (ser)	Aspartic acid (asp)	Glutamic acid (glu)
Leucine (leu)	Isoleucine (ile)	Threonine (thr)	Cysteine (cys)	**Basic (positively charged at pH 7)**	
Proline (pro)	Phenylalanine (phe)	Tyrosine (tyr)	Asparagine (asn)	Histidine (his)	Lysine (lys)
Tryptophan (trp)	Methionine (met)	Glutamine (gln)		Arginine (arg)	

A B C

FIGURE 3-18 **Structure of Amino Acids. A,** Every amino acid is composed of an amino group, carboxyl group, and side group (R). The side group can be simple or complex, depending on the amino acid. **B,** Alanine is an example of an amino acid with a simple side group. **C,** Tryptophan has a more complex side group.

protein molecules into their amino acid components. These free amino acids are, for the most part, transported to the liver via the bloodstream of the **hepatic portal system.** The liver then assists in determining the type and amount of amino acids released into the blood for supply to nonhepatic tissues.

Essential Amino Acids

Some amino acids cannot be synthesized by the body and must be provided in the diet. These amino acids are therefore called the **essential amino acids.** Most species have 10 essential amino acids, but some animals have more than 10. Cats, for example, require taurine in their diet and therefore have 11 essential amino acids. Because dogs, horses, and oxen are able to manufacture taurine themselves, it is considered a **nonessential amino acid** in these species. Similarly, chickens and turkeys require dietary glycine, but mammals do not because they can manufacture it themselves (Box 3-1).

Structure of Proteins

Proteins are composed of amino acids that are linked to one another by covalent links called *peptide bonds.* A molecule with many amino acids linked together is therefore called a **peptide.** The amino group of one amino acid is linked to the carboxyl group of another amino acid to form a long peptide chain known as the **primary structure.** The genetic material contained within the nucleus of the cell determines the sequence of amino acids in the primary structure, and this sequence determines the function of the protein. Proteins such as **adrenocorticotropic hormone (ACTH)** are a single linear peptide.

In more complex proteins, the primary structure is coiled or forms a pleated appearance (Figure 3-19). These formations are collectively known as the **secondary structure.** The coil, which is called the **alpha helix,** is held together by **hydrogen bonds** connecting the oxygen atom of the carboxyl group of one amino acid with the amino group of another amino acid. The pleat formation, known as the **beta pleat,** is held together by hydrogen bonds between atoms of the spine of the polypeptide chain. R groups extend above and below the pleated plane. Proteins that assume the secondary structure are generally fibrous proteins that are important in maintaining structural aspects of the body. Collagen, which is the primary constituent of tendon, is an example of a fibrous protein.

In still other proteins, hydrophobic R groups tend to cluster toward the center of the molecule, whereas hydrophilic R groups tend to extend outward into solution. In addition, oppositely charged portions of the molecule are attracted to one another, and those areas with like charges are repelled. These forces cause the formation of a twisted, three-dimensional complex called the **tertiary structure.** Tertiary proteins are globular proteins that are stabilized by **disulfide bonds** between amino acids. Many of the proteins that regulate chemical reactions in the body, such as enzymes, and antibodies are examples of globular proteins.

Many proteins, such as the hormone insulin, are composed of more than one polypeptide chain. As a group, these large, complex proteins are called **multimeric.** Those that contain two polypeptide chains are called **dimers,** those that contain three chains are **trimers,** and those that contain four are called **tetramers.** The level of organization of a protein that is composed of two or more polypeptide chains is called the **quaternary structure.** The formation of multimeric proteins is held by disulfide and hydrogen bonds, by hydrophobic and hydrophilic forces, and by the positive and negative charges within the molecule.

Protein Catabolism

In addition to the multiple roles that proteins play in the structural and functional maintenance of the body, proteins

Box 3-1 Essential Amino Acids

Arginine	Methionine
Glycine*	Phenylalanine
Histidine	Taurine†
Isoleucine	Threonine
Leucine	Tryptophan
Lysine	Valine

*Only in poultry.
†Only in cats.

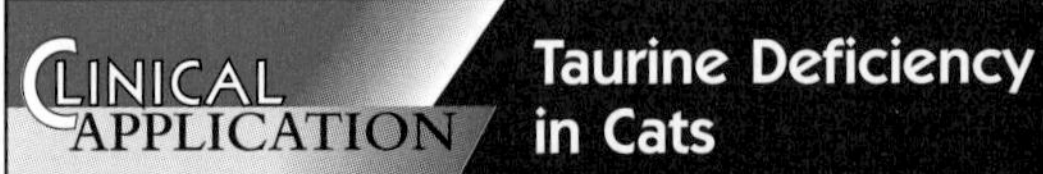

Taurine Deficiency in Cats

Taurine is an essential amino acid in cats and is found in high quantities in meat and fish, but it is virtually nonexistent in plant-based foods, such as dog food. Therefore cats that are fed dog food or home-cooked vegetarian diets develop taurine deficiency after several months. The result is a progressive, irreversible **retinal degeneration** that ultimately leads to blindness. In addition, taurine deficiency has been associated with **dilated cardiomyopathy,** a condition in which the heart enlarges because of dilation of the cardiac chambers. In some cases, the walls of the ventricles become very thin and the ability of the heart to pump blood efficiently is altered. Cats may exhibit signs of heart failure such as depression, shortness of breath, decreased exercise tolerance, and coughing. Fortunately, cardiomyopathy caused by taurine deficiency is reversible and affected cats recover with nutritional supplementation.

Queens that are taurine deficient may appear clinically normal but may have diminished reproductive success, including problems with abortion, early embryonic death, and malformations of **neonates.** An examination of the eyes in these cats usually reveals some degree of retinal degeneration.

Kittens that are born to taurine-deficient queens and fed deficient diets often die. Those that do survive exhibit neurologic signs, including **cerebellar dysfunction** and **paresis** in the hind legs, which frequently splay outward.

Occasionally, even cats that are fed diets adequate in taurine develop clinical signs of deficiency. In these cases, a biochemical disturbance in the retinal cells is thought to prevent normal taurine uptake and use.

may also be catabolized and used to make energy (ATP). Although amino acid catabolism occurs in most tissues, it is of particular importance in the intestinal mucosa, kidney, brain, liver, and skeletal muscle, where the amino acid molecules may undergo one of two processes: **deamination** or **transamination.** These processes occur in the mitochondria and require **pyridoxine,** a coenzyme derivative of vitamin B_6 (Figure 3-20).

In transamination, the amine group (—NH_2) is transferred to another carbon chain to form a different amino acid. These newly constructed amino acids then diffuse across the mitochondrial membranes into the surrounding cytosol, where they become the building blocks for other proteins.

In deamination, the amine is removed from the carbon chain and becomes an ammonia molecule. Because ammonia is toxic, even in small quantities, most deamination reactions occur in the liver, where specialized enzymes are present to convert ammonia to urea—a nontoxic water-soluble molecule that is excreted in urine. After the amine is removed in deamination, the remaining carbon chain may enter the Krebs cycle at one of several locations, resulting in the formation of ATP. Some of the pathways, for example, enter the Krebs cycle from the formation of acetyl-coenzyme A, whereas others enter much later. As a result, deamination may give rise to a variable amount of ATP, depending on where the cycle was entered. If energy is not immediately required, the carbon chains may not enter the Krebs cycle but instead will be converted to glucose or fat (Figure 3-21).

TEST YOURSELF

1. Can you list six different types of protein according to their function?
2. What is the principal building block unit of proteins? How are these units arranged?
3. What are the four basic components of an amino acid molecule? Which part(s) of the molecule change to create the different kinds of amino acids?
4. Some amino acids cannot be synthesized in the body and must be provided in the diet. What are these amino acids called? Can you give an example of one in the cat? Can you give an example of one in birds?
5. How does the arrangement of amino acids influence the function of a protein?
6. Describe the four structural levels of protein organization.
7. What two processes are involved in the breakdown of amino acids? Can you describe them?

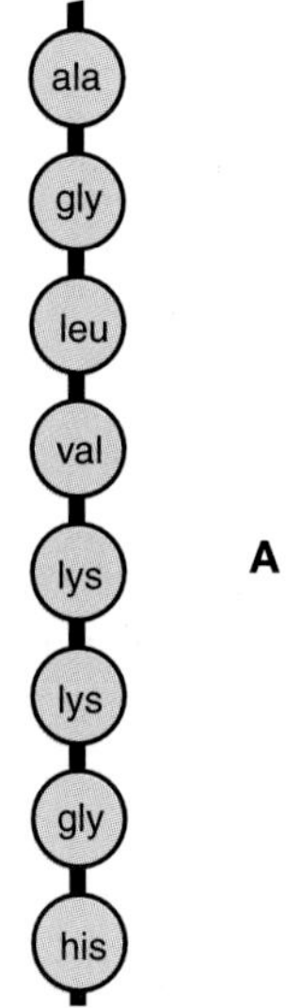

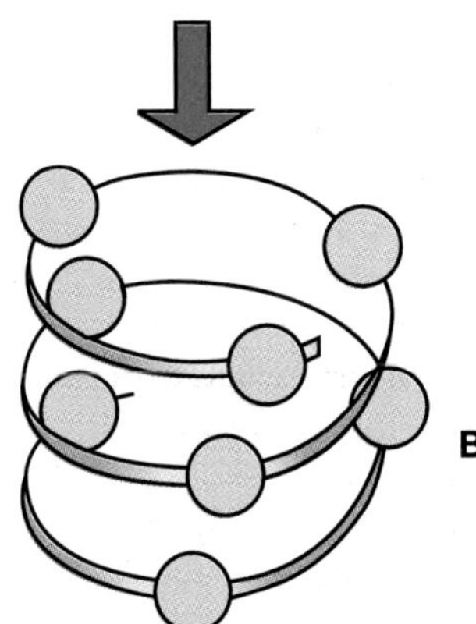

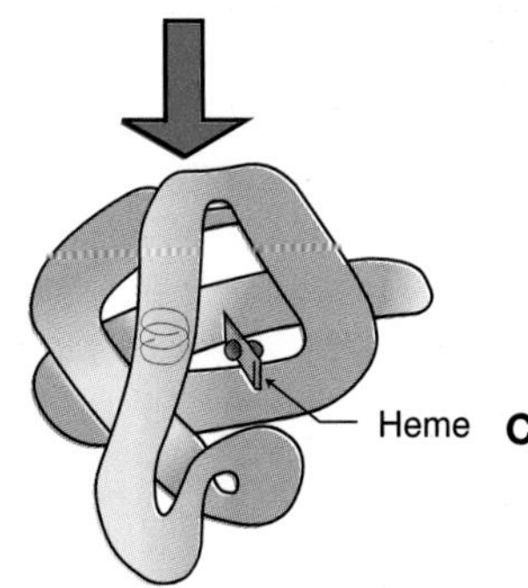

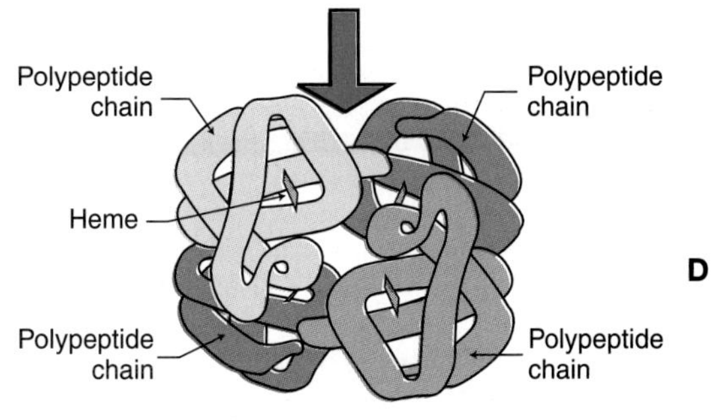

FIGURE **3-19** **Levels of Organization of Proteins. A,** The primary structure of proteins consists of sequence of amino acids. Amino acids are linked to one another like beads in a necklace. **B,** The secondary structure can be either helical (as shown) or pleated. The secondary structure is held by hydrogen bonds between nearby amino and carboxyl groups. **C,** The tertiary structure consists of either folded alpha helixes (as shown) or beta pleats. **D,** The quaternary structure refers to the combination of more than one polypeptide chain, which unites to form the complete protein molecule.

Proteins from foods
Hydrolysis
Amino acids
Deamination
Deaminated portions
+
NH_2 groups
NH_3 ammonia
Urea
By various pathways
Acetyl coenzyme A
Krebs cycle
Energy
+ CO_2 + H_2O
ATP
Heat

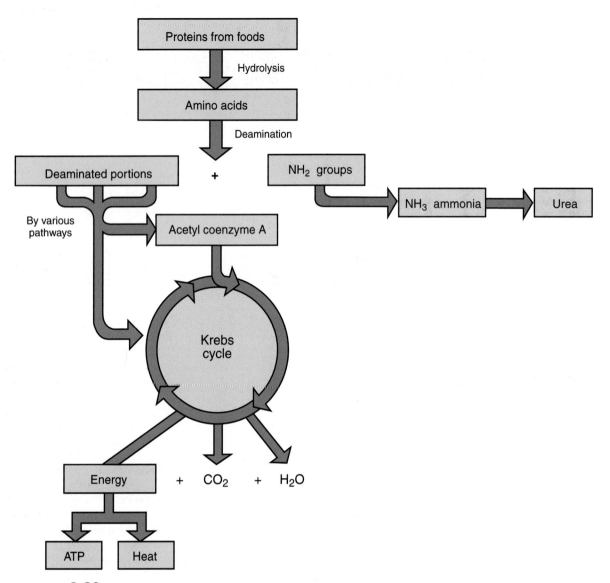

FIGURE **3-20** **Overview of Protein Metabolism.** Protein from food is digested into amino acids, but before they are completely catabolized, the amine group (NH_2) is removed and converted to ammonia, which is later excreted in urine. The remainder of the deaminated portion is then converted to acetyl-CoA and subsequently is used to generate ATP.

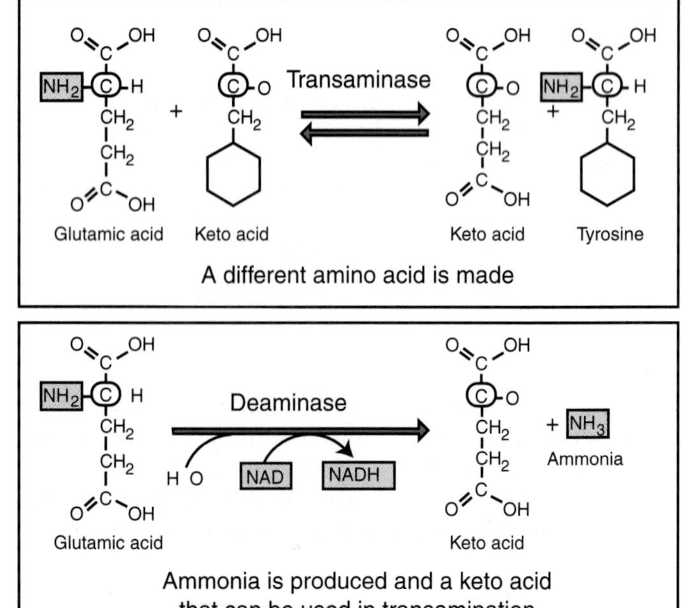

FIGURE **3-21** **Transamination and Deamination. A,** During transamination, amine group of an amino acid is transferred to another molecule by the enzyme transaminase, and a different amino acid is subsequently formed. When stripped of its amine group, an amino acid becomes a keto acid. **B,** During deamination, amine group is removed from an amino acid by the enzyme deaminase. Amino acid then becomes a keto acid, which can be reused in transamination reactions, as shown in **A.** Amine group is converted to ammonia, a toxin. Liver subsequently converts ammonia to nontoxic molecule called *urea.*

Clinical Application: Liver and Kidney Failure

During protein catabolism, ammonia is produced. Because ammonia is toxic, it is converted by the liver to a nontoxic molecule called *urea*. Urea is a type of nitrogenous waste in that it is a compound that contains nitrogen and is excreted. Nitrogenous waste is normally pulled out of the bloodstream by the kidney and put into urine. When the kidney becomes diseased, however, it is sometimes unable to excrete urea effectively. The urea therefore builds up in the bloodstream, causing a condition called *uremia*. Uremia can be detected by a blood test that evaluates the blood urea nitrogen (BUN) level of the patient. Veterinarians look for this in the blood chemistry profiles of sick animals. Similarly, if the BUN is abnormally low, the veterinarian might suspect liver disease because the liver is responsible for converting ammonia to urea. If the liver is not functioning normally, it cannot carry out this conversion. Can you guess what might happen to the ammonia level in an animal with liver disease?

Clinical Application: Starvation: A Threat to Life

We have all marveled at the fortitude of wild animals that survive severe winters, drought, and food deprivation. Neglected domestic animals may also endure inadequate shelter, food supplies, and access to water. For them, food deprivation and subsequent starvation are a threat to their lives. Fortunately, evolution has dictated physiological adaptations that extend the time animals can live without food. Except for the terminal phase, starvation is reversible, and the reproductive capacity of the animal is preserved for as long as possible. How does the body do this?

The process of starvation can be organized into the three stages that follow.

Stage I

Initially, the body tries to balance the animal's energy expenditure with energy intake by lowering the basal metabolic rate. In this way, the animal needs less food for maintenance but may feel weak, dizzy, and tired. Although many tissues can use nutrients other than glucose, certain tissues such as blood cells, the kidney, and nervous tissue (brain and spinal cord) are normally glucose dependent. The body therefore uses glycogen stores in the liver to provide glucose to these important tissues. However, the glycogen stores are depleted after several hours, and the body must turn to other sources of energy. Glycerol and fatty acid stores from fat and amino acids from body proteins are catabolized next to produce glucose. Ketone bodies are released as a product of fatty acid metabolism, causing the blood levels of ketone bodies and glucose to rise.

Stage II

After 1 to 2 weeks, depending on the species, a change occurs in the body that allows the brain and other tissues to use ketones and glucose for energy. Stored body fat therefore becomes the primary source of energy as the body breaks down fatty acids into ketone bodies. This process continues until fat reserves are depleted. The length of this stage varies among individual animals, depending on the amount of body fat that is available for catabolism. Generally, this stage lasts for several weeks. Because body fat serves primarily as an energy storage tissue, an insulator, and protector of internal organs, progressive loss of adipose does not threaten normal body functions or survivability until the stores are nearly depleted.

Stage III

Once fat reserves are used up, protein becomes the principal metabolic fuel. Even during the first stages of starvation, the body catabolizes protein to produce glucose. However, the level of protein catabolism remains high after the fat reserves are depleted. Initially, liver and plasma proteins are used, followed by protein from the gastrointestinal tract, heart, and skeletal muscle. These structures decrease dramatically in size, and critical body functions are lost. Decreases in plasma proteins, for example, lead to changes in oncotic pressure, and fluid subsequently leaks into the abdominal cavity, causing abnormal distention (called *ascites*). Loss of muscles between ribs and in the diaphragm may lead to respiratory failure. The heart, which can lose 50% of its mass, may simply stop beating. Gastric emptying and intestinal transit times are prolonged, and the absorption of fat and, later, protein is impaired as the inner layers of the intestine degenerate. Diarrhea and nausea may result. In addition, malnourished animals are immunocompromised and often develop pneumonia and other infections. Only the skeletal system seems remarkably unaffected by starvation.

Treatment

Warm intravenous fluids in conjunction with antibiotics and parenteral nutrition are important in the treatment of end-stage starvation cases. In addition, malnourished animals are less able to maintain adequate body temperature and should be given a warm environment in which to recover. Good nursing care is important in these cases because animals will need thick, soft bedding and care of any decubital ulcers or sores that may have developed from prolonged recumbency. After the animal is stabilized through the use of parenteral nutrition, high-protein liquid diets would be given by mouth initially until semisolid foods could be tolerated.

Protein Anabolism

A single cell contains the information to make over 100,000 different types of proteins. However, only a few hundred kinds of protein are actually made by any one cell. The type of proteins made is determined by the *function* of the cell. Note that *all* of the somatic cells in an animal contain the same genetic information, that is, the same DNA; however, a single cell cannot and does not make use of all of it.

DNA and RNA Molecules. Protein synthesis begins in the nucleus, where the instructions for building them are contained within the molecule DNA. Although amino acids are assembled in the cytoplasm, DNA does not leave the nucleus. Instead, the valuable instructions for protein synthesis are transferred to a messenger molecule that carries the information out of the nucleus and into the cytoplasm. The messenger is a special type of ribonucleic acid (RNA) called **messenger RNA (mRNA).**

Just as proteins are composed of chains of amino acids, DNA and RNA are made up of chains of **nucleotides.** Unlike an amino acid, however, a nucleotide is composed of three subunits: a nitrogenous base, a five-carbon sugar, and a phosphate group. In DNA, the sugar is deoxyribose, and in RNA, the sugar is ribose. DNA and RNA nucleotides are linked in such a way as to form a "backbone" of alternating sugar and phosphate groups. The nitrogenous bases project out of this backbone, and in DNA, they are weakly bonded to nitrogenous bases on an opposing strand. In this way, DNA forms a double-stranded molecule, the basic structure of which is analogous to a twisted ladder in which the vertical poles are composed of alternating sugar and phosphate groups and the horizontal rungs are paired nitrogenous bases. DNA's molecular structure is therefore called the **double helix** (Figure 3-22). RNA, however, is a single-stranded molecule that has no opposing strand. The single strand of RNA is similar in structure to each of the strands found in DNA.

Four kinds of nitrogen bases are found in DNA and RNA nucleotides (Figure 3-23). Three that are found in *both* RNA and DNA are **adenine (A), cytosine (C),** and **guanine (G).** However, only DNA contains **thymine (T),** and only RNA contains **uracil (U).** In addition, the structure of each nitrogenous base permits the bonding of only certain pairs of nucleotides. For example, thymine can only bond to adenine, and cytosine can only bond to guanine. Uracil, the RNA base, can only bond to the DNA base adenine. These nitrogenous bases and their corresponding bonding parameters are the foundation for the storage of genetic information.

The sequence of nitrogenous bases along the length of the DNA strand can be translated into the sequence of amino acids that make up a protein. Three nitrogenous bases represent one amino acid. This sequence is called the **genetic code.** The triplet CGT, for example, codes for the amino acid alanine, and the triplet GTA codes for the amino acid histidine. When the genetic code is transferred to the mRNA, these same amino acids would be coded as GCA and CAU, respectively.

DNA molecules are divided into subunits called **genes.** Each gene carries all of the information necessary to make one peptide chain. The beginning and ending of the gene are each delineated by a nucleotide triplet. For example, TAC on DNA codes for "start here," and ATT codes for "stop here." The start signals are called **promoters,** and the stop signals are called **terminators.** In this way, the sequence of nucleotides on the DNA molecule not only defines the sequence of amino acids within a protein molecule but also indicates where to start and stop protein synthesis.

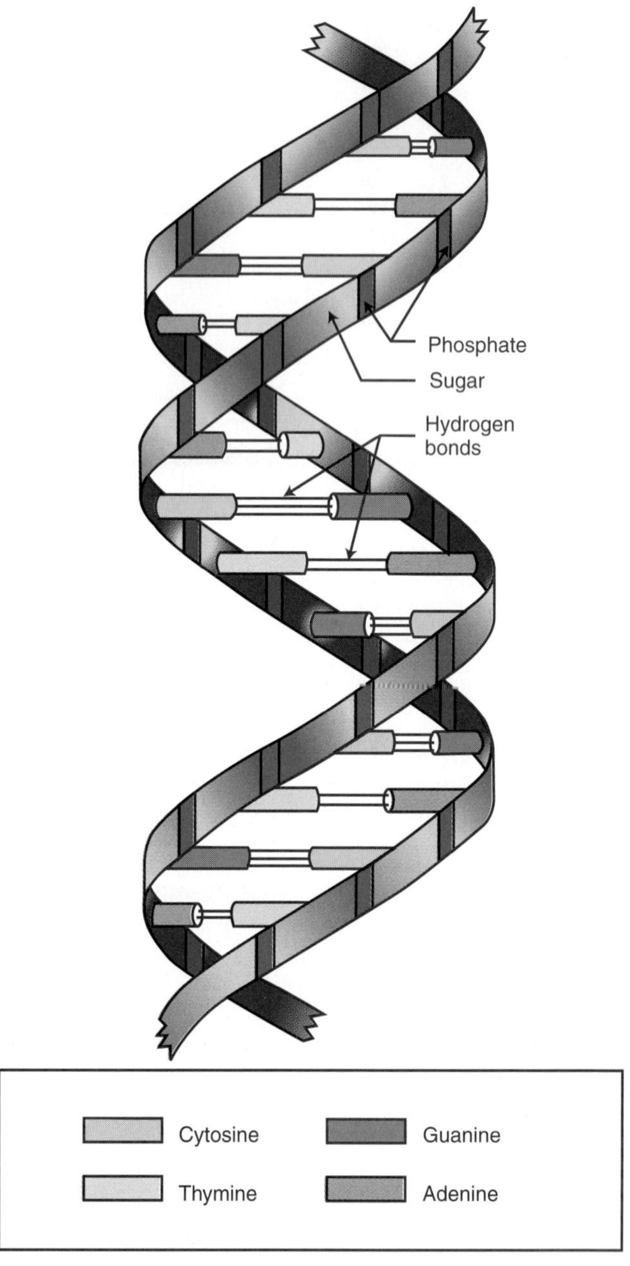

FIGURE **3-22** **Structure of DNA: Double Helix.** Deoxyribonucleic acid (DNA) looks like a spiraling ladder. Vertical portion of "ladder" is composed of alternating phosphate and sugar groups, and rungs of the ladder are composed of nitrogenous bases.

Transcription. As mentioned earlier, DNA does not leave the nucleus, but the genetic information it contains is copied onto a carrier molecule called *mRNA* and transported out of the nucleus to the cytoplasm, where it is used to make protein. The formation of mRNA in the nucleus is called **transcription** (Figure 3-24).

mRNA is assembled one nucleotide at a time. Normally, RNA nucleotides drift freely in the nucleoplasm, but during transcription, a special enzyme called **RNA polymerase** binds to a DNA molecule and coordinates bonding between DNA nitrogenous bases and circulating nucleotides. When RNA polymerase bonds to the DNA molecule, it initiates separation of the double helix and causes the nitrogenous bases of a particular gene to be exposed. Transcription begins at the promoter: the first segment of the gene. As RNA polymerase

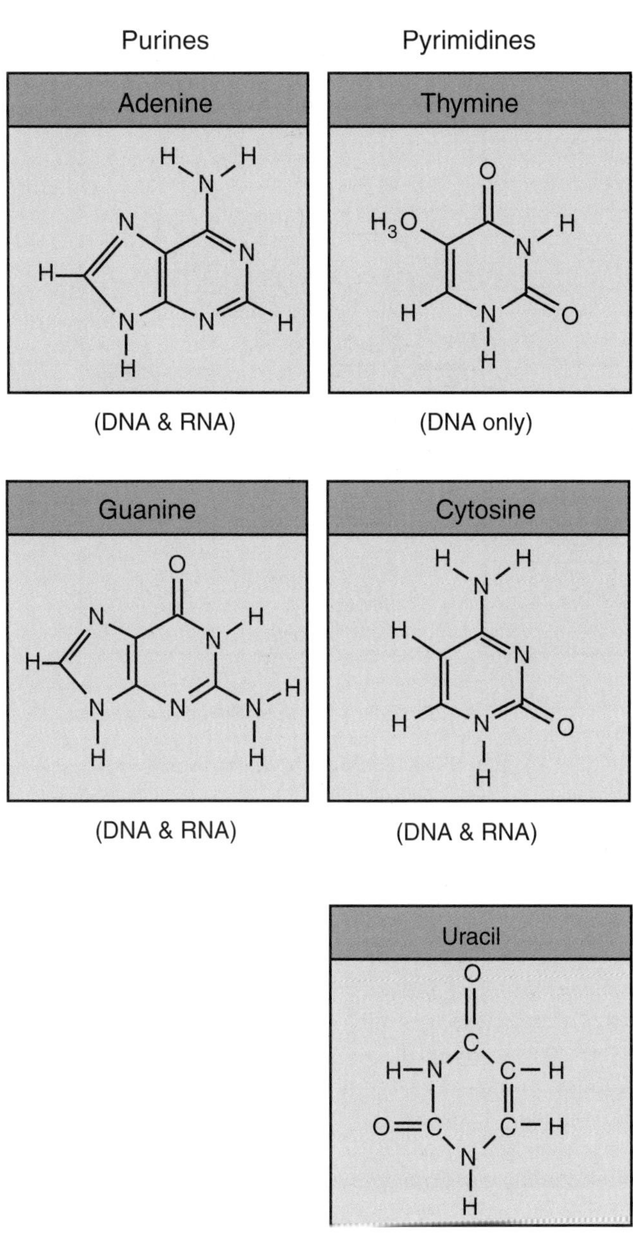

FIGURE 3-23 **Nitrogenous Bases.** DNA and RNA are composed of two types of nitrogenous bases: purines and pyrimidines. Purine molecules each have two rings and are found in both DNA and RNA. Pyrimidines, in contrast, are single-ringed molecules. Cytosine is the only pyrimidine that occurs in both RNA and DNA. Thymine occurs only in DNA, and uracil occurs only in RNA.

moves along the exposed strand of DNA, a molecule of mRNA forms as the enzyme systematically pairs each DNA nucleotide with its corresponding RNA nucleotide. For example, U is bonded to A, and C is bonded to G. A DNA code that reads T, C, A, A, T, C, C, A is transcribed as A, G, U, U, A, G, G, U in the developing mRNA molecule. Each group of three RNA nucleotides, such as "A, G, U," for example, is called a **codon.** Each codon represents a different amino acid. Therefore the order of the codons will translate into the order of the amino acids in the protein (Table 3-2).

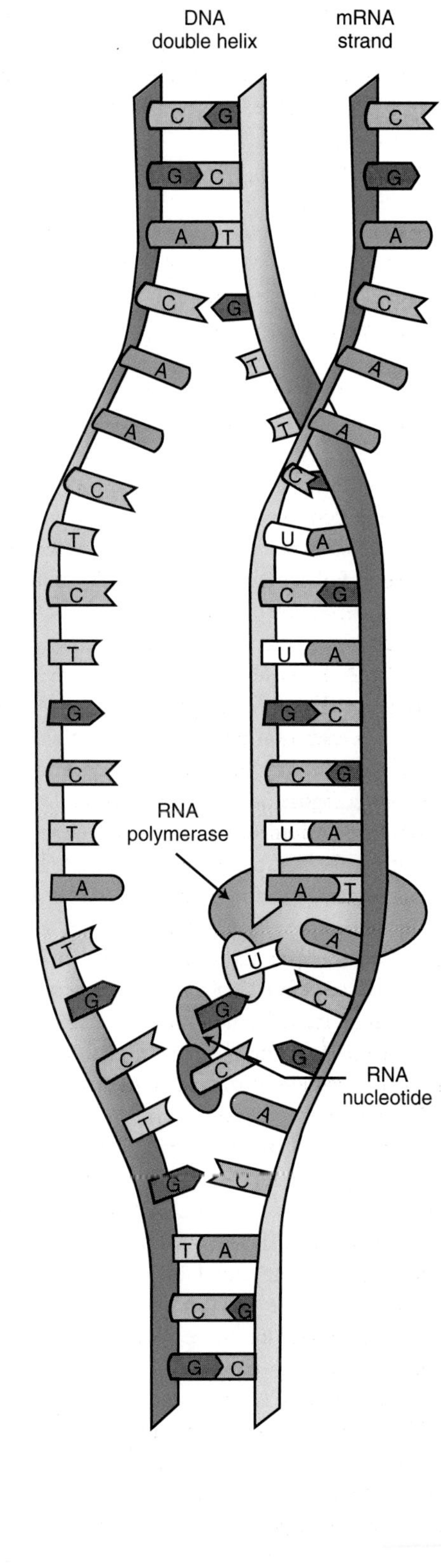

FIGURE 3-24 **Transcription.** In the nucleus, the enzyme RNA polymerase initiates separation of the double helix so that a single strand of DNA is exposed. It then coordinates pairing and bonding of circulating RNA nucleotides to corresponding DNA nucleotides. In this way, mRNA is assembled one nucleotide at a time. When transcription is complete, two strands of DNA reunite and the newly formed mRNA molecule leaves the nucleus to convey its important genetic message to the cytoplasm.

Table 3-2 Examples of Codons in the Genetic Code

Amino Acid	DNA Sequence	RNA Sequence
Alanine	CGT	GCA
Aspartic acid	CTA	GAU
Cysteine	ACA	UGU
Glutamine	GTT	CAA
Histidine	GTA	CAU
Isoleucine	TAG	AUC
Phenylalanine	AAA	UUU
Tryptophan	ACC	UGG
Valine	CAA	GUU

A, Adenine; *C*, cytosine; *G*, guanine; *T*, thymine; *U*, uracil.

When RNA polymerase reaches the terminator, the transcription is finished and the new strand of mRNA is complete. At this time, RNA polymerase detaches from the DNA molecule, and the two complementary strands of DNA reconnect to form a double helix once again.

DNA has noninformational or "nonsense" triplets called **introns** that separate informational triplets called **exons.** The first strand of mRNA that is manufactured from transcription therefore contains noninformational codons that must be removed from the mRNA molecule before it can be used for protein synthesis. Special RNA-protein complexes found in the nucleus form assembly lines called **spliceosomes** to remove the "nonsense" portions of the mRNA molecule. The complexes, called **small ribonucleoproteins,** cut out the introns and splice together the exons in the order in which they occurred in the DNA gene (Figure 3-25). After this editing process is complete, the mRNA molecule leaves the nucleus and enters the cytoplasm by passing through a nuclear pore.

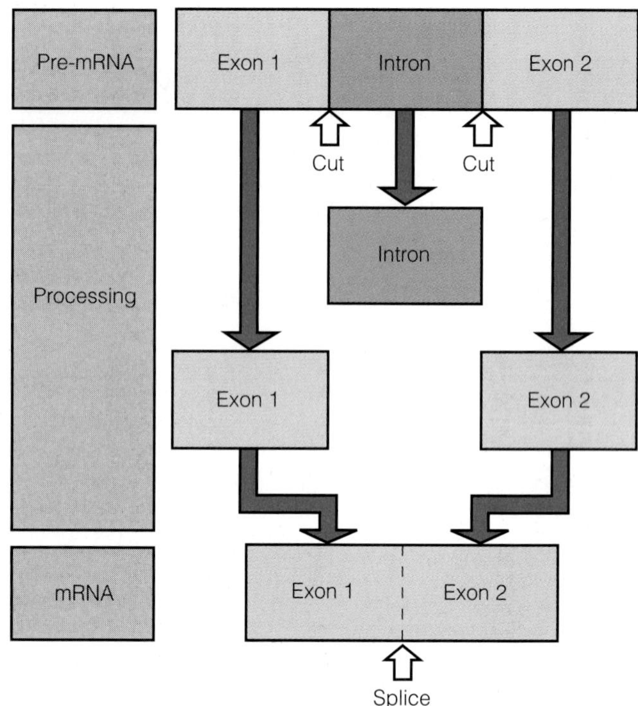

FIGURE **3-25** **"Fine-Tuning" After Transcription.** In the last stage of mRNA production, final "edits" in the genetic code are completed. Here an intron is cleaved from between two exons and discarded. Exons are subsequently bonded together.

Translation: Protein Synthesis. The process of building a new protein using the information on the mRNA molecule is known as **translation** because information is translated from one language (nucleotides) into another (amino acids). After leaving the nucleus, mRNA enters the cytoplasm, where one or more ribosomes bond to the mRNA strand. The ribosomes act as "translation stations." Carrier molecules bring amino acids to the ribosome, where the amino acids are linked together to form a peptide chain using the sequence mapped out on the **mRNA** molecule. Several ribosomes can bond to one mRNA molecule at once, and translation can occur simultaneously at different sites along the strand to form multiple copies of the same protein (Figure 3-26).

Ribosomes are composed of protein and a second type of RNA called **ribosomal RNA (rRNA).** The protein and rRNA molecules are interwoven to form two unequally sized globular units. Protein synthesis begins when the two ribosomal units interlock around the initial codon of an mRNA strand. The larger ribosomal unit contains an **active site** that serves as a "docking site" for a third type of RNA called **transfer RNA (tRNA).** The active site has room for only two tRNA molecules at a time.

tRNA is a small, clover leaf–shaped molecule and consists of approximately 80 nucleotides. There are at least 20 different kinds of tRNA in a cell, one for each type of amino acid. Each tRNA binds to a specific amino acid found in the cytoplasm and subsequently transports the amino acid to the active site of a ribosome bound to mRNA. At this time, a trio of nitrogenous bases on tRNA, called the **anticodon,** binds to the mRNA codon. Bonds between mRNA and tRNA molecules occur only if the nitrogenous bases in the codon and anticodon are complementary. In this way, transfer RNA provides the link between the forming protein and the mRNA molecule because part of it binds to an amino acid and another part binds to a particular codon on mRNA.

After tRNA binds to the active site, enzymes on the ribosome break the link between the tRNA molecule and the amino acid that it is carrying. A peptide bond is then created to link the amino acid to its new neighbor on the active site. The tRNA molecule, now free of its amino acid, disembarks from the active site on the ribosome and ventures into the cytoplasm, where it may collect another amino acid. Subsequently, the ribosome moves to the next codon on the mRNA strand and receives another amino acid–carrying tRNA molecule. A peptide chain is created from the successive

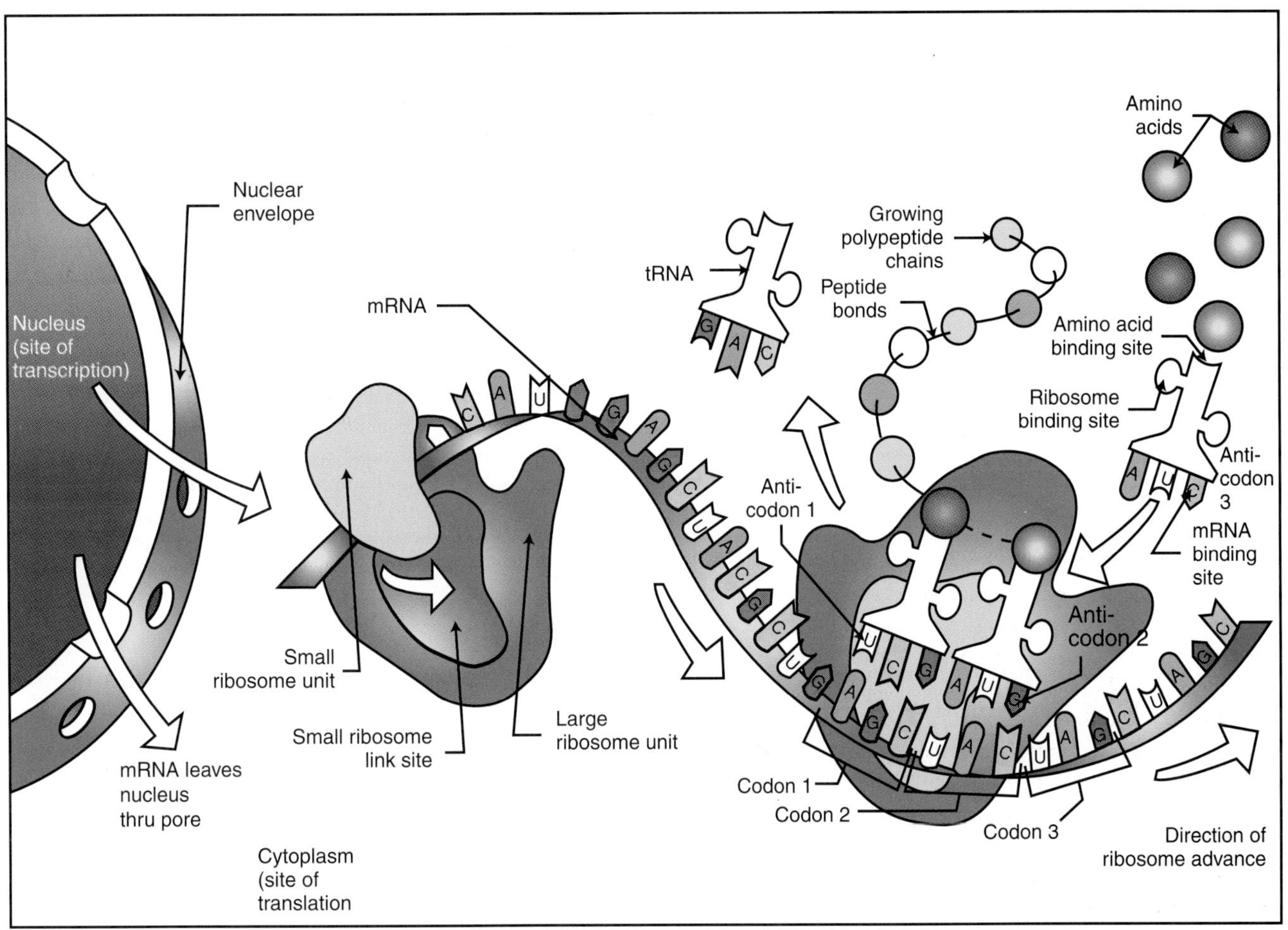

FIGURE **3-26** **Translation: Protein Synthesis.** Messenger RNA (mRNA) molecules carry genetic information from DNA in nucleus, through the nuclear envelope, to the cytoplasm, where it is used to make protein. In cytoplasm, ribosomal subunits attach to the beginning of the mRNA strand and begin the process of translation. Transfer RNA (tRNA) molecules transport specific amino acids to the mRNA molecule as prescribed by codon sequence on the mRNA. A codon of mRNA is paired with the corresponding anticodon of tRNA. As tRNA molecules line up next to one another along the mRNA strand, they bring attached amino acids into close proximity to one another. This allows peptide bonds to form between the amino acids so that a long chain of amino acids is subsequently formed (a *polypeptide*). Some proteins are composed of several polypeptide chains bonded together.

additions of amino acids to a chain of increasing length. The order of the amino acids is determined by the sequence of nucleotides in mRNA. See Box 3-2 for a summary of protein synthesis.

Replication of DNA. The bodies of animals are composed of cells that are continually replicating to maintain body tissues, to heal wounds, or to enable growth. However, before each cell can divide, a perfect copy of the DNA must be created to pass onto the daughter cells. This replication occurs during the interphase of the cell's life cycle.

DNA replication is initiated by the separation of the double helix. Bonds that link the complementary base pairs are broken, and the double-stranded molecule pulls apart, exposing the nitrogenous bases of each nucleotide. An enzyme called **DNA polymerase** links the four types of circulating DNA nucleotides to their complementary organic bases, and a new strand forms along each of the original strands. As a result, two complete DNA molecules are formed, each with one strand from the original molecule and one new strand (Figure 3-27).

During the initial phase of mitosis, DNA condenses, combines with protein, and forms chromosomes. In this form, one molecule of DNA is passed on to each daughter cell during mitosis.

TEST YOURSELF

1. Of all of the thousands of different proteins that a cell could make, how many does it actually produce? Why?
2. Where does protein synthesis begin?
3. What is a nucleotide and how is it structured?
4. Compare and contrast the structures of DNA and RNA.
5. What are the nucleotides found in DNA? In RNA?
6. What is the term for mRNA formation?
7. What are codons and what role do they play in transcription?
8. Can you describe the events that occur in translation?
9. When in the cell cycle does DNA replication occur?

Box 3-2 Protein Synthesis: Transcription and Translation

NUCLEUS

Transcription

1. RNA Polymerase binds to a DNA molecule and initiates separation of the double helix. A specific section of DNA (called a *gene*) is exposed.
2. RNA polymerase moves along the DNA strand and coordinates the pairing of RNA nucleotides to corresponding DNA nucleotides. The RNA nucleotides are linked to one another to form a strand of mRNA.
3. When RNA polymerase reaches the end of the gene, the newly formed mRNA molecule is released and travels through the nuclear envelope to the cytoplasm.
4. The separated strands of DNA are reunited to form a double helix once again.

CYTOPLASM

Translation

1. A ribosome binds to the beginning of the mRNA strand.
2. Transfer RNA molecules move into the vicinity of the ribosome. The tRNA anticodon is paired with the appropriate codon on the mRNA molecule.
3. The amino acid carried by the tRNA molecule is released and linked to the neighboring amino acid.
4. The ribosome continues to move along the mRNA molecule until all of the codons have been paired.
5. As the developing chain of amino acids lengthens, it coils and folds into the structure of a functional protein.
6. When translation is complete, the new protein is released and later modified. The ribosome, tRNA, and mRNA are free to repeat the process and form more of the same type of protein.

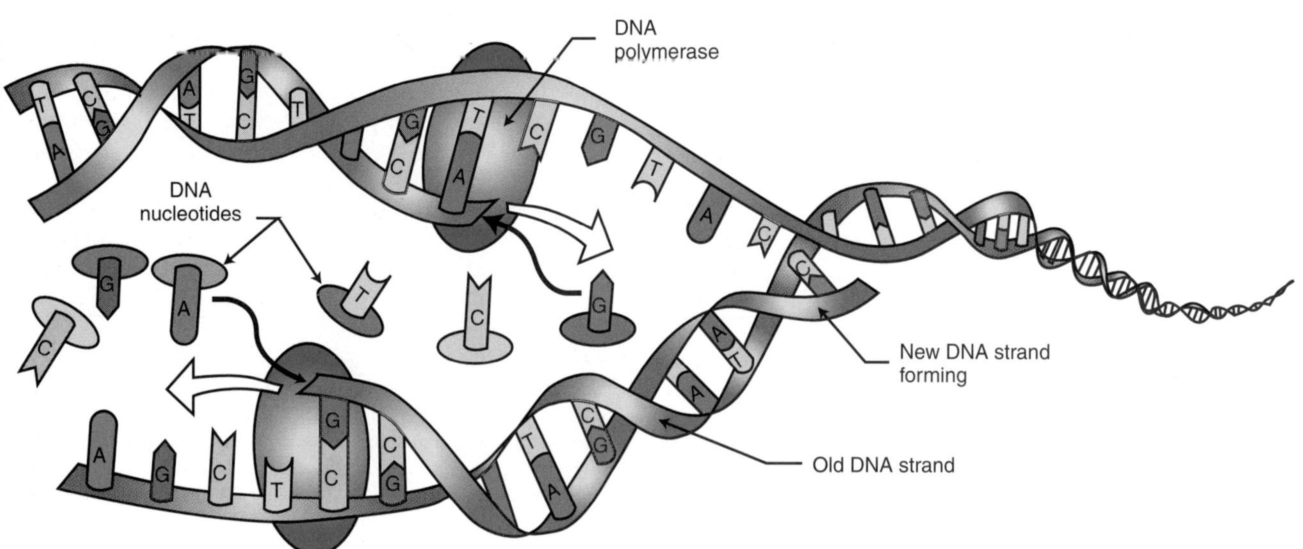

FIGURE **3-27** **DNA Replication.** Before a cell divides, it makes an identical copy of its genetic material. To do this, DNA uncoils and the double helix separates. The enzyme DNA polymerase coordinates pairing of free nucleotides with exposed bases. Note that there is an obligatory pattern of base pairing; for example, adenine (A) pairs with thymine (T), and cytosine (C) pairs with guanine (G). After the strands of DNA have been replicated, the cell is ready to divide. An identical copy of the genetic material is passed onto each of the daughter cells.

Genetic Mutations

The body of a large dog is composed of trillions of cells and each cell is derived from the division of the parent cell. The number of cell divisions, therefore, that are made within the lifetime of a dog is staggering. The process of DNA replication must not only be efficiently orchestrated, but it must be highly accurate as well. Given the enormous amount of information held within a single chromosome, it is not surprising that genetic mistakes occasionally occur in the countless replications of DNA. These errors lead to alterations in genetic material, and if the cell is able to survive such an error, it may pass on the genetic misinformation to future generations of cells. A genetic error is called a **mutation.**

Mutations can be caused by a wide variety of factors. Some of them seem to arise spontaneously, but others have been associated with some kinds of viruses, ionizing radiation and certain chemicals. These factors are called **mutagens**.

Mutagens can affect genetic material in several ways. For example, sections of DNA may be left out during the replication process, a gene may be spliced into the wrong position, or the wrong nucleotide may be paired to a nitrogenous base. Ionizing radiation such as x-rays and ultraviolet light is most likely to cause adjacent nucleotides to bond to one another or to cause a single strand of DNA to break apart. Chemical mutagens tend to cause bases to be left out, as well as the abnormal formation of linkages between strands. There are

CLINICAL APPLICATION Chemotherapeutic Drugs

Many drugs are currently used to fight cancer in animals. These drugs are called *chemotherapeutic drugs*, and they work by blocking cell division and protein synthesis. The cell cannot repair itself or divide and subsequently dies without leaving behind daughter cells. Chemotherapeutic drugs may be either specific for a certain phase of cell division or nonspecific, affecting all phases of cell division. These drugs are particularly effective against rapidly dividing cells, such as tumor cells, but may also affect rapidly dividing normal cells as well. For example, cells that line the intestinal tract, young blood cells that form in bone marrow, and the active cells in hair follicles are all normal cells that are often affected by chemotherapeutic drugs. Therefore it is not surprising that some of the side effects of chemotherapy include nausea, diarrhea, hair loss, and decreased production of blood cells. Unfortunately, some tumors that do not grow quickly are not as affected by chemotherapeutic agents. In these cases, chemotherapy may need to be extended for long periods or the veterinarian may consider using other forms of cancer treatment, such as surgery and radiation therapy.

Some chemotherapeutic drugs are extremely toxic to the tissues that lie outside of blood vessels, so technicians must be very careful to administer the drugs intravenously. Placing a catheter in the vein is a good way to ensure that the chemotherapeutic agent is administered properly. Extravascular administration of vincristine, for example, will cause necrosis (tissue death) and sloughing of the perivascular tissue. Any attempt to irrigate the tissue or dilute the drug by injecting saline spreads the drug and increases the area of tissue that sloughs.

The six major classes of chemotherapeutic drugs are alkylating agents, antimetabolites, plant alkaloids, antibiotics, hormonal agents, and miscellaneous agents.

HOW DO THEY WORK?

Alkalating agents such as cyclophosphamide (Cytoxan), cisplatin (Platinol), carboplatin (Paraplatin), chlorambucil (Leukeran), and melphalan (Alkeran) stop cell division by causing strands of DNA to cross-link and in doing so inhibit DNA replication. A cell cannot divide or make proteins if the DNA is abnormally linked together. Without the necessary proteins and enzymes required for metabolic function, the cell quickly dies. The antibiotic doxorubicin (Adriamycin) works in a similar manner as it binds DNA and inhibits mitotic activity.

Antimetabolites such as cytosine arabinoside, 5-fluorouracil, and methotrexate are analogues of the DNA bases purines and pyrimidines. They are incorporated into the DNA molecule during DNA replication and subsequently inhibit protein and enzyme synthesis.

Plant alkaloids, such as vincristine, are phase specific and affect only the M phase of the cell cycle by inhibiting mitosis. They bind to the proteins in microtubules and interrupt the formation of the mitotic spindle. Without a spindle, the chromosomes cannot be separated properly, cell division is halted, and the cell subsequently dies.

In high doses, corticosteroids, such as prednisone and prednisolone, interfere with the cell division of lymphocytes. This lympholytic activity makes them particularly useful in treating lymphoid cancers such as lymphoma. They have an added benefit of increasing appetite and therefore are often used in conjunction with other chemotherapeutic agents.

The best known miscellaneous agent in veterinary use is asparaginase, which as its name implies, is an enzyme that breaks down asparagine, an amino acid used by cancer cells. It has no effect on normal cells and usually is used in combination with other chemotherapeutic drugs.

Example

A chemotherapeutic treatment protocol for a cat with lymphosarcoma might include vincristine, prednisone, and Cytoxan. Can you explain why each of these drugs is used?

many ways in which an error can be made, but no matter how the mutation occurs, the consequence is the same; an alteration in genetic information.

Some mutations are so severe that the cell is not able to survive. For example, if the gene that codes for the production of RNA synthetase is left out of the DNA, the cell will die. But mutations can also have relatively little effect. For example, if a cell is unable to manufacture an enzyme that is relatively unimportant, the cell can continue to function normally. The mutations that cause the greatest harm are those that fall in between these two extremes. These mutations do not kill the cell or preclude cellular reproduction, but they affect the normal function of the cell in ways that can be harmful. In time, the increasing numbers of mutant cells may cause structural and functional abnormalities in the tissues and organs they comprise.

It is important to recognize that the effect of mutations is more severe in young animals than it is in adults. A mutation in a growing embryo, for example, will produce large numbers of abnormal cells that may occur in multiple tissue systems. In addition, a mutation that occurs in a fertilized egg would effect every cell in the animal's body and would, therefore, have the most extreme consequences. A mutant cell in an adult, on the other hand, is surrounded by normal cells and may go undetected.

Fortunately, cells are equipped with special "repair" enzymes that can detect certain kinds of errors in the newly forming DNA strands. These enzymes are able to detach defective nucleotides and replace them with the correct complement to those nucleotides on the opposite strand. Unfortunately, the repair enzymes are unlikely to correct errors in a mutation that involves both strands of the DNA at the same region. If the cell survives, this type of mutation is likely to be passed on to future generations of cells.

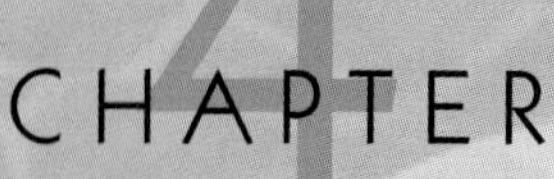

CHAPTER 4

Tissues: Living Communities

Joanna M. Bassert

A unicellular organism, such as a **paramecium,** can live as an individual. It can feed itself, respire, grow, and produce or find all of the biochemical substances that it needs without the assistance of other cells. The cells that compose multicellular organisms, however, cannot survive independently. These cells have **differentiated** to form a wide range of cell types, each with its own characteristic structural feature and distinct function. In the course of their differentiation, they have lost the ability to perform all of the metabolic functions required to sustain life as an isolated entity. Consequently, the cells that compose animals and all multicellular organisms exist within cooperative living communities. Many different types of communities are found in any single animal. These communities differ from one another based on the types of cells that compose them and on the role that they play in the organism as a whole. In this way, cells of similar type and function are clustered into layers, sheets, or groups called **tissues.** Tissues are classified into the following four primary types:

1. Epithelial tissue
2. Connective tissue
3. Muscle tissue
4. Nervous tissue

Although each classification can be divided further into subgroups, each with its own special purpose, we can review the main functions of each tissue classification. In general, **epithelial tissue** *covers* and *lines,* **connective tissue** *provides support,* **muscle tissue** *enables movement,* and **nervous tissue** *controls work.* Because each type completes a specific purpose, the tissues must work collaboratively to meet the vital needs of the animal as a whole. Thus tissues are clustered to form organs, such as the liver, spleen, or kidney. All four tissue types can be found in most organs. The heart, for example, is a powerful *muscle* that moves blood throughout the body. Blood vessels, such as the coronary arteries, provide pathways for blood to reach the heart muscle. The vessels are composed of *connective* and *epithelial tissue.* Nerves and *nervous tissue* are threaded throughout the muscle of the heart to govern coordinated contractions of the ventricular and atrial chambers. These chambers are covered and lined with layers of *epithelia.* In this chapter, epithelial and connective tissues are the primary focus. Muscle and nervous tissues are discussed in greater detail in subsequent chapters.

GROSS AND MICROSCOPIC ANATOMY

The study of anatomical structures that can be seen with the naked eye is called **gross anatomy.** This includes learning the names and locations of bones, muscles, arteries, veins, and nerves throughout the body. Therefore anatomists must have excellent memories because hundreds if not thousands of isolated structures can be examined. The study of the microscopic structures of tissues and organs is called **histology,** or **microanatomy.** This chapter represents an introduction to the study of microanatomy: a discipline that beautifully complements the study of gross anatomy and gives a structural basis for understanding the physiology of each anatomical system. Let's begin.

EPITHELIAL TISSUE

Epithelial tissue is composed of sheets of cells that cover and line other tissues. For example, it lines the bladder, mouth, blood vessels, thorax, and all of the body cavities and ducts in the body. Although well grounded to underlying structures, epithelia have an exposed surface that affords access to the surrounding environment or to the inner openings of chambers and ducts. Epithelial tissue acts as an interface layer that separates and defines the beginning and ending of different types of tissues. It is protective of underlying tissues and frequently acts as a filter of biochemical substances. In addition, epithelia may be absorptive; for example, the epithelia that line the gastrointestinal tract absorb nutrient molecules from the gut, which are then placed into circulation. Epithelia can detect changes in the environment and play an important role in the reception of sensory input. Epithelial cells on the tongue, for example, are sensitive to touch, temperature, and taste. The eyes, ears, and nasal passages also are assisted by the presence of specialized epithelia that provide the sensations of sight, sound, and smell. The sensory information collected by these cells is conveyed to the nervous system.

Another common function of epithelial tissue is the secretion or excretion of biochemical substances. Epithelia that engage in the manufacture and release of substances are called **glandular epithelia.** Glandular epithelial cells may occur as individuals, such as the **goblet cells** found in the intestine, or they may occur as organized glands, such as those found in the pancreas. Some of the substances produced by glandular epithelia lubricate parts of the body, such as the mucus secreted in the colon, whereas others play a vital role in producing biochemical substances that influence physiological events. Hormones, enzymes, milk, sweat, and musk are all examples of substances produced by glandular epithelia. Substances that ultimately leave the body (excreted), such as sweat, urine, and feces, are called **excretions,** and substances that remain within the body, such as regulatory molecules and mucus, are termed **secretions.**

In these ways, epithelia perform vital functions in the body of animals. The functions of epithelial tissue are summarized as follows:

1. Protects, covers, and lines
2. Filters biochemical substances
3. Absorbs nutrients
4. Provides sensory input
5. Manufactures secretions
6. Manufactures excretions

GENERAL CHARACTERISTICS OF EPITHELIA

Epithelial cells are organized into tightly packed groups that form sheets of tissue. These sheets may be composed of either a single layer or multiple layers of cells depending on where they are located in the body. Although the size and shape of the cells vary, epithelia share certain common characteristics.

1. Epithelial cells are **polar,** that is, they have a sense of direction relative to surrounding structures. Each epithelial cell has an **apical surface** and a **basal surface,** which are quite different from one another. The apical surface is the side of the cell that faces the lumen or body cavity, and the basal surface is the side of the cell that faces the underlying connective tissue.
2. Epithelial cells have lateral surfaces that are connected to neighboring cells by **junctional complexes.** These junctions bring the cells into close apposition to one another, leaving little room for extracellular matrix. The matrix that surrounds epithelia therefore exists in very small quantities, if at all.
3. All epithelial cells lack blood vessels or capillaries. They are **avascular** and rely on underlying connective tissue to provide oxygen and nutrients.
4. Although some epithelia, such as those in the stomach, intestines, and cervix, lack nerves, most epithelial cells are **innervated** and provide valuable sensory input.

Cellular Attachments

Epithelial cells are held together many ways. Their lateral surfaces, for example, are wavy and fit together like pieces of a jigsaw puzzle. Between the plasma membranes of adjacent cells are matrix-filled channels, which transport nutrients from underlying connective tissue. These passages act as distribution routes for biological supplies and as elimination routes for waste. In addition, the plasma membranes of epithelial cells are joined to form specialized attachments, or junctional complexes, that give epithelial tissue surprising strength even though the attachments only involve a small portion of the cell membrane. Three major types of cellular junctions found between epithelial cells are tight junctions, desmosomes, and gap junctions (Figure 4-1).

A **tight junction** is formed by the fusion of the outermost layers of the plasma membranes of adjoining cells. Therefore the matrix-filled space between cells is lost at the site of a tight junction. For centrally placed cells, the fusion occurs as a strip that wraps around the entire circumference of the cell like a belt. In this way, an impenetrable barrier is formed that prevents the passage of substances from the luminal end to the basal end of the cell and vice versa. Only by passing through the body of the cell can substances pass through the epithelial layer. Tight junctions are found in tissues in which there can be no leaks, such as (1) in the urinary bladder, where urine is held, or (2) in the digestive tract, where they play a critical role in preventing the leakage of digestive enzymes into the bloodstream.

A **desmosome** is a strong, welded **plaque,** or thickening,

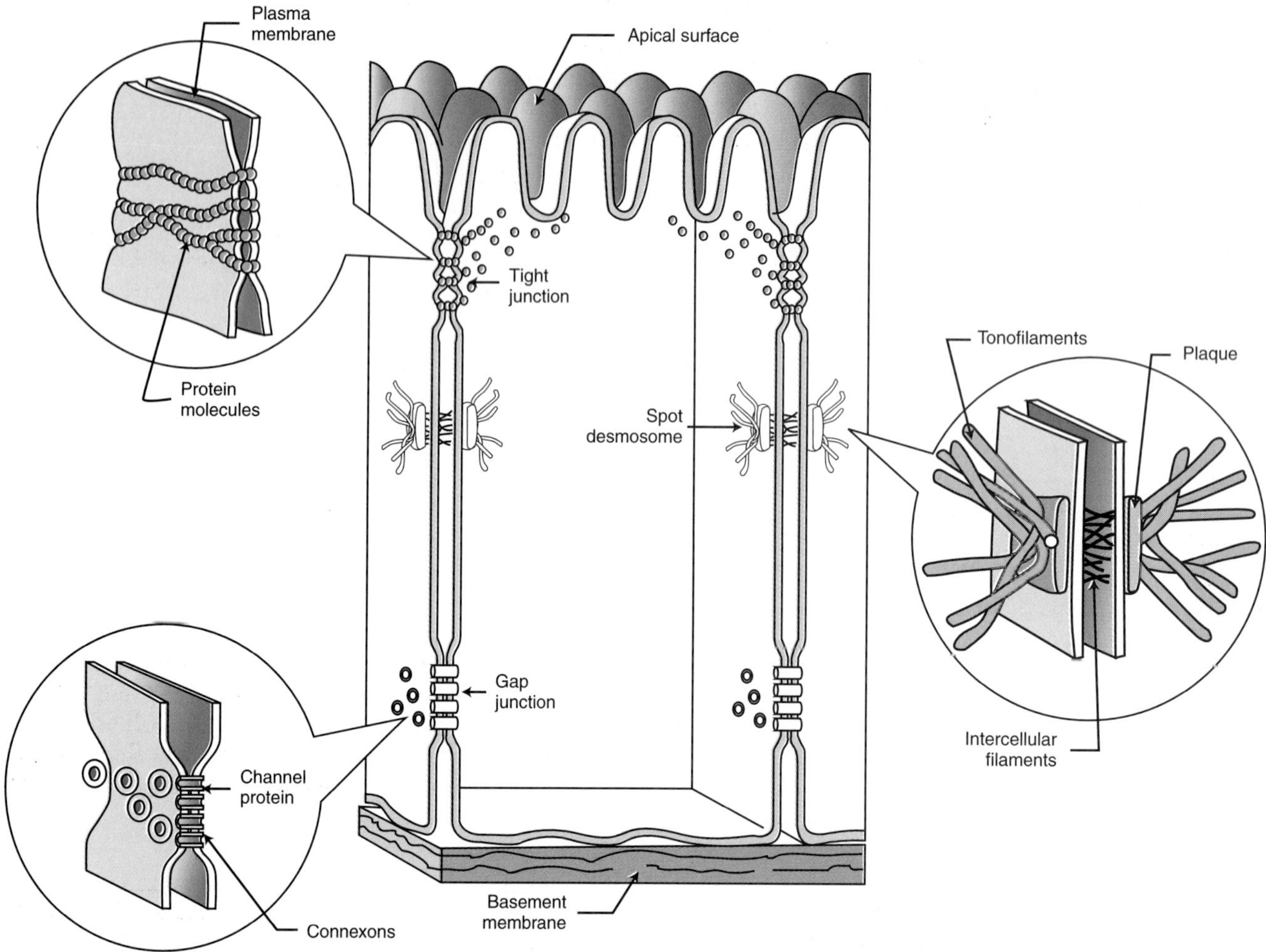

FIGURE **4-1** **Intercellular Junctions.** An interesting feature of epithelial cells is the varied way in which they bond together. These intercellular junctions are both functionally and structurally different from one another. Three main types of intercellular connections are tight junctions, gap junctions, and spot desmosomes. A simplified form of these junctions is depicted here.

that connects the plasma membranes of adjacent cells. The bond is a mechanical coupling formed by filaments that interlock with one another, just as plastic fibers do in Velcro. In addition to these linkages, **tonofilaments,** or intermediate filaments, extend from the plaque into the cytoplasm of each cell like anchors, forming stabilizing bases for the membrane junction. In this way, desmosomes form tough bonds between cells and therefore are found most commonly in tissues that undergo repeated episodes of tension and stretching, such as the skin, heart, and uterus. Junctions that look like half-desmosomes, called **hemidesmosomes,** link epithelial cells to the basement membrane.

Cells that are connected by **gap junctions** are linked by tubular channel proteins, called **connexons** (ko-NEK-sonz), that extend from the cytoplasm of one cell to the cytoplasm of the other. These transmembrane proteins allow the exchange and passage of ions and nutrients, such as nucleotides, sugars, and amino acids, from one cell to the other. Gap junctions are most commonly found in intestinal epithelial cells, the heart, and smooth muscle tissue. Although the exact function of gap junctions in epithelial cells is not yet fully understood, their role in cardiac and smooth muscle cells centers around their ability to quickly transport electrical signals from one cell to another. In this way, they coordinate the contraction of cardiac and smooth muscle.

Basement Membrane

The **basement membrane** is the foundation of the epithelial cell. It is a nonliving meshwork of fibers that cements the epithelial cell to the underlying connective tissue. Its strength and elasticity help to prevent the cell from being torn off by intraluminal pressures, such as stretching or erosion caused by the rubbing of luminal material. The basement membrane (also called *basal lamina*) is manufactured and laid down by epithelial cells in varying degrees of thickness. The basement membrane in skin, for example, is thin, but in the trachea, it is much thicker. Oxygen and nutrient molecules are supplied to the epithelial cells by diffusing through the basement membrane from capillaries in the underlying connective tissue. Similarly, nutrient substances that are absorbed and waste that

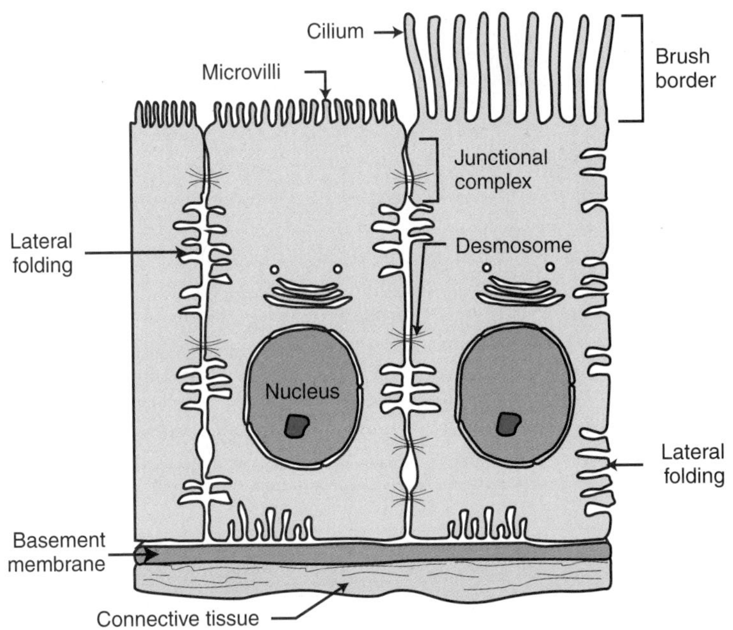

FIGURE **4-2** **Epithelial Cell Specializations.** In addition to forming unique intercellular connections, epithelial cells vary in their cell surfaces. Some cells are smooth and flat, whereas others have elaborate brush borders of microvilli designed to expand surface area to maximize the absorption or secretion of substances. In addition, epithelial cells may be covered with long, hairlike structures called *cilia* that beat in a rhythmic fashion to propel mucus and other materials across the cell's apical border. Elaborate folds of plasma membrane are also evident along the lateral sides of the cell, as well as on the surface. These are important in providing space for those materials that pass between cells from apical to basal ends and vice versa.

is excreted by the epithelium diffuse across the basement membrane into the blood supply of the connective tissue. In this way, the basement membrane acts as a partial barrier between the epithelial cell and the underlying connective tissue. Cancerous epithelia do not respect this boundary and aggressively invade the connective tissue layer underneath.

Surface Specialization

The surfaces of epithelial cells vary depending on where the epithelium is located in the body and, more importantly, what role it plays in the function of the tissue. The epithelia that line blood vessels, for example, have smooth surfaces to allow the easy passage of blood cells. However, other epithelia have irregular surfaces and may be covered with many fingerlike projections, called **microvilli,** or thousands of tiny hairs, called **cilia** (Figure 4-2).

The surface of a cell covered with microvilli is called the **brush border.** The brush border greatly increases the surface area of the cell surface, thereby increasing the absorptive ability of the cell. For this reason, microvilli usually occur on cells that are involved in absorption or secretion, such as the epithelia in the intestinal and urinary tracts. Remarkably, a cell with microvilli has about *20 times* the surface area of a cell without them.

Cilia are also found on the free surface of cells, usually in the respiratory and urogenital tracts. In the trachea, for example, the cilia help to propel mucus and debris up and away from the lungs toward the mouth. In the opening of the **oviduct,** called the **infundibulum,** cilia encourage newly ovulated ova into the oviduct. Ciliary movement occurs in coordinated "beats," which enable the efficient transport of material. This coordinated action is brought about by an electrical potential that moves through junctional complexes connecting adjacent cells. The movement crosses the entire epithelial surface as a perfectly synchronized wave.

Epithelial cells of the skin become filled with a protective, waterproof substance called **keratin.** The accumulation of keratin occurs as the cell matures and moves from the basal layer to the superficial layer of the integument. These cells are called *keratinized epithelium* and are discussed in greater detail in Chapter 6.

TEST YOURSELF

1. What are the four primary types of tissue?
2. What is histology?
3. List seven functions performed by epithelial cells.
4. What four attributes characterize epithelial tissue in general?
5. List four types of cellular junctions. Can you describe them?
6. How does the basement membrane act as a partial barrier between the epithelial cell and the underlying connective tissue?
7. Why do some epithelial cells have cilia and microvilli? What role do they play? Where are the cells with these specialized surfaces found in the body?

Classifications of Epithelia

Epithelial tissue is classified according to the following three characteristics (Figure 4-3).

1. *Number of layers of cells.* If there is only a single layer of epithelial cells, the tissue is classified as *simple.* If there is more than one layer of cells, the tissue is called *stratified.* Simple epithelia provide little protection to the underlying connective tissue and therefore are found in protected areas of the body, such as internal compartments, ducts, vessels, and passageways. Stratified epithelia, on the other hand, are thicker and stronger than

CLINICAL APPLICATION Parvovirus: Killer of Intestinal Epithelia

Feline panleukopenia and **canine parvoviral enteritis** are two life-threatening diseases that affect cats and dogs, respectively. The virus is highly contagious and is carried on clothing, shoes, and toys. It is shed in the feces and other excretions of affected animals and can be easily tracked into your house by riding on the soles of your shoes! Fortunately, most cats and dogs are **immunized** against **parvovirus** and therefore never contract the disease.

However, for those animals that do contract parvovirus, mortality is high, particularly in young animals. The virus attacks and kills cells that are actively engaged in mitosis. Thus tissues that are continually renewing themselves, such as epithelial tissue, may be devastated by parvovirus. The small intestine, for example, is lined with epithelial tissue that helps to absorb nutrient molecules from the lumen of the gut. During **infections,** the epithelial cells die and slough in sheets. Therefore animals develop diarrhea, vomit, and can become severely dehydrated in a short time. In addition, the sudden loss of epithelial tissue causes bleeding into the intestine, which creates a distinctively noxious, foul-smelling, hemorrhagic diarrhea. A simple laboratory test of the stool may indicate the presence of the virus and, in this way, offers a definitive diagnosis.

Treatment centers on combating dehydration and includes intravenous fluid therapy with electrolyte supplements, antibiotics, and antivomiting medications. Animals that are alive after 3 to 4 days of illness generally survive but continue to shed the virus for several months. Because of the highly contagious nature of parvoviral diseases, every effort should be made to isolate affected animals.

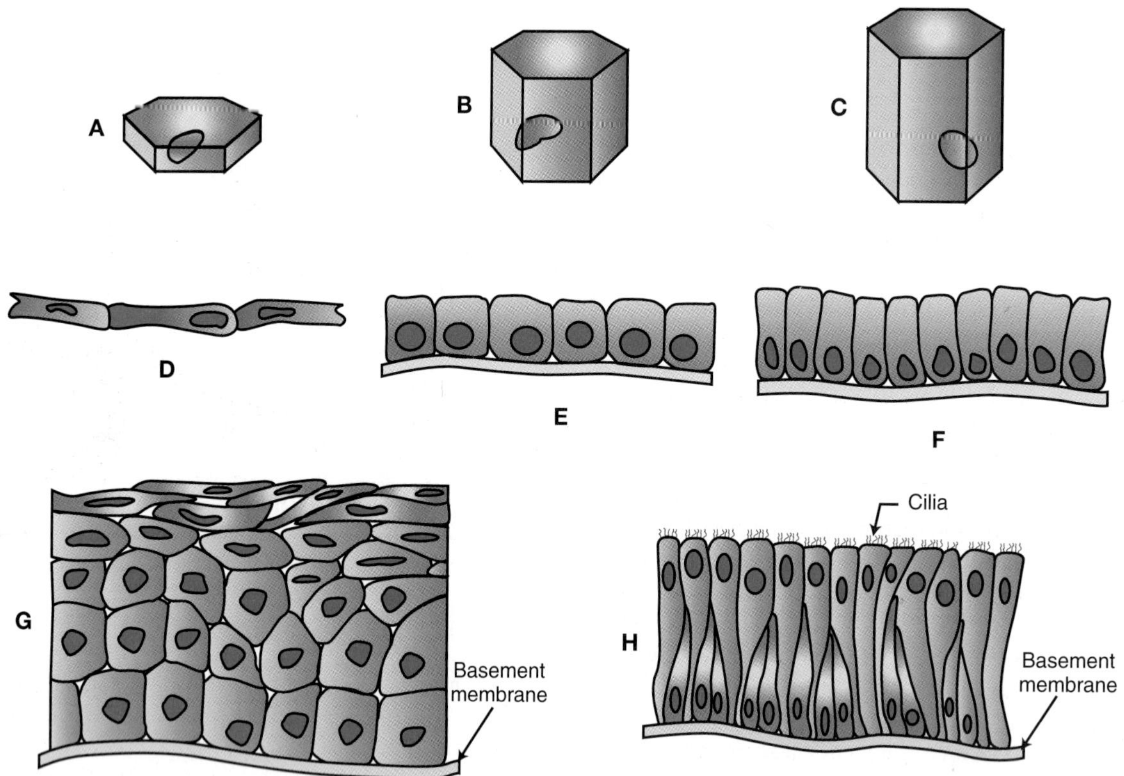

FIGURE **4-3** **Classification of Epithelia.** Epithelial tissues are classified according to shape of the cell and the way in which cells are arranged. Stratified epithelial tissues are composed of many layers of cells, and each layer of cells may have a different shape. In these cases, tissue is classified according to the shape of the cells on the surface, in the outermost layer. **A,** Squamous; **B,** cuboidal; **C,** columnar; **D,** simple squamous; **E,** simple cuboidal; **F,** simple columnar; **G,** stratified (squamous); **H,** pseudostratified.

simple epithelium and are found in areas of the body that are subjected to mechanical and chemical stress.

2. *Shape of the cells.* In cross section, epithelial cells may take on many shapes, such as squamous, cuboidal, and columnar. In **stratified epithelium,** many different cell shapes are visible within the same tissue, but the classification is based on the shape of the cell that resides on the *exposed or luminal* surface of the tissue. In stratified squamous epithelium, for example, **cuboidal cells** are visible near the basement membrane, but **squamous cells** are found at the luminal surface; therefore the tissue is called *stratified squamous,* not *stratified cuboidal.*
3. *Presence of surface specializations.* Terms for surface specializations, such as "cilia" and "keratinized," may be added to the classifications of epithelia to indicate an increased level of specialization. Stratified squamous

epithelium, for example, may be classified as keratinized stratified squamous epithelium (found in the skin) or nonkeratinized stratified squamous epithelium (found in the lining of the mouth).

TYPES OF EPITHELIA

Simple Squamous Epithelium

Simple squamous epithelia are delicate and thin. They are often found lining surfaces involved in the passage of either gas or liquid. Therefore they are found (1) in the inner lining of the lung, where oxygen is absorbed and carbon dioxide released, and (2) in the filtration membranes of kidneys, where water and other small molecules are excreted as urine (Figure 4-4, *A*). The fragile nature of simple squamous epithelium requires that it occur only in protected regions of the body, such as in the lining of the chest and abdominal cavities. Because simple squamous epithelia are flat and smooth, they are important in reducing friction and are found in the lining of blood and lymphatic vessels. Simple squamous epithelia have been given special names depending on where they are located in the body. For example, the epithelium that lines the pleural (chest), pericardial (around the heart), and peritoneal (abdominal) cavities is called *mesothelium*. The epithelium that lines blood and lymphatic vessels is called *endothelium*.

Simple Cuboidal Epithelium

Simple cuboidal epithelium is composed of a single layer of cubical cells (see Figure 4-4, *B*). On microscopic examination, one finds their round, dark-staining nuclei aligned in a single row that resembles a string of pearls. Like simple squamous epithelium, simple cuboidal epithelium provides little protection from abrasion. Therefore it occurs in sheltered regions of the body where secretion and absorption take place. It is found on the surface of ovaries; in the secretory portions of glands, such as the thyroid; and in the lining of the ducts of the liver, pancreas, kidney, and salivary gland. Some simple cuboidal epithelia in kidney tubules are covered with microvilli, attesting to their absorptive function. Others are smooth surfaced and associated with secretory glands.

Simple cuboidal epithelium plays an important role in both endocrine and exocrine tissue. Exocrine ducts lined with simple cuboidal epithelium, for example, carry saliva from the salivary gland to the oral cavity, and enzymes secreted by the pancreas are transported to the duodenum. In addition, the thyroid gland, an endocrine structure, contains chambers lined by a single row of cuboidal cells and secretes the hormone thyroxine that is carried throughout the body via the bloodstream.

Simple Columnar Epithelium

Simple **columnar epithelial cells** are elongated and closely packed together, making the epithelia relatively thick and more protective than the simple squamous and cuboidal epithelia (see Figure 4-4, *C*). Their nuclei are not centrally located, as they are in cuboidal cells, but rather are aligned in a row at the base of the cell near the basement membrane. Simple columnar epithelia line the length of the gastrointestinal tract from the stomach to the rectum. Like simple cuboidal, they are associated with absorption and secretion and are found in many **excretory ducts,** as well as in the digestive tract. Two types of cells make up the gut lining. The most numerous is the absorptive cell, whose apical surface is blanketed by dense microvilli, which maximize absorption by increasing surface contact with the nutrient-filled lumen. The other cell is called

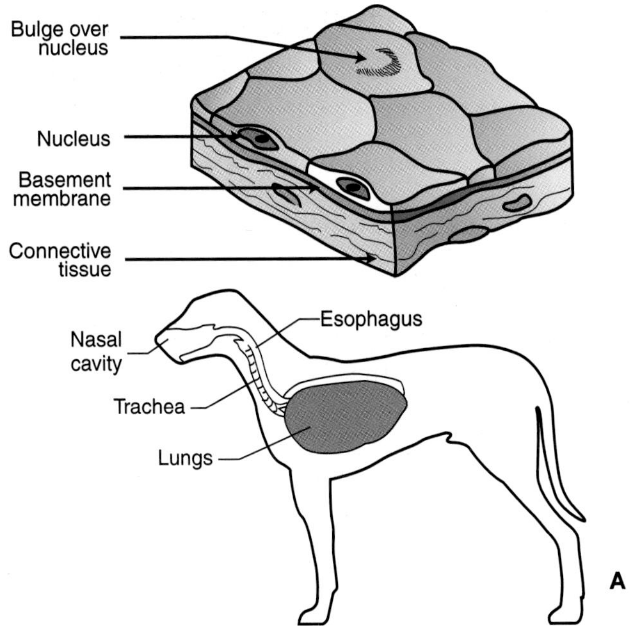

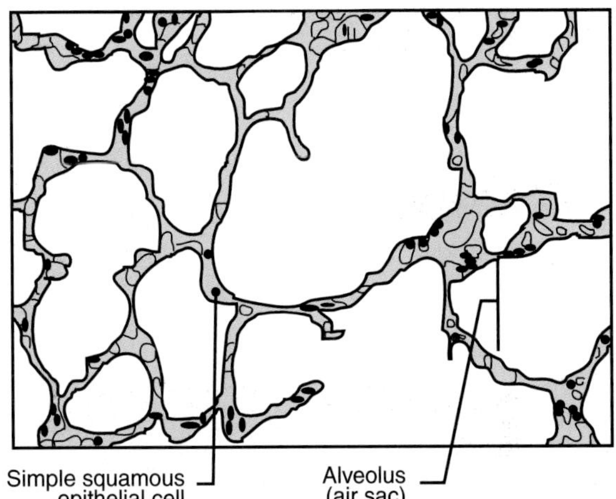

FIGURE **4-4 Types of Epithelial Tissue.**
A, Simple Squamous Epithelium.
Description: A single layer of flattened, hexagonal-shaped cells. The nuclei are disk shaped and centrally located. They often appear as raised bumps in the center of the flattened cell, giving cells a fried egg appearance.
Location: Alveoli of lungs, lining in blood and lymphatic vessels, lining in heart and major body cavities, filtration units (glomeruli) in kidney.
Function: In regions of the body where protection is not important, simple squamous epithelium allows diffusion, filtration, secretion, and absorption.
Microanatomy: Simple squamous cells make up the walls of air sacs in the lung. *Continued*

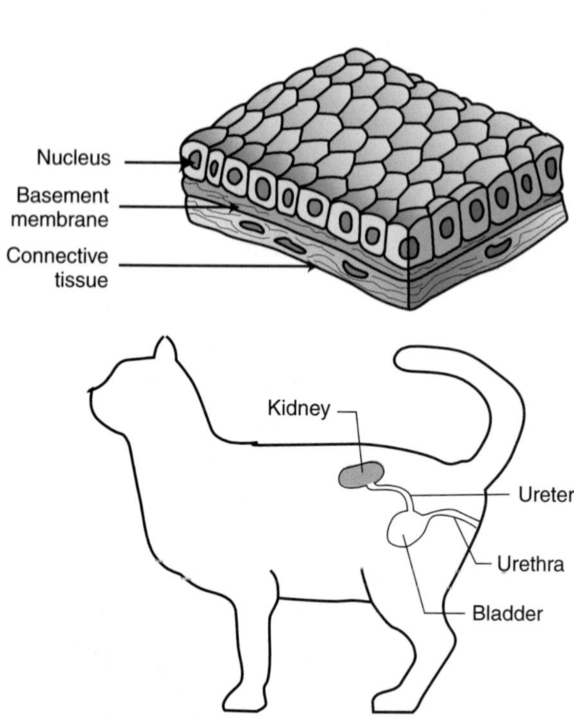

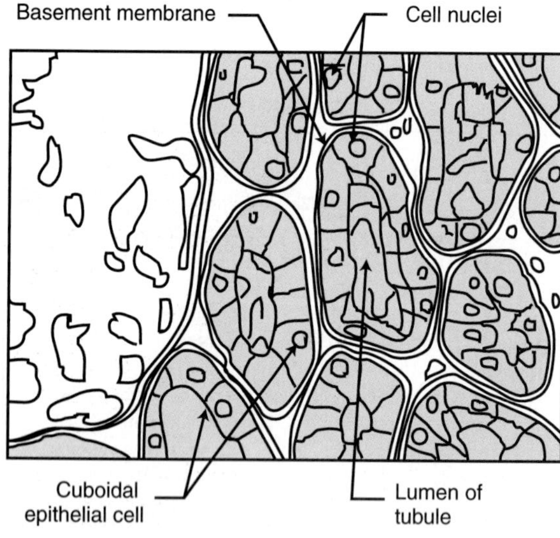

FIGURE **4-4, cont'd**

B, Simple Cuboidal Epithelium.

Description: A single row of tightly packed, cubelike cells, each of which contains a round, centrally located nucleus.

Location: Tubules of kidney, terminal bronchioles in lungs, choroid plexus of brain, glands, and their ducts, surface of ovaries.

Function: Cells in kidney are engaged in absorption and secretion; cells in bronchioles are ciliated and assist with movement of particles away from lungs. Cells in choroid plexus and in glands secrete substances.

Microanatomy: Simple cuboidal epithelium lines tubules in the kidneys.

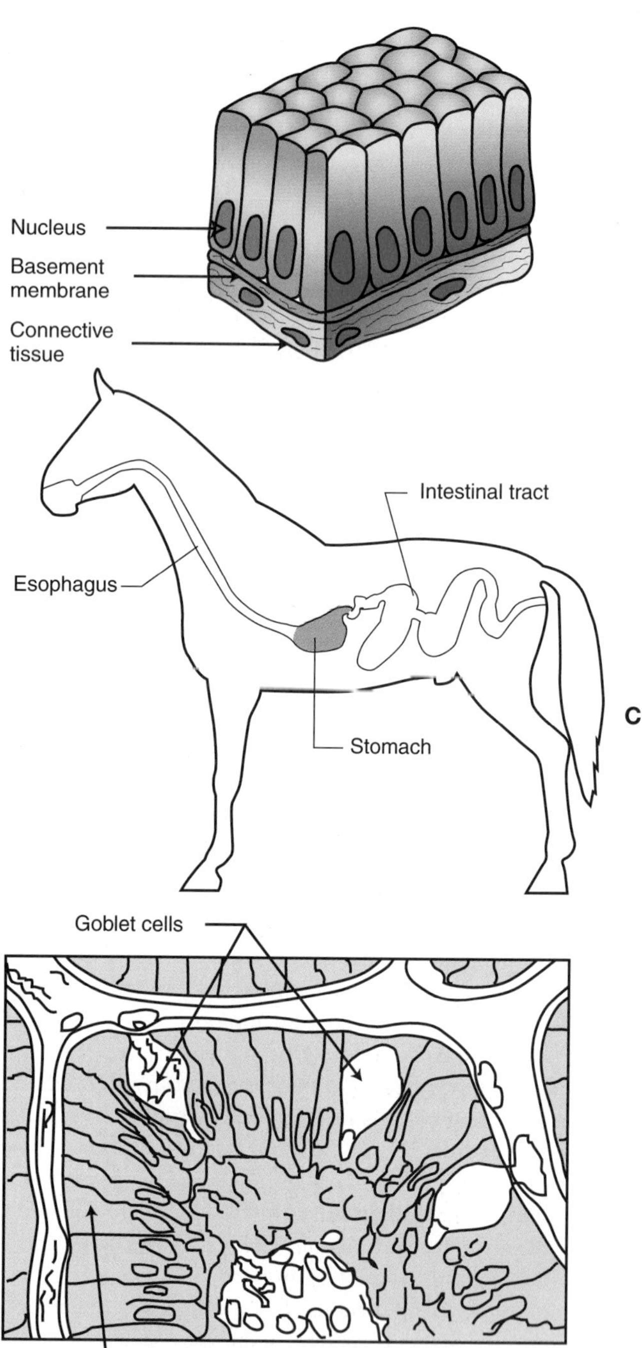

FIGURE **4-4, cont'd**

C, Simple Columnar Epithelium.

Description: A single row of tall, slender cells with oval nuclei. Nuclei are generally located near basal border. Surface may or may not be ciliated. Goblet cells can be seen interspersed among cells.

Location: Nonciliated variety lines the digestive tract from stomach to rectum, gallbladder, and excretory ducts of some glands; ciliated cells are found in uterine tubes, uterus, and small bronchi of lungs.

Function: Absorption in intestine and secretion in stomach, glands, and intestines. Ciliated cells assist with movement of particles out of the lungs and with movement of the oocyte through uterine tubes.

Microanatomy: Simple epithelium lines the stomach.

Continued

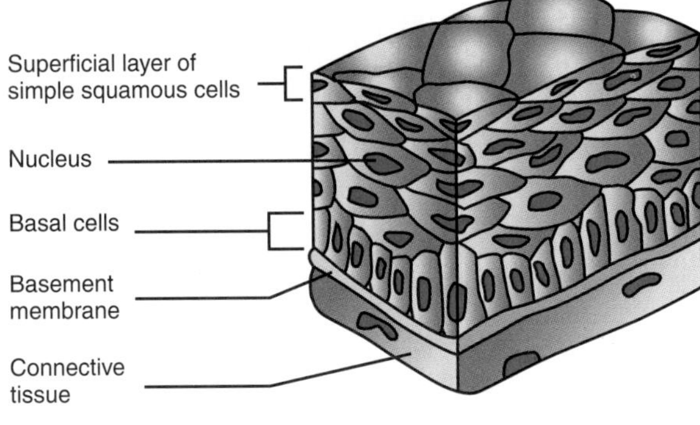

D

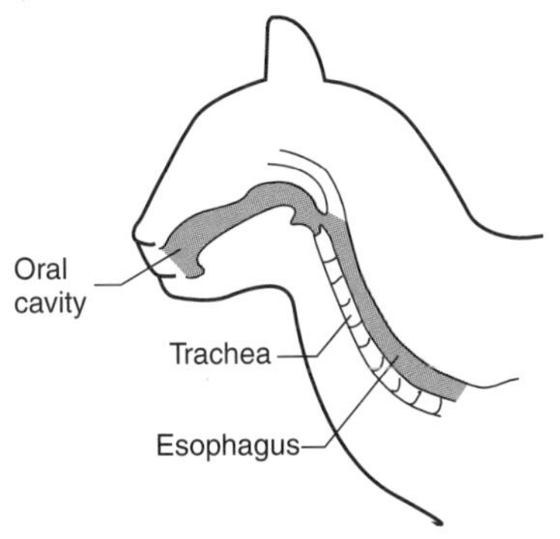

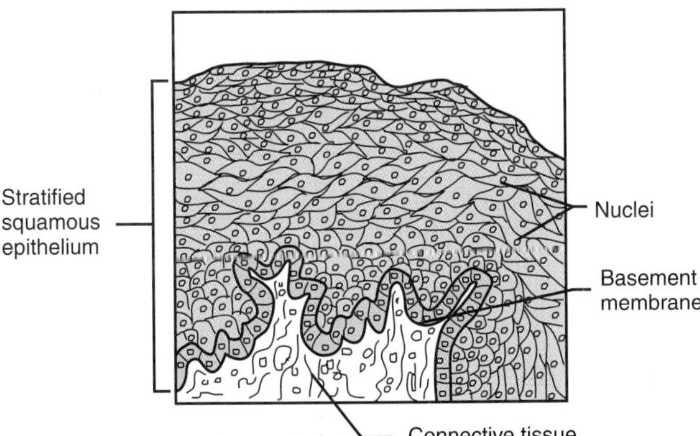

FIGURE **4-4, cont'd**

D, Stratified Squamous (Keratinized and Nonkeratinized) Epithelium.

Description: A multilayered tissue in which cells along basement membrane are metabolically active and dividing. These basal cells are cuboidal or columnar, and as they mature, they are pushed to the surface, lose their organelles, and flatten into thin flakes. In skin, maturing cells fill with keratin.

Location: Lining of mouth, esophagus, and vagina. Keratinized cells are found in epidermis.

Function: In areas that are prone to abrasion, stratified squamous protects underlying tissues.

Microanatomy: Thick membrane that lines mouth and esophagus is stratified squamous.

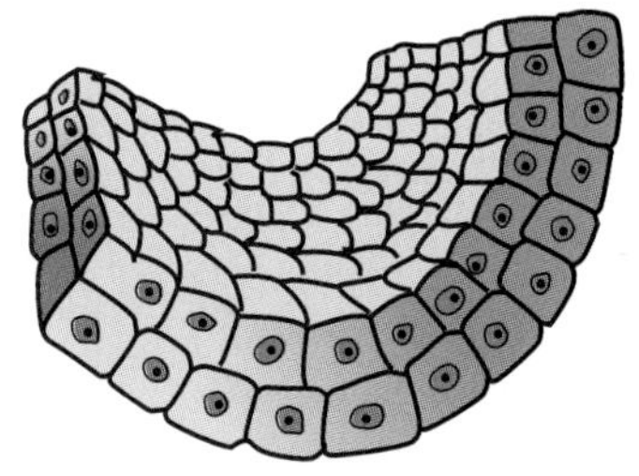

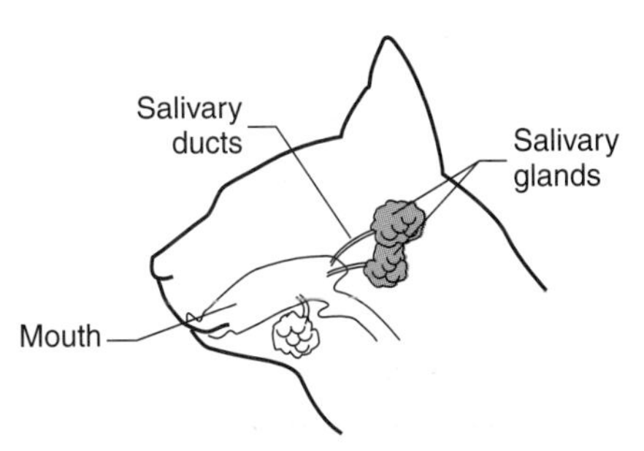

E

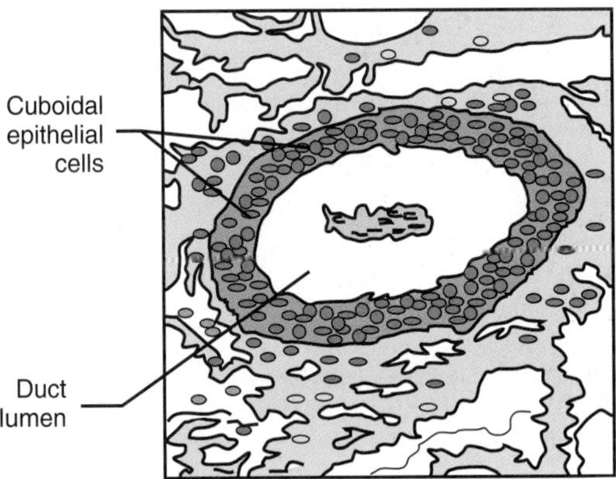

FIGURE **4-4, cont'd**

E, Stratified Cuboidal Epithelium.

Description: Generally, two layers of cuboidal cells.

Location: Ducts of mammary glands, sweat glands, and salivary glands.

Function: Secretion, absorption, and protection.

Microanatomy: Stratified cuboidal epithelia located in salivary gland.

Continued

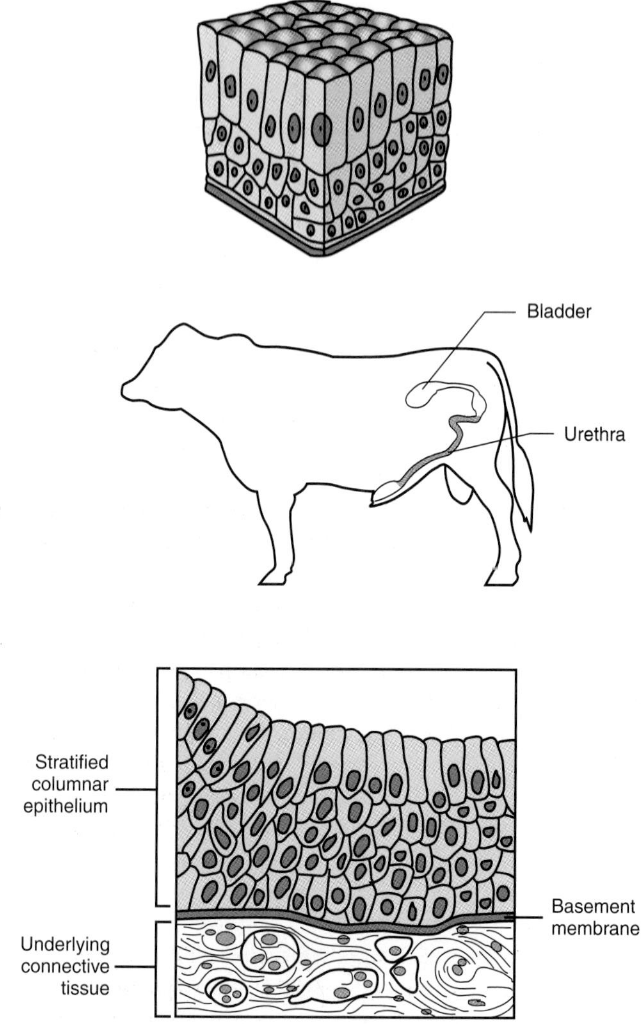

FIGURE **4-4, cont'd**
F, Stratified Columnar Epithelium.
Description: Several layers of cells in which basal cells are cuboidal and superficial cells are columnar.
Location: Large ducts of mammary gland and in small portion of urethra of some male animals. This type of epithelium is rare.
Function: Secretion and protection.
Microanatomy: Stratified columnar epithelium is found in urethra.

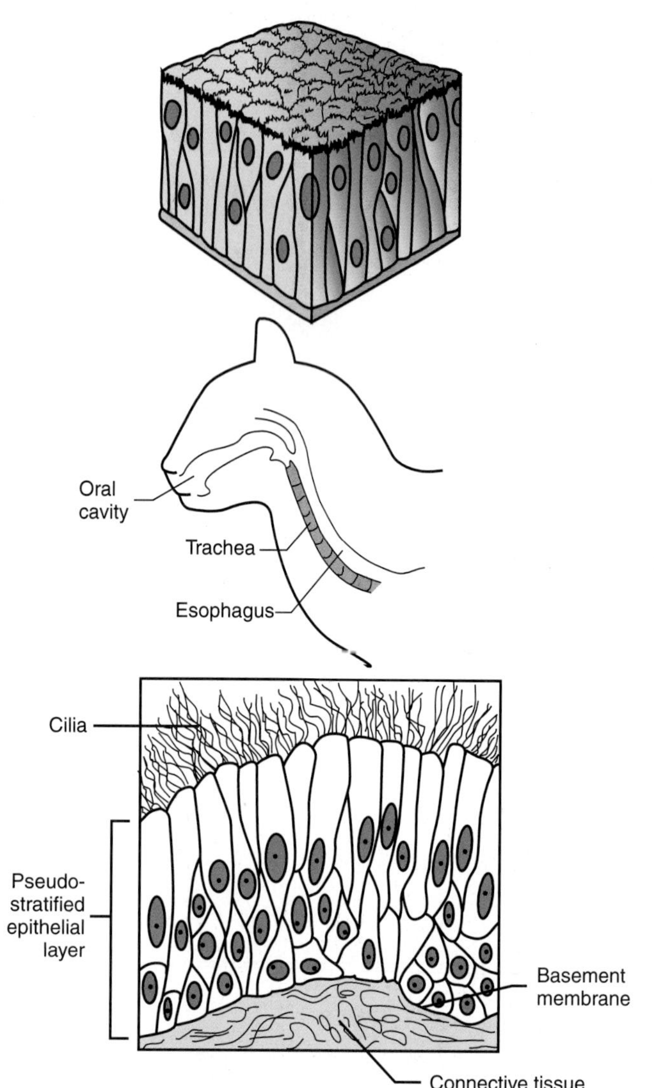

FIGURE **4-4, cont'd**
G, Pseudostratified Epithelium.
Description: Pseudostratified epithelium appear stratified but are not. Each cell is attached to basement membrane, but not all of them reach luminal surface. Cells vary in shape and height. Their nuclei occur at different distances from basement membrane. Cells are generally ciliated and are often associated with goblet cells.
Location: Respiratory tract, including nasal cavity, larynx, pharynx, trachea, and bronchi.
Function: Surface layer of mucus traps particles, which are moved away from lungs by beating cilia.
Microanatomy: Ciliated pseudostratified epithelium lines trachea.

Continued

a **goblet cell** because of its wineglass shape. Goblet cells manufacture and store lubricating mucus that is secreted onto the luminal surfaces of the epithelia.

Some less common epithelia are covered with cilia on their apical surfaces. These cells are called **simple ciliated columnar epithelia,** and they line the uterine tubes and respiratory tracts.

Stratified Squamous Epithelium

Stratified squamous epithelium consists of various cell layers (see Figure 4-4, *D*). It occurs in regions of the body that are subject to mechanical and chemical stresses, such as the lining of the mouth, esophagus, vagina, and rectum. The epithelial cells that make up the outer surface are continually being worn away or sheared off, but they are replaced at an equal rate by cells from deeper layers. Cuboidal cells form the base of stratified squamous epithelium. They are attached to the basement membrane and are continually dividing to keep up with the cell losses from the luminal surface. As the young cuboidal cells mature, they are progressively pushed to the surface away

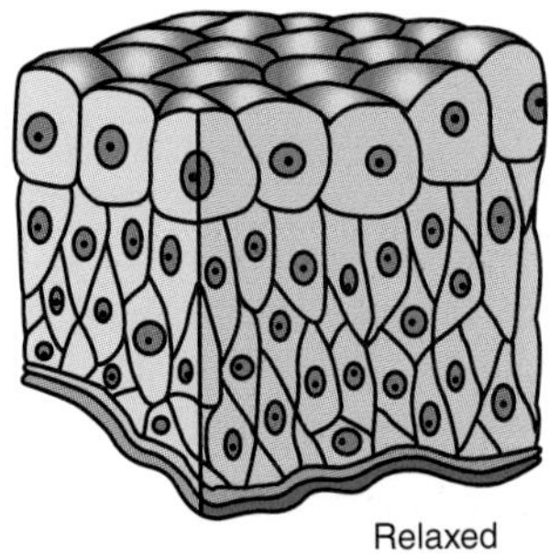

H

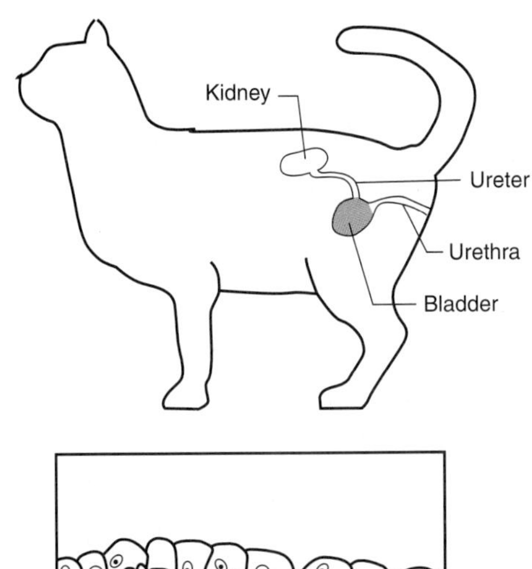

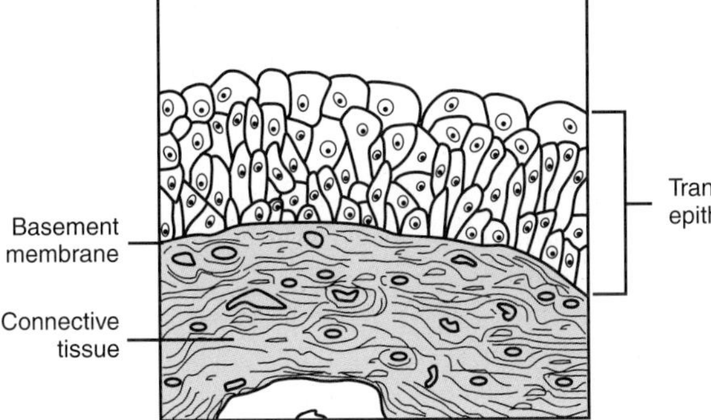

FIGURE **4-4, cont'd**
H, Transitional Epithelium.
Description: Stratified epithelium in which basal layer is composed of cuboidal or columnar cells. Superficial layer is composed of cuboidal or squamous cells, depending on level of distension in tissue.
Location: Urinary bladder, ureters, and urethra.
Function: Transitional epithelium is flexible to accommodate fluctuations in amount of urine in bladder, ureters, and urethra. It forms permeable barrier that holds liquid and protects underlying tissues from caustic effects of urine.
Microanatomy: Transitional epithelium in bladder.

from the nutrient sources provided by the underlying connective tissue. During this movement, the cells lose their cytoplasm and nuclei, take on a squamous shape, and eventually become paperlike sheets that slough.

Stratified Cuboidal Epithelium

Stratified cuboidal epithelium generally occurs as two layers of cuboidal cells and is found primarily along large excretory ducts, such as those of sweat glands, mammary glands, and salivary glands (see Figure 4-4, *E*). This type of epithelium is important in protecting the delicate tissues in deeper layers.

Stratified Columnar Epithelium

Stratified columnar epithelium is rare and is found only in select parts of the **respiratory, digestive,** and **reproductive systems** and along some excretory ducts (see Figure 4-4, *F*).

Pseudostratified Columnar Epithelium

Pseudo- means "false"; therefore **pseudostratified columnar epithelium** is an epithelial layer that is *not* truly stratified. The epithelial cells appear to be stratified because the nuclei are found at different levels across the length of the tissue layer. In addition, not all of the cells reach the luminal surface; therefore the cells *appear* to be at different levels as though stratified. In reality, each cell forms a distinct attachment, however subtle, with the basement membrane. In this way, pseudostratified columnar epithelium forms a single layer and therefore is considered a *simple* epithelium (see Figure 4-4, *G*).

Most pseudostratified columnar epithelium is ciliated and is found in the respiratory tract and in portions of the male reproductive tract. In the trachea, for example, the epithelium is coated with a layer of mucus that is propelled by cilia across the luminal surface toward the mouth. This assists in preventing debris from entering the lungs. The mucus is also fortified with protective **immunoglobulins,** disease-fighting molecules that help to protect animals from **pathogens** (bacteria and viruses) that have been inhaled.

Transitional Epithelium

Transitional epithelium has the remarkable ability to stretch. It is found in regions of the body that are required to expand and contract as part of their normal function. Thus transitional epithelium is found in portions of the urinary tract where great changes in volume occur, such as the urinary bladder, ureters, urethra, and calyxes of the kidney. The histological appearance of transitional epithelia varies depending on how much it is stretched. For example, in an empty bladder the epithelial layer is thick and multilayered and has rounded, domelike cells on the luminal surface. When the bladder is filled, greater pressure is applied to the epithelial layer, making it stretch and thin out. The extent to which the membrane stretches depends on how full the bladder is and how much force is applied to the epithelia. As epithelia stretch, they may thin out from six to three cell layers, and the apical cells become flattened and squamous. The ability of transitional cells to change shape in the urine-holding tissues allows greater volumes of urine to be transported, stored, and excreted (see Figure 4-4, *H*).

In addition to its ability to stretch, transitional epithelium forms a leakproof membrane that prevents the diffusion of potentially scalding urine into the delicate environment of the abdominal cavity.

TEST YOURSELF

1. Epithelial tissue is characterized as simple, stratified, or pseudostratified. What does this mean?
2. What are the three basic shapes of epithelial cells?
3. Draw a picture of each of the following types of epithelia and give an example of where each of them can be found in the body.
    - Simple squamous
    - Simple cuboidal
    - Simple columnar
    - Stratified squamous
    - Pseudostratified columnar
    - Transitional

GLANDULAR EPITHELIA

A gland is a cell or group of cells that have the ability to manufacture and discharge a secretion. Secretions are specialized protein molecules that are produced in the rough endoplasmic reticulum, packaged into granules by the Golgi apparatus, and discharged from the cell. Thus typical glandular epithelial cells are recognized by their prominent endoplasmic reticulum, Golgi apparatus, and secretory granules. Some of the secretions produced by glandular epithelia are used locally, whereas others are needed in distant regions of the body.

During embryonic development, multicellular glands form from an infolding of a layer of epithelial cells. Initially, these invaginations form ducts and tubules that maintain contact with the surface epithelium. In the course of development, some of the glands lose the ducts and become separated from the parent epithelial sheet (Figure 4-5). In this way, glands are derived from epithelium.

Glands can be classified in many ways. For example, we can organize them based on the following factors:

1. Presence or absence of ducts (endocrine or exocrine)
2. Number of cells that compose them (unicellular or multicellular)
3. Shape of the secreting ducts (simple or compound)
4. Complexity of the glandular structure (tubular, acinar, or tubuloacinar)
5. Type of secretion they produce (mucoid or serous)
6. Manner in which the secretion is stored and discharged (merocrine, apocrine, or holocrine)

Each of these classifications is discussed.

Endocrine Glands

Glands that do not have ducts or tubules and whose secretions are distributed throughout the body are called **endocrine glands.** They produce and secrete regulatory chemicals, known as **hormones,** into the bloodstream or the lymphatic system, where they are carried to many regions of the body. Endocrine glands are part of a complex, biochemical network known as the **endocrine system.** The pituitary gland in the brain and the adrenal gland near the kidney are examples of

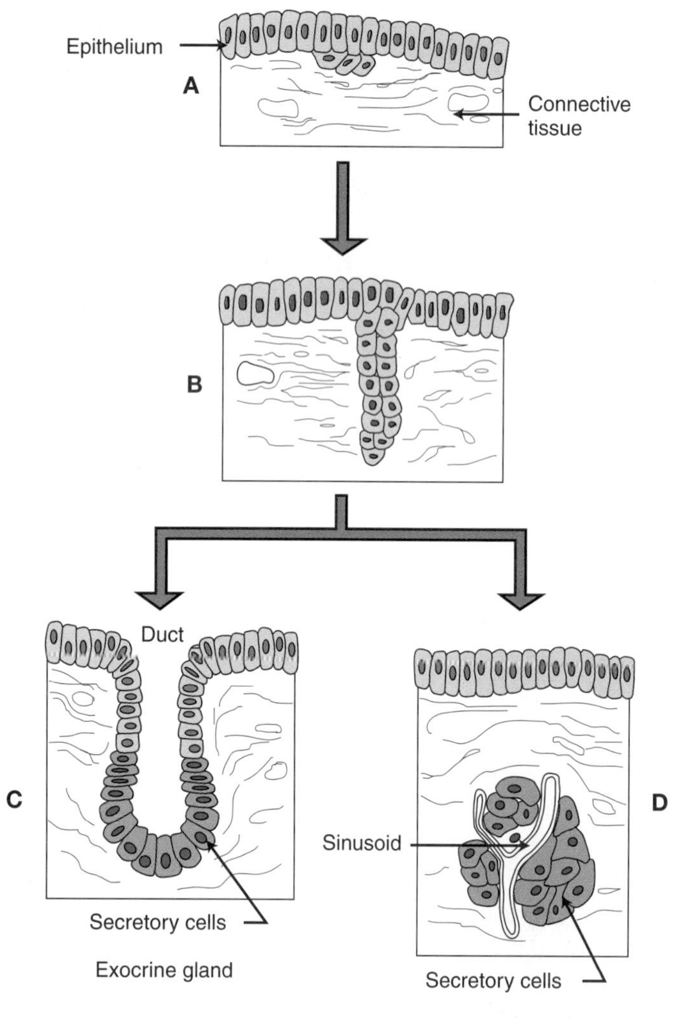

FIGURE **4-5 Development of Glands.** Exocrine and endocrine glands develop from epithelium during the maturation of a fetus (**A** and **B**). Surface epithelial cells grow down into the underlying connective tissue. Exocrine glands develop when the connection between deep and superficial layers of cells form a duct. The deepest cells become secretory **(C).** Endocrine glands form when connecting cells die. Secretions of the gland are transferred to sinusoids and then into the circulatory system rather than through a duct **(D).**

endocrine glands. The endocrine system and the glands it includes are discussed in detail in Chapter 14.

Exocrine Glands

With the exception of the goblet cell, **exocrine glands** possess ducts. They are more common than endocrine glands and act by discharging secretions via their ducts directly into local areas, where they may, for example, cover cell surfaces or empty into body cavities. Unlike those of endocrine glands, the secretions of exocrine glands act locally and do not normally enter the circulation. A wide variety of exocrine glands are found in animals, including hepatoid, musk, sweat, and salivary glands. Other examples can be found in the liver and pancreas, where exocrine glands

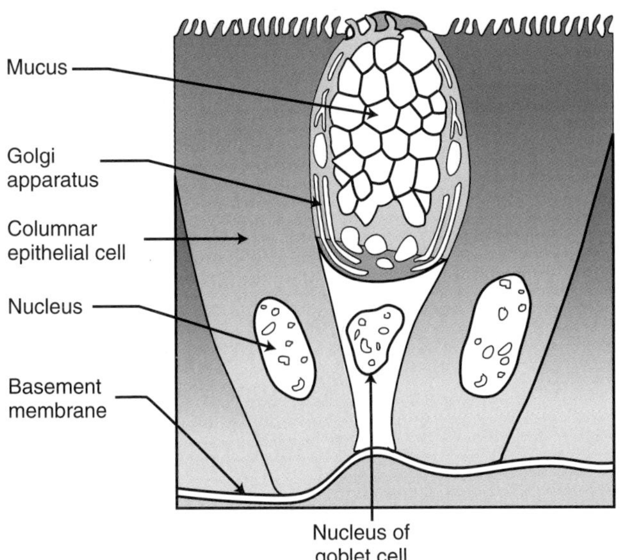

FIGURE **4-6** **Goblet Cell.** A unicellular goblet cell occurs among simple and pseudostratified epithelia that line the respiratory and digestive tracts. Mucus is contained within the cytoplasm at the luminal end of the cell, and the nucleus is located in the basal end of the cell, near the basement membrane. A goblet cell releases its stored mucus onto the tissue surface.

secrete bile and digestive enzymes, respectively. The pancreas possesses endocrine and exocrine properties because it is responsible for producing many hormones and secreting digestive enzymes.

Unicellular Exocrine Glands. The only example of a **unicellular exocrine gland** is the ductless goblet cell, so named because of its resemblance to the drinking goblet (Figure 4-6). The goblet cell is a modified columnar epithelial cell and is found interspersed among the **columnar cells** of the respiratory and digestive tracts and in the conjunctiva of the eye. Goblet cells secrete **mucin:** a thick, sticky mixture of glycoproteins and **proteoglycans** that when mixed with water becomes mucus. The mucus functions in two ways: it helps protect the apical surface of the epithelial layer, and it assists with the entrapment of microorganisms and foreign particles.

Multicellular Exocrine Glands. Multicellular exocrine glands are made up of two distinct components: a **secretory unit** in which secretions are produced by secretory cells and a **duct** that carries the secretion to the deposition site. In most glands the secretory unit is surrounded by connective tissue that is rich in blood vessels and nerve fibers. It not only nourishes the secretory unit but also provides structural support and may extend into the gland to form distinct lobes. In some exocrine glands the secretory unit is surrounded by contractile cells called **myoepithelial cells** that assist with the discharge of secretions into the glandular duct. The rate of secretion production and discharge is controlled by hormonal and nervous influences.

We begin the classification of exocrine glands with examination of the glandular ducts (Table 4-1). If the main duct is *unbranched*, the gland is considered to be **simple.** If the main duct is *branched*, the gland is called **compound**. Next, we examine the secretory portions of glands. If the secretory cells form a long channel of even width, the gland is called **tubular.** If the secretory unit forms a rounded sac, the gland is called **alveolar,** or **acinar.** Glands with secretory units that possess both tubular and alveolar qualities are called **tubuloalveolar,** or **tubuloacinar** (Figure 4-7).

Glands are classified further according to the way in which they secrete their products. How much of the cell is sacrificed in the act of secretion determines whether the gland is **merocrine, apocrine,** or **holocrine** (Figure 4-8). The majority of glands package their secretions into granular units and release them via exocytosis as they are manufactured. These glands are called *merocrine* because the secretory cells remain intact during the secretory process. The pancreas, sweat glands, and salivary glands are examples of merocrine glands. Secretion in apocrine glands involves the loss of the **apex** of the secretory cell. The secretory cells in apocrine glands do not release their granules as they are manufactured. Instead, they store the granules until the apex of the cell is full. Then the cell pinches in two and releases the top part of the cell (the apex) into the duct system. Later, the cell repairs the damage and repeats the process. Apocrine glands can be found in mammary tissue and are represented by some sweat glands. Like apocrine glands, holocrine glands also store granules in the secretory cells until they are needed. However, in holocrine glands, the entire secretory cell is destroyed in the act of releasing its secretory product. The subsequent degeneration of the cell allows the release of the granules. Holocrine secretion occurs principally in sebaceous glands.

We can also categorize glands according to the type of secretion they produce. **Serous secretions** are watery and contain a high concentration of enzymes, whereas **mucous secretions** are thick, viscous, and composed of glycoproteins. Secretory cells that manufacture both types of secretions are common in the digestive and respiratory tracts. **Mixed exocrine glands** contain both mucous and serous components.

TEST YOURSELF

1. What is a gland?
2. How did glands develop embryologically?
3. What is the difference between endocrine and exocrine glands? Can you give examples of each?
4. Where are goblet cells found? What type of secretion do they produce?
5. In general, how are multicellular exocrine glands constructed?
6. Can you describe merocrine, apocrine, and holocrine glands? How do they differ from one another?
7. How are serous and mucous secretions different?

Table 4-1 Classification of Multicellular Exocrine Glands

Shape of Gland	Type of Gland	Location of Gland
Tubular (single, straight)	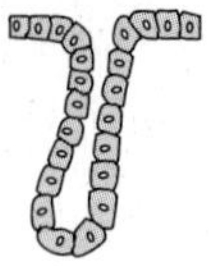 Simple tubular	Stomach, intestine
Tubular (coiled)	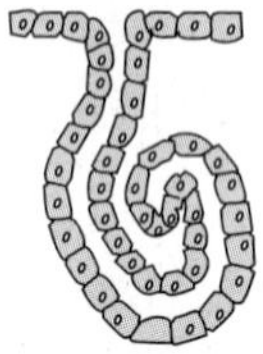 Simple coiled tubular	Sweat glands
Tubular (multiple)	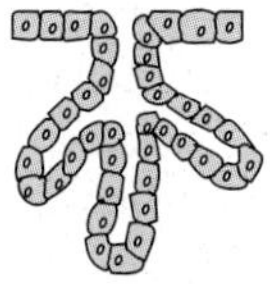 Simple branched tubular	Stomach, mouth, tongue, esophagus
Alveolar (single)	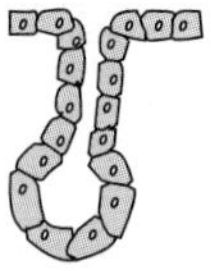 Simple alveolar	Sebaceous glands
Alveolar (multiple)	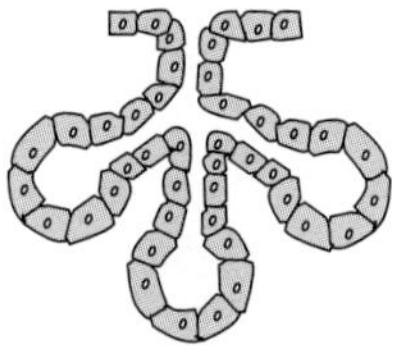 Branched alveolar (acinar)	Sebaceous glands
Tubular (multiple)	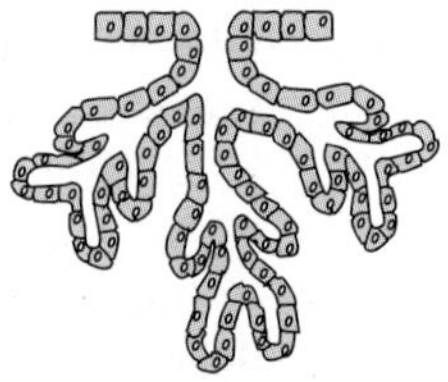 Compound tubular	Bulbourethral glands, mammary glands, kidney tubules, testes, mucous glands of the mouth
Alveolar (multiple)	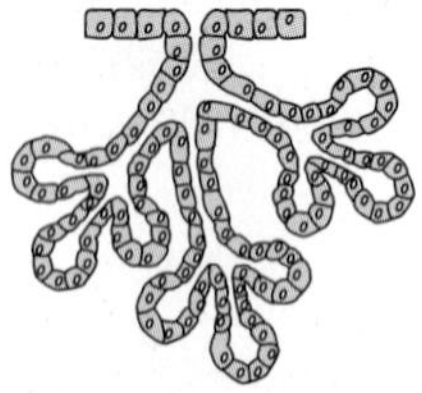 Compound alveolar (acinar)	Mammary glands
Some tubular; some alveolar	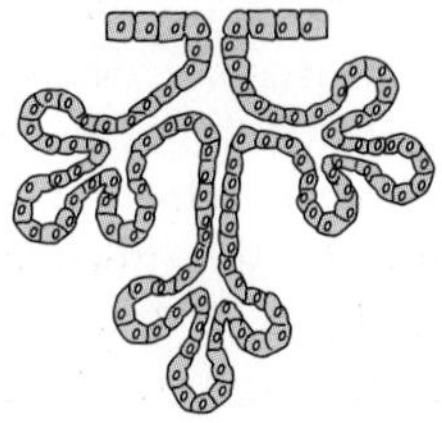 Compound tubuloalveolar	Salivary glands, pancreas, respiratory passages

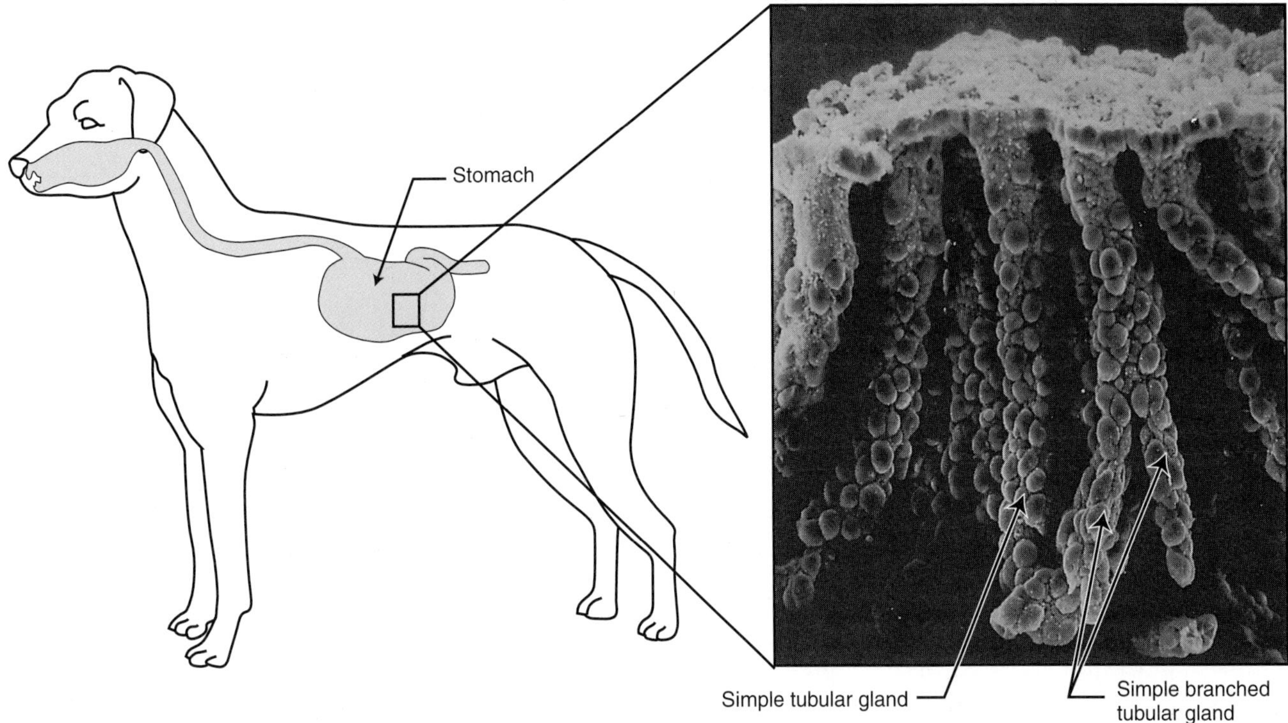

FIGURE **4-7** **Exocrine Glands in Canine Stomach.** Exocrine glands are structured in many different ways and occur in diverse regions of the body. In the lining of the stomach, for example, exocrine glands occur as simple straight, simple coiled, and compound (or branched) tubular glands. These gastric glands produce a mixture of water, enzymes, acid, and mucus, which together forms an important digestive "juice."

CONNECTIVE TISSUE

GENERAL CHARACTERISTICS

Connective tissue is found everywhere in the body and represents the most abundant tissue type by weight. Some organ systems, such as the skeletal and integumentary systems, are composed almost exclusively of connective tissue, whereas others, such as the neurological system, contain very little. Connective tissue is derived from **mesoderm** and, unlike epithelial tissue, is composed primarily of nonliving **extracellular matrix.** The matrix surrounds and separates the cells, and it provides important structural and nutritional support that enables connective tissue cells to exist farther apart than epithelial cells. In addition, unlike epithelial tissue that has no direct blood supply, connective tissue is **vascularized** although the level of vascularity varies among different connective tissue types. Loose connective tissue and adipose connective tissue, for example, possess good blood supplies, whereas dense connective tissue is poorly vascularized.

All connective tissue is composed of three distinct components: **extracellular fibers, ground substance,** and cells. The mixture of fiber and ground substance is called the *extracellular matrix*. Variations in the ground substance, fibers, and cellular components have given rise to a wide range of connective tissue types (Figure 4-9). Blood, tendon, fat, cartilage, and even bone are all examples of connective tissue even though their textures and appearances are different from one another. Variations in the type of ground substance and in the type of fiber enable the tissue to take on many different qualities. It can be elastic and flexible, rigid, semisolid, and liquid. Blood, for example, is a highly cellular connective tissue with a liquid matrix containing relatively little fiber. In contrast, bone is composed of a solid **calcified** matrix. Tendon contains a matrix that is primarily fibrous with little ground substance. These variations give connective tissue the ability to withstand a wide range of forces, such as direct pressure, abrasion, and shearing forces, that would destroy other tissue types.

As with all living structures, form and function are intertwined. Thus the plethora of forms that characterize connective tissue gives rise to a wide range of functions. In general, as its name implies, connective tissue forms metabolic and structural connections between other tissues; however, it serves many other important roles as well. For example, connective tissue forms a protective sheath around organs and helps insulate the body. It acts as a reserve for energy, provides the frame that supports the body, and composes the medium that transports substances from one region of the body to another. In addition, connective tissue plays a vital role in the healing process and in the control of invading microorganisms.

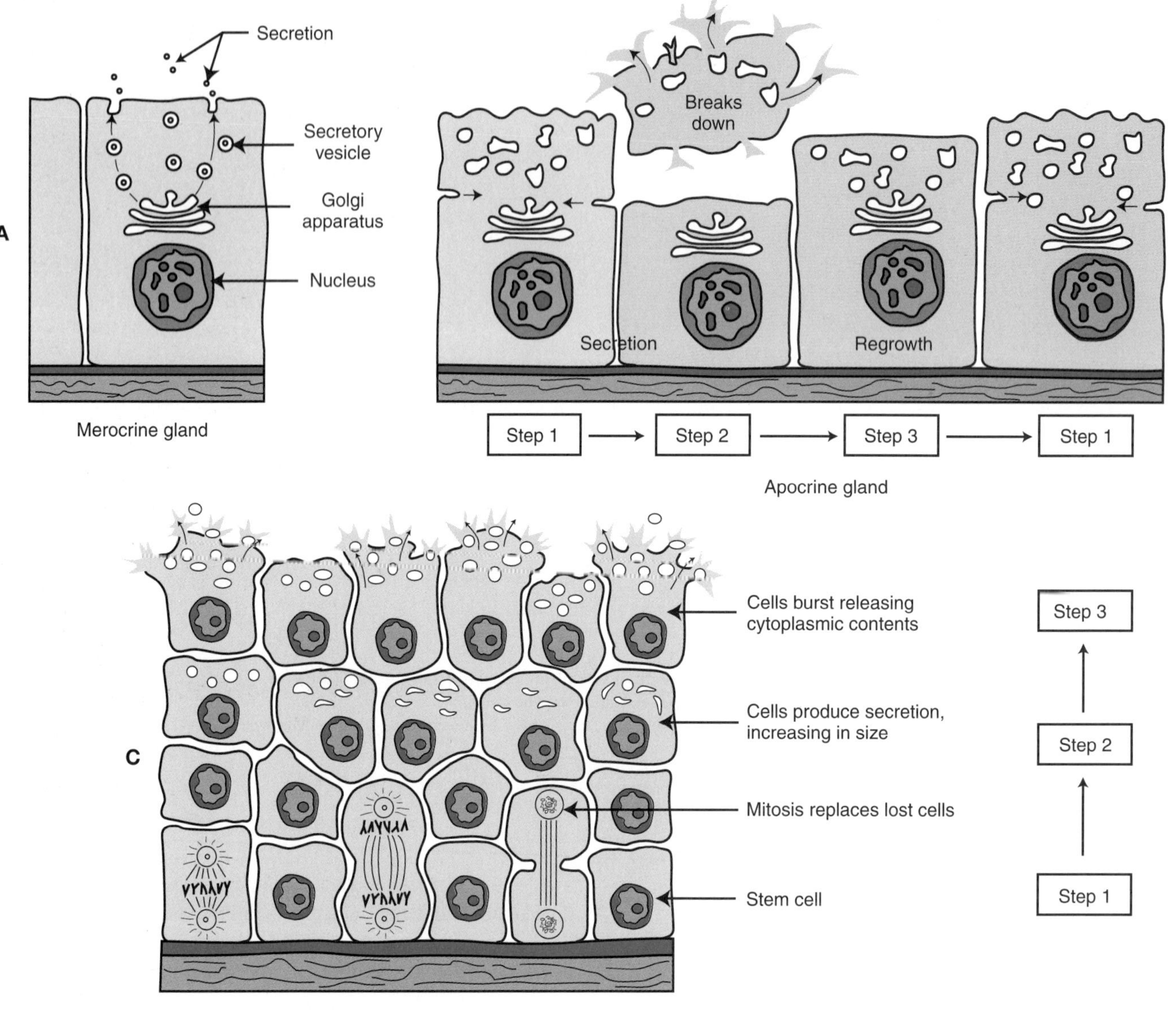

FIGURE **4-8** **Secretion Styles of Exocrine Glands. A,** Cells of merocrine glands store substances intended for excretion in vesicles in their cytoplasm. The vesicles are transported to the surface of the cell, where they release their contents. A cell can continue to produce and excrete substances throughout its life and is not in any way harmed by the secretory process. **B,** Cells of apocrine glands also store secretory substances within vesicles. However, secretion occurs as the luminal end of the cell is detached from the basal portion. Cytosol, inclusions, and other cytoplasmic components are discharged along with the secretory vesicles. The cell must take time to regrow lost portions of itself before it can secrete again. **C,** Holocrine secretion involves release of the entire contents of the cell. In this process, the cell is killed and is replaced by new cells that have moved up from deeper layers.

COMPONENTS OF CONNECTIVE TISSUE

The major components of connective tissue are summarized in Box 4-1.

Ground Substance

The **ground substance** in connective tissue is an **amorphous, homogeneous** material that ranges in texture from a liquid or gel to a calcified solid. In soft connective tissues, it is composed of unbranched chains of glycoproteins called **glycosaminoglycans (GAGs).** The most commonly found GAG in connective tissue is hyaluronic acid combined with 2% protein. These large molecules help to orient the formation of fibers within the tissue.

Ground substance is the medium through which cells exchange nutrients and waste with the bloodstream. It acts as a shock-absorbing cushion and helps to protect the more delicate cells that it envelopes. In addition, its thick texture serves as an effective obstacle for invading microorganisms although some microbes have developed the ability to produce the enzyme hyaluronidase, which degrades hyaluronic acid and enables the **microbe** to move with greater ease through the tissue.

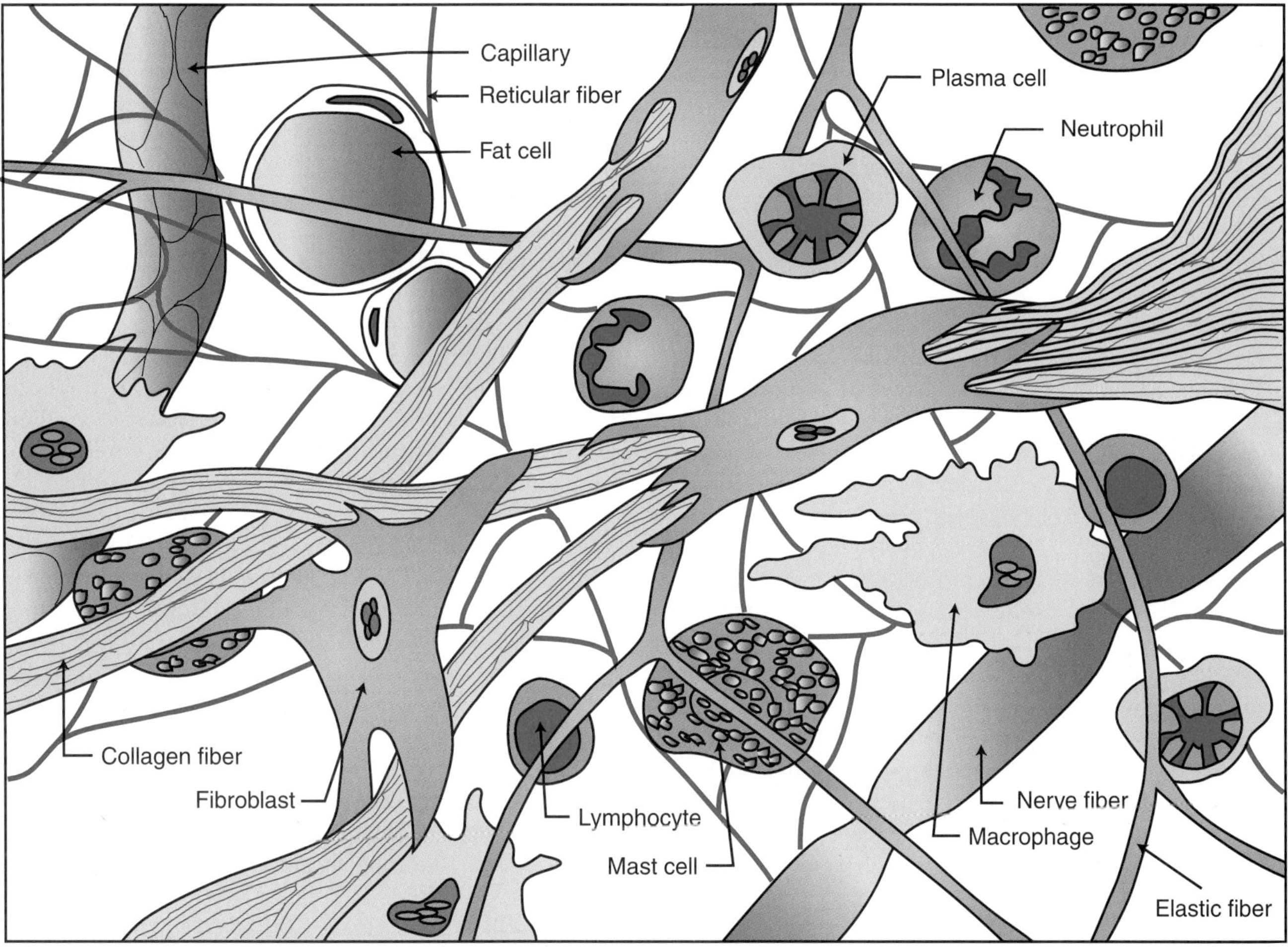

FIGURE **4-9** **Loose or Areolar Connective Tissue.** Loose or areolar tissue is a model-type of connective tissue because it contains all three types of fibers (elastic, collagen, and reticular) and a wide variety of cells (lymphocytes, mast cells, neutrophils, fibroblasts, adipocytes, and plasma cells) suspended in ground substance. These three components—fibers, cells, and ground substance—are found in varying amounts in all connective tissue.

Fibers of Connective Tissue

Connective tissue contains three types of fibers: collagenous, reticular, and elastic. Although these fibers exist in all connective tissue, their proportions vary from one type of connective tissue to another. Collagenous fibers are by far the most commonly found in the body.

Collagenous fibers are strong, thick strands composed of the structural protein collagen. Collagen fibers are organized into discrete bundles of long, parallel fibrils, which in turn are composed of bundled microfibrils. Because it possesses tremendous tensile strength, enabling it to resist pulling forces, collagenous fibers are found in tendons and ligaments that are continually being pulled and stretched. When not under pressure, collagenous fibers look wavy. The fiber itself is white, and the tissue it forms when the fibers are packed closely together is also white. Therefore it is not surprising, that collagenous fibers are sometimes known as the *white fibers.* The density and arrangement of collagen fibers can vary depending on the function of the tissue as a whole. Thus collagenous connective

Box 4-1 Major Components of Connective Tissue

MATRIX (EXTRACELLULAR COMPONENTS)
Ground substances (ranges from liquid to gel to solid)
Fibers
- Collagenous
- Reticular
- Elastic

CELLS
Fixed cells
- Fibroblasts
- Adipocytes (fat cells)
- Reticular cells

Wandering cells
- Mast cells
- Leukocytes (white blood cells)
- Macrophages (can be fixed, as well as wandering)

tissue can range from loose, as in the loose connective tissue that surrounds and protects organs, to dense arrangements seen in tendons. The tissue forms when collagen proteins are secreted into the extracellular environment, where they are arranged into formation. If subjected to heat, collagen denatures and turns into a soft gel. This is why meat, which is rich with collagenous fibers, softens when cooked for long periods in soups and stews. At the same time, collagen can be fortified with tannic acid, as is evident in leather that has been strengthened by tanning.

Reticular fibers, like collagenous fibers, are composed of collagen, but they are not thick. Instead, they are thin, delicate, and branched into complicated networks. Reticular fibers form a kind of "mist net" (*rete* is Latin for "net") that provides support for highly cellular organs, such as endocrine glands, lymph nodes, spleen, bone marrow, and liver. Reticular fibers are also found around blood vessels, nerves, muscle fibers, and capillaries.

Elastic fibers are composed primarily of the protein elastin. Like reticular fibers, elastic fibers are branched and form complex networks, but they lack the tensile strength of collagenous fibers. Elastic fibers are composed of bundles of microfibrils, and because they are coiled, they can stretch and contract like a rubber band. Therefore elastic fibers tend to occur in tissues that are commonly subjected to stretching, such as the vocal cords, lungs, skin, and walls of blood vessels. Because of their color, elastic fibers are sometimes referred to as the *yellow fibers.*

Major Cell Types

Although connective tissue contains a wide variety of cell types, they can be organized into two major categories: those that remain in the connective tissue, called "fixed cells," and those that pass in and out of the connective tissue, called **transient cells.** Fixed cells remain in the connective tissue and are usually involved in the production and maintenance of the matrix. Transient cells, on the other hand, do not have a permanent residence in the tissue but move in and out of it as needed. Transient cells generally are involved in the repair and protection of the tissue.

Fixed Cells. The most noteworthy **fixed cell** is the **fibroblast.** These are large, irregularly shaped cells that manufacture and secrete both the fibers and the ground substance characteristic of their particular matrix. Fibroblasts can reproduce and are metabolically very active. Each type of connective tissue is characterized by a predominant fibroblast. For example, cartilage contains **chondroblasts,** bone contains **osteoblasts,** and connective tissue contains fibroblasts. As the cells mature and the matrix is formed, the cells adopt a less active role. When this occurs, the name of the cell adopts the suffix *-cyte,* such as **chondrocyte, osteocyte,** or **fibrocyte,** depending on the tissue in which they are found. If additional matrix is required later, the cells can convert back to the *-blast* form.

Fat cells are found throughout connective tissue and are known as **adipose cells,** or **adipocytes.** As young cells, adipocytes resemble fibroblasts, but as they mature, they fill with lipid and become swollen, pushing their nuclei to one side. When adipocytes cluster into groups, they become a tissue in their own right, known as *adipose tissue.* Adipose tissue is found throughout the body but is particularly evident under the skin (particularly on the ventrum between the hind legs in cats), behind the eyes, around the kidneys and in the omentum of the abdominal cavity.

Reticular cells are flat, star-shaped cells with long, outreaching arms that touch other cells, forming netlike connections throughout the tissue they compose. The function of reticular cells is debated, but most agree that they are involved in the immune response and in the manufacture of reticular fibers. It is not surprising therefore that reticular cells are found primarily in tissues that are part of the immune system, such as lymph nodes, spleen, and bone marrow.

Wandering Cells. **Leukocytes** are commonly known as *white blood cells.* They are found in blood and move into connective tissue in large numbers during times of infection. Although they are relatively large and round, compared with red blood cells, they can squeeze through the walls of tiny blood vessels to enter the surrounding tissue. This process is called **diapedesis.** Leukocytes are important members of the defensive immune system. There are five different types of leukocytes, but most protect the body by engulfing and digesting (phagocytizing) invading microbes. Other kinds, however, defend against infection by manufacturing **antibodies** that attach to microbes and destroy them.

Mast cells are oval cells that are easily identified by the large number of dark-staining granules stored in the cytoplasm. These granules contain **histamine** and **heparin,** potent biochemicals that when released into the tissue initiate an inflammatory response. Histamine increases blood flow to the area by making the capillaries leaky, and heparin prevents blood from clotting and ensures that the pathways for increased blood flow remain open. Mast cells tend to be found near blood vessels, where they can release their contents directly into the bloodstream and where they can most effectively guard against foreign proteins or microbes. When stimulated by the presence of these invaders, mast cells burst open, releasing hundreds of stored granules. This begins the complex events of allergic and inflammatory reactions, a process that is discussed in greater detail later in this chapter.

Macrophages are massive, irregularly shaped phagocytizing scavengers that may be either fixed or transient in connective tissue. They engulf microbes, dead cells, and debris that are subsequently digested in the macrophage's lysosomes. Mobile macrophages are drawn to sites of infection or inflammation, where they move aggressively through the affected area to engulf microinvaders. In this way, they are an important part of the immune system and help tissues fight infection. Macrophages are given different names depending on the tissue. For example, they are called **Kupffer cells** in the liver, **microglial cells** in the brain, and **histiocytes** in loose connective tissue.

TEST YOURSELF

1. How is connective tissue and epithelial tissue similar? How are they different?
2. What are the three basic constituents of connective tissue?
3. List seven functions of connective tissue.
4. What are GAGs and what role do they play in connective tissue? Why do you suppose animals with joint injuries are sometimes given dietary supplements of GAGs?
5. Compare and contrast collagenous, reticular, and elastic fibers.
6. What are fibroblasts and what role do they play in connective tissue?
7. Can you give three examples of cells that are transient in connective tissue? Can you describe their form and function?

TYPES OF CONNECTIVE TISSUE

As already mentioned, all connective tissue is made up of three major components; ground substance, cells, and fibers. Many different types of connective tissue are formed by the variety of textures of ground substance, the number and type of cells, and the number and type of fibers present in the tissue. By varying the three major constituents, a wide range of connective tissue types are generated (Figure 4-10).

In general, connective tissue is divided into two broad categories: **connective tissue proper** and **specialized connective tissue**.

Connective Tissue Proper

Connective tissue proper is the largest classification and contains every subtype of connective tissue except bone, cartilage, and blood. The two subclasses of connective tissue proper are **loose connective tissue** and **dense connective tissue.** Loose connective tissue includes areolar, adipose, and reticular, and dense connective tissue includes dense regular, dense irregular, and elastic.

Loose Connective Tissue

Areolar Tissue. **Areolar connective tissue** is a beautiful tangle of randomly placed fibers and cells suspended in a thick, translucent ground substance. The tissue appears relaxed with a myriad of round and star-shaped cells placed among crisscrossing fibers. The predominant cell is the fibroblast, a large spindle-shaped cell that manufactures the elastic, reticular, and collagenous fibers found throughout the tissue. Areolar tissue acquires its name from the Latin *areola*, which means "small open space."

Areolar tissue is the most common type of connective tissue and is found everywhere in the body. It acts generally as packing material to support and cushion organs and other delicate structures of the body. It surrounds every organ; forms the subcutaneous layer that connects skin to muscle; envelopes blood vessels, nerves, and lymph nodes; and is present in all mucous membranes as the **lamina propria.** It is supportive to body structures but is flexible and soft to enable organs the freedom to move within their position. Thus areolar tissue is

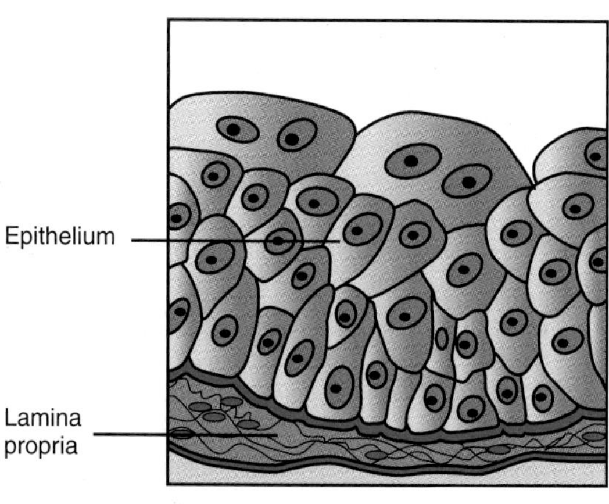

A

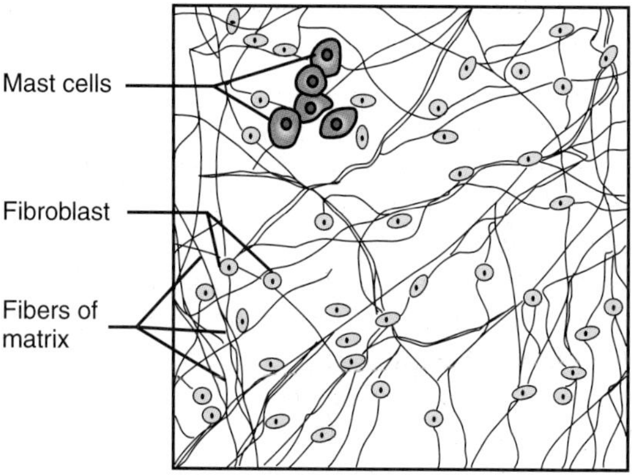

FIGURE **4-10** **Types of Connective Tissue.**
A, Loose or Areolar Connective Tissue.
Description: Loose array of fibers suspended in gel-like ground substance. Includes all three types of fibers and many cells, such as macrophages, fibroblasts, mast cells, and some white blood cells.
Location: Throughout the body under epithelial basement membranes; between glands, muscles, and nerves; surrounding capillaries and many organs. It is also found under skin and helps to attach it to underlying tissues.
Function: Provides nutrients to tissues that it surrounds and supports. Important as a loose packing material.
Microanatomy: Areolar tissue is soft padding for many organs.

Continued

moderately elastic but tears easily compared with the other types of connective tissue.

The "small open spaces" in areolar tissue are filled with a mixture of body fluids and ground substance. The ground substance is thick and is composed primarily of **hyaluronic acid,** which serves as a medium through which nutrients, gases, and waste can be easily transported to and from the bloodstream. In addition, the viscous texture of the ground substance is an effective barrier against most invading microorganisms because it inhibits their movement through the tissue. Some white blood cells have developed the ability to produce **hyaluronidase,** an enzyme that liquefies the matrix and allows them to pass through the matrix with greater ease. This adaptation has improved the ability of white blood cells to perform their duties in loose connective tissue. Unfortu-

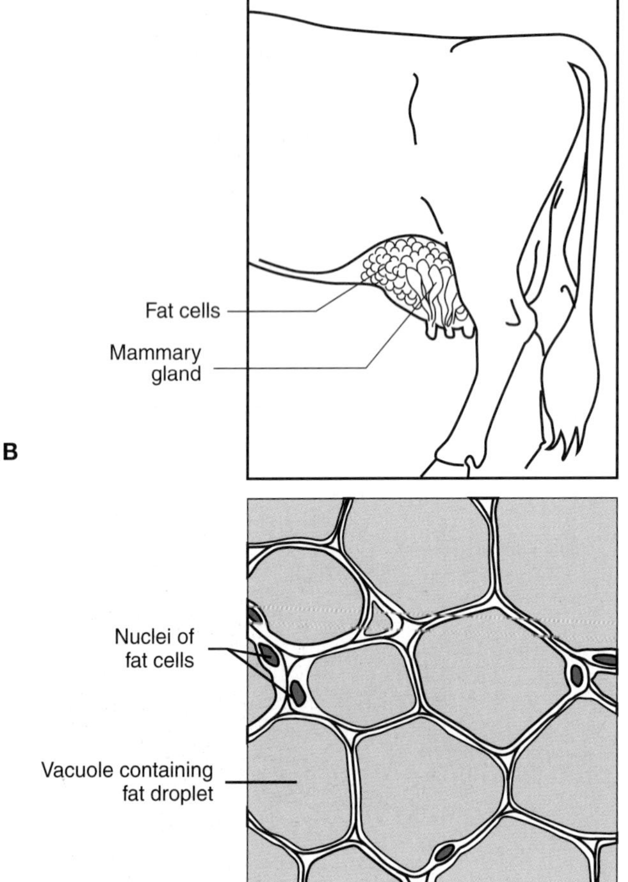

FIGURE **4-10, cont'd**
B, Adipose Tissue.
Description: Adipose tissue is fat. The tissue has little extracellular material and is composed primarily of closely packed adipocytes filled with lipid. The nucleus is pushed to periphery of the cell to accommodate sizable lipid stores.
Location: Throughout the body, under skin, around heart and kidneys, within mesenteries and omentum and around colon.
Function: Thermoinsulator; protects organs and other tissues it surrounds.
Microanatomy: Adipose tissue is composed of fat cells.

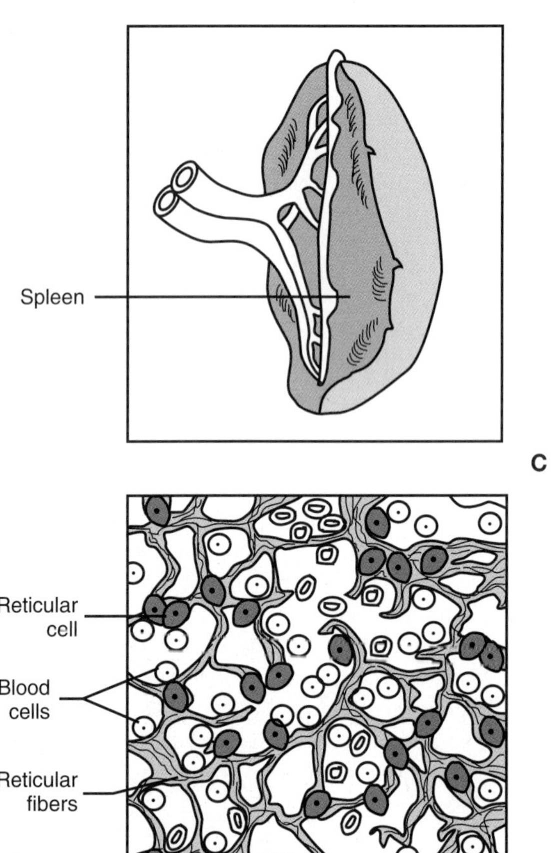

FIGURE **4-10, cont'd**
C, Reticular Connective Tissue.
Description: Reticular cells supported by fine network of irregularly arranged reticular fibers.
Location: Spleen, lymph nodes, and bone marrow.
Function: Provides internal skeleton for hematopoietic and lymphatic tissue.
Microanatomy: Reticular fibers stain darkly. They surround and support cells of the spleen. *Continued*

nately, some microbes have also developed the ability to produce hyaluronidase, which facilitates the spread of infection throughout the tissue.

During trauma or other pathological states, the spaces in loose connective tissue can fill with an excessive amount of body fluid. This condition is called **edema**, and the connective tissue is said to be *edematous*. You can see this condition in cats that have a swollen paw caused by an insect bite or in dogs that have fractured a bone in their leg. Sometimes, the edema will remain compressed in an area after pressing on it with your thumb. This is called **pitting edema** because the tissue, rather than springing back after being compressed, leaves impressions or "pits" in the tissue.

Adipose Tissue. **Adipose tissue** is commonly known as *fat*. It is areolar tissue in which adipocytes or fat cells predominate. Adipose tissue is found beneath the skin, in spaces between muscles, behind the eyeballs, on the surface of the heart, surrounding the joints, in bone marrow, and among the omentum of the abdomen. Its cells expand and wither depending on the amount of lipid that is being stored within them. Not surprisingly, the rate of lipid storage and use is based on the amount of calories being consumed by the animal relative to the amount of energy exerted. In addition, the sympathetic nervous system, certain hormones, and genetic influences may also profoundly affect fat metabolism. Adipose tissue is highly vascularized so that the lipid droplets contained within adipocytes are accessible to the enzymes responsible for triglyceride breakdown and to a bloodstream that readily transports the glycerol and free fatty acid products to other parts of the body. Thus adipose tissue represents an important energy store for animals. It also acts as a thermal insulator under the skin, prevents heat loss from the body, and acts as a mechanical shock absorber around organs, such as the kidneys.

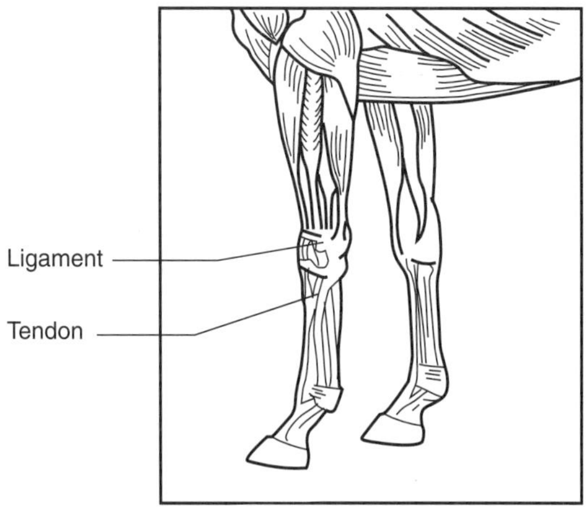

D

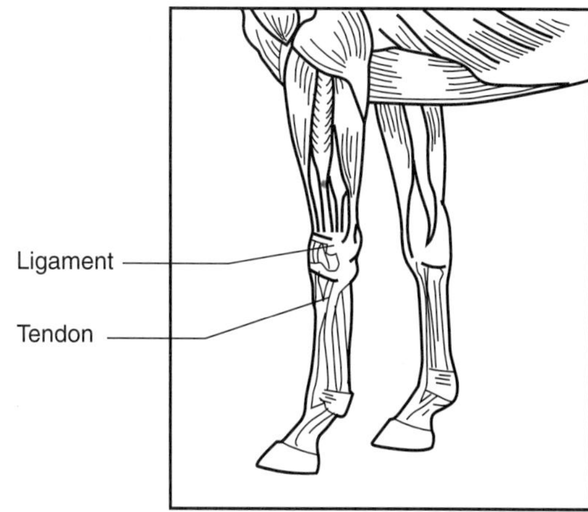

E

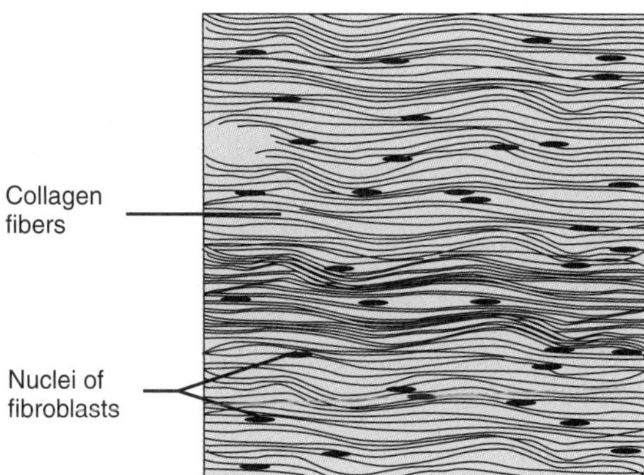

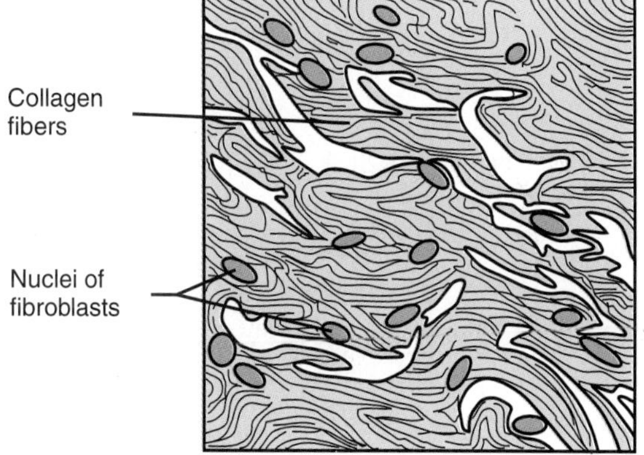

FIGURE **4-10, cont'd**
D, Dense Regular Connective Tissue.
Description: Primarily parallel collagen fibers. Occasional fibroblast interspersed among the fibers.
Location: Tendons and ligaments. Tendons attach muscle to bone, and ligaments attach bones to one another.
Function: Resists strong pulling forces. Has great capacity for stretch resistance in the direction of the muscle fibers.

FIGURE **4-10, cont'd**
E, Dense Irregular Connective Tissue.
Description: Sheets of collagen that run in different directions or sheets of parallel fibers stacked in alternating directions.
Location: Dermis of skin, organ capsules, submucosa of digestive tract.
Function: Designed to withstand pulling forces in all directions.

Continued

The two main types of adipose tissue are **white adipose tissue** and **brown adipose tissue.** White adipose is found throughout the body, particularly in the deep layers of the skin. Initially, white adipocytes resemble fibroblasts, but as they fill with lipid, the organelles and nuclei are pushed to one side and the cells become large spheres with eccentrically placed nuclei. As the cells swell, the cytosol is compressed into a thin, barely visible rim that surrounds the lipid droplet. Despite the compact condition of the cytoplasm, it continues to house all of the organelles normally found in cells. During tissue preparation for microscopic examination, the lipid content of the adipocyte is extracted, leaving a large unstained space in the center of the cell. This, combined with the densely cellular nature of adipose tissue, lends itself to the "chicken wire" appearance that is evident microscopically.

Brown adipose tissue is found in newborn animals and in animals that **hibernate** during the winter. It is a highly specialized form of adipose and plays an important part in temperature regulation because it is a site of heat production. In brown fat, as in white adipose, the nucleus is eccentrically placed; however, the cytoplasm in brown fat is clearly visible, and lipid is stored in multiple small vesicles rather than in a single large droplet. The energy derived from the oxidation of lipids and that released from electron transport are dissipated as *heat* in brown fat, not adenosine triphosphate (ATP). For this reason, brown fat contains an exceptionally high number of mitochondria (the site of electron transport), which become darkly stained in the cytoplasm. This dark coloration gives brown fat its name. In addition, brown fat is also more vascular than white fat. Its rich vascular network helps to dissipate the heat to many areas of the body. In this way, neonatal animals and hibernating animals can generate enough body heat during the vulnerable periods (after birth and during the winter) to survive. Histologically, brown fat looks glandular and therefore sometimes is called the **hibernating gland.**

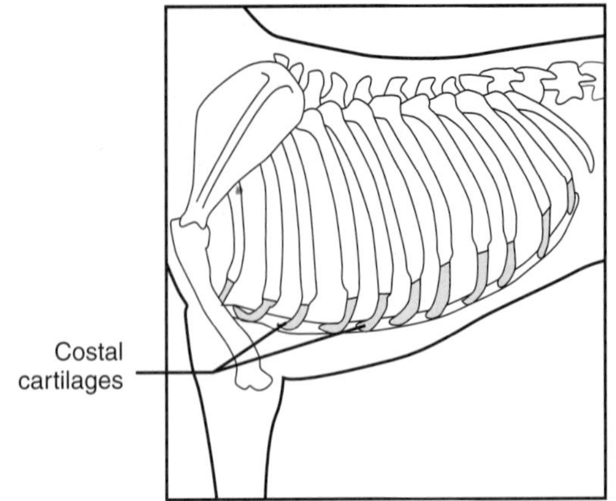

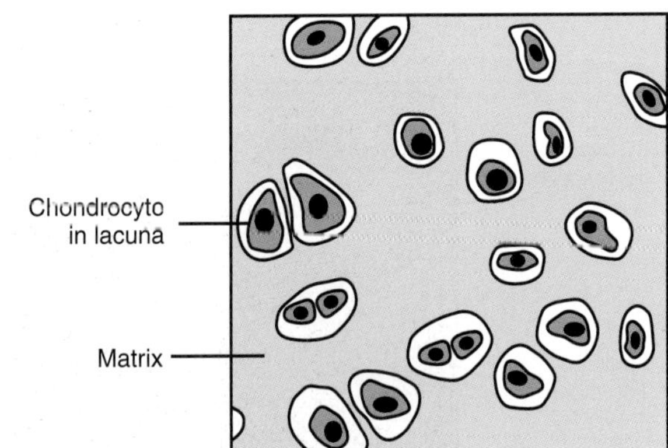

FIGURE **4-10, cont'd**
F, Hyaline Cartilage.
Description: Collagen fibers are evenly distributed throughout a rigid matrix. Cartilage cells or chondrocytes sit in spaces within the matrix called *lacunae.*
Location: Articulating surfaces of bones; costal cartilages of ribs; cartilages in nose, trachea and larynx; most of embryonic skeleton.
Function: Provides both structural rigidity and flexibility at once. Cushions joints during compressive forces.
Microanatomy: Hyaline cartilage from the chondral region of the sternum in a horse.

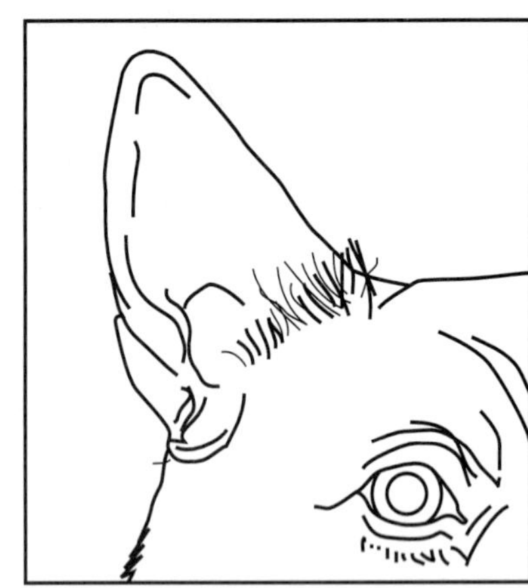

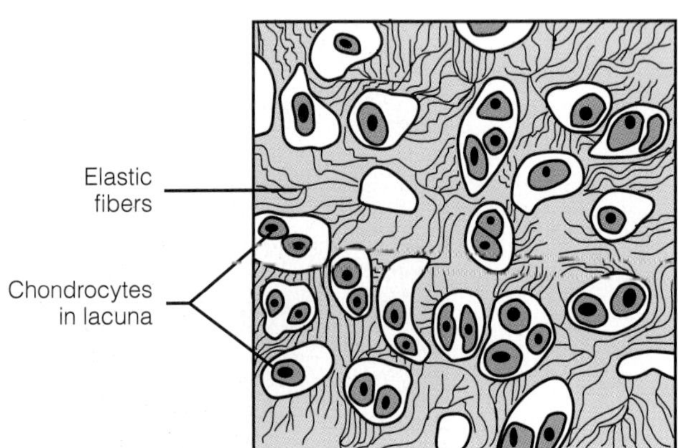

FIGURE **4-10, cont'd**
G, Elastic Cartilage.
Description: Elastic fibers suspended in firm matrix. Chondrocytes arranged in lacunae.
Location: External ear (pinna), auditory tubes, and epiglottis.
Function: Provides support and even more flexibility than hyaline cartilage.
Microanatomy: Elastic cartilage of the canine ear.

Continued

Reticular Connective Tissue. Reticular connective tissue is composed of a complex, three-dimensional network of thin reticular fibers. It resembles areolar connective tissue in that it contains loosely arranged fibers and many fibroblasts suspended in a supportive ground substance. Unlike areolar connective tissue, however, reticular connective tissue contains only one type of fiber: reticular fibers. Together, the cellular and matrix components form a network called **stroma,** which constitutes the framework of several organs, such as the liver, spleen, lymph node, and bone marrow. Although reticular fibers are found throughout the body, reticular connective tissue is found in a limited number of sites.

Dense Fibrous Connective Tissue. Dense fibrous connective tissue is characterized by its densely packed arrangement of collagen fibers. Because little room is available for ground substance and cells, they are found in smaller quantities than in loose connective tissue. Nevertheless, as in loose connective tissue, fibroblasts can be found intermingled with fibers, where they play out their important role of manufacturing fibers and ground substance. The three major types of dense fibrous connective tissue are *dense regular, dense irregular,* and *elastic.*

Dense Regular Connective Tissue. Dense regular connective tissue is composed of tightly packed, parallel collagen fibers. The fibers lie in the direction of the force that is exerted on them, thereby giving the overall tissue tremendous tensile strength but only in one direction. Dense regular connective tissue is silvery or white. It is relatively avascular and therefore is very slow to heal because restorative nutrients and building molecules have difficulty reaching the damaged tissue. Fibroblasts form rows along the crowded fibers and devote most of their energy toward the manufacture of fibers. Little ground substance is produced. Dense connective tissue makes up the tendons that attach muscles to bone and the ligaments that hold bones together at joints. It also composes the broad, fibrous ribbons that sometimes cover muscles or connect one muscle to another structure. In addition, dense connective

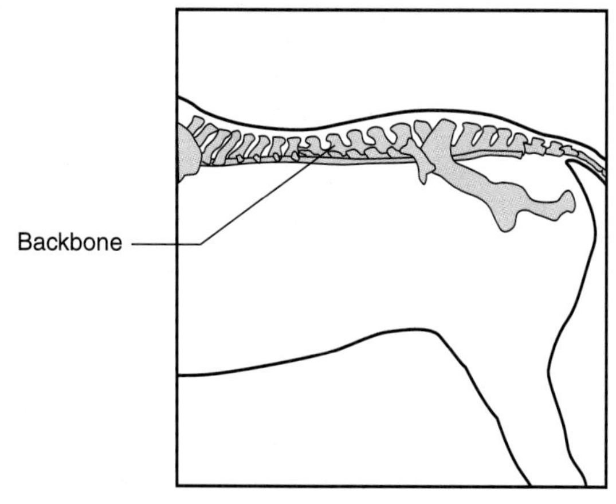

H

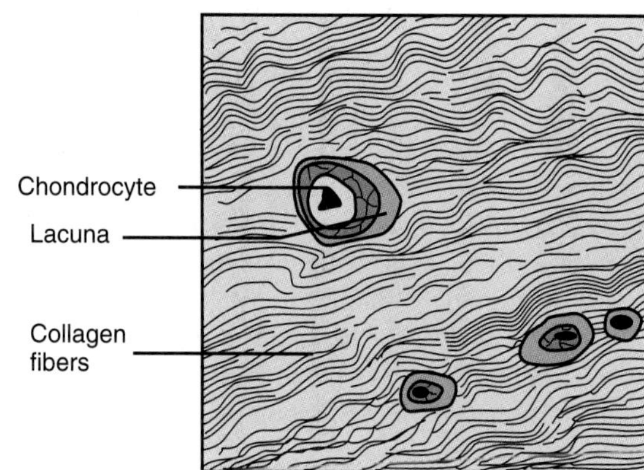

FIGURE **4-10, cont'd**
H, Fibrocartilage.
Description: Similar to hyaline cartilage, but collagen fibers are more numerous and are arranged in thicker bundles. Matrix is less firm.
Location: Pubic symphysis, intervertebral disks, disks in stifle and knee joints. Also found in temporomandibular joint of jaw.
Function: Withstands compressive forces.
Microanatomy: Fibrocartilage from the spine of a horse.

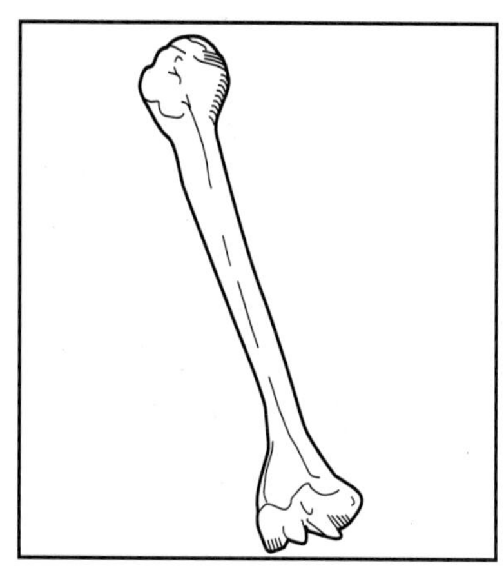

I

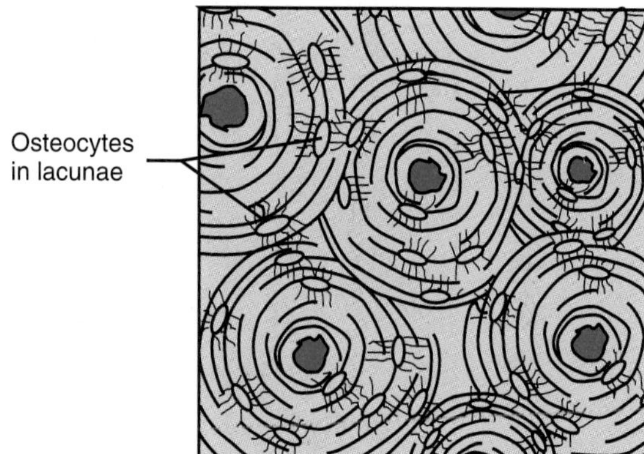

FIGURE **4-10, cont'd**
I, Compact Bone.
Description: Hard matrix dominates this tissue and is organized into concentric rings that surround central canal. Chambers (called *lacunae*) and tunnels (called *canaliculi*) form spaces in hard matrix to accommodate bone cells (osteocytes) and their long cytoplasmic projections.
Location: Bones of skeleton.
Function: Provides support and protection; blood is produced in bone marrow; provides storage depot for calcium and other types of minerals.

Continued

tissue can be found in fascial sheets that cover muscles. These sheets are stacked into layers, one on top of another, but the direction of the fibers in one fascial layer may be different from the direction of the fibers in another layer. This helps to create an overall structure **(fascia)** that can withstand forces from more than one direction.

Dense Irregular Connective Tissue. Dense irregular connective tissue is composed primarily of collagen fibers that are arranged in thicker bundles than those found in dense regular connective tissue. The fibers are interwoven randomly to form a single sheet that can withstand forces from many different directions. It is found in the **dermis** of the skin and in the fibrous coverings of organs such as the kidney, testes, liver, and spleen. It also forms the tough capsule of joints.

Elastic Connective Tissue. Ligaments can stretch more than tendons because of the larger number of elastic fibers contained within them. The massive nuchal ligament in the neck of horses, for example, has a particularly high concentration of elastic fibers and is therefore extremely flexible, enabling horses to lower their heads for long periods while grazing. Dense connective tissue that is primarily composed of elastic fibers, rather than collagen fibers, is called **elastic connective tissue.**

Elastic connective tissue is found in relatively few regions of the body, such as in the spaces between vertebrae in the backbone. It also occurs in regions of the body that require stretching, such as in the walls of arteries, stomach, large airways (bronchi), bladder, and regions of the heart. It lies beneath the transitional epithelium in the urinary tract and in the ligament suspending the penis. As its name implies, elastic connective tissue consists primarily of yellow elastic fibers. These fibers may be arranged in parallel or in an interwoven pattern with fibroblasts and collagenous fibers interspersed.

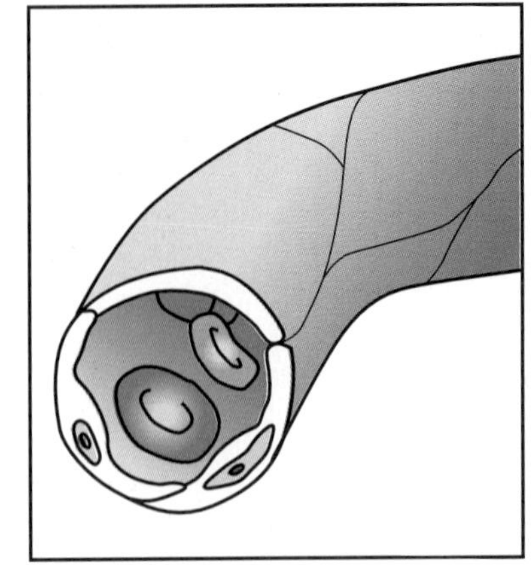

J

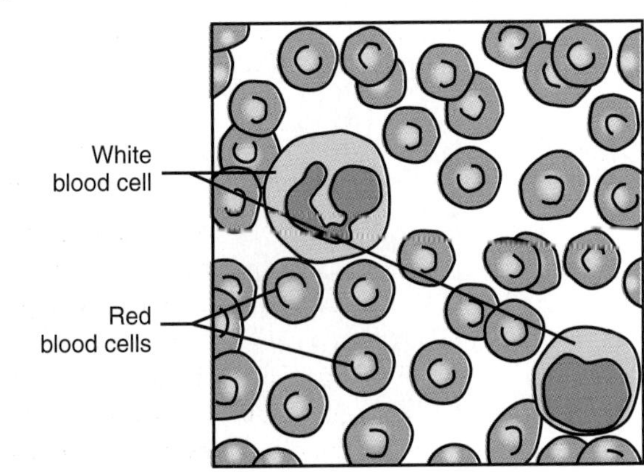

FIGURE **4-10, cont'd**
J, Blood.
Description: Cells in fluid matrix.
Location: Found in blood vessels and heart.
Function: Carries oxygen and nutrients to tissues; transports waste products and gases for disposal.

Specialized Connective Tissues

Cartilage. **Cartilage** is a tough, specialized connective tissue that is commonly called **gristle.** It is more rigid than dense connective tissue but is more flexible than bone. Cartilage is found in joints and helps to prevent the sensitive outer layers of bone from rubbing against one another. Because cartilage does not contain nerves, it can tolerate a great deal of compression without causing pain to the animal. Thus animals normally can walk and run pain free. Imagine the compressive forces in the legs of an elephant! In addition to joints, cartilage is found in the ear, nose, and vocal cords and forms a vital framework on which bone is formed in growing animals.

Like other forms of connective tissue, cartilage is composed of cells and matrix. The cells, called *chondrocytes,* live in hollowed-out pockets in the matrix, called **lacunae.** The ground substance of the matrix is a firm gel containing two different types of glycosaminoglycans—**chondroitin sulfate** and hyaluronic acid—and an adhesion protein called **chondronectin.** It also contains an unexpectedly large amount of tissue fluid. The fluid is held within the matrix and is important in transporting nutrients to the chondrocytes. It also gives cartilage its flexible resiliency and its ability to withstand compression. Collagen fibers are most commonly found in the matrix, but elastic fibers are also present in varying amounts.

Cartilage is avascular and therefore is very slow to heal. It receives its nutrition from a surrounding membrane, called the **perichondrium,** which is rich with tiny blood vessels. Nutrients diffuse from the perichondrium through the matrix to the chondrocytes. Therefore the chondrocytes that are farthest away from the perichondrium are potentially less well nourished than cells that are close to it. For this reason, the thickness of cartilage is limited.

Three types of cartilage that vary from one another based on the type of fiber found in the matrix are hyaline cartilage, elastic cartilage, and fibrocartilage.

Hyaline Cartilage. **Hyaline cartilage** is the most common type of cartilage found in the body. It is composed of closely packed collagen fibers that make it tough but more flexible than bone. Grossly, hyaline cartilage resembles a blue-white, frosted, ground glass. It is found as **articular cartilage** at the ends of long bones in joints and connects the ribs to the sternum. In addition, it forms supportive rings in the trachea and composes most of the embryonic skeleton. In growing animals, it is found in the growth plates of long bones, where it supports continued bone development and the extension of the length of the bone. Hyaline cartilage is the most rigid type of cartilage and is enclosed within a perichondrium.

Elastic Cartilage. Histologically, **elastic cartilage** is similar to hyaline cartilage but contains a plethora of elastic fibers, which form dense branching bundles that appear black microscopically. These fibers give elastic cartilage tremendous flexibility so that it can withstand repeated bending. Elastic cartilage is found in the epiglottis of the larynx and in pinnae (the external ears) of animals.

Fibrocartilage. **Fibrocartilage** usually is found merged with hyaline cartilage and dense connective tissue. It contains thick bundles of collagen fibers like hyaline cartilage, but it has fewer chondrocytes and lacks a perichondrium. Fibrocartilage is particularly well designed to take compression and therefore is found in the spaces between vertebrae of the spine, between bones in the pelvic girdle, and in the knee joint.

Bone. Bone, or osseous connective tissue, is the hardest and most rigid type of connective tissue. Its specialized matrix is a combination of organic collagen fibers and inorganic calcium salts, such as calcium phosphate and calcium carbonate. The calcium salts alone would render bone brittle, but when combined with collagen fibers, bone becomes more flexible and has greater strength. Despite the rigidity of its matrix, bone, unlike cartilage, is well vascularized. A central **haversian canal** contains both a vascular and a nerve supply. In addition, tiny channels exist within the matrix that support the passage

Box 4-2 Organization of Connective Tissue

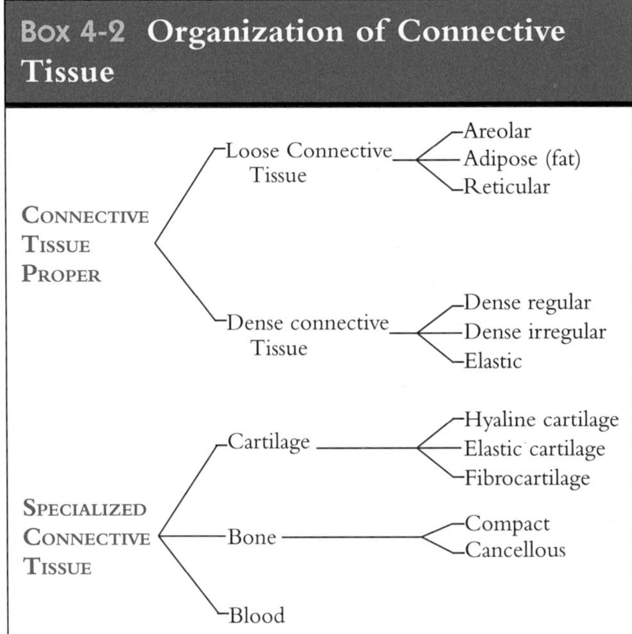

of blood vessels into deeper portions of the tissue. Bone cells, such as osteoblasts and **osteoclasts,** collaborate to remodel bone in response to the stresses that are placed on the tissue. This involves a well-orchestrated combination of laying down new bone and taking away bone that is not needed. Osteoblasts, like other fibroblasts, manufacture the fibers that are part of the matrix. Although mature osteocytes reside individually in chambers called *lacunae,* they possess long cellular extensions that pass through tiny threadlike channels called **canaliculi.** These chambers and canals are created as the osteoblasts surround themselves with the bony matrix they manufacture. Later they mature to become osteocytes. In this way, the cells not only create their own living spaces but also maintain connections with other cells.

Bone forms the skeletal frame of animals. It protects vital organs, such as the brain and heart, and acts as a calcium reserve for the body. In addition, bone marrow is the site of blood cell production and fat storage. A discussion of the development, structure, and function of bone is found in Chapter 5.

Blood. The red fluid that passes through vessels and that carries nutrient molecules and gases throughout the body is the most atypical type of connective tissue. The liquid component of blood is called **plasma** and constitutes the matrix. The fibrous component of the matrix is an array of protein molecules that are suspended in solution and are visible only when blood clots. Blood is rich with a variety of cell types, such as **erythrocytes** (red blood cells), leukocytes (white blood cells), and **thrombocytes (platelets)**. Blood is discussed in greater detail in Chapter 9. Box 4-2 summarizes the organization of connective tissue.

TEST YOURSELF

1. Connective tissue is divided into two broad categories. What are they?
2. What are the components of areolar tissue?
3. What is the common term for adipose tissue?
4. Both in terms of its form and function, how is brown fat different from white fat?
5. What are three subtypes of dense connective tissue?
6. Give three examples of specialized connective tissue. How are they similar to connective tissue proper? How are they different?
7. Why is cartilage limited in thickness and slow to heal?
8. Describe three types of cartilage. What are their differences and similarities?
9. Even though blood and bone appear to be very different grossly, they both represent types of connective tissue. Why?

MEMBRANES

Epithelial and connective tissue may be collaboratively linked to form membranes in the body. Membranes are thin, protective layers that line body cavities, separate organs, and cover surfaces. They are composed of a multicellular epithelial sheet that is bound to an underlying layer of connective tissue proper. Commonly, the epithelium is bathed in a wet solution of mucus or transudate or, in the case of the bladder, in urine. Four common types of epithelial membranes are mucous, serous, cutaneous, and synovial (Figure 4-11, *A*).

MUCOUS MEMBRANES

Mucous membranes, or **mucosae,** are characterized by their position in the body because they are always found lining the organs with connections to the outside environment. These organs are part of the digestive, respiratory, urinary, and reproductive tracts and include the mouth, esophagus, stomach, intestines, colon, nasal passages, trachea, bladder, and uterus, to name a few. The epithelial layer in mucous membranes is usually composed of either stratified squamous or **simple columnar epithelium,** and it covers a layer of loose connective tissue called the *lamina propria*. Another connective tissue layer, called the *submucosa,* usually connects the mucosa to underlying structures.

With the exception of the mucosae of the urinary tract, mucosae in general can produce large quantities of protective and lubricating mucus. Goblet cells or multicellular glands may be found throughout the tissue. These structures are responsible for the production and secretion of mucus that consists primarily of water, electrolytes, and a protein called *mucin*. The mucus is slippery and therefore can decrease friction and assist with the passage of foodstuffs or waste. Because of its rich supply of antibodies, as well as its viscous consistency, the mucus produced by mucosae is also helpful in the entrapment and disposal of invading pathogens and foreign particles. This is particularly apparent in the nasal passages, where microorgan-

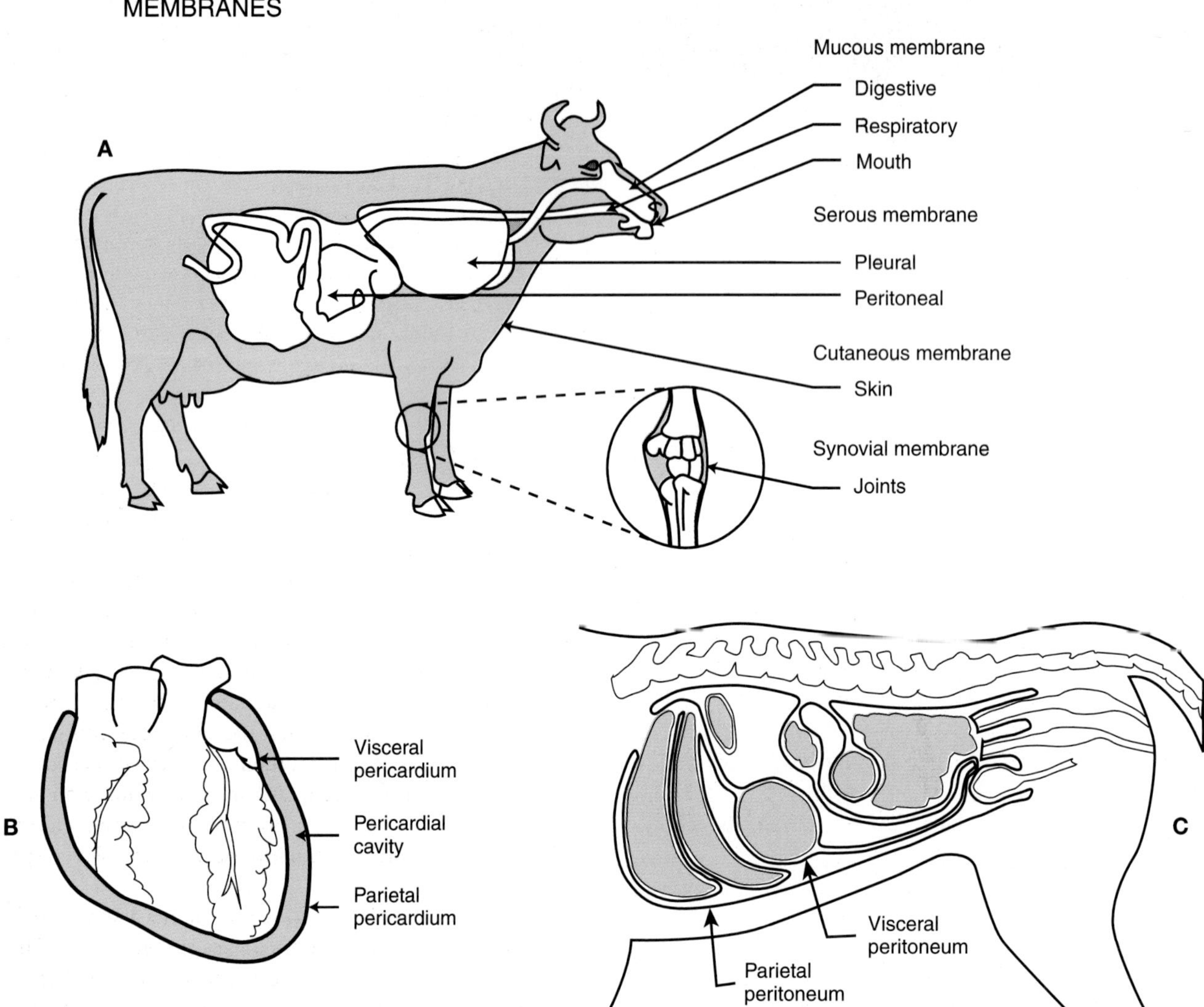

FIGURE **4-11** **Types of Membranes. A,** Mucous, serous, cutaneous, and synovial membranes are found throughout the body. *Mucous* membranes line body cavities, such as the anus, mouth, and nares, that are exposed to the outside. Membranes often contain glands, which secrete mucus. *Serous* membranes line body cavities that have no connection with the outside. Although they do not contain glands, they secrete serous fluid, which helps lubricate and prevent adhesions within body cavities. The *cutaneous* membrane is the dermis, or skin, which covers the outer region of the body. *Synovial* membranes line cavities that surround joints. **B,** The heart is covered by serous membrane called the *pericardium.* The pericardium folds back on itself, forming two layers with a space or cavity in between. The layer closest to the heart is called *visceral pericardium,* whereas the outer layer is called the *parietal pericardium.* **C,** The serous membrane in abdominal cavity is called the *peritoneum.* Visceral peritoneum covers organs, and parietal peritoneum lines the peritoneal, or abdominal, cavity.

isms and debris are inhaled and trapped by mucus. We may find, for example, accumulations of black debris in our noses after we have been near a sooty campfire. When we have a "cold," we find that the amount of mucus produced and secreted by the mucosae increases and a "runny nose" develops. Some mucosae also can absorb, as well as secrete. For example, the epithelial layer in the intestine is specially designed for rapid and efficient transfer of nutrient molecules from the intestinal lumen to the underlying connective tissue and its blood supply. The mucosa therefore plays an important role in monitoring and controlling what enters the body. Thus mucous membranes form an important barrier between the outside environment and the delicate inner workings of underlying tissues. Their secretory and absorptive qualities make them particularly well suited for this role.

Serous Membranes

Serous membranes are also called **serosae.** They line the walls and cover the organs that fill closed body cavities, such as the chest cavity or thorax and the abdominal and pelvic (abdominopelvic) cavities (see Figure 4-11). Serosa is characterized as a continuous sheet that is doubled over on itself to form two layers with a narrow space in between them. The portion of the membrane that lines the cavity wall is called the **parietal layer,** and that which covers the outer surface of organs is called the **visceral layer.**

CLINICAL APPLICATION: Mucous Membranes: Keys to a Diagnosis

When animals are sick, they show signs of illness in many ways. We know that they may become depressed and lethargic. They may stop eating and drinking, vomit, have diarrhea or bloody urine, or stop urinating entirely. Another way in which animals show signs of illness is through changes in the appearance of their mucous membranes. The easiest mucous membranes to examine in an animal are those located on the inside of the mouth; they are also known as the "gums." Here a veterinarian or veterinary technician can gain clues about the general status of the animal. For example, dehydrated animals have dry, tacky mucous membranes. However, animals with wet mouths are less likely to be dehydrated.

The *color* of mucous membranes is also very important. A yellow tinge, for example, may indicate an elevation of bilirubin in the blood. This condition is known as **icterus,** and the yellow appearance of an animal is called **jaundice.** There are many causes of increased levels of bilirubin, such as liver failure and **hemolytic anemia.** For this reason, additional tests would be run to determine the cause of the jaundice. Blue mucous membranes occur in animals that cannot provide their tissues with adequate amounts of oxygen. These animals develop a condition called **hypoxia** (*hypo-* meaning "below normal"; *oxia* meaning "oxygen"). Animals with tracheal obstructions, severe pneumonia, or circulatory collapse may all show signs of hypoxia. Bright red mucous membranes may be evident in animals that are hyperperfused: a condition in which blood flow to peripheral tissues is increased. Febrile and hypertensive animals, for example, and animals undergoing an allergic reaction may have **hyperemia,** or bright red mucous membranes. In contrast, pale or white mucous membranes may indicate anemia, shock, or hypothermia.

Finally, the gums of an animal may give the clinician additional clues about the status of the circulatory system by examining the **capillary refill time (CRT)**. If you press firmly on a pink region of a dog's gum, for example, the gum blanches white. When you remove your finger, you will notice that the gum changes from white back to pink relatively quickly. The time that it takes for the blood to return to the capillaries and turn the gum pink again is the CRT. Normal CRT is 1 to 2 seconds. In animals that have compromised cardiac output, low blood pressure, or severe peripheral **vasoconstriction,** the CRT will be prolonged and will be longer that 2 seconds. Animals with high blood pressure and those in hypercompensatory states may have shortened CRTs (less than 1 second).

Thus examination of the mucous membranes in an animal is very important and may lead to a greater understanding of the animal's condition.

The serosa is composed of a sheet of simple squamous epithelium bound to an underlying layer of loose connective tissue. This histological organization allows a great deal of permeability and enables interstitial fluid to pass through the membrane into the narrow spaces between the serosal layers. In this way, serosal fluid is a **transudate** and, unlike the thick mucoid secretion of mucous membranes, is thin and watery. It contains electrolytes but no mucin. By coating the parietal and visceral layers, serosal fluid creates a moist and slippery surface, which reduces friction between adjacent organs and between the organs and the cavity wall. Transudates take on different names depending on where they are located in the body. A transudate in the thorax, for example, is called **pleural fluid;** in the abdomen, **peritoneal fluid;** and in the region around the heart, **pericardial fluid.**

The consistency of serous fluid may vary and change during pathological conditions. For example, if an animal fractures a rib, blood cells, as well as fluid, may leak from ruptured capillaries into the pleural space, creating a **hemothorax.** When cells, protein, and other solid material mix with serous fluid, it becomes denser than a transudate and is called an **exudate.**

Normally the amount of serous fluid found in body cavities is small, but during trauma or some pathological conditions, such as in hemothorax, the amount of fluid may become excessive. When an abnormally large amount of fluid enters a body cavity, the fluid is known as an **effusion. Ascites,** for example, is the presence of an effusion in the peritoneal space of the abdominopelvic cavity and can be caused by a wide range of pathological conditions, such as congestive heart failure, **nephrosis,** malignant neoplastic disease, and **peritonitis.**

Sometimes if the serous membranes are damaged, production of serous fluid is impeded and abnormal connections called *adhesions* may form between the parietal and visceral layers. These connections may alter the normal function of the organs involved and can cause excruciating discomfort to the patient, particularly if the adhesions occur in the pleural space of the thoracic cavity.

In the abdominopelvic cavity, the visceral layers of serosa merge to form supportive ligaments called *mesenteries.* These ligaments secure organs to the body wall and form a framework for the passage of blood vessels and nerves. The stomach, for example, is connected to the abdominal wall by mesentery called the **omentum,** and the uterus is similarly attached via the **broad ligament**.

CUTANEOUS MEMBRANES

The **cutaneous membrane** is also called *integument,* or, more simply, *skin.* It is an organ that is perpetually exposed to the outside environment and therefore possesses unique features that distinguish it from the other membrane types. It is composed of an outer **keratinized stratified squamous epithelium,** or **epidermis.** Keratin is a waxy substance that fills the cells of the epidermal layer as they make their developmental migration from the basement membrane to the outermost layer. It is responsible for the waterproof quality of skin and aids in the prevention of desiccation. Keratinized squamous epithelium is also durable and is partly responsible for the skin's ability to withstand abrasive forces.

The epidermis is attached to an underlying layer of dense irregular connective tissue called the *dermis.* The dermis is rich with collagenous, reticular, and elastic fibers, which enable skin to be both strong and elastic. The structural and functional properties of skin are discussed further in Chapter 6.

Clinical Application: Histopathology: An Introduction

Histopathology is the microscopic study of disease in tissues (*histo-* means "tissue"; *pathology* means "the study of disease"). The normal microanatomy of tissues is altered by pathological disorders in many ways. For example, in mammary tissue that contains a malignant tumor, abnormally large, immature mammary cells may be evident microscopically. The nuclei of these cells are abnormally large, and many of the cells may be actively dividing. Other diseases, such as viral and bacterial infections, may cause cell death and create regions within the tissue that are dead, or **necrotic.** Still other diseases may cause the abnormal accumulation of fluid leading to a condition called *edema,* or may involve the accumulation of a waxlike glycoprotein called **amyloid.** Thus pathological disease or illness may be seen microscopically as the abnormal increase or decrease in cell numbers, cell size, and cell shape and as abnormal changes in the architecture of the tissue's support structures.

Although the pathological nature of diseased tissue is often evident under microscopic examination, grossly the tissue may appear normal. For this reason, a definitive diagnosis often can be made only through the microscopic examination of the tissue. This is done by taking a **biopsy** of the tissue in question. Sometimes aspirating cells from the tissue can lead to a diagnosis also.

A biopsy is the removal of a small piece of tissue from an organ or other part of the body. This may involve the insertion of a special kind of biopsy needle into the tissue, or it may involve cutting out or **excising** a piece of tissue with a scalpel. Some biopsy samples are obtained using special grasping attachments on the exploratory end of endoscopes; others may be acquired using a "cookie cutter" type of instrument called a *biopsy punch.* No matter how the sample is obtained, it must be handled with care and prepared in a special way before it can be examined.

Samples should be sliced so that each piece is no thicker than 1 cm and should be placed in a fixative solution of 10% buffered formalin. The ratio of the volume of formalin to the volume of tissue should be approximately10:1. If the specimen is too large, it cannot absorb enough fixative to preserve it in its thickest regions. For example, if a large section of heart from a Doberman pinscher is stuffed into a small container of formalin, the fixative may not be able to penetrate the tissue adequately. The heart will therefore degenerate, the architecture of the muscle will be lost, and a potential diagnosis of dilated cardiomyopathy will be impossible to confirm. Encapsulated or very fibrous tissues are also difficult to fix. Conversely, samples that are extremely small are sometimes invisible within a sea of formalin and are *seemingly* lost. In these cases, reports of "no sample found" are returned to the clinician.

Biopsy samples are harvested from the normal-abnormal tissue borders if possible. In addition, because the tissues are delicate, they should be cut with sharp instruments, such as scalpels, and maneuvered with **tissue forceps,** not **dressing forceps,** so that the microanatomy is not crushed.

The preserved tissue is transported to a clinical pathology laboratory, where it is removed from its container and prepared for sectioning. Many tissues are prepared by imbedding them in a fine, soft wax called **paraffin.** The paraffin provides support to the tissue and enables it to be sliced into very thin sections using a special cutting device called a **microtome.** These paper-thin sections are floated in liquid and carefully placed onto microscope slides. They are then stained and prepared for examination by a veterinary pathologist. Veterinary pathologists are specially trained to examine and evaluate tissue samples for possible disease.

Synovial Membranes

Synovial membranes line the cavities of joints. Unlike the other membrane types, synovial membranes have no epithelium. They are composed exclusively of connective tissue. Grossly, the synovial membrane is smooth, shiny, and white. Histologically, the membrane is composed of loose connective tissue and adipose tissue covered by a layer of collagen fibers and fibroblasts. Synovial membranes manufacture the synovial fluid that fills the joint spaces and, together with hyaline cartilage, reduces friction and abrasion at the ends of the bones.

Test Yourself

1. Membranes are composed of what two tissue types?
2. Where are mucous membranes found? What functions do they perform?
3. What portion of a serous membrane covers the outer surface of organs?
4. What is an effusion? What is ascites?
5. What is another name for "cutaneous membrane"?
6. Where are synovial membranes found? How are they different from other membrane types?

MUSCLE TISSUE

Muscle cells or muscle fibers are uniquely designed for contraction. The fibers are composed of specialized proteins called *actin* and *myosin,* which are arranged into microfilaments. Contraction, or shortening, of the muscle cell occurs when the microfilaments slide over one another like the bars in an old-fashioned slide ruler. In this way, the cells change shape and can be made shorter or longer. As the muscles contract, they move the bones, blood, and soft tissue structures that are associated with them. Thus blood is circulated, legs are made to run, and foodstuffs are moved slowly through the intestine. Three types of muscle tissue are skeletal, smooth, and cardiac (Figure 4-12).

Skeletal Muscle

Skeletal muscle contains numerous large cells that may be a foot or more in length. Because of their large size and heavy metabolic requirements, the cells contain hundreds of nuclei and mitochondria needed to maintain cellular homeostasis. Skeletal muscle is responsible for an animal's ability to walk, run, kick, bite, and have facial expressions. Unlike cardiac and smooth muscle, skeletal muscle is usually controlled through conscious efforts and therefore is called **voluntary muscle.** In

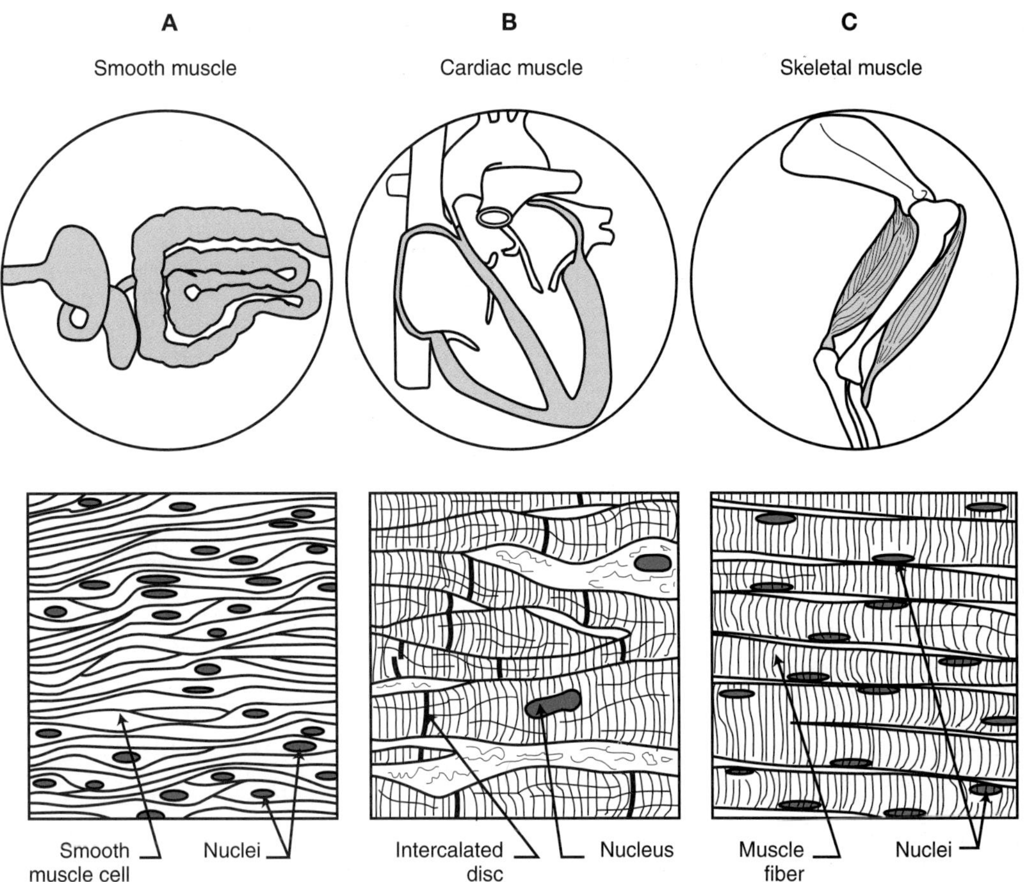

FIGURE **4-12** **Types of Muscle Tissue.**
A, Smooth Muscle.
Description: Nonstriated, involuntary; composed of small, spindle-shaped cells that lack striations or bands and therefore appear "smooth." Each cell has a centrally located nucleus.
Location: In the walls of hollow organs such as the esophagus, stomach, intestine, colon, blood vessels, and bladder; also in skin attached to hair and in the iris of the eye.
Function: It moves food through the digestive tract, regulates the size of an organ, controls light entering the eye, moves fluid through vessels, and causes hair to stand erect.
B, Cardiac Muscle.
Description: Striated, involuntary; cells are cylindrical and branched with a single centrally located nucleus. Cells form an intricate network and are connected by intercalated disks (specialized type of gap junction)
Location. Found only in the heart.
Function: Pumps blood through the vascular system.
C, Skeletal Muscle.
Description: Striated, voluntary; cells are striped, long, and cylindrical, each one with multiple, eccentrically placed nuclei.
Location: Attached to bone and occasionally to skin, eyeballs, and upper part of the esophagus.
Function: Voluntary movement of body, including movement of the eyes and the initial part of swallowing.

other words, the animal can control its movement through conscious thought. In addition, skeletal muscle cells are **striated,** or striped, because histologically they have alternating bands of light and dark across them. Thus skeletal muscle is referred to as *striated, voluntary* muscle.

The cells of skeletal muscle are essentially fibers that are clustered into bundles and held together by loose connective tissue. The collagen fibers that surround the cells merge with the collagen fibers in tendons. In this way, muscle is firmly attached to bone. Muscle cells are stimulated to contract by the action of nerve fibers that are attached to them and located throughout the entire muscle belly. If the nerves are damaged, the ability of the muscle to contract is impaired, and the muscle is said to be **paretic,** or **paralyzed.** In this way, all of the actions that an animal can normally control, such as walking, running, eating, and moving the head and arms, depend on a healthy nervous system, as well as a healthy muscular system.

SMOOTH MUSCLE

Smooth muscle is composed of small, spindle-shaped cells that lack striations or bands and therefore appear "smooth." Like skeletal muscle, smooth muscle may be stimulated to contract by the action of nerves, but unlike skeletal muscles, the contractions cannot be consciously controlled. Smooth muscle is therefore called **nonstriated involuntary muscle.** It is found in the walls of hollow organs, such as blood vessels, urinary bladder, uterus, intestines, and stomach. It is also found in exocrine glands and along the respiratory tract. It is responsible for **peristalsis** in the gastrointestinal tract, for the constriction of blood vessels, and for the emptying of the bladder. Because smooth muscle cells are relatively small, they require only one centrally located nucleus.

Cardiac Muscle

Cardiac muscle exists only in the heart and possesses the remarkable ability to contract even when neural input has been altered. Specialized pacemaker cells within the heart muscle supply the signal for the heart to contract at regular intervals. This input is entirely involuntary and is responsible for initiating the pumping force, which propels blood through blood vessels. Thank goodness we do not need to *concentrate* on keeping our hearts beating!

As in smooth muscle, the cells of cardiac muscle are relatively small and contain only one nucleus. However, unlike smooth or skeletal muscle, cardiac muscle branches to form a complex network. The cardiac muscle cells are striated and are connected to one another at each end via a specialized intercellular junction called an *intercalated disk.* These disks occur only in cardiac muscle. Thus cardiac muscle is classified as an *involuntary, striated* tissue.

NERVOUS TISSUE

Nervous (or neural) tissue is uniquely designed to receive and transmit electrical and chemical signals throughout the body (Figure 4-13). It is found in the brain, spinal cord, and peripheral nerves and is composed primarily of two general cell types: **neurons** and supporting **neuroglial cells**.

Neurons are the longest cells in the body and may reach up to a meter in length. They are composed of three primary parts: a cell body called a **perikaryon,** short cytoplasmic extensions called **dendrites,** and a long, single extension called an **axon.** The cell body contains the nucleus, which controls the metabolism of the cell. The dendrites *receive* impulses from other cells, whereas the axon conducts impulses away from the cell body. The neuron forms connections with many other tissues, such as muscle, **viscera,** glands, and other neurons. In this way, a complex network is formed that controls and regulates many body functions. The neuron is exquisitely sensitive to electrical and chemical changes in its environment and may respond by transmitting nerve impulses along its axon to other tissues. These electrical impulses, which carry information and instructions, are transmitted through conductive membranes on the neurons.

Neuroglial cells are found in greater numbers in neural tissue than are neurons. They do not transmit impulses but rather serve to support the neurons. Some specialized types of neuroglial cells function to isolate the conductive membranes, others provide a supportive framework that helps to bind the components of neural tissue together, and still others **phagocytize** debris or help supply nutrients to neurons by connecting them to blood vessels. The gross anatomy and physiology of nervous tissue are discussed in Chapter 7.

Box 4-3 summarizes tissues.

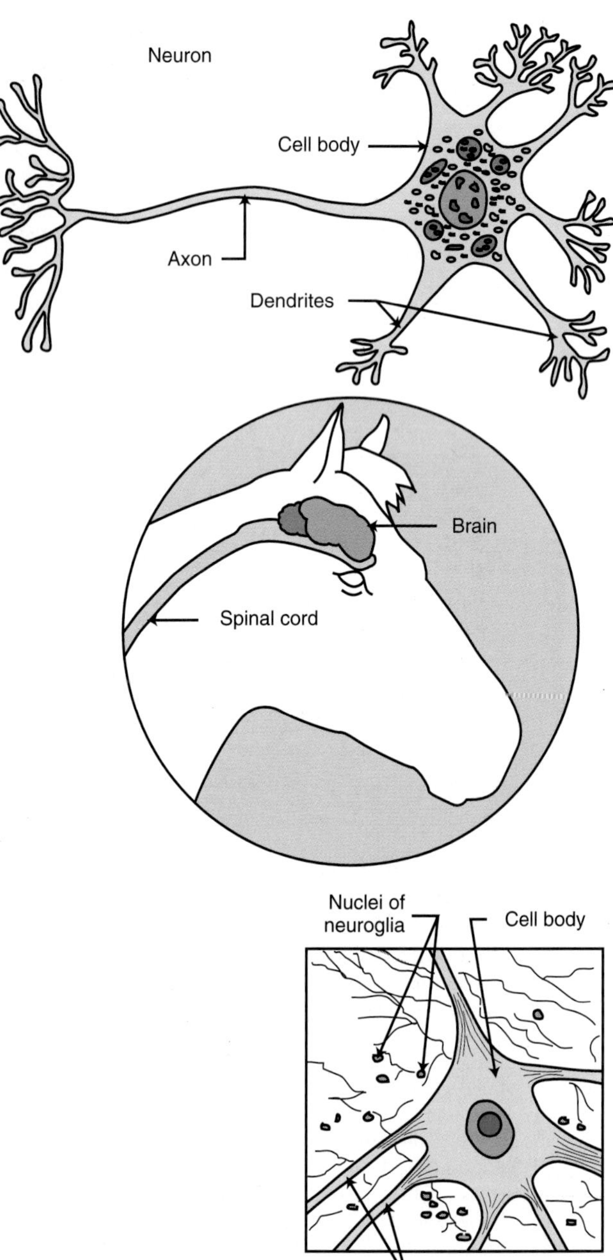

FIGURE **4-13** **Nervous Tissue.**
Description: Composed of neurons and supportive neuroglial cells. A neuron may be multipolar (as shown) or unipolar. Each multipolar neuron is composed of: a cell body, which contains a nucleus; multiple short, branched dendrites; and a single long axon. A unipolar neuron is composed of a cell body and one branched axon.
Location: Brain, spinal cord, and nerves.
Function: To conduct electrical signals, store information, and evaluate data; to transmit sensory information to spinal cord and brain.

Box 4-3 Summary of Tissues

I. Epithelial tissue
   A. Simple squamous
   B. Simple cuboidal
   C. Simple columnar
   D. Stratified squamous
   E. Stratified cuboidal
   F. Stratified columnar
   G. Transitional
   H. Pseudostratified
II. Connective tissue
   A. Connective tissue proper
      1. Loose connective tissue
         a. Areolar tissue
         b. Adipose tissue
         c. Reticular tissue
      2. Dense connective tissue
         a. Dense regular
         b. Dense irregular
         c. Elastic tissue
   B. Specialized connective tissue
      1. Cartilage
         a. Hyaline cartilage
         b. Elastic cartilage
         c. Fibrocartilage
      2. Bone
         a. Compact
         b. Cancellous
      3. Blood
III. Muscle tissue
   A. Skeletal (striated, voluntary)
   B. Cardiac (striated, involuntary)
   C. Smooth (nonstriated, involuntary)
IV. Nervous tissue

TISSUE HEALING AND REPAIR

Injuries occur in many ways. Animals may experience trauma from being hit by a car or falling out of a window. They may be bitten, scratched, or kicked by other animals and may experience broken bones and wounds that later become infected by pathogens. The body's initial response to these injuries is **inflammation,** a series of events that develop quickly to limit further damage and eliminate any harmful agents. Repair occurs more slowly and involves the *organization* of granulation tissue and the *regeneration* of lost tissue or the formation of scar tissue. Many of these processes occur simultaneously, making the injured area a busy workplace for cells. Let's take a closer look at what is happening during the healing process. A summary of tissue repair is illustrated in Figure 4-14.

INFLAMMATION: THE FIRST STEP

Whenever a tissue is injured, it causes an immediate inflammatory response. The affected area becomes red, swollen, hot, and tender. Sometimes there is decreased function of the injured body part. Inflammation is the body's attempt to limit the damage caused by the injury, to isolate the area, and to prevent further damage. *Note that inflammation does not imply infection.* Infection is inflammation caused by viruses, bacteria, and fungi. Injuries such as chemical burns, broken bones, and pulled muscles do not necessarily involve the invasion of these microorganisms. *Inflammation therefore is a nonspecific reaction to injury or disease.* The inflammatory process is the same regardless of the type of disease or injury. The extent of inflammation, however, depends on the type of tissue involved and on the severity of the injury or illness.

Steps in the Process of Inflammation

1. Inflammation begins with a 5- to 10-minute period of vasoconstriction, followed by a sustained period of **vasodilation.** The initial constriction occurs in the small vessels of the injured tissue and aids in the control of **hemorrhaging.** Histamine and heparin molecules subsequently are released from mast cells, which stimulate vasodilation and increase permeability of the capillaries. Blood flow to the area is increased, which in turn causes the clinical signs of heat and redness. It also increases the supplies of oxygen and nutrients to the active cells of the damaged tissue.
2. Fluid from plasma, composed of enzymes, antibodies, and proteins, pour into the affected area, causing swelling of the soft tissue structures. This swelling irritates delicate nerve endings and causes pain and tenderness in the affected area.
3. Clot formation begins to take place, which slows bleeding. The clot also helps to isolate the wound from the invasion of pathogens and helps to prevent bacteria and toxins from spreading to surrounding soft tissue structures. A clot first forms when platelets become sticky and clump together. **Fibrinogen,** which is found in rich quantities in the swollen tissue, is converted to an insoluble protein called **fibrin.** The fibrin is woven into a netlike structure that surrounds the platelets and provides support and stability to the newly formed clot. It also forms a framework to support the movement of cells throughout the site. Clots that form on external surfaces, such as skin, eventually dry and become known as *scabs.*
4. Large cells, such as macrophages and **neutrophils** (a type of white blood cell), move through blood vessels and can squeeze through dilated capillaries to assist in the removal of debris and microinvaders. The phagocytic cells are short lived, however, and can function for only a few hours before dying. Pus, which is an accumulation of dead and degenerated neutrophils and macrophages, may therefore collect in the injured area.
5. With increased blood flow, histamine and heparin are dispersed, and their levels drop in the affected area. The decrease in these molecules causes the return of normal capillary size and permeability. When capillaries return to normal size, blood flow and fluid leakage into the affected area abate. Swelling, heat, and redness begin to subside.

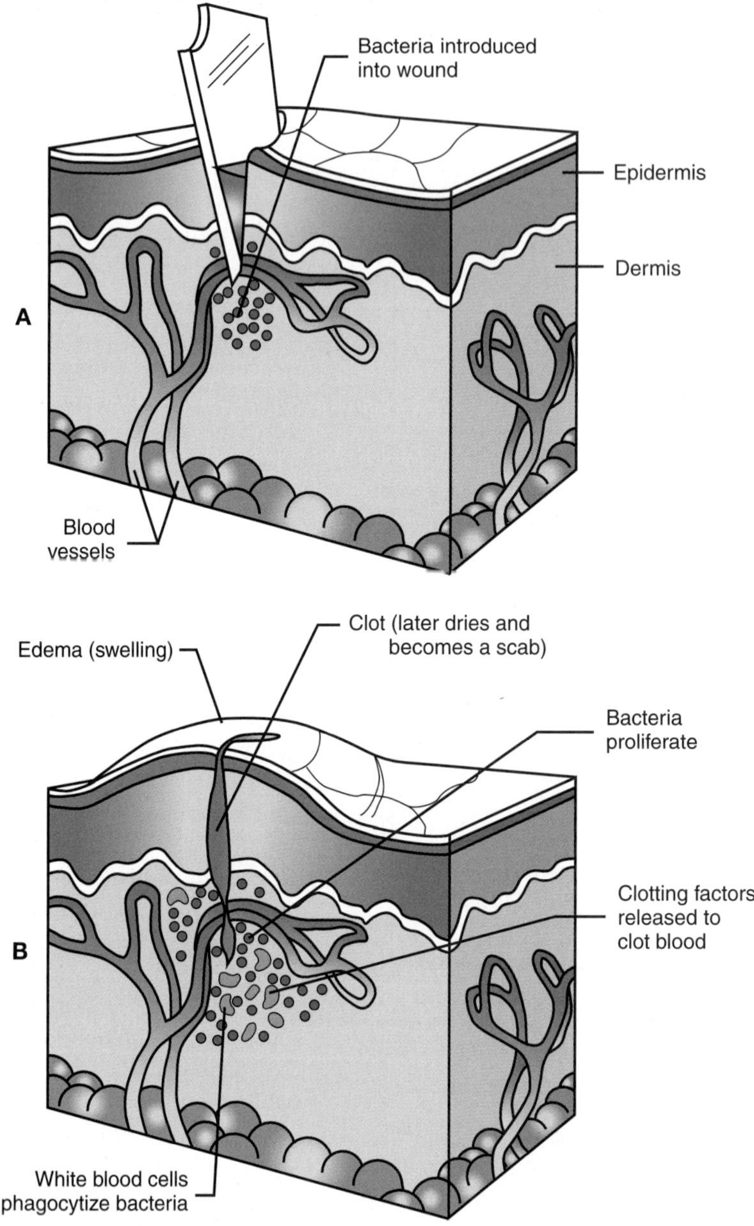

FIGURE **4-14** **Tissue Repair of Minor Skin Wound. A,** Injury: A piece of glass forms a cut (laceration) in the skin. **B,** Inflammation: Blood vessels dilate and become more permeable, causing redness in the tissue around the wound. Fluid leaks into the tissue from dilated capillaries and causes swelling. A blood clot forms (later becomes a scab) at the wound opening. Pressure of fluid on nerve endings causes pain. *Continued*

Organization: The Formation of Granulation Tissue

Wound repair begins soon after the injury occurs and continues while dead cells and debris are removed from the area. In wounds that are infected, neutrophils and macrophages play a particularly critical role in the healing process because they are responsible for phagocytizing and disposing of invasive microorganisms. The presence of pathogens inhibits healing.

As macrophages work to clear debris, a new, bright pink tissue, called **granulation tissue,** forms beneath the overlaying blood clot or scab. Granulation tissue is composed of a layer of collagen fibers that has been manufactured by fibroblasts. It is richly infiltrated with small permeable capillaries that have

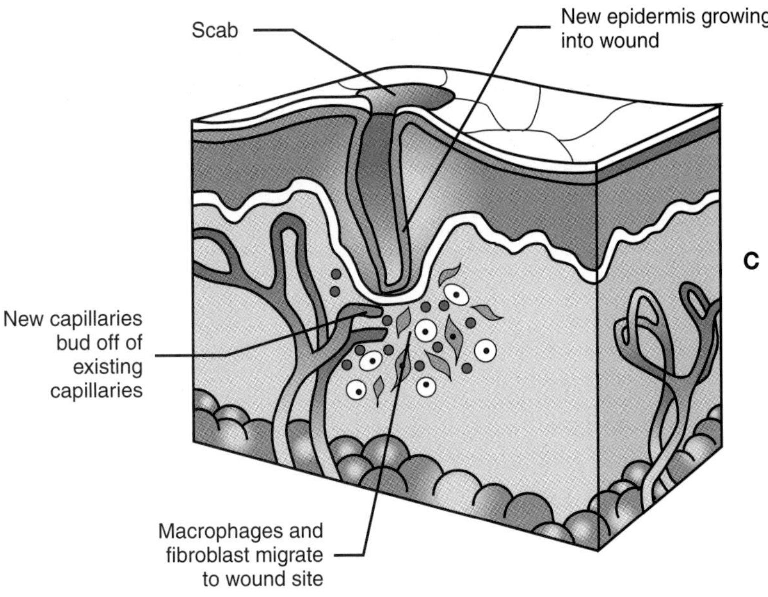
ORGANIZATION: bacterium-inhibiting substances are produced
Scab
New epidermis growing into wound
C
New capillaries bud off of existing capillaries
Macrophages and fibroblast migrate to wound site

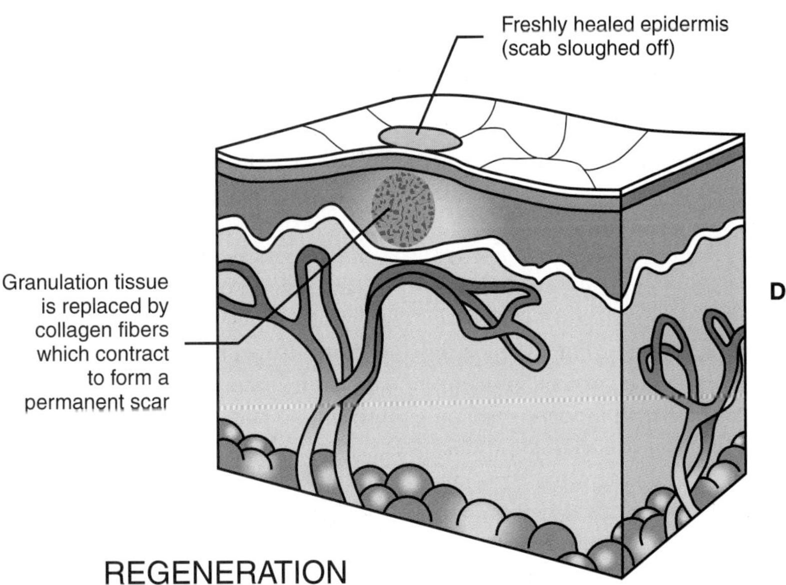
Freshly healed epidermis (scab sloughed off)
D
Granulation tissue is replaced by collagen fibers which contract to form a permanent scar
REGENERATION

FIGURE **4-14, cont'd** **C,** Organization: Granulation tissue forms below the scab. Fibroblasts lay down collagen fibers while macrophages engulf foreign debris and invading microorganisms. **D,** Regeneration or fibrosis: Epithelial cells around wound edges proliferate and cover granulation tissue. Scab is pushed off. Granulation tissue becomes fibrous scar tissue, which contracts and pulls wound edges together.

branched off of existing capillaries in the deeper layers of the damaged tissue. These new tiny vessels push up into the bed of collagen fibers and provide rich supplies of nutrients and oxygen to hard-working cells such as fibroblasts, macrophages, and neutrophils. Grossly, the capillaries appear to be minute *granules* and therefore account for the name "granulation tissue." Granulation tissue produces bacterium-inhibiting substances, which make it highly resistant to infection.

In some cases, granulation tissue becomes *too* thick and stands out above the epithelial layer. This is known as **proud flesh** and may be surgically cut down to facilitate closure of the epithelial layer. Proud flesh is commonly seen in equines that have sustained skin wounds.

CLINICAL APPLICATION: The Clinical Patient and Healing

Some tissue types heal more readily than others. Epithelial tissues, for example, skin and mucous membranes, heal rapidly. Smooth muscle and dense regular connective tissue, on the other hand, have limited regenerative ability. Cardiac muscle and nervous tissue in the brain and spinal cord have essentially no regenerative ability and only can be replaced by scar tissue. In addition, some patients heal more easily than other patients. For example, old, **immunosuppressed,** debilitated, or sick animals heal more slowly than young, healthy, well-nourished animals. In this way, the age, health status, and nutrition of patients are important factors in the rate and extent of healing. This is why elective surgery is avoided in unhealthy animals and why intravenous nutrition may be used in critically ill patients. Some animals, for example, may have a disease in which they produce too much cortisol hormone. High levels of cortisol can inhibit an animal's ability to heal; incision sites may take weeks rather than days to close, and wounds from even superficial injuries may become chronic nightmares. In addition, some drugs, such as prednisone, can also delay healing if blood levels are high. Thus the clinician must consider the entire health status and medical history of an animal before carrying out a procedure, such as surgery, which subsequently requires the healing of tissue.

REGENERATION OR FIBROSIS

Epithelialization Occurs, and Granulation Tissue Is Replaced by Scar Tissue

While organization is occurring, epithelial cells around the wound edges actively divide to lay down a new layer of epithelial tissue over the granulation tissue. This process is called **epithelialization.** Connections between the scab and the thickening epithelial layer are weakened, and the scab subsequently falls off. Fibroblasts in the granulation tissue continue to manufacture collagen fibers and ground substance, which are used to replace lost tissue and bridge the wound. Slowly the granulation tissue is completely replaced by fibrous scar tissue, which contracts and assists in pulling the wound closed. When epithelialization is complete, the underlying scar may or may not be visible, depending on the severity of the injury and on the extent of scar formation.

Although scar tissue is strong, it is less flexible than normal tissue and cannot perform the function of the damaged tissue. With time, scar tissue shrinks, but its presence can still have detrimental effects on the organ as a whole. For example, if scar tissue forms in the wall of the heart, it can interrupt electrical pathways, weaken contractile capability, and result in decreased cardiac function. Similarly, if it occurs in the wall of the intestine or esophagus, it can decrease the diameter of the lumen and subsequently incur an obstruction or occlusion. For this reason, dogs that have undergone esophageal surgery to remove a foreign body are likely to have a repeated episode. The site of the first incision in the esophagus often heals with a thick fibrous scar, which narrows the esophageal lumen and increases the possibility that another foreign body, such as a piece of bone or chew toy, will once again become lodged.

In the abdominal and thoracic cavities, healing is often associated with the formation of fibrous adhesions and tags, which cover organs and form connections between multiple structures. Reentry into the abdomen to repeat a surgical procedure or to correct a complication therefore can be more difficult because of the formation of adhesions. Adhesions can obscure visibility of important structures. They can restrict normal shifting of bowel loops and can bind organs to the body wall or to the omentum. In addition, adhesions can be painful to the animal if they cause tension between well-innervated structures.

CLASSIFICATIONS

Wound repair may be classified as first, second, or third intention, depending on the mechanism of healing and the proximity of the wound edges. Wounds that heal via first intention are those in which the edges of the wound are held in close apposition. These wounds may be superficial scratches or wounds that have been sutured or held closed with special bandages. During **first-intention healing,** the skin forms a primary union without the formation of granulation tissue or significant scarring. Healing by **second intention** and third intention occurs in wounds in which the edges are separated from one another, in which granulation tissue forms to close the gap, and in which scarring results. **Third-intention healing** occurs more slowly than that of second intention because larger, more extensive wounds (gaps) are usually involved.

TEST YOURSELF

1. In what ways are muscle fibers uniquely adapted for contraction?
2. List three types of muscle. How do they differ from one another?
3. What are the two basic cell types that make up neural tissue?
4. What is the most important function of neural tissue?
5. Describe the process of inflammation. What causes the clinical signs of heat, swelling, redness, and tenderness?
6. When does the healing process begin?
7. What is granulation tissue? Why is it important in the healing process?
8. Describe first-, second-, and third-intention wound repair.

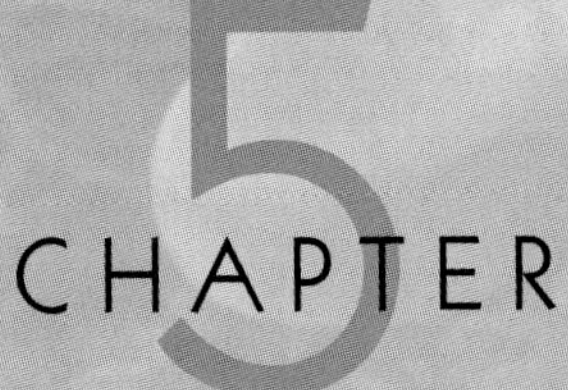

CHAPTER 5

The Skeletal System

Thomas Colville

Try to imagine what an animal's body would be like without a skeleton. Picture a furry sac of semisoft, gelatin-like material lying on the ground twitching. That's about what it would look like. The other connective tissues would hold the cells together, and the muscles would still contract and attempt to move the body. However, without bones to support it and give the muscles leverage to move it, the body would lie on the ground, unable to accomplish anything useful.

The skeleton is the framework of bones that supports and protects the soft tissues of the body. Besides making up the skeleton, the bones also serve a variety of other important functions. Before discussing the parts of the skeleton, let's take a look at bone—what it is, what it does, and some of its common characteristics.

BONE

Bone Terminology

The terms *os* and *osteo-* generally refer to bone. For example, the *os* penis is a bone in the penis of dogs and *osteo*cytes are bone cells.

Bone Characteristics

Bone is one of the most fascinating body tissues. It is the second hardest natural substance in the body—only the enamel of the teeth is harder. Despite its dead, rocklike appearance, bone is a vital, living tissue with an excellent capacity to repair itself after injury. All that is usually necessary for broken bones to heal is for the broken ends to be brought together in some reasonable sort of alignment and then kept from moving for a few weeks or months. (See the Clinical Application on fracture repair for more information.)

Bone is composed of a few cells embedded in an intercellular (between cells) substance called the *matrix* that starts out soft and then becomes hardened when calcium and phosphate crystals are deposited in it. The cells that produce bone are called **osteoblasts** (*osteo-*, "bone"; *-blast,* a cell that produces something). The osteoblasts first secrete the soft, flexible matrix. The matrix is composed of collagen fibers embedded in a gelatin-like "ground substance" made of protein and polysaccharides (complex carbohydrates). The osteoblasts harden the matrix through a process called **ossification.** When ossification takes place, the matrix is infiltrated with calcium and phosphate in the form of hydroxyapatite crystals. These hydroxyapatite crystals give bone its characteristic hardness. As they create areas of bone, the osteoblasts become trapped in spaces in the ossified matrix called **lacunae.** Once they are surrounded by bone, the former osteoblasts get a new identity (kind of like people in the witness protection program). They are now called **osteocytes,** or "bone cells." Osteocytes live out their days in their little, cell-like lacunae. Their only contact with each other and their blood supply is through threadlike cellular processes in tiny channels through the bone called **canaliculi.** The canaliculi are sort of like slots in jail cell doors through which the "prisoners," the osteocytes, get food and can talk with other prisoners.

FUNCTIONS OF BONES

Support

The most basic function of bone is to support the animal body. The cells and tissues that make up the rest of the body are fairly soft and do not have much inherent strength. The bones serve as "scaffolding" to support them. The rest of the body either hangs from or is attached directly to the bones.

Protection

The bones also have an important protective function. Their firm strength protects many delicate, vital organs and tissues by surrounding them partially or completely. Good examples of this are the bones of the skull, which protect the soft brain and the delicate structures of the eye and ear.

Leverage

The bones act as levers for the skeletal muscles to move the body. Attachment of skeletal muscles to the bones via the tendons allows the muscles to move the joints. This lets the animal move around in its environment.

Storage

The bones act as storage sites for minerals, particularly calcium. Bones act as a reservoir or "bank" for calcium, enabling the body to deposit and withdraw it as needed to precisely control the level of calcium in the bloodstream. Calcium plays many important roles in many body functions, including muscle contraction, blood clotting, milk secretion, and skeleton formation and maintenance. Its level in the blood must be kept within a narrow range for these functions to proceed without difficulty. Two hormones—**calcitonin** from the thyroid gland and **parathyroid hormone** from the parathyroid glands—act as "cashiers" at the calcium bank. Calcitonin helps prevent hypercalcemia (too high a level of calcium in the blood) largely by depositing excess calcium in the bones. Parathyroid hormone does the opposite. It helps prevent hypocalcemia (too low a level of calcium in the blood) in part by withdrawing calcium from the bones. This depositing and withdrawing of calcium go on constantly as the body's needs and the contents of its food supply change. (Chapter 14 explains this process more fully.)

Blood Cell Formation

Some of the bones serve as sites for blood cell formation **(hematopoiesis)** in the bone marrow that fills their interiors. More information about this is provided shortly.

BONE STRUCTURE

The two main types of bone are light, spongy **cancellous bone** and heavy, dense **compact bone.**

Cancellous Bone

Cancellous bone is sometimes called *spongy bone* because it looks like a sponge (Figure 5-1). It consists of tiny "spicules" of bone that appear randomly arranged with lots of spaces between them, like a bunch of "pick-up-sticks" that have been tossed into a pile. In life the spaces between the spicules are occupied by bone marrow. To the naked eye, the many spicules and spaces give cancellous bone its spongy appearance. It is light, but amazingly strong. It helps lighten the bones of the skeleton without significantly reducing their strength. The organization of the spicules of cancellous bone appears random, but they are actually arranged to stand up to the forces the bone is subjected to. Muscles, gravity, and other bones all push and pull on bones constantly. The makeup of cancellous bone helps keep the bones light while also preventing them from being damaged by all the forces acting on them.

Compact Bone

Compact bone is very heavy, dense, and strong. It makes up the shafts of long bones and the outside layer of all bones. It is composed of tiny, tightly compacted cylinders of bone called **haversian systems** (see Figure 5-1). Each haversian system runs lengthwise with the bone and consists of a laminated (multilayered) cylinder composed of concentric layers of ossified bone matrix arranged around a central **haversian canal.** The haversian canal contains blood and lymph vessels and nerves that supply the osteocytes. The osteocytes are located at the junctions between the layers of bone that make up each haversian system. In cross section, these layers of bone look like the growth rings of a tree. Tiny channels through the bone, called *canaliculi,* allow osteocytes to contact each other and exchange nutrients and wastes via tiny cellular processes.

Except for their **articular** (joint) **surfaces,** the outer surfaces of bones are covered by a membrane called the **periosteum.** The outer layer of the periosteum is composed of fibrous tissue, and its inner layer contains bone-forming cells (osteoblasts). This inner bone-forming layer enables bones to increase in diameter. It is also involved in the healing of bone fractures. Another membrane, the **endosteum,** lines the hollow interior surfaces of bones. It also contains osteoblasts.

BONE CELLS

Three types of cells that make up bone are osteoblasts, osteocytes, and **osteoclasts.** Osteoblasts are the cells that form bone. They secrete the matrix of bone and then supply the minerals necessary to ossify (harden) it. (This aspect is discussed shortly.) Once the osteoblasts become trapped in the ossified matrix that they have created, they are called **osteocytes.** Talk about painting yourself into a corner! The osteocytes are always ready to revert to their former lives as osteoblasts and form new bone if an injury makes that necessary. Osteoclasts are the "evil twins" of osteoblasts; instead of forming bone, they eat it away. Actually, they are not evil at all. Bones are dynamic structures that must be remodeled constantly. Osteoclasts are necessary for remodeling to take place by removing bone from where it is *not* needed while osteoblasts form new bone in areas where it *is* needed. Osteoclasts also allow the body to withdraw calcium from the bones when it is needed to raise the calcium level in the blood.

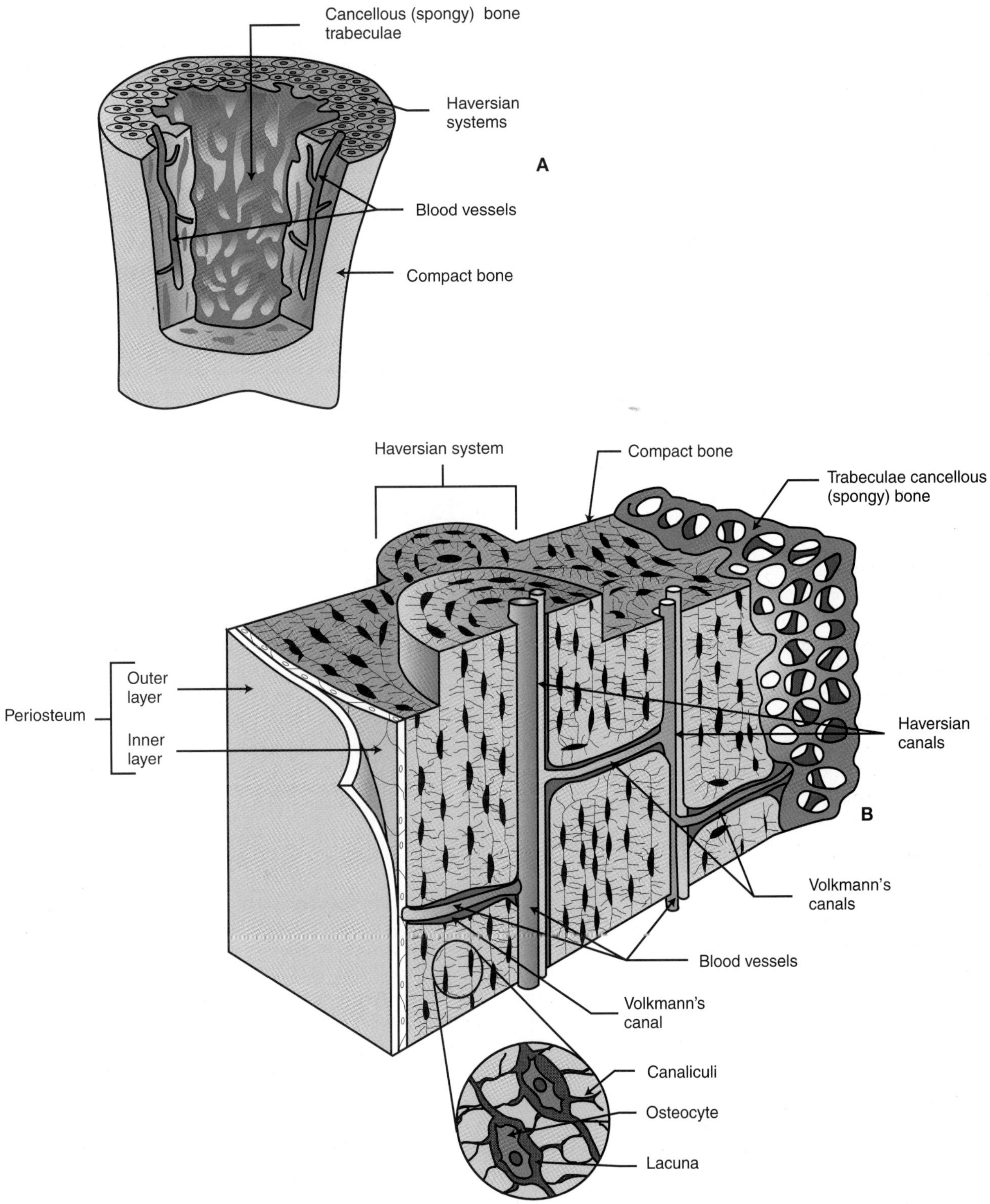

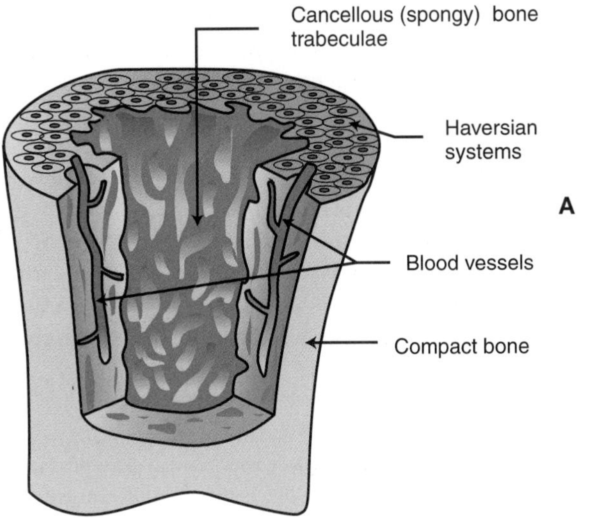

FIGURE **5-1** **Structure of Compact and Cancellous Bone. A,** Section through the long bone showing outer compact and inner cancellous bone. **B,** Enlarged view showing components of each type of bone.

TEST YOURSELF

1. Besides supporting the other tissues of the body, what else do bones do?
2. What are the three kinds of bone cells? What role does each play in the life of a bone?
3. What is the matrix of bone made of? Why is it so hard?
4. What are the main differences between the structures of cancellous bone and compact bone? Why does the body need these two different types of bone?

Blood Supply to Bone

Most of the blood supply to bones comes from countless tiny blood vessels that penetrate in from the periosteum. The vessels pass through tiny channels through the bone matrix called **Volkmann's canals.** The Volkmann's canals come in at right angles to the long axis of the bone and at right angles to the haversian canals. The blood vessels in the Volkmann's canals join with the blood vessels in the haversian canals and bring nutrition to the osteocytes in the haversian systems.

Large blood vessels, along with lymph vessels and nerves, also enter many large bones (especially long bones) through large channels called **nutrient foramina.** These large vessels primarily carry blood into and out of the **bone marrow.** The locations of the larger nutrient foramina on long bones are fairly predictable. Seen from the side on a radiograph (x-ray picture), a nutrient foramen can resemble a crack-type fracture of the **bone cortex.** This is a good example of why a thorough knowledge of anatomy is necessary to properly interpret radiographs.

Bone Formation

Bone is formed in the body by one of two mechanisms: It either (1) grows into and replaces a cartilage model, called **endochondral** (or "cartilage") **bone formation,** or (2) develops from fibrous tissue membranes, called **intramembranous** (or "membrane") **bone formation.**

Most of the bones in the body develop by the endochondral method. When bones form by this method, the body first creates a cartilage "template" that is subsequently replaced by bone. Most bones start out as rods of cartilage in the developing fetus. These cartilage rods are prototypes of the bones that will eventually replace them. In **long bones,** such as the **femur** (thigh bone), bone begins developing in the shaft **(diaphyses)** of the cartilage rod in what is called the **primary growth center.** Cartilage is removed as bone is created, and the growth center expands, gradually replacing the cartilage with bone. Additional growth centers, called **secondary growth centers,** develop in the ends **(epiphyses)** of the bone. By the time of birth, most of the cartilage prototypes have been replaced by bone.

Just two areas of a long bone remain as cartilage when an animal is born. They are two plates of cartilage located between the shaft (diaphysis) of the bone and the ends (epiphyses) of the bone. They are called the **epiphyseal** or **growth plates.** They are the sites where the creation of new bone allows the long bones to lengthen as the animal grows. In each growth plate, cartilage cells create new cartilage on the epiphyseal (outside) surface of the plate, and osteoblasts replace the cartilage on the diaphyseal (inside) surface of the plate with bone. By this mechanism the bone gradually gets longer as the animal grows. When the bone has reached its full size, the epiphyseal plates completely **ossify,** that is, all of the cartilage is replaced by bone. This stops the growth of the bone. Remodeling continues to take place, but the bone is as long as it is going to get.

The intramembranous method of bone formation only occurs in certain skull bones. Bone forms in the fibrous tissue membranes that cover the brain in the developing fetus. This process creates the flat bones of the **cranium** (the bones that surround the brain).

CLINICAL APPLICATION — Fracture Repair

Bones are among the best healing tissues in the body. Three steps that are necessary for optimal healing to occur when bones are fractured (broken) are alignment, immobilization, and time. The fractured ends must be brought close together in reasonable anatomical alignment and kept from moving from that position so that the healing processes have adequate time to do their thing. Aligning the fracture fragments is called "setting" or "reducing" the fracture, and the immobilization is called "fixation" of the fracture. External fixation devices, such as splints and casts, can be used, or internal devices, such as pins, wires, screws, or plates, can be surgically implanted. The length of time that the fixation device must be kept in place varies with the type and location of the fracture and the physical characteristics of the animal. Factors such as the species, age, physical condition, and size of the animal affect the speed of healing. The whole process might only take a couple of weeks in a young, small critter, or it might take several months or more in an older, larger animal.

Regardless of the type and location of the fracture, the basic healing processes are the same. The large blood supply of bones results in considerable bleeding (hemorrhage) at the fracture site. After the blood clots, forming what is called the *fracture hematoma,* it is gradually invaded by healing cells and tissues over the next few weeks and months. Osteoblasts from the area begin forming the healing tissue, called the **callus,** that gradually bridges the fracture gap. The callus can be felt as a "lump" at the fracture site. The size of the callus is an indicator of how much movement has been occurring between the fracture fragments. The less movement, the smaller the callus, and vice versa. Fractures with small calluses generally heal faster, which is usually our treatment goal. Once the callus is fully formed and mineralized, the basic healing of the fracture is complete. However, what occurs after that is very important. Over the next few months, the body slowly remodels the bone at the fracture site according to the mechanical stresses that are placed on it. Hopefully, this will return the bone to its original size, shape, and strength.

Bone Shapes

Bones come in four basic shapes—long, short, flat, and irregular.

Long Bones

As their name implies, long bones are relatively longer than they are wide. Most bones of the limbs are long bones. The basic parts of a long bone are illustrated in Figure 5-2. The ends of a long bone are called the *epiphyses;* each long bone has a proximal epiphysis and a distal epiphysis. They consist primarily of light cancellous bone covered by a thin layer of compact bone. The main part of a long bone, the shaft, is called the *diaphysis.* It is composed of strong compact bone. Between the epiphyses and the diaphysis of a young animal are the plates of cartilage called the *epiphyseal plates.* The epiphyseal plates are more commonly called the *growth plates* because they are the sites of bone growth that allow long bones to get longer as the animal grows. They are also weak areas of the bone. Fractures through epiphyseal plates are common in young animals. These are called *epiphyseal fractures.* When an animal reaches its full adult size, the epiphyseal plates ossify (are converted to solid bone).

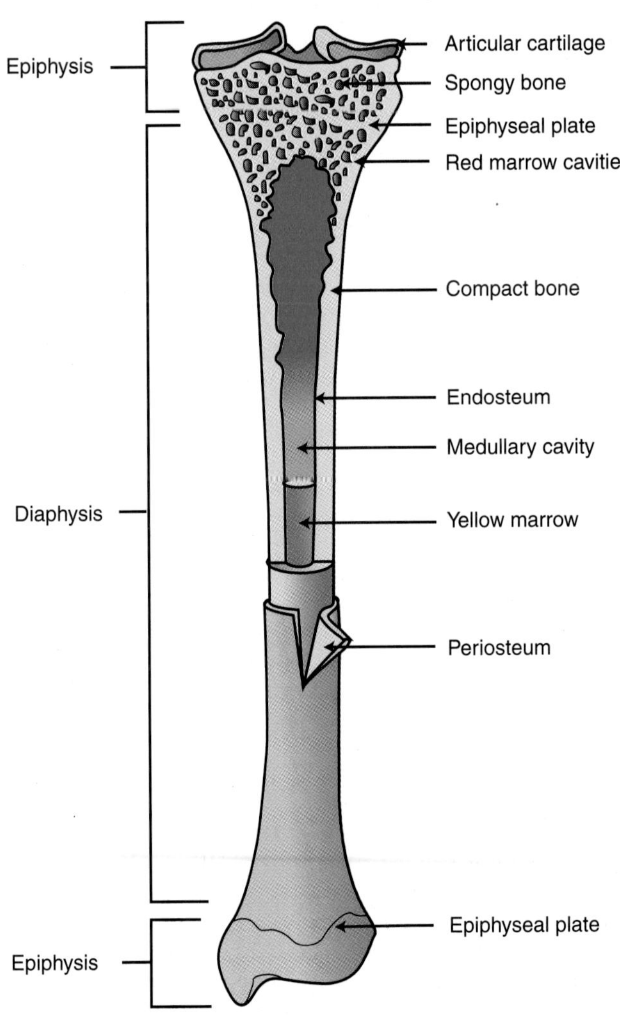

FIGURE **5-2** **Long Bone.** Structure of long bone (tibia).

Short Bones

Short bones are shaped like small cubes or marshmallows. They consist of a core of spongy bone covered by a thin layer of compact bone. Examples include the carpal and tarsal bones.

Flat Bones

Flat bones, as their name implies, are relatively thin and flat. Their structure is kind of like a cancellous bone sandwich in that they consist of two thin plates of compact bone separated by a layer of cancellous bone. Many of the skull bones are flat bones, as are the scapulas (shoulder blades) and pelvic bones.

Irregular Bones

The term **irregular bones** is the anatomist's version of a miscellaneous category. Irregular bones don't fit into the long, short, or flat categories. They either have characteristics of more than one of the other categories or just have a truly irregular shape. The bones of the spine (the vertebrae) are irregular bones, as are some of the strangely shaped skull bones. **Sesamoid bones** are also included in this category. Sesamoid bones got their name because early anatomists thought their shapes resembled sesame seeds. You have to give the early anatomists credit for their active imaginations! Sesamoid bones are present in some tendons where they change direction markedly over the surfaces of joints. The **patella** (kneecap) is the largest sesamoid bone in the animal body, but typically several others are found also. (We'll discuss some of the clinically important sesamoid bones later in the section on the appendicular skeleton.)

Bone Marrow

Bone marrow fills the spaces within bones. This includes the spaces between the spicules of cancellous bone and the large spaces within the diaphyses of long bones. It comes in two basic types—**red bone marrow** and **yellow bone marrow.**

Red Bone Marrow

Red bone marrow is **hematopoietic tissue.** *Hemato-* refers to blood, and *-poiesis* means to form something. Red bone marrow forms blood cells. It makes up the majority of the bone marrow of young animals but only a small portion of the marrow of older animals. In older animals it is confined to a few specific locations, such as the ends of some long bones and the interiors of the pelvic bones and the sternum.

Yellow Bone Marrow

Yellow bone marrow consists primarily of adipose connective tissue (fat). It is the most common type of marrow in adult animals. Yellow bone marrow does not produce blood cells, but it can revert to red bone marrow if the body needs to churn out larger than normal numbers of blood cells.

This might be necessary if an animal were suffering from chronic low-level blood loss caused by numerous blood-sucking parasites.

TEST YOURSELF

1. What is the difference between a haversian canal and a Volkmann's canal?
2. By which mechanism of bone formation do most of the bones in the animal body develop before birth and how does the process take place?
3. What is the difference between the primary growth center of a bone and a secondary growth center?
4. Where would you find an epiphyseal plate and what would you find it doing?
5. What is bone marrow and what is the difference between the red kind and the yellow kind?

Common Bone Features

The roles that particular bones fill often become clear when their lumps, bumps, grooves, and holes are examined. These features show us where bones form joints with each other, where muscles attach to move them, where tendons press on their surfaces, and where they are pierced by blood vessels and nerves. We can learn a lot about a bone just by looking at its shape and surface features.

Articular Surfaces

Articular surfaces are joint surfaces—smooth areas of compact bone where bones come in contact with each other to form joints. Each articular surface is covered by a smooth, thin layer of hyaline cartilage called **articular cartilage.** The smooth articular surface and its smooth and slightly softer articular cartilage covering help reduce friction and wear in joints.

Condyle. A **condyle** is usually a large, round articular surface. Condyles have, in the creative imagery of anatomists, a somewhat *cylindrical* shape. The major condyles of the body are located on the distal end of the humerus and femur and on the occipital bone of the skull, where it joins the spinal column to attach the head to the neck.

Head. A **head** is a somewhat spherical articular surface on the proximal end of a long bone. Heads are found on the proximal end of the humerus, femur, and rib. The heads of the humeri and femurs form the ball portion of the **ball-and-socket** shoulder and hip **joints.** The head of a bone is united with the main portion (shaft) of the bone by an often narrowed region called the **neck.**

Facet. A **facet** is a flat articular surface. The joint movement between two facets is a kind of rocking motion. Facets are found on many bones, such as carpal and tarsal bones, vertebrae, and long bones, such as the radius and ulna.

Processes

A **process** is a general term that includes all the lumps, bumps, and other projections on a bone. Some processes, such as *heads* and *condyles,* have articular (joint-forming) functions. They have very smooth surfaces. Other processes are not part of joints. They have rough, irregular surfaces. They are usually sites where muscles (or more accurately, tendons) attach. In general, the larger the process, the more powerful the muscular pull on that area of the bone. This can help us figure out how and in what direction(s) the bone usually moves and how powerful the movement usually is. This principle is often used by paleontologists to explain the functions that fossilized dinosaur bones probably had when the animals were alive.

Unfortunately, processes are given a variety of names depending on their location. Sometimes they are simply called *processes,* such as the spinous process of a vertebra. On other bones they have a variety of names, such as *trochanter* on the femur, *tubercle* on the humerus, *tuber* on the ischium, *spine* on the scapula, *crest* on the tibia, and *wing* on the atlas. Such is the complex language of anatomy.

Holes and Depressed Areas

Foramen. A hole in a bone is called a **foramen** (*plural,* foramina). Usually something important, such as a nerve or blood vessel, passes through a foramen in a bone. As usual, there are exceptions; for example, no major structures pass through the two large obturator foramina of the pelvis. They merely exist to lighten the pelvis.

Fossa. A **fossa** is a depressed or sunken area on the surface of a bone. Fossae are usually occupied by muscles or tendons. Paleontologists use the fossae of dinosaur bones to infer the sizes and actions of some of the animals' tendons and muscles.

AXIAL SKELETON

The bones of the skeleton can be conveniently divided into two main groups—the bones of the head and trunk and the bones of the limbs. Because the bones of the head and trunk are located along the central axis of the body, they are referred to as the **axial skeleton.** The bones of the limbs (appendages of the trunk) are collectively called the **appendicular skeleton.** Some animals may have a third category of bones—the **visceral skeleton.** These are bones formed in soft organs (the viscera). (These are discussed in more detail after the two main groups.) Figure 5-3 is a generic "word" skeleton that shows the locations of the main bones of the axial and appendicular portions of the skeleton. Figures 5-4 and 5-5 show the bones that make up the skeletons of the horse and dog.

The components of the axial skeleton are the skull, the hyoid bone, the spinal column, the ribs, and the sternum. All the bones of the axial skeleton lie on or near the median plane of the body.

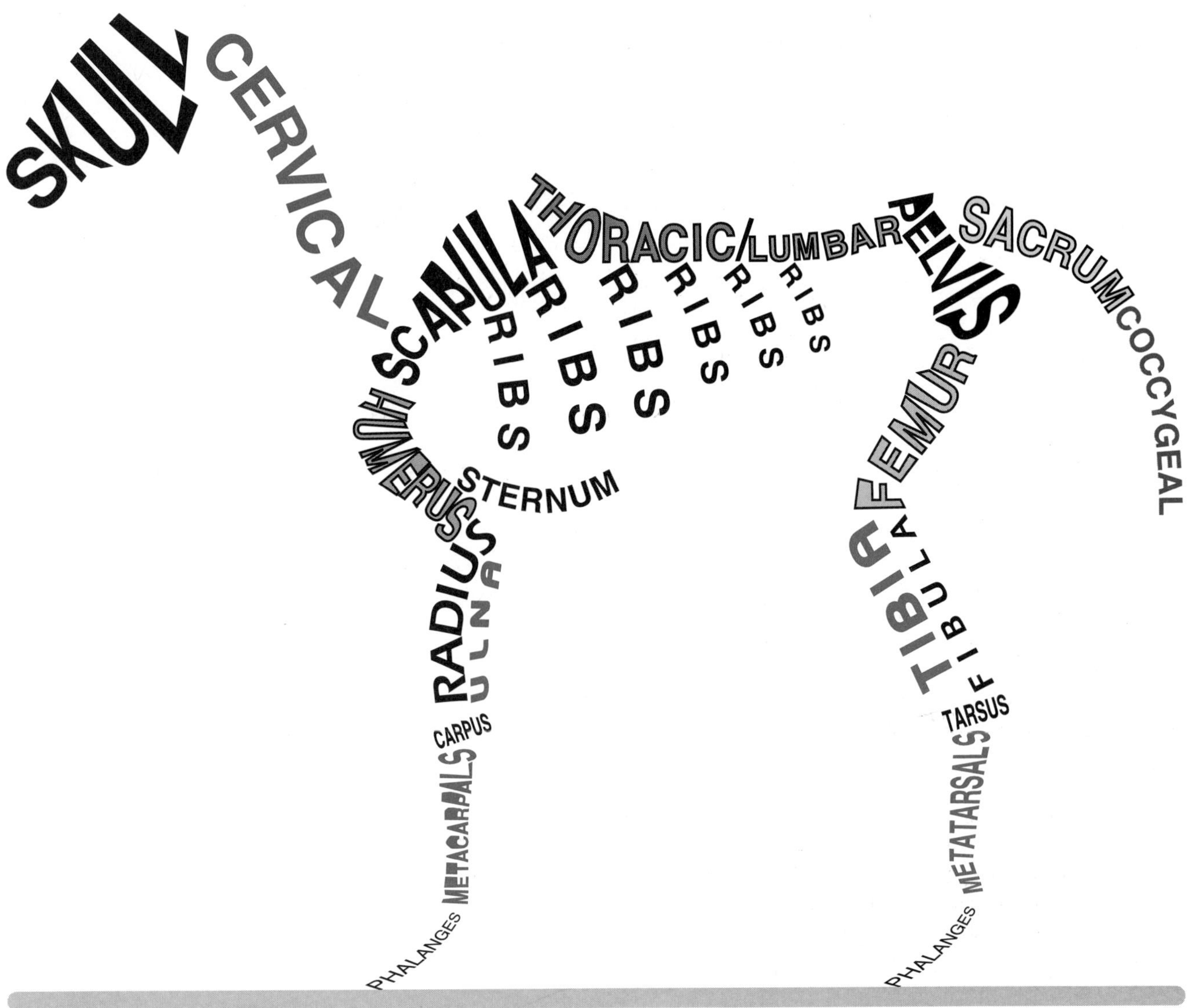

FIGURE **5-3** **Word Skeleton.** Word skeleton showing main bones of axial and appendicular portions of the skeleton.

Skull

The **skull** is the most complex part of the skeleton. At first glance it looks like one big bone (or two if you count the mandible), but in most domestic animals it consists of 37 or 38 separate bones. Most of the skull bones are united by jagged, immovable, fibrous joints called **sutures.** Only the mandible (the lower jaw) is connected to the rest of the skull by a freely movable **synovial joint.** Figures 5-6 through 5-8 show the externally visible skull bones of horses, cattle, and cats.

Author's suggestion: If you have access to a skull and a live animal of the same species, locate each of the external skull bones on the skull and find the comparable regions on the head of the live animal. Anatomy is a lot more fun and useful if we find the structures we are discussing on live animals.

Because of its complexity, we group the skull bones into regions: the bones of the cranium, the bones of the ear, and the bones of the face. Table 5-1 lists the skull bones in each region.

External Bones of the Cranium

The **cranium** is the portion of the skull that surrounds the brain. In most domestic animal species, 11 bones form the cranium. To make things a little easier, we can divide the **bones of the cranium** into external and internal bones. External bones are at least partially visible on the surface of an intact skull. We can use them as landmarks to describe the locations of features on the heads of living animals. Internal bones are hidden and cannot be seen without disassembling the skull.

Starting at the caudal (rear) end of the skull and working our way rostrally (forward), the external bones of the cranium are the occipital bone, the interparietal bones, the parietal bones, the temporal bones, and the frontal bones.

Occipital Bone. The **occipital bone** is a single bone that forms the "base" (caudoventral portion) of the skull. It is the most caudal skull bone and is very important because (1) it is

Text continued on p. 106

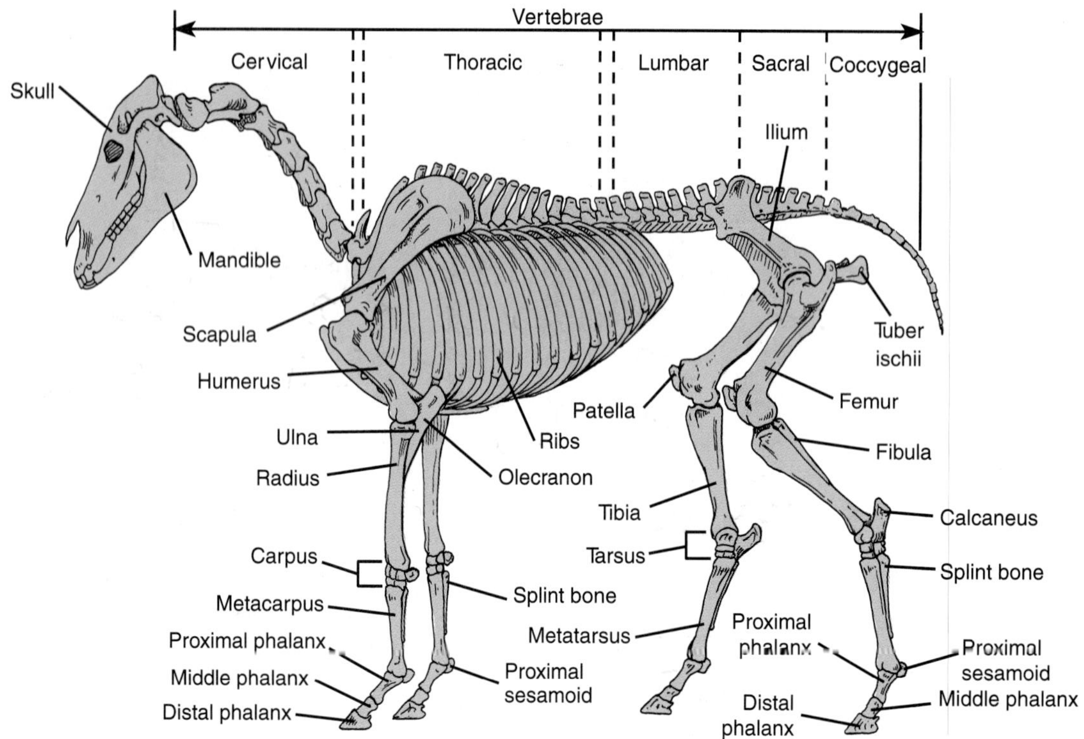

FIGURE **5-4** **Equine Skeleton.** (From McBride DF: *Learning veterinary terminology,* ed 2, St Louis, 2002, Mosby.)

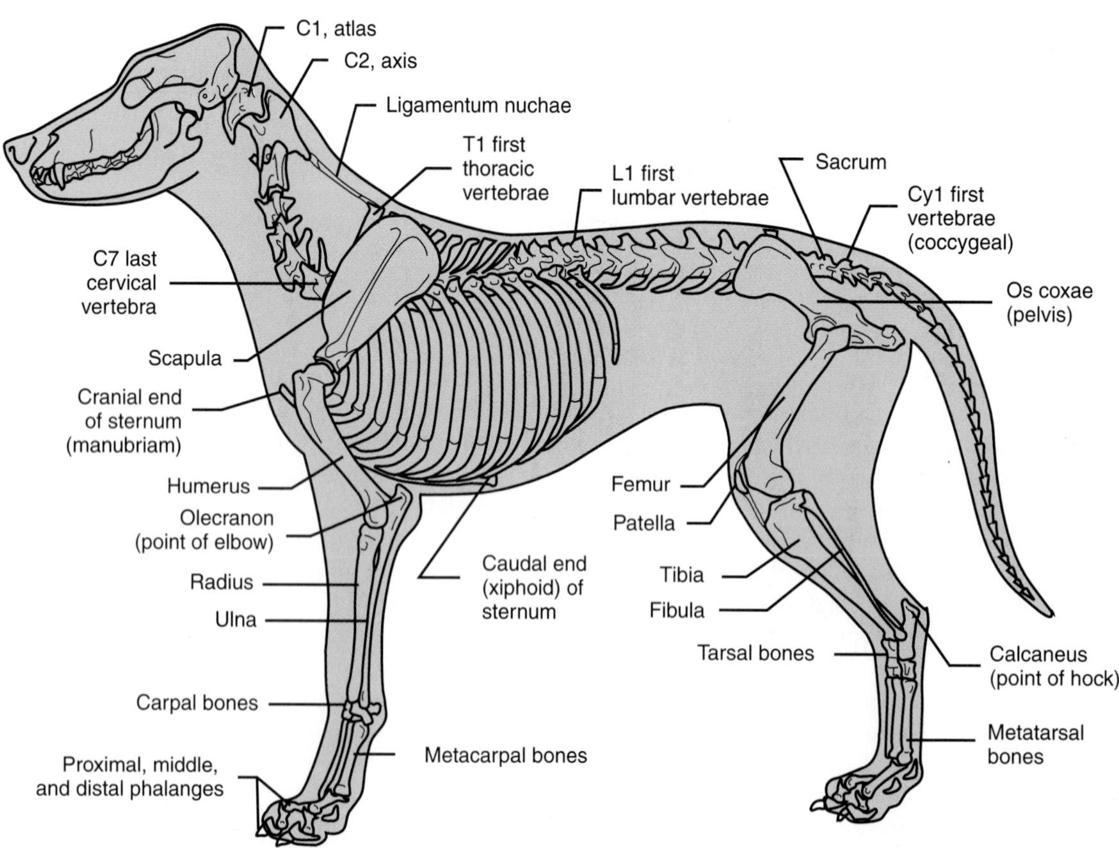

FIGURE **5-5** **Canine Skeleton.**

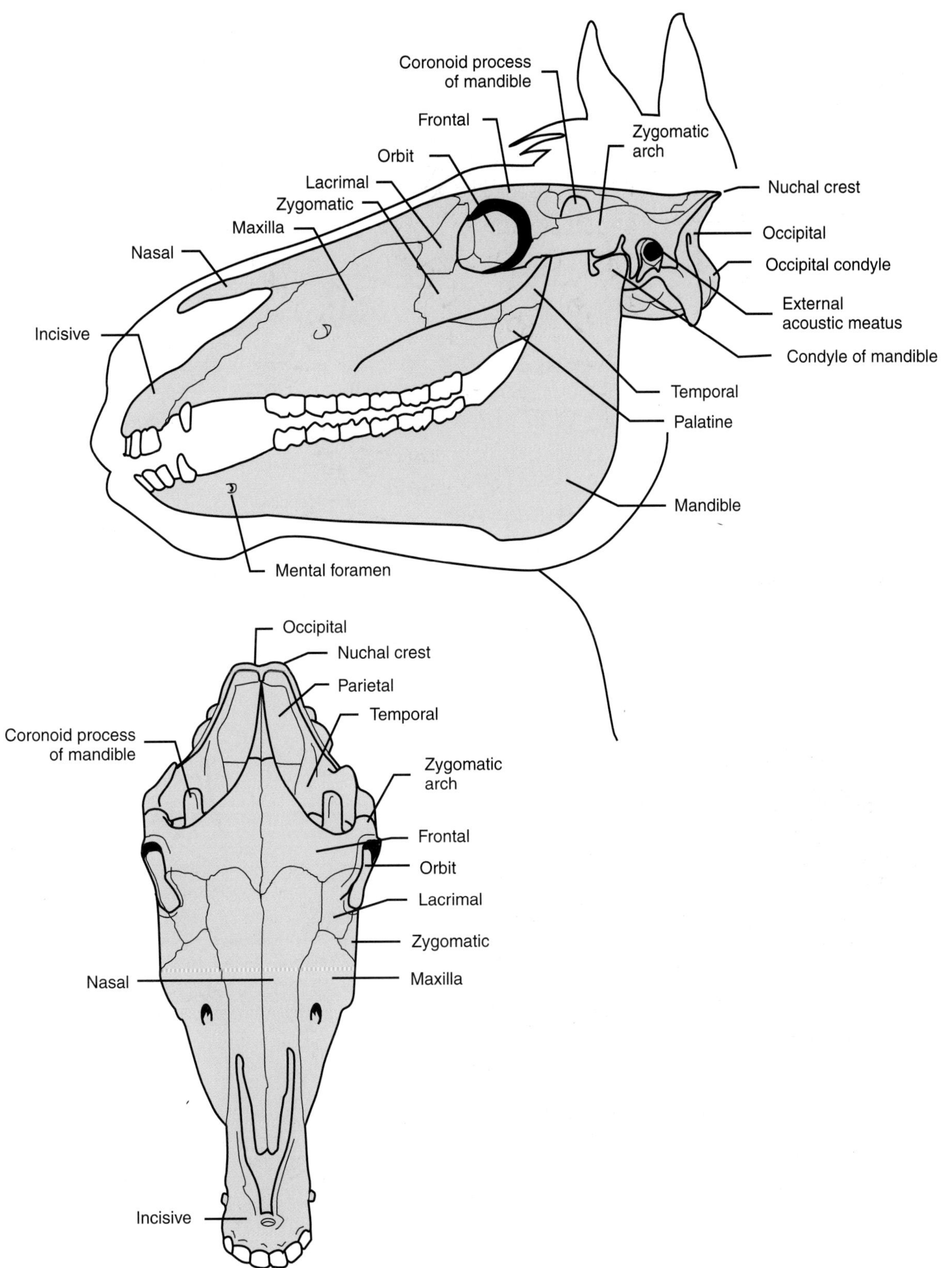

FIGURE **5-6** **Skull of the Horse.**

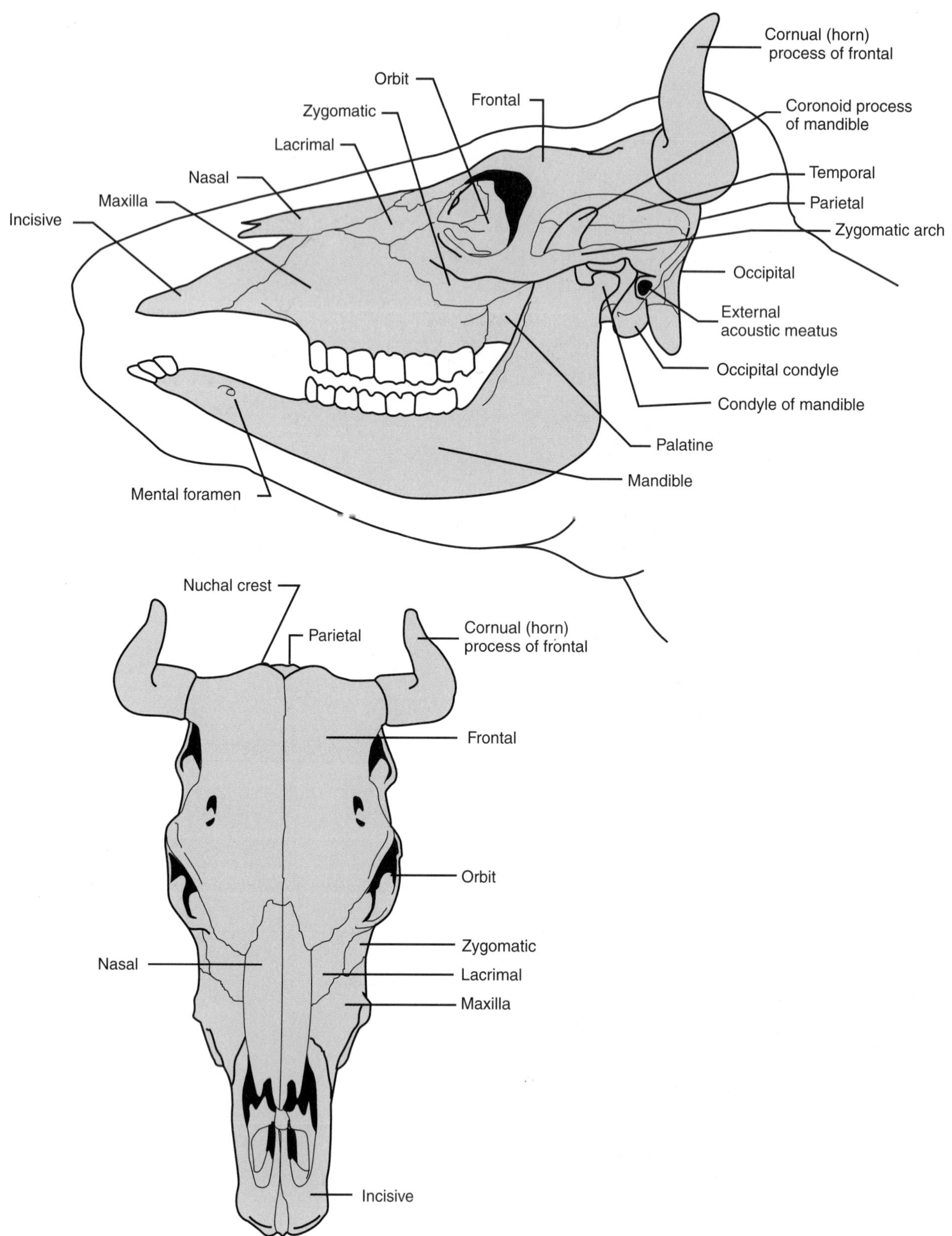

FIGURE **5-7** **Skull of the Cow.**

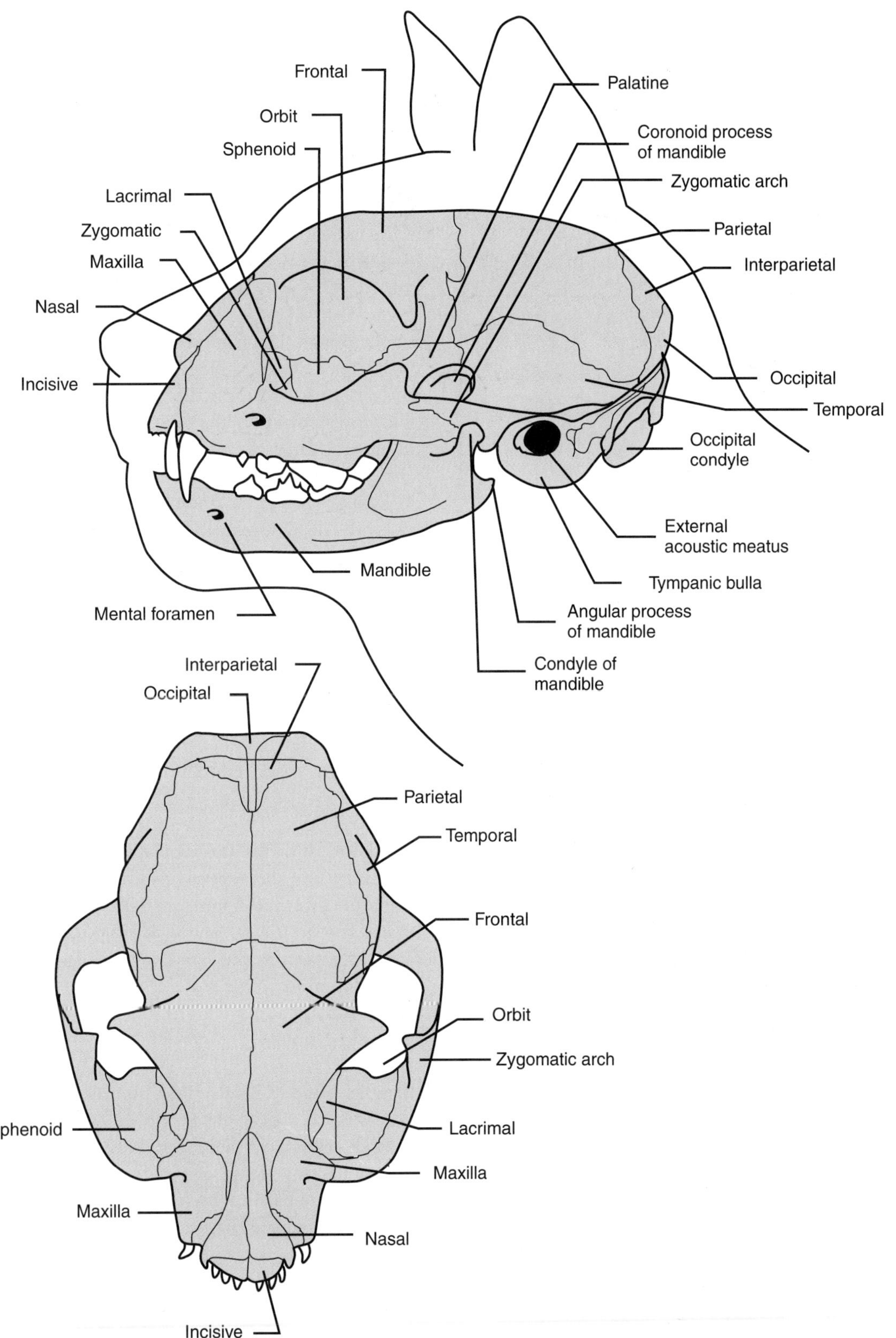

FIGURE **5-8** **Skull of the Cat.**

Table 5-1 Skull Bones*

External (Landmarks)	Internal (Hidden)
Bones of the Cranium	
Frontal bones (2)	Ethmoid bone (1)
Interparietal bones (2)	Sphenoid bone (1)
Occipital bones (1)	
Parietal bones (2)	
Temporal bones (2)	
Bones of the Ear	
None	Incus (2)
	Malleus (2)
	Stapes (2)
Bones of the Face	
Incisive bones (2)	Palatine bones (2)
Lacrimal bones (2)	Pterygoid bones (2)
Mandible (1 or 2)	Turbinates (4)
Maxillary bones (2)	Vomer bone (1)
Nasal bones (2)	
Zygomatic bones (2)	

*Bones are listed in alphabetical order.

where the spinal cord exits the skull and (2) it is the skull bone that articulates (forms a joint) with the first cervical (neck) vertebra. A large hole, the **foramen magnum,** is in the center of the occipital bone. It is where the spinal cord exits the skull. On either side of the foramen magnum are the **occipital condyles**—articular (joint) surfaces that join with the first cervical vertebra (the atlas) to form the atlantooccipital joint (the joint that connects the head with the neck). As you might imagine, injuries to the occipital bone are serious because of its location and the vital structures it encloses. Fortunately, it is well protected by muscles, tendons, and ligaments, so injuries to the occipital bone are rare.

Interparietal Bones. The **interparietal bones** are two small bones located on the dorsal midline between the occipital bone and the parietal bones. They are usually clearly visible in young animals. In older animals they may fuse together into one bone, or they may fuse to the parietal bones and become indistinguishable.

Parietal Bones. The two **parietal bones** form the dorsolateral walls of the cranium. They are large and well developed in the dog and cat (and human) but are relatively small in horses and cattle.

Temporal Bones. The two **temporal bones** are located ventral to (below) the parietal bones. The temporal bones are important for several reasons. They form the lateral walls of the cranium, they contain the middle and inner ear structures, and they are the skull bones that form the **temporomandibular joints** (TMJs) with the mandible (lower jaw). The ear structures are contained within the temporal bone, and most are not visible from the outside. The only ear structure that is visible from the outside is the **external acoustic meatus**—the bony canal that leads into the middle and inner ear cavities. In the living animal it contains the external ear canal. By looking into the external acoustic meatus, we can see the middle ear cavity. Ventral to (below) the external acoustic meatus on each side is the concave articular (joint) surface that receives the condyle of the mandible to form the TMJ. These articular surfaces are located on the ventral (bottom) surface of each of the temporal bones.

Frontal Bones. The **frontal bones** form the "forehead" region of the skull. They are located just rostral to (ahead of) the parietal bones and form the rostrolateral portion of the cranium and a portion of the orbit (the concave socket that holds the eye). A large **paranasal sinus,** the **frontal sinus,** is contained within the frontal bone. In horned breeds of cattle, the **cornual process** of the frontal bone is the "horn core" around which the horn develops. This process is hollow and communicates with the frontal sinus. When adult cattle are dehorned, the cornual processes are sawed off and we can look right down into the frontal sinus. This is a really good reason to dehorn cattle when they are young, before the "horn buds" have united with the frontal bone.

Internal Bones of the Cranium

The two hidden bones of the cranium are the sphenoid bone and the more rostral ethmoid bone.

Sphenoid Bone. The single **sphenoid bone** forms the ventral part (bottom) of the cranium and contains a depression (the **pituitary fossa**) that houses the pituitary gland—an important endocrine (hormone-producing) gland. The sphenoid bone is located just rostral to (ahead of) the occipital bone. If it is removed from the skull and examined, the sphenoid bone looks kind of like a bat with its wings and legs extended. The sphenoid bone of most animals contains a paranasal sinus (the **sphenoidal sinus**).

Ethmoid Bone. The **ethmoid bone** is a single bone located just rostral to (ahead of) the sphenoid bone. It contains the sievelike **cribriform plate** through which the many branches of the olfactory (sense of smell) nerve pass from the upper portion of the nasal cavity to the olfactory bulbs of the brain. Horses (and humans) have a small paranasal sinus, the **ethmoidal sinus,** in the ethmoid bone.

Bones of the Ear

The three tiny but very important pairs of ear bones are hidden away in the middle ear. Known as the **ossicles,** the bones (from outside in) are the **malleus** (hammer), the **incus** (anvil), and the **stapes** (stirrup). Their function is to transmit vibrations from the **tympanic membrane** (eardrum) across the middle ear cavity to an inner ear structure called the *cochlea*. In the cochlea, receptor cells for hearing convert the vibrations to nerve impulses that are interpreted by the brain as sound. The characteristics and functions of the ossicles are covered more completely in Chapter 13.

External Bones of the Face

The **bones of the face** make up the rest of the skull. We can also divide them into external (landmark) bones and internal (hidden) bones.

Starting at the rostral (front) end of the skull and working caudally (toward the rear), the external bones of the face are the incisive bones, the nasal bones, the maxillary bones, the lacrimal bones, the zygomatic bones, and the mandible.

Incisive Bones. The two **incisive bones** (sometimes called the *premaxillary bones*) are the most rostral (forward) skull bones. In all common domestic animals except ruminants, such as cattle, sheep, and goats, the incisive bones house the upper incisor teeth. Our ruminant friends do not have upper incisor teeth; they have a hard dental pad instead.

Nasal Bones. The two **nasal bones** form the "bridge" of the nose, that is, the dorsal (upper) part of the nasal cavity. Considerable variety is seen in the relative size and shape of the nasal bones, depending on the species and breed of animal. The length of the animal's face is the main influence on the nasal bones. In animals with long faces, such as horses and **dolichocephalic** (long-faced) dog breeds (such as collies), the nasal bones are long and thin. In animals with short faces, such as cats and **brachycephalic** (short-faced) breeds of dogs (such as Pekinese), the nasal bones are short and more triangular.

Maxillary Bones. The two **maxillary bones** make up most of the upper jaw. (The incisive bones make up the rest.) They house the upper canine teeth, if present, and all of the cheek teeth (premolars and molars). They also contain the **maxillary sinuses.** Along with the palatine bones, the maxillary bones form the **hard palate,** which is the bony separation between the mouth and the nasal cavity that we call the "roof of our mouth." The maxillary bones form the rostral (forward) portion of the hard palate, and the palatine bones form the caudal (rear) part.

Lacrimal Bones. The **lacrimal bones** are two small bones that form part of the medial portion of the orbit of the eye. A space within each lacrimal bone houses the lacrimal sac (part of the tear drainage system of the eye) in the living animal.

Zygomatic Bones. The two **zygomatic bones** are also known as the *malar bones.* They form a portion of the orbit of the eye and join with a process from the temporal bones to form the **zygomatic arches** on either side of the skull. The caudal (rear)–facing temporal process of the zygomatic bone joins with the rostral (forward)–facing zygomatic process of the temporal bone (do you sense a pattern here?) to form the zygomatic arch on each side. The zygomatic arches are easily palpable, bony landmarks below and behind the eyes that form the widest part of the skull in dogs and cats.

Mandible. The **mandible** is the lower jaw. It houses all the lower teeth and is the only movable skull bone. It forms the TMJ with the temporal bone on each side. In some species, such as dogs, cats, and cattle, the two sides of the mandible are separate bones that are united by a cartilaginous joint, the **mandibular symphysis,** at their rostral (front) ends. Because the symphysis is the weakest part of the mandible, separation of the bones can occur at that site from blunt-force trauma to the face. This is called a *mandibular symphyseal fracture.* This is the most common type of mandibular fracture in dogs and cats. Fortunately, it usually is easy to repair also. In adult horses and swine the two halves of the mandible fuse together into one solid bone. The two main regions of the mandible are the **shaft** and the **ramus.** The shaft is the horizontal portion that houses all the teeth. At its caudal end is the vertical portion of the mandible, the ramus. This is where the powerful jaw muscles attach and where the articular condyles that form the TMJs with the temporal bones are located.

Internal Bones of the Face

The internal bones of the face are the palatine bones, the pterygoid bones, the vomer bone, and the turbinates.

Palatine Bones. The two **palatine bones** make up the caudal portion of the hard palate (the bony part of the roof of the mouth). The palate separates the mouth from the nasal cavity. The rest of the hard palate (the rostral portion) is made up of part of the maxillary bones.

Pterygoid Bones. The two small **pterygoid bones** support part of the lateral walls of the pharynx (throat).

Vomer Bone. The single **vomer bone** is located on the midline of the skull and forms part of the **nasal septum**—the central "wall" between the left and right nasal passages.

Turbinates. The **turbinates** are also called the **nasal conchae.** They are four thin, scroll-like bones that fill most of the space in the nasal cavity. Each side has a dorsal and a ventral turbinate. In the living animal the turbinates are covered by the moist, very vascular soft-tissue lining of the nasal passages. The scroll-like shape of the turbinates forces air inhaled through the nose to pass around many twists and turns as it passes through the nasal cavity. This helps warm and humidify the air and also helps trap any tiny particles of inhaled foreign material in the moist surface of the nasal epithelium. This process helps "condition" the inhaled air before it reaches the delicate lungs. (I'll bet you didn't know you had air conditioners in your nose.)

TEST YOURSELF

1. Name the skull bones that make up each of these groups:
   External bones of the cranium
   Internal bones of the cranium
   Bones of the ear
   External bones of the face
   Internal bones of the face
2. In which skull bones are each of the following structures found?
   Cribriform plate
   External acoustic meatus
   Foramen magnum
   Frontal sinus
   Lacrimal sac
   Lower teeth
   Pituitary fossa
   Upper incisor teeth
   Upper cheek teeth
3. Which would likely be a greater threat to an animal's well-being, a fracture of the mandible or a fracture of the occipital bone? Why?

HYOID BONE

The **hyoid bone,** also called the **hyoid apparatus,** looks somewhat like an "H" that has had its two legs bent back to form a U-shaped structure. It is located high in the neck just above the larynx between the caudal ends of the mandible. It supports the base of the tongue, the pharynx, and larynx and helps the animal swallow. It is usually referred to as a single bone, but it is composed of several individual portions united by cartilage. It is attached to the temporal bone by two small rods of cartilage. Some authors include the hyoid bone as a skull bone for convenience, but its location and attachments seem to indicate that it is a separate bone of the axial skeleton.

SPINAL COLUMN

The **spinal column,** also called the **vertebral column,** is made up of a series of individual irregular bones called **vertebrae** (*singular,* vertebra) that extend from the skull to the tail. The spinal column is divided into five regions—cervical (neck), thoracic (chest), lumbar (abdomen), sacral (pelvis), and coccygeal (tail). Most vertebrae do not have individual names. Instead, they are numbered within each region from cranial to caudal. A shorthand way of referring to particular vertebrae is the abbreviation for the region (*C* for cervical, *T* for thoracic, *L* for lumbar, *S* for sacral, and *Cy* for coccygeal) followed by the number of the vertebra within that region. For example, C5 is the fifth cervical vertebra, and L2 is the second lumbar vertebra. The usual numbers of vertebrae within each region, the vertebral formulas, for some common species are listed in Table 5-2.

Vertebrae Characteristics

A typical vertebra consists of a body, an arch, and a group of processes (Figure 5-9). The body of a vertebra is the main, ventral portion of the bone. It is the strongest, most massive portion. The bodies of adjacent vertebrae are separated by little cartilage "shock absorbers"—the **intervertebral disks.**

Dorsal to the body of a vertebra is the hollow arch. When the arches of all the vertebrae are lined up, they form a long, flexible "tunnel" called the **spinal canal** that houses and protects the spinal cord.

Vertebrae usually have some combination of three kinds of processes. The single, dorsally projecting **spinous process** and the two laterally projecting **transverse processes** vary in size among vertebrae and act as sites for muscle attachment and leverage to move the spine and trunk. The **articular processes** are located on the cranial and caudal ends of the vertebral arches and help form the joints between adjacent vertebrae. Each intervertebral joint allows only very limited movement, but, taken as a whole, the entire spinal column has considerable flexibility. Cats demonstrate this flexibility by the strange positions that they can get their bodies into, especially when they are lying in a sunbeam. *Author's note:* As I was writing this section, one of our cats, Bogie, was doing a spinal flexibility demonstration beside my computer by lying on his back with his front end facing one direction and his back end facing the other.

Cervical Vertebrae

The **cervical vertebrae** are in the neck region. A quick look at Table 5-2 will show that seven cervical vertebrae are found in all common domestic animals and humans. Actually, nearly all

Table 5-2 Vertebral Formulas for Some Common Species

	Cervical	Thoracic	Lumbar	Sacral	Coccygeal
Cat	7	13	7	3	5-23
Cattle	7	13	6	5	18-20
Dog	7	13	7	3	20-23
Goat	7	13	7	5	16-18
Horse	7	18	6	5	15-21
Human	7	12	5	5	4-5
Pig	7	14-15	6-7	4	20-23
Sheep	7	13	6-7	4	16-18

mammals have seven cervical vertebrae. Even the long-necked giraffe has only seven v-e-r-y l-o-n-g cervical vertebrae. This is the only group of vertebrae that has a constant number across most species.

The first two cervical vertebrae are somewhat unusual in shape and have specific names (Figure 5-10). The first (C1) is called the **atlas** because, like the mythical figure Atlas who holds up the world, this vertebra "holds up" the head. The atlas has two large, winglike transverse processes (called the *wings of the atlas*) that can be **palpated** (felt) just behind the skulls of most animals. The next time you are around a dog or cat, feel the wings of the atlas right behind the skull. The atlas is unique in that it has no vertebral body. It just consists of a bony ring that the spinal cord passes through with the two wings sticking out laterally. Just caudal to the atlas is the second cervical vertebra (C2)—the **axis.** Its most prominent features are its large, bladelike spinous process that projects up dorsally and the peglike **"dens"** that fits into the caudal end of the atlas. The rest of the cervical vertebrae are fairly normal looking and are just numbered like the rest of the vertebrae.

Thoracic Vertebrae

The **thoracic vertebrae** are located dorsal to the thorax. Their number varies among species and can even vary

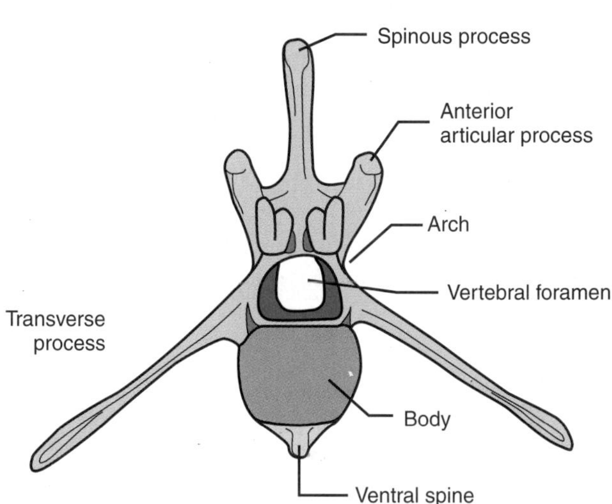

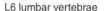

FIGURE **5-9** **Basic Anatomy of Vertebra.**

CLINICAL APPLICATION: Fun Facts About Human Intervertebral Disks

Because we walk upright, gravity compresses our intervertebral disks slightly when we're up moving around during the day. At night when we lie down and sleep, the compression stops and the disks expand back to their original size. The compression and expansion of each individual disk are very slight, but when combined, the variation in the total length of the spine is measurable. We are tallest in the morning—by as much as ½ to 1 inch! We proceed to get shorter throughout the day. For astronauts living in the microgravity environment of space, the result is even more impressive. After just a few days in space, their spines can expand by 2 inches or more. Some astronauts report soreness in their backs during the first few days in space because of this spinal expansion stretching the muscles around the spinal column. This dramatic increase in height is temporary, however. Astronauts quickly return to their normal terrestrial height when they return to earth.

CLINICAL APPLICATION: Intervertebral Disk Disease

Normal intervertebral disks have a soft, cushioning center of gelatinous material (the nucleus pulposus) surrounded by tough fibrocartilage. On their sides and bottoms, intervertebral disks are surrounded by tough ligaments and dense muscles that support the spinal column and join the vertebrae together. The only thing dorsal to (above) them, however, is the spinal cord, which is tightly encased in the bony spinal canal.

Intervertebral disk disease results when one or more intervertebral disks degenerates. When an intervertebral disk becomes diseased, normal mechanical forces on the spine often result in degenerated disk material being squeezed out. The ligaments and muscles on the sides and bottom of the disk prevent the material from moving in any of those directions. The only direction it can protrude is dorsally, that is, up into the spinal cord. Because the spinal cord is surrounded by bone, the protruded material compresses it. This causes the common clinical signs of intervertebral disk disease: pain, numbness, weakness, and paralysis.

Intervertebral disk disease can occur in any species of animal but is seen most often in dogs, particularly long-backed breeds such as dachshunds. It usually occurs in one of two sites: the cervical (neck) region or the thoracolumbar (midback) region. Cervical disk disease usually causes severe pain. The neck muscles go into spasm, and the animal holds its head and body very rigidly and does not like being touched. Disk disease back in the thoracolumbar region usually causes weakness (paresis) and numbness of the hind legs that can progress to complete paralysis. Treatment options include exercise restriction (cage rest), medical treatment with drugs intended to reduce pressure on the spinal cord, and surgery to directly decompress the spinal cord. The prognosis depends on the location, extent, and duration of the damage to the spinal cord.

Author's note: I once had a dachshund patient with thoracolumbar disk disease whose rear legs remained paralyzed despite weeks of intensive treatment. His owners reluctantly decided to **euthanize** the dog and have him buried in a nearby pet cemetery. The afternoon before the scheduled euthanasia, a representative from the pet cemetery came to our hospital to measure the dog for a coffin. This apparently got the dog's attention because the next morning when the time came to do the regrettable deed, we noticed some slight movement of his rear legs. We canceled the euthanasia, of course, and the dog went on to make a full recovery. I guess he just needed the right kind of motivation.

within a species. Usually, however, the number of thoracic vertebrae is the same as the number of pairs of ribs the animal has. The most characteristic features of thoracic vertebrae are their tall spinous processes and their lateral articular facets, which form joints with the heads of the ribs.

Lumbar Vertebrae

The **lumbar vertebrae** are dorsal to the abdominal region. Like the thoracic vertebrae, their number varies among species and even within a species. The lumbar vertebrae are the most massive-looking bones of the spinal column. Their bodies are large and bulky because they have to support all the weight of

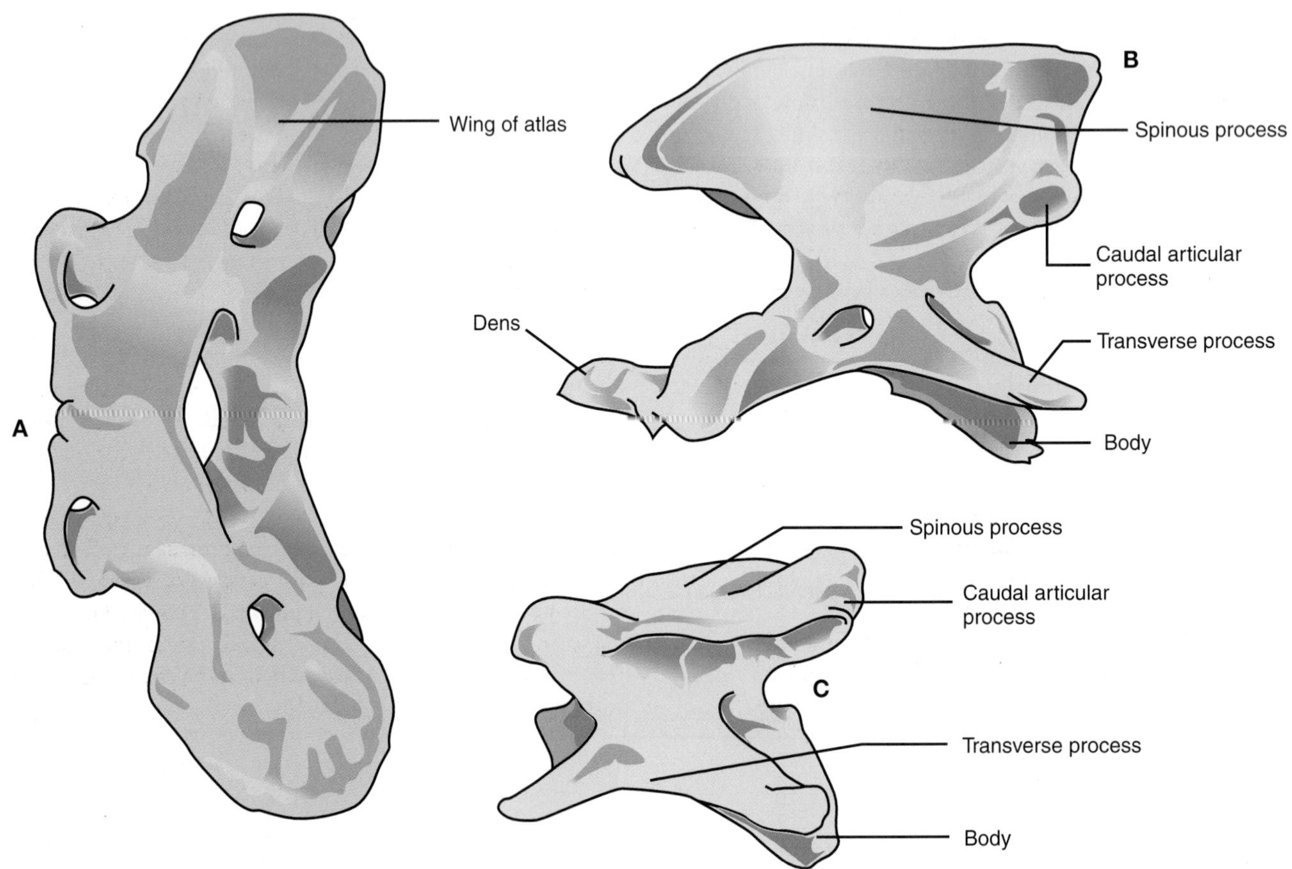

FIGURE 5-10 **Cervical Vertebrae of the Dog. A,** Atlas (C1), dorsal view. **B,** Axis (C2), lateral view. **C,** Fifth cervical vertebra, lateral view.

CLINICAL APPLICATION: Wobbler Syndrome

Wobbler syndrome occurs most commonly in certain breeds of dogs (basset hounds, borzois, Doberman pinschers, and Great Danes) and horses (thoroughbreds). It results from a narrowing of the spinal canal in the cervical region that compresses the spinal cord. The narrowing can result from physical abnormalities (malformations) of cervical vertebrae or improper articulations (joints) between them (malarticulations). The precise cause is not known, but inherited (genetic) factors and nutritional factors seem to be involved. Clinical signs typically develop slowly and gradually, starting with weakness and **ataxia** (incoordination). The name "wobbler syndrome" comes from the wobbly, uncoordinated gait seen in affected animals. The disease can progress to complete paralysis. Medical treatments may be attempted to decrease the compression of the spinal cord, but surgery is often necessary. The prognosis for recovery is usually guarded at best.

CLINICAL APPLICATION: The Anticlinal Vertebra

Dogs are the animal species in which clinical intervertebral disk disease is most commonly seen in most veterinary practices. As a result, veterinary personnel take a lot of spinal radiographs of dogs. The bones of the spine can be confusing to look at when we are trying to identify the precise location of a lesion. The **anticlinal vertebra** is a convenient landmark that can help us. It is the eleventh thoracic vertebra (T11) in the dog and is called *anticlinal* because its spinous process, unlike those of the vertebrae ahead of and behind it, projects straight up vertically. The spinous processes of the first 10 thoracic vertebrae all tilt backward (caudally), and the last two (T12 and T13) incline forward (cranially). So, T11 looks kind of odd sitting there by itself and is easily identified. The anticlinal vertebra in some other animals is T11 in the cat, T16 in the horse, T13 in cattle, T13 in sheep, and T10 in swine.

the abdominal organs and structures without the aid of the ribs, which help support the thoracic contents.

Sacral Vertebrae

The **sacral vertebrae** are unique in that they fuse to form a single solid structure—the **sacrum** (Figure 5-11). The number of vertebrae fused in the sacrum varies among species (see Table 5-2). The sacrum is located dorsal to the pelvic region and forms a joint with the pelvis on each side—the **sacroiliac joint.**

Coccygeal Vertebrae

The **coccygeal vertebrae** are the bones of the tail. Their number varies a lot not just between species but even within a species, and their appearance varies quite a bit even within an individual animal. The first few coccygeal vertebrae have the usual characteristics of vertebrae, such as bodies, arches, and processes, but further caudally, they are reduced to simple little rods of bone. In humans the coccygeal vertebrae are fused into a single bone called the **coccyx,** or what we commonly call our *tailbone.*

RIBS

The **ribs** are long bones that form the lateral walls of the thorax (Figure 5-12). The number of pairs of ribs (one on each side) usually equals the number of thoracic vertebrae that the animal has. At their dorsal ends the heads of the ribs articulate (form joints) with the thoracic vertebrae. These freely movable joints help the process of ventilation (the movement of air in and out of the lungs). By swiveling the ribs at their dorsal ends, the ventilatory muscles can enlarge or diminish the size of the thorax, depending on the direction of the muscle contraction.

The ventral ends of the ribs are a lot more variable. Each rib actually has two parts—a dorsal part made of bone and a ventral part made of cartilage. The cartilaginous part is called the **costal** (rib) **cartilage,** and its junction with the bony part is called the **costochondral junction.** The costal cartilages either directly join the sternum or join the costal cartilage ahead of them (Figure 5-13). The ribs whose cartilages join the sternum are called **sternal ribs** and make up the cranial part of the thorax. The ones that join the adjacent costal cartilage are called **asternal ribs** and make up the caudal part of the thorax. The cartilage of the last rib or two on each side may not join anything at all. It may just end in the muscles of the thoracic wall. These "nonattached" ribs are called **floating ribs.**

STERNUM

The **sternum,** also called the *breastbone,* forms the floor of the thorax. It is made up of a series of rodlike bones called **sternebrae** (see Figure 5-13). Only the first and last sternebrae are named and used as landmarks. The others are numbered from cranial to caudal. The first, most cranial, sternebra is called the **manubrium** (full name, manubrium sterni). The last, most caudal, sternebra is called the **xiphoid** (full name, xiphoid process). A piece of cartilage, the xiphoid cartilage, extends caudally from the xiphoid process and is easily felt in most animals at the caudal end of the sternum.

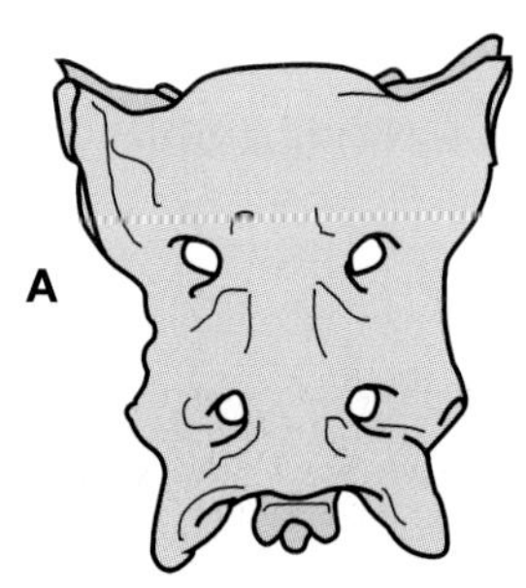

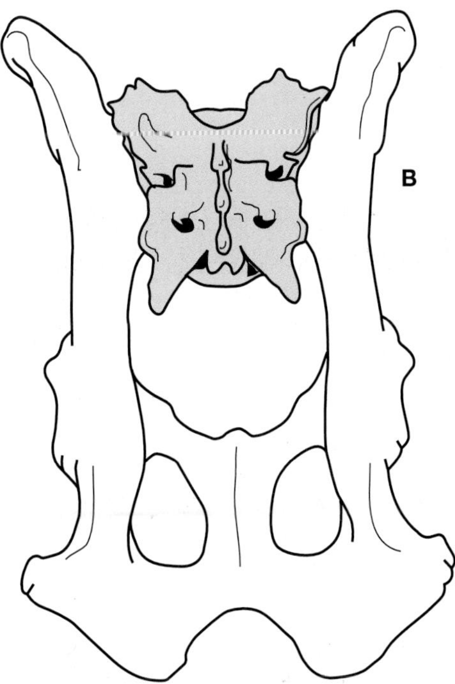

FIGURE **5-11** **Canine Sacrum. A,** Ventral view. **B,** Dorsal view.

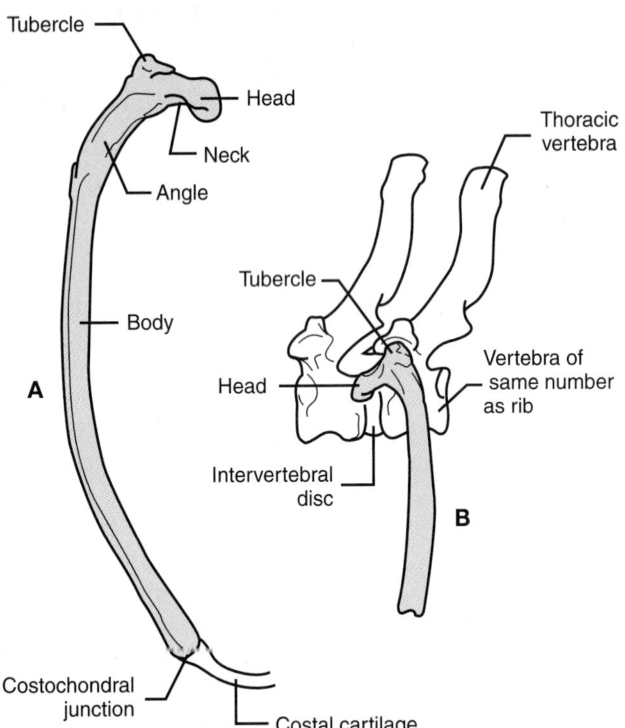

FIGURE **5-12** **Canine Rib. A,** Caudal view of rib. **B,** Lateral view of rib articulating with vertebrae.

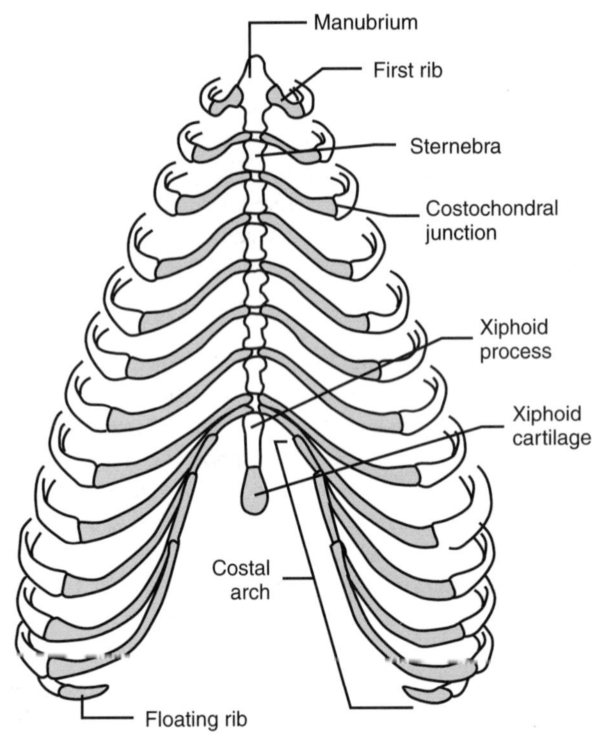

FIGURE **5-13** **Canine Costal Cartilages and Sternum.** Ventral view.

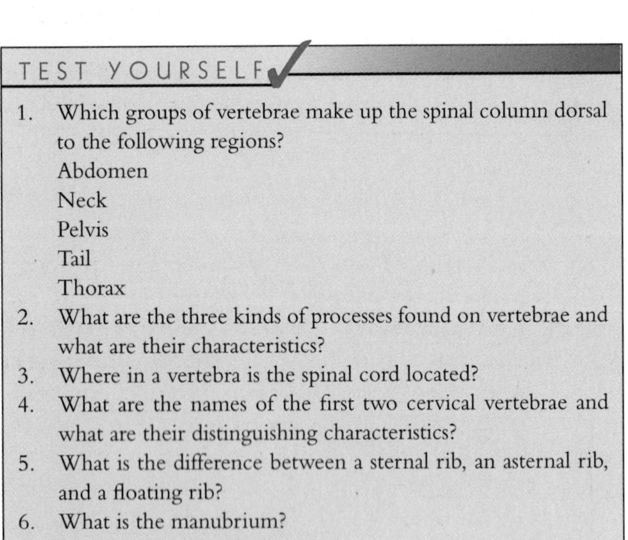
TEST YOURSELF

1. Which groups of vertebrae make up the spinal column dorsal to the following regions?
   Abdomen
   Neck
   Pelvis
   Tail
   Thorax
2. What are the three kinds of processes found on vertebrae and what are their characteristics?
3. Where in a vertebra is the spinal cord located?
4. What are the names of the first two cervical vertebrae and what are their distinguishing characteristics?
5. What is the difference between a sternal rib, an asternal rib, and a floating rib?
6. What is the manubrium?
7. What is the xiphoid?

Table 5-3 Bones of the Limbs (Proximal to Distal)

Thoracic Limb	Pelvic Limb
Scapula	Pelvis
	Ilium
	Ischium
	Pubis
Humerus	Femur
Radius	Tibia
Ulna	Fibula
Carpal bones (carpus)	Tarsal bones (tarsus)
Metacarpal bones	Metatarsal bones
Phalanges	Phalanges

APPENDICULAR SKELETON

The appendicular skeleton is made up of the bones of the main appendages of the animal body, that is, the limbs. In anatomical terms, the front leg is the **thoracic limb,** and the hind leg is the **pelvic limb** (Table 5-3).

Author's suggestion: Find the bones discussed in the following section on skeletons and also identify the bones in living animals. Sometimes they are not where we might think they are.

THORACIC LIMB

In common domestic animals the thoracic limb has no direct bony connection with the axial skeleton. This is in contrast with primates, such as humans, that have a clavicle (collar bone) that joins the scapula (shoulder blade) with the sternum. Instead, the forelegs support the weight of the body by a slinglike arrangement of muscles and tendons. Some animals, such as the dog and cat, may have a small remnant of the clavicle embedded in a tendon in the shoulder region, but it does not articulate with the axial skeleton and is of little or no clinical significance.

Scapula

The **scapula** (shoulder blade) is the most proximal bone of the thoracic limb. It is a flat, somewhat triangular bone with a prominent longitudinal ridge on its lateral surface—the spine of the scapula. At its distal end it forms the socket portion of the ball-and-socket shoulder joint. This fairly shallow, concave articular surface is called the **glenoid cavity.** It is connected with the main part (body) of the scapula by a narrowed area (the neck).

Humerus

The **humerus** is the long bone of the "upper arm," or **brachium.** On its proximal end is the ball portion of the ball-and-socket shoulder joint—the head of the humerus, which is joined to the shaft by a neck. Opposite the head on the proximal end are some large processes, the tubercles, where the powerful shoulder muscles attach. The largest one is called the *greater tubercle.* The shaft of the humerus extends down to the distal end that forms the elbow joint with the radius and ulna. The distal articular surfaces of the humerus are referred to collectively as the *condyle.* To be more precise, the medial articular surface is the *trochlea,* which articulates with the ulna, and the lateral one is the *capitulum,* which articulates with the radius. Just above the condyle on the back surface of the humerus is a deep indentation called the *olecranon fossa* (this is discussed later with the ulna). The nonarticular "knobs" on the medial and lateral surfaces of the condyle are called the *medial* and *lateral epicondyles.* They are easily palpated and can be used as landmarks on living animals.

Author's note: Note the spelling of *humerus.* It looks a lot like the word *humorous,* which might lead you to believe that it is the "funny bone." It is not. Actually, the "funny bone" is not a bone at all. It is the ulnar nerve, which is located fairly superficially as it passes through the elbow joint region. When we bump it, we experience that distinctive "funny bone" tingle.

Radius

Two bones form the "forearm," or **antebrachium**—the radius and the ulna. The **radius** is usually the main weight-bearing bone and along with its partner, the ulna, forms the elbow joint with the distal end of the humerus. On its proximal end the radius has a large, concave articular surface, where it joins with the distal end of the humerus, and facets that articulate with the proximal end of the ulna. The shaft of the radius varies from fairly straight in cats and cattle to somewhat bowed in dogs, horses, and swine. At its distal end the radius has several facets and a pointed process (the styloid process) that articulate with the carpus.

Ulna

The **ulna,** the other bone of the "forearm" (antebrachium), forms a major portion of the elbow joint with the distal end of the humerus. Several interesting structures can be found on its proximal end. The large **olecranon process** forms the point of the elbow. It is the site where the tendon of the powerful triceps brachii muscle attaches. The trochlear notch is a half moon–shaped, concave articular surface that wraps around part of the humeral condyle to help make the elbow joint a very tight, secure joint. At the proximal end of the trochlear notch is a beak-shaped process known as the **anconeal process.** When the elbow is extended (straightened), the anconeal process tucks into the olecranon fossa on the distal end of the humerus. Facets on the proximal end of the ulna articulate with the radius. The shaft of the ulna extends down to the carpus in all common species but the horse. Its shape parallels the straight or curved shape of the radius. In the horse the ulna only consists of the proximal portion that joins with the radius about midshaft. In the other species the distal end of the ulna consists of a pointed process (the styloid process) that articulates with the carpus.

CLINICAL APPLICATION: Ununited Anconeal Process in the Dog

The anconeal process of the ulna develops from a secondary growth center that is separate from the primary growth center in the ulnar shaft. Normally in dogs it fuses to the rest of the ulna by about 6 months of age. Sometimes, particularly in large and giant dog breeds, mechanical forces in the elbow break down the fusion process and prevent the anconeal process from uniting with the rest of the bone. This results in elbow joint instability that damages the joint surfaces and leads to secondary **osteoarthritis.** The affected animal gradually becomes lame. The diagnosis can be confirmed by taking a lateral radiograph of the elbow in the flexed position. This will show the unattached process. Treatment usually involves surgical removal of the ununited anconeal process.

Carpal Bones

The **carpus** consists of two rows of short bones—the **carpal bones.** The two rows of bones are arranged parallel to each other in a proximal row and a distal row. In humans the carpus is our wrist, and in horses it is referred to as the knee. Considerable variety is seen among the species in the precise makeup of the carpus, but a basic naming convention holds true across species lines. The bones of the proximal row are given individual names. All common species have a radial carpal bone, an ulnar carpal bone, and, protruding backward, an accessory carpal bone. Some species also have an intermediate carpal bone. The bones of the distal row of the carpus are given numbers instead of names, starting at the medial side and working laterally. Figure 5-14 shows the distal bones of the horse leg from the carpus on down, and Figure 5-15 shows the comparable bones of the dog.

Metacarpal Bones

The **metacarpal bones** extend distally from the distal row of carpal bones to the proximal phalanges of the digits. In humans, metacarpal bones are the bones of our hands. They extend from our wrists down to our first knuckles and are numbered from medial to lateral. The metacarpal of our

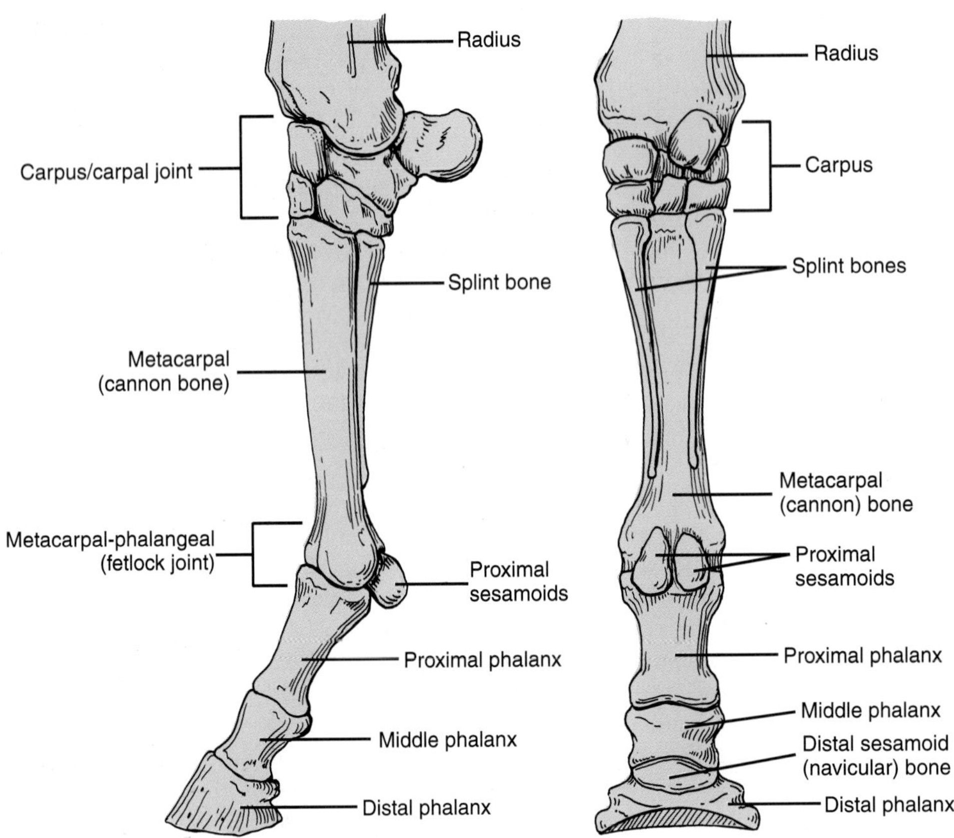

FIGURE **5-14** **Distal Limb Bones of Equine Front Leg.** (From McBride DF: *Learning veterinary terminology,* ed 2, St Louis, 2002, Mosby.)

thumb is metacarpal I, and the one of our little finger is metacarpal V. The flexibility of the joint between the metacarpal bone of our thumb and our wrist makes our thumb apposable with the rest of our hand. This gives us a great grasping advantage over many other animal species. In other animals the appearance of the metacarpal bones is determined largely by what kind of foot the animal has.

Horses have a simple foot consisting of only one digit (toe). Therefore they have only one large metacarpal bone supporting their weight in each leg (see Figure 5-14). This large metacarpal bone is referred to as the **cannon bone** by lay people. Actually, a horse has three metacarpal bones in each leg—one large metacarpal and two smaller, **vestigial** metacarpal bones (the **splint bones**). According to the fossil evidence, ancestors of the modern horse had multiple toes. Over many millennia, those animals became increasingly specialized for speed and eventually developed into the modern horse that walks on only one toe. The large metacarpal bone of the horse is assumed to be what is left of metacarpal III, and the smaller splint bones on either side of it are designated as metacarpals II and IV. There is no remnant of digits I or V. The splint bones do not support any weight and only extend one half to two thirds of the way down the shaft of the large metacarpal. They do, however, sometimes cause problems for horses. They can suffer various kinds of injuries, including fractures. Most commonly, though, the ligaments joining them to the large metacarpal bone become inflamed. This condition is referred to as "splints" and can be quite painful for the horse. Treatment ranges from rest to surgery.

The feet of cattle are like horse feet split in two (Figure 5-16). Cattle walk on two toes. Accordingly, they have two metacarpal bones (bones III and IV), but the two bones are fused into a single bone. A longitudinal groove running down the metacarpal bone clearly shows its two-bone origin, however.

Dogs and cats have paws that are structurally similar to our hands. They typically have five digits (toes) making up their front paws. Figure 5-15 shows the bones of the canine forepaw. The bones of the cat are quite similar. Note that, like us, dogs have five metacarpal bones that are numbered from medial to lateral. Metacarpal I is part of what is usually termed the **dewclaw,** and the others are numbered II, III, IV, and V. Metacarpal V is the lateral-most metacarpal.

Phalanges

We need to clarify and differentiate a couple of terms used to describe animal feet. The anatomical term **digit** means the same as the common term *toe* (and, in our case, *finger*). Each digit is made up of two or three bones called phalanges (*singular,* **phalanx**). So the phalanges are the individual bones that make up the digits.

Horses have one digit on each limb. It is composed of three

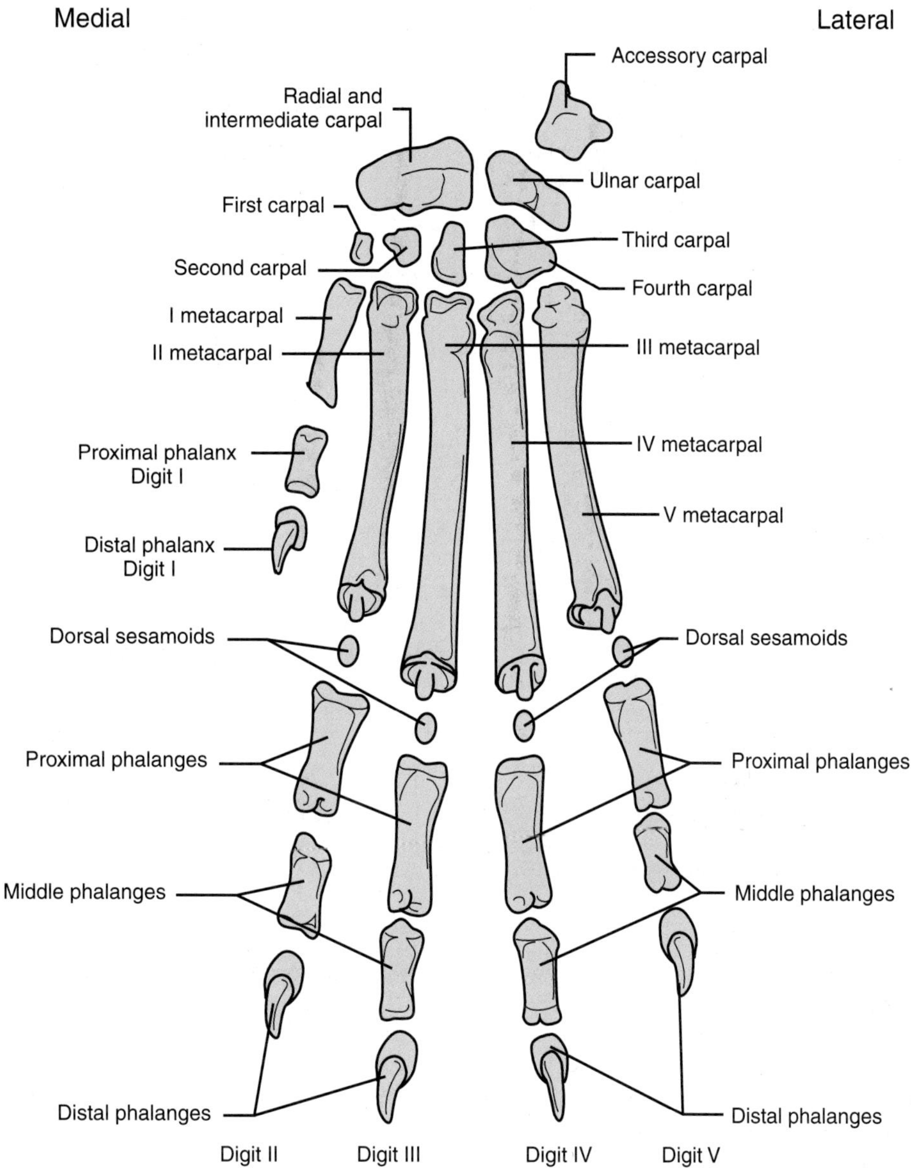

FIGURE **5-15** **Distal Limb Bones of Canine Front Leg.**

phalanges and three sesamoid bones. The phalanges are named according to their position. They are the proximal phalanx (common name, long pastern bone), middle phalanx (common name, short pastern bone), and distal phalanx (common name, coffin bone). In some older anatomy texts the phalanges are numbered from proximal to distal instead of being named. This method works okay in the horse that has only one digit but becomes confusing in animals with multiple digits that are, themselves, numbered. For clarity, we ignore that particular identification scheme.

The digit of the horse also contains two proximal sesamoid bones and one distal sesamoid bone. You may recall that sesamoid bones are irregular bones that are found in some tendons, where they change direction suddenly over the surfaces of joints. They act as "bearings" over the joint surfaces to allow muscles to exert powerful forces on the bones without the tendons wearing out from the constant back-and-forth movement over the joint. The sesamoid bones of the horse digit are important in allowing the spindly, little horse foot to support and propel the large horse body around. The two **proximal sesamoid bones** are located behind the joint between the large metacarpal bone and the proximal phalanx in the large digital flexor tendons. This joint is referred to as the **fetlock joint** by lay people. The **distal sesamoid bone** is located deep in the hoof behind the joint between the middle and distal phalanges where the digital flexor tendon attaches to the distal phalanx. Some imaginative early anatomist thought this distal sesamoid bone resembled a tiny boat. This led to its common name, **navicular bone.** Proximal and distal sesamoid bones are found in both the front and hind digits of the horse.

Cattle have four digits on each limb—two that support weight (the third and fourth) and two that are vestiges (the

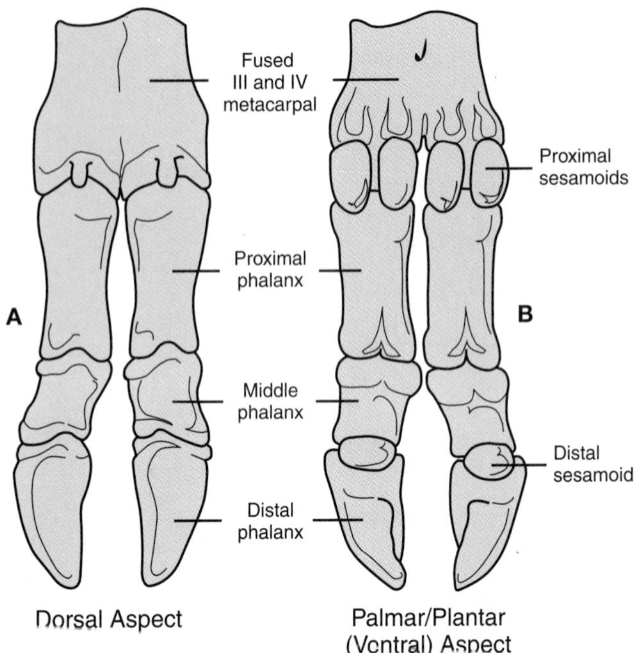

FIGURE **5-16** **Digit of the Cow. A,** Dorsal view. **B,** Palmar/plantar (ventral) view.

CLINICAL APPLICATION **Navicular Disease in the Horse**

Because of its location deep in the hoof where powerful forces are placed on it with each step, the navicular (distal sesamoid) bone is subject to chronic wear and injury. This is particularly true in the front feet because of their more upright position. When the bone starts to undergo chronic, painful degeneration, the condition is called "navicular disease." Despite its name, navicular disease is not one specific disease with one specific cause. It is a complex syndrome that involves many factors, including damage to the bone itself, damage to the bone's blood supply, and damage to surrounding structures, such as bursas, tendons, and ligaments. The net result is a lameness that starts out intermittent and progressively gets worse. The animal tries to shift weight off the heel area of the affected foot where the damaged navicular bone is located. This changes the animal's gait and can lead to secondary problems. The signs of navicular disease can sometimes be managed, but the condition is usually not curable. Some pain relief sometimes can be provided through corrective hoof trimming and shoeing, and through drug therapy.

second and fifth). The two vestigial digits are called the **dewclaws,** and each contains one or two small bones that do not articulate with the rest of the bones of the foot. Figure 5-16 shows the structure of the weight-bearing bones of the bovine foot. As you can see, each digit has a proximal, middle, and distal phalanx, as well as two proximal sesamoid bones and one distal sesamoid bone.

Dog and cat forepaws contain bones that are very similar to our fingers. As you can see in Figure 5-15, digit I, the **dewclaw,** contains only two bones: a proximal phalanx and a distal phalanx. This is similar to our thumb, which contains only two phalanges. Digits II to V each contain three bones: a proximal phalanx, a middle phalanx, and a distal phalanx. Each distal phalanx contains a pointed **ungual process** that is surrounded by the claw in the living animal. The digits of dogs and cats also contain tiny sesamoid bones, but they are rarely of clinical significance except in performance dogs, such as racing greyhounds.

TEST YOURSELF

1. Name the bones of the thoracic limb from proximal to distal.
2. What is the anatomical name for the shoulder blade?
3. What are the brachium and the antebrachium and which bones form them?
4. On which bone is the olecranon process found? What is its purpose?
5. What are the anatomical names for the cannon bone and the splint bones in a horse?
6. Which digit is the dewclaw on the front leg of a dog?
7. What is the common name for the distal sesamoid bone in the horse?

PELVIC LIMB

Unlike the thoracic limb, the pelvic limb is directly connected to the axial skeleton through the sacroiliac joint that unites the pelvis with the spinal column. This eliminates the need for large, slinglike muscles in the rear quarters to support the weight of the caudal part of the body. This allows room for all the reproductive, urinary, and digestive system structures that are present between and behind the rear legs.

Pelvis

The **pelvis** is sometimes referred to anatomically as the *os coxae.* It starts developing as three separate bones on each side that eventually fuse into a solid structure. The two halves of the pelvis are joined ventrally by a cartilaginous joint—the **pelvic symphysis.** Dorsally the pelvis joins the axial skeleton at the left and right sacroiliac joints.

Even though the bones that make up the pelvis fuse together, the names of the individual bones are still used to designate the main regions of the pelvis—the **ilium,** the **ischium,** and the **pubis** (Figure 5-17).

Ilium. The ilium is the forward-most bone of the pelvis. When we put our hands on our hips, the ilium on each side is the bone we have our hands on. It projects up in a dorsocranial direction and is the bone that forms the sacroiliac joints with the sacrum. In dogs and cats the smooth "wing" of the ilium projects forward and is easily felt as a landmark in living animals. In cattle and horses the cranial end of the ilium on each side has large medial and lateral processes. The tuber sacrale projects medially and joins with the sacrum to form the sacroiliac joint. The tuber coxae projects laterally and is called the "point" of the hip.

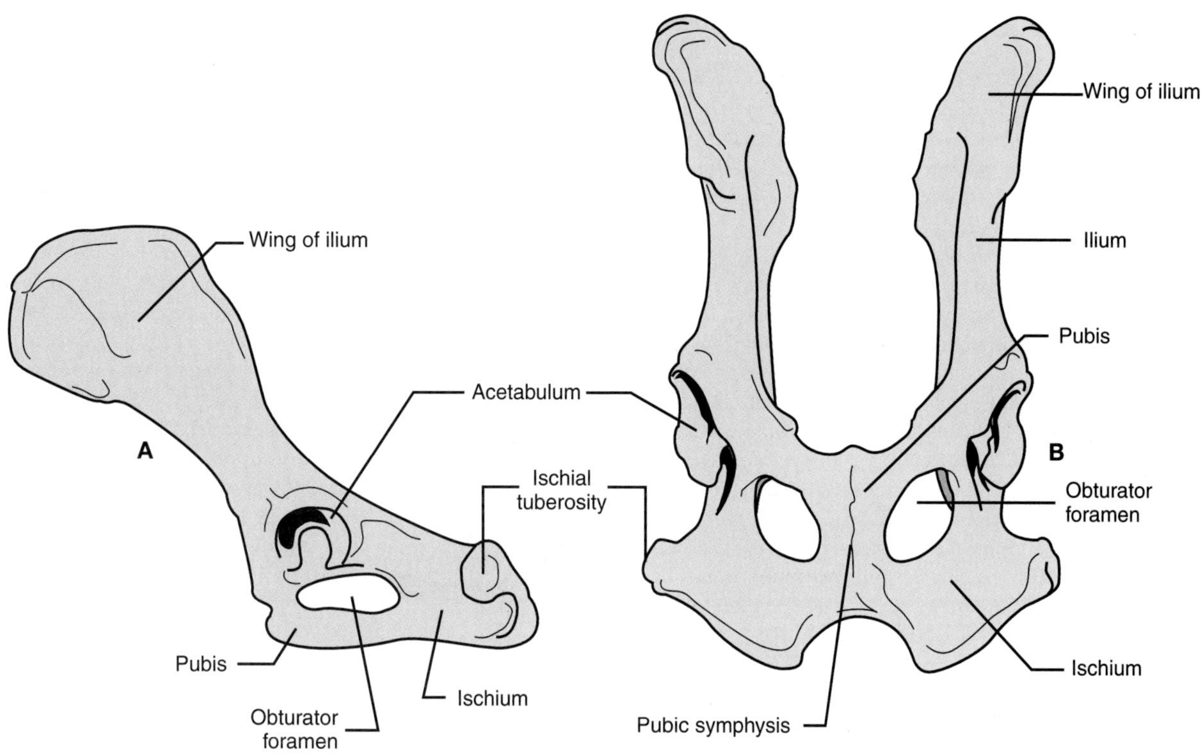

FIGURE **5-17** **Canine Pelvis.** **A,** Lateral view. **B,** Ventral view.

Ischium. The ischium is the caudal-most pelvic bone. If you are sitting down as you are reading this, you are sitting on your ischia. The main rear-projecting process of the ischium is the ischial tuberosity.

Pubis. The pubis is the smallest of the three pelvic bones. It is located medially and forms the cranial portion of the pelvic floor. (The ischium forms the caudal part.)

The three bones that make up each side of the pelvis come together at the socket portion of the ball-and-socket hip joint—a concave area called the **acetabulum.** The acetabulum is a deep socket that tightly encloses the head of the femur to form the quite stable hip joint.

Located on either side of the pelvic symphysis are two large holes—the **obturator foramina.** Usually a big hole in a bone would allow something large and important to pass through it; however, that is not the case here. Nothing but a few small blood vessels and nerves pass through the obturator foramina. Their primary function is to lighten the pelvis. Drag racers use this same principle when they drill numerous holes in many of the chassis components of their race cars to lighten them.

Femur

The femur is the long bone of the "thigh." On its proximal end is the ball portion of the ball-and-socket hip joint (the head of the femur), which is attached to the shaft by a neck. In contrast to the large, round head of the humerus, the head of the femur is smaller and nearly spherical. It normally fits very deeply and securely into the acetabulum of the pelvis. Opposite the head on the proximal end are some large processes, the trochanters, where strong hip and thigh muscles attach. The largest one is called the *greater trochanter.* The shaft of the femur is fairly straight and extends down to the distal end, which forms the stifle joint with the patella and tibia. Three articular surfaces on the distal end of the femur are the two condyles toward the rear and the trochlea on the front. The medial and lateral condyles articulate with the condyles on the proximal end of the tibia. The trochlea is a smooth articular groove in which the patella (kneecap) rides. Like the humerus, the femur has nonarticular "knobs" medial and lateral to the condyles called the *medial* and *lateral epicondyles.* They are easily palpated and can be used as landmarks on living animals.

Patella

The patella, or kneecap, is the largest sesamoid bone in the body. It is formed in the distal tendon of the large quadriceps femoris muscle on the front of the stifle joint. It helps protect the tendon as it passes down over the trochlea of the femur to insert on the tibial crest.

Fabellae

The fabellae are two small sesamoid bones located in the proximal gastrocnemius (calf) muscle tendons just above and behind the femoral condyles of dogs and cats. They are not present in cattle or horses.

CLINICAL APPLICATION: Canine Hip Dysplasia

Canine **hip dysplasia** is an abnormal "looseness" (laxity) of the hip joint(s) of some dogs that leads to joint instability and degenerative bony changes. Many factors contribute to its development, including "overnutrition" leading to too rapid growth, exercise, and genetic factors. Puppies of dysplastic parents are more likely to develop clinical hip dysplasia than are puppies of normal parents, and larger breeds are affected more often than small. In a dysplastic animal the normally tight-fitting hip joint is much looser, allowing the femoral head to "rattle around" in the acetabulum. This damages the joint surfaces, leading to degenerative changes and osteoarthritis development. Movement of the diseased hips is painful, especially after exercise. Definitive diagnosis of canine hip dysplasia usually requires pelvic radiographs. Treatment can range from weight reduction and exercise restriction to medical treatments with antiinflammatory drugs to a variety of surgical procedures. The best treatment for canine hip dysplasia is to attempt to prevent its development by only breeding hip dysplasia–free parents.

CLINICAL APPLICATION: Patellar Luxation in Dogs

Normally the patella rides securely in the deep groove of the trochlea on the distal end of the femur. The pull of the quadriceps tendon is normally directly in line with the trochlea. Sometimes physical abnormalities cause the pull of the tendon to be off-line, or one rim of the trochlear groove is not high enough to hold the patella securely in place. When that occurs the patella can "luxate," or pop out of the trochlea, usually toward the medial side. The most common type of patellar luxation occurs in small and miniature dog breeds and results in the patella popping out of the medial side of the trochlear groove when the animal plants its foot wrong. This causes pain when the animal tries to flex the **stifle joint** to take its next step, and the animal often carries the affected leg (holds it up) for a step or two until the patella pops back into place. This causes a periodic, skipping-type gait that is characteristic of this disorder. The condition is easily diagnosed by extending the stifle joint and palpating the easily displaced patella. Treatment usually consists of any of several surgical corrections.

Tibia

The **tibia** is the main weight-bearing bone of the lower leg. It forms the **stifle joint** with the femur above it and the hock with the tarsus below it. When viewed from above, the proximal end of the tibia appears triangular with the apex of the triangle facing forward. The tibial condyles on top of the proximal end articulate with the condyles of the femur. The forward-facing point of the triangle is the tibial tuberosity, which continues distally as a ridge (the **tibial crest**). The patellar tendon attaches to the tibial tuberosity. The shaft of the tibia is triangular at the proximal end and fairly round further distally. At its distal end the articular surface of the tibia consists of grooves that articulate with the tibial tarsal bone. Medial to the distal articular surface of the tibia is a palpable process called the *medial malleolus.* The "knob" on the medial side of our ankle is our medial malleolus (the distal end of our tibia). If you start at the tibial crest just below the front of your knee, you can trace down the tibia (shinbone) to your medial malleolus.

Fibula

The **fibula** is thin but complete bone in the dog and cat that parallels the tibia and consists of a proximal extremity, a shaft, and a distal extremity. It does not support any significant weight. It mainly serves as a muscle attachment site. In horses and cattle, only the proximal and distal ends of the fibula are present. The shaft is not present. At its distal end, the fibula forms a palpable process called the *lateral malleolus.* The lateral "knob" of our ankle is our lateral malleolus.

Tarsal Bones

The **tarsus** is what we call our ankle or the **hock** of a four-legged animal. It consists of two rows of short bones known as the **tarsal bones.** Like the carpus, the proximal row of bones is named, and the distal row is numbered. The two largest proximal tarsal bones are the tibial tarsal bone and the fibular tarsal bone. A smaller central tarsal bone is tucked behind the two larger bones. The tibial tarsal bone has a large trochlea that articulates with the distal end of the tibia to form the most movable part of the hock joint. The **calcaneal tuberosity** of the fibular tarsal bone projects upward and backward to form the point of the hock. It acts as the point of attachment for the tendon of the large gastrocnemius (calf) muscle and corresponds to our heel. The distal row of tarsal bones is numbered from medial to lateral, much like the distal row of carpal bones.

Metatarsal Bones

The **metatarsal bones** are almost exactly the same as the metacarpal bones. The only major differences are in the dog and cat. Usually only four digits make up the paw on each hind leg, so there are usually only four metatarsal bones: metatarsals II to V. Like the front leg, horses have a large metatarsal bone (the cannon bone) and two small metatarsal bones (the splint bones) on each hind leg. Our metatarsal bones are the bones of our feet.

Phalanges

The phalanges of the pelvic limb are almost exactly like the phalanges of the thoracic limb. The only major difference is, again, in the dog and cat. Usually only four digits make up the paw on each hind leg (digits II to V).

TEST YOURSELF

1. Name the bones of the pelvic limb from distal to proximal.
2. What three pairs of bones make up the pelvis? What region of the pelvis does each form?
3. What is the largest sesamoid bone in the animal body?
4. Which bone is larger and supports more of an animal's weight, the tibia or the fibula?
5. On which bone of the pelvic limb is the calcaneal tuberosity found? What is its purpose?

VISCERAL SKELETON

The visceral skeleton consists of bones that form in soft organs (viscera). It is the strangest division of the skeleton and the most variable. Not all animals have visceral bones. As a matter of fact, they are pretty unusual. Three examples include the **os cordis, os penis,** and **os rostri.** The os cordis is a bone in the heart of cattle and sheep that helps support the valves of the heart. The os penis is a bone in the penis of dogs (as well as beaver, raccoons, and walruses) that partially surrounds the penile portion of the urethra. The os rostri is a bone in the nose of swine that strengthens the snout for the rooting behavior of pigs, whereby they dig into the ground with their snouts. In Europe, pigs are used to find and root out rare and expensive "truffles," a type of underground fungus used in gourmet cooking.

JOINTS

Joints are the junctions between bones. Some of them are completely immovable, some are slightly movable, and some are free movable. When we think of joints, we usually think of freely movable joints, such as the elbow or the hip; however, the immovable sutures that hold most of the skull bones together are joints also.

JOINT TERMINOLOGY

The terms *arthro-* and *articular* refer to joints. For example, the study of joints is *arthrology,* and the smooth bony surfaces that come together to form freely movable joints are called *articular* surfaces.

The terminology of arthrology can be confusing. The meanings of many anatomical terms used to describe types of joints are obscure and cryptic to many of us. In our discussions of joints, we use the clearer terms commonly used in clinical veterinary medicine. The more complex anatomical terms are mentioned in case you wish to consult other, more in-depth anatomical references.

TYPES OF JOINTS

The three general classifications of joints in the animal body are the immovable **fibrous joints,** the slightly movable **cartilaginous joints,** and the freely movable **synovial joints.**

Fibrous Joints

The anatomical term for fibrous joints is **synarthroses.** (See what I mean about that obscure terminology?) Fibrous joints are immovable in that the bones are firmly united by fibrous tissue. Some examples include the sutures that unite most of the skull bones and the fibrous union of the splint bones of horses with the large metacarpal and metatarsal bones.

Cartilaginous Joints

Slightly movable cartilaginous joints are termed **amphiarthroses.** They are capable of only a slight rocking movement. Examples include the intervertebral disks between the bodies of adjacent vertebrae in the spine and the symphyses between the two halves of the pelvis and between the two sides of the mandible in some animals.

Synovial Joints

Synovial joints are what we usually think of when we hear the word *joint.* They are freely movable joints, such as the shoulder joint and the stifle joint. The anatomical term for synovial joints is **diarthroses.**

The rest of our discussion of joints centers on synovial joints.

SYNOVIAL JOINT CHARACTERISTICS

Synovial joints all share some common characteristics. These include articular surfaces on the bones, articular cartilage covering the articular surfaces, and a fluid-filled **joint cavity** enclosed by a **joint capsule.** Firm connective tissue bands called **ligaments** may help stabilize the bones and hold the joint together.

Articular surfaces are the very smooth joint surfaces of bones where they rub together in a joint. They consist of a smooth, thin layer of compact bone over the top of cancellous bone.

Articular cartilage is a thin, smooth layer of hyaline cartilage that lies on top of the articular surface of a bone. The articular cartilage functions like a Teflon coating on the joint surfaces to aid the smooth movement between joint surfaces and reduce friction.

The joint cavity, called the **joint space,** clinically is a fluid-filled potential space between the joint surfaces. A multilayered joint capsule surrounds it. The outer layer of the joint capsule is fibrous tissue, and the lining layer is called the *synovial membrane.* The synovial membrane produces the **synovial fluid** that lubricates the joint surfaces. Synovial fluid is normally transparent and has the viscosity of medium-weight motor oil. When joint disease is suspected, a joint "tap" is often done. This involves doing a surgical skin prep, inserting a sterile needle into the joint cavity, and withdrawing synovial fluid for examination, analysis, and possible bacterial culture.

Ligaments are bands of fibrous connective tissue that are present in and around many synovial joints. They are similar to tendons but differ in that they join bones to other bones. Tendons join muscles to bones. They are not present in all synovial joints, but when they are present, they are often vital to the joint's effective operation.

The ligaments of the stifle joint offer a nice model of how important ligaments can be to normal joint function. The arrangement of the joint surfaces of the stifle joint, between the distal end of the femur and the proximal end of the tibia, make it an inherently unstable joint. No deep sockets or closely fitting heads are present to hold it together or to allow only the desired hingelike movements between the bones. The round condyles of the femur sit on top of the flattish condyles of the tibia, supported only by two shallow, concave, half moon–shaped cartilage structures called the medial and lateral **meniscus.** Proper function of the stifle joint depends on a large tendon and a group of four ligaments. The patellar tendon,

Clinical Application: Cranial Cruciate Ligament Rupture

Sometimes, particularly in dogs, a wrong step can result in tearing (rupture) of the cranial cruciate ligament (CCL). The other ligaments are damaged less often than the CCL. This can occur in athletic dogs if they plant their foot wrong while running and turning, or it can occur in overweight, sedentary dogs if they land wrong as they jump off the couch. The result is instability of the stifle joint. Instead of just hinging on each other like they are supposed to, the femur and tibia also slide forward and backward relative to each other. This can damage other joint structures, such as the menisci, and lead to osteoarthritis in the joint. CCL rupture is diagnosed by palpating the stifle joint and producing what is called "anterior drawer movement"—an abnormal forward and backward movement of the femur and tibia relative to each other. Therapy of CCL rupture can range from exercise restriction and weight reduction to any of several surgical repair techniques.

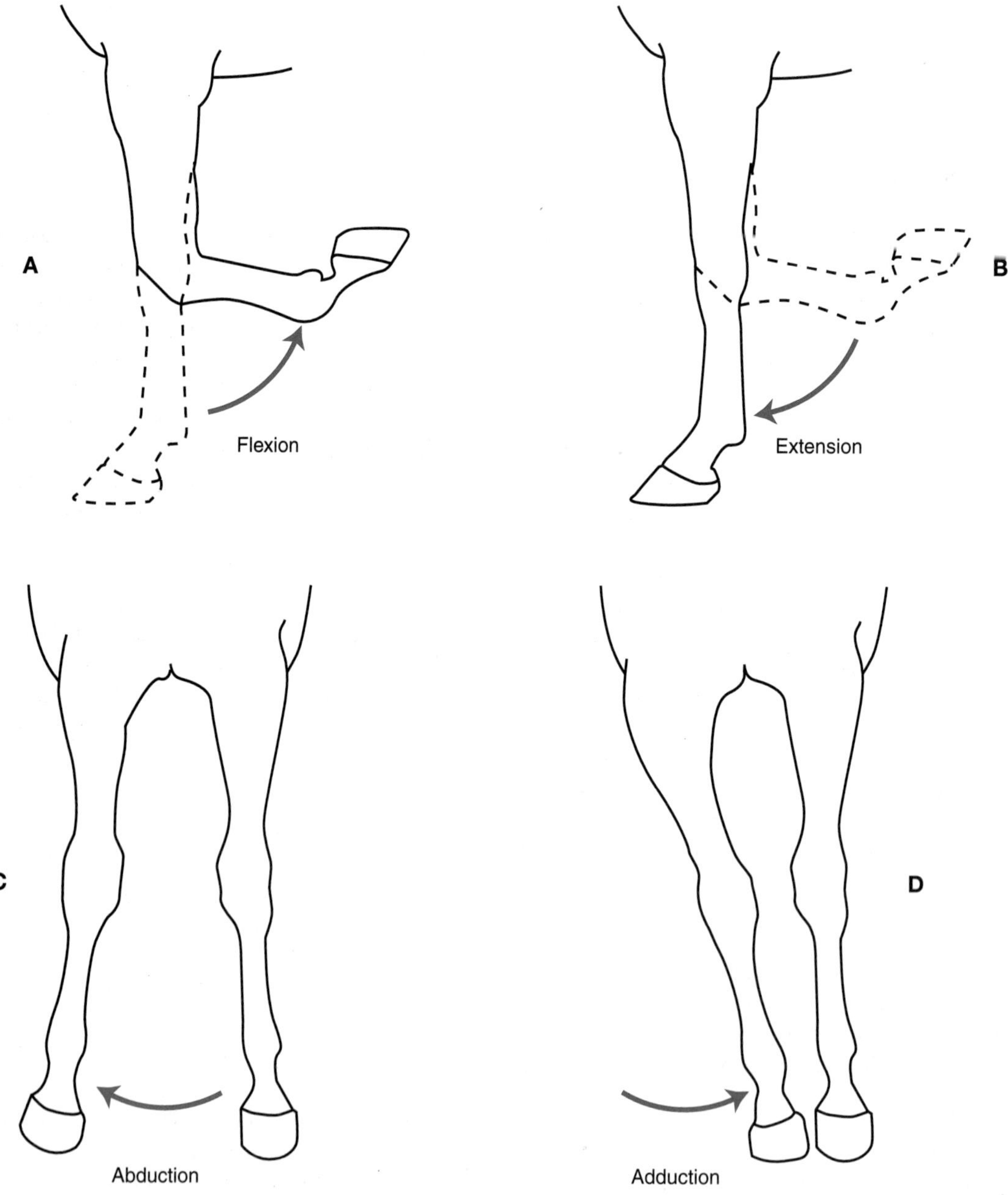

FIGURE **5-18** **Movements of Equine Front Leg. A,** Flexion, lateral view. **B,** Extension, lateral view. **C,** Abduction, cranial view. **D,** Adduction, cranial view.

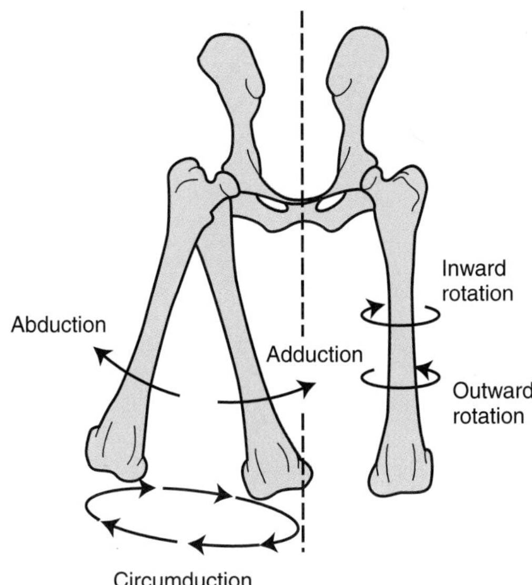

FIGURE **5-19** **Movements of Canine Femurs.** Cranial view.

which is sometimes called the *patellar ligament,* provides support on the front of the joint. On the medial and lateral sides of the joint, two straplike collateral (meaning "on both sides") ligaments connect the femur and the tibia. Inside the joint are two ligaments that cross each other in an "X" shape. They are called the cranial and caudal cruciate (X-shaped) ligaments. They help prevent the bones of the stifle from sliding back and forth as the joint bends and straightens.

Synovial Joint Movements

The range of movements possible in synovial joints are illustrated in Figures 5-18 and 5-19. They are **flexion, extension, adduction, abduction, rotation** and **circumduction.**

Flexion and extension are opposite movements. Flexion decreases the angle between two bones. Picking a horse's front foot up for examination flexes the carpus joint. Extension is the opposite movement—an increase in the angle between two bones. Straightening a bent (flexed) elbow joint extends the joint.

Adduction and abduction are also opposite movements. They involve movement of extremities relative to the median plane of the body. Adduction is the movement of an extremity toward the median plane, and abduction is a movement away from the median plane. One way to keep them straight is to remember that to *abduct* something is to take it *away.*

Rotation is a twisting movement of a part on its own axis. If you hold your arm out with your palm down and move it so your palm is up, that movement is rotation.

Circumduction is the movement of an extremity so that the distal end moves in a circle. You can produce this movement by extending your arm and moving your hand in a circle.

Types of Synovial Joints

Synovial joints can be categorized according to the type of joint surfaces and the movements that are possible. Most of the joints of the body can be classified into one of four basic joint types: **hinge joints, gliding joints, pivot joints,** and **ball-and-socket joints.**

Hinge Joints

Hinge joints are also called **ginglymus joints.** One joint surface swivels around another. The only movements possible are flexion and extension. The elbow joint is a good example of a hinge joint.

Gliding Joints

The complicated name for gliding joints is **arthrodial joints.** Actually, "rocking joints" would be more descriptive. The joint surfaces of a gliding joint are relatively flat. The movement between them is a rocking motion of one bone on the other. The main movements possible are flexion and extension, but some abduction and adduction may also be possible. The carpus is a good example of a gliding joint. Note that you can flex and extend your wrist (carpus), but you can also move your hand side to side (abduction and adduction). Most four-legged animals can only do the flexion and extension part.

Pivot Joints

Pivot joints are also known as **trochoid joints.** One bone pivots (rotates) on another. The only movement possible is rotation. Only one true pivot joint is found in the bodies of most animals, that being the joint between the first and second cervical vertebrae. Some anatomists with a sense of humor refer to this as the "no" joint because the only movement it allows is a rotation of the head back and forth in a "no" movement. The movement is actually occurring between the vertebrae, but the head goes along with the first cervical vertebra as it pivots on the second cervical vertebra.

Ball-and-Socket Joints

Ball-and-socket joints are also called **spheroidal joints.** They allow the most extensive movements of all the joint types—basically, all the synovial joint movements. Ball-and-socket joints permit flexion, extension, abduction, adduction, rotation, and circumduction. The shoulder and hip joints are ball-and-socket joints.

TEST YOURSELF

1. What are the main characteristics of fibrous joints, cartilaginous joints, and synovial joints?
2. What is synovial fluid and why is it important to the functioning of a synovial joint?
3. What is the difference between a tendon and a ligament?
4. Make the following joint movements with your own body: abduction, adduction, circumduction, extension, flexion, and rotation.
5. Name some examples of each of these kinds of synovial joints:
   Ball-and-socket joint
   Gliding joint
   Hinge joint
   Pivot joint

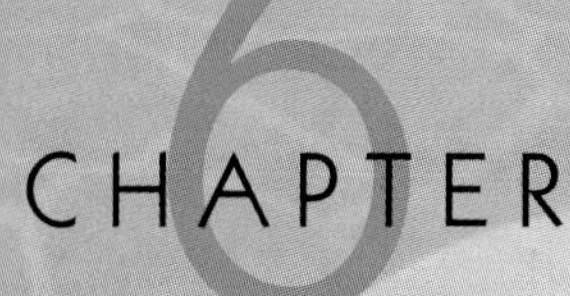

CHAPTER 6

The Integument and Related Structures

Joanna M. Bassert

THE INTEGUMENT

The **integument** is one of the largest and most extensive organ systems in the body. Composed of all four tissue types, it covers and protects underlying structures and forms a critical barrier between the delicate inner workings of the body and the harsh elements of the external world. Its surface is constantly being rubbed, scratched, attacked by microbes, irritated by external parasites and subjected to environmental chemicals and ultraviolet radiation. The skin, together with related structures, forms the **integumentary system** or "common integument." This system involves every inch of the external animal and includes hair, hooves, horns, claws, and various skin-related glands. It is contiguous with the mucous membranes that line the mouth, anus, and nostrils and has a remarkable ability to regenerate and heal.

Although derived from living germinal layers, the outer shell of an animal or person is entirely dead. Remarkably, everything you see from the hair to the skin is composed of dead cells. Once alive in histologically deeper layers and in earlier stages of development, these cells gave up vital organelles and nuclei to make room for the tough, protective substance called *keratin*. It is during this process, called **keratinization,** that the cell expires.

The integument carries out a plethora of protective and regulatory duties. As already mentioned, it prevents desiccation and reduces the threat of injury. In addition, it assists in the maintenance of normal body temperature and excretes water, salt, and organic wastes. It is an important sensory organ that takes in information from the environment via touch and pressure and conveys this input to regions of the central nervous system. It is also engaged in the synthesis of **vitamin D** and in the storage of nutrients.

The thickness of skin varies among species and its location in the body. The thinnest skin, for example, tends to occur around the eye and in the scrotum, whereas some of the thickest layers can be found in the center of the back, between the shoulder blades, and on the paw pads.

Histologically, skin forms two distinct layers: the **epidermis** and the underlying **dermis** (also known as the *corium*). These layers are separated by an epithelial basement membrane. In some species, this membrane is wavy and undulates, creating infoldings and outpouchings. The downward folds of the epidermis interdigitate with the upward projections of the dermis, which are called **dermal papillae.** These interdigitations help to cement the epidermis and the dermis together and are therefore most pronounced in areas where there is a great deal of friction.

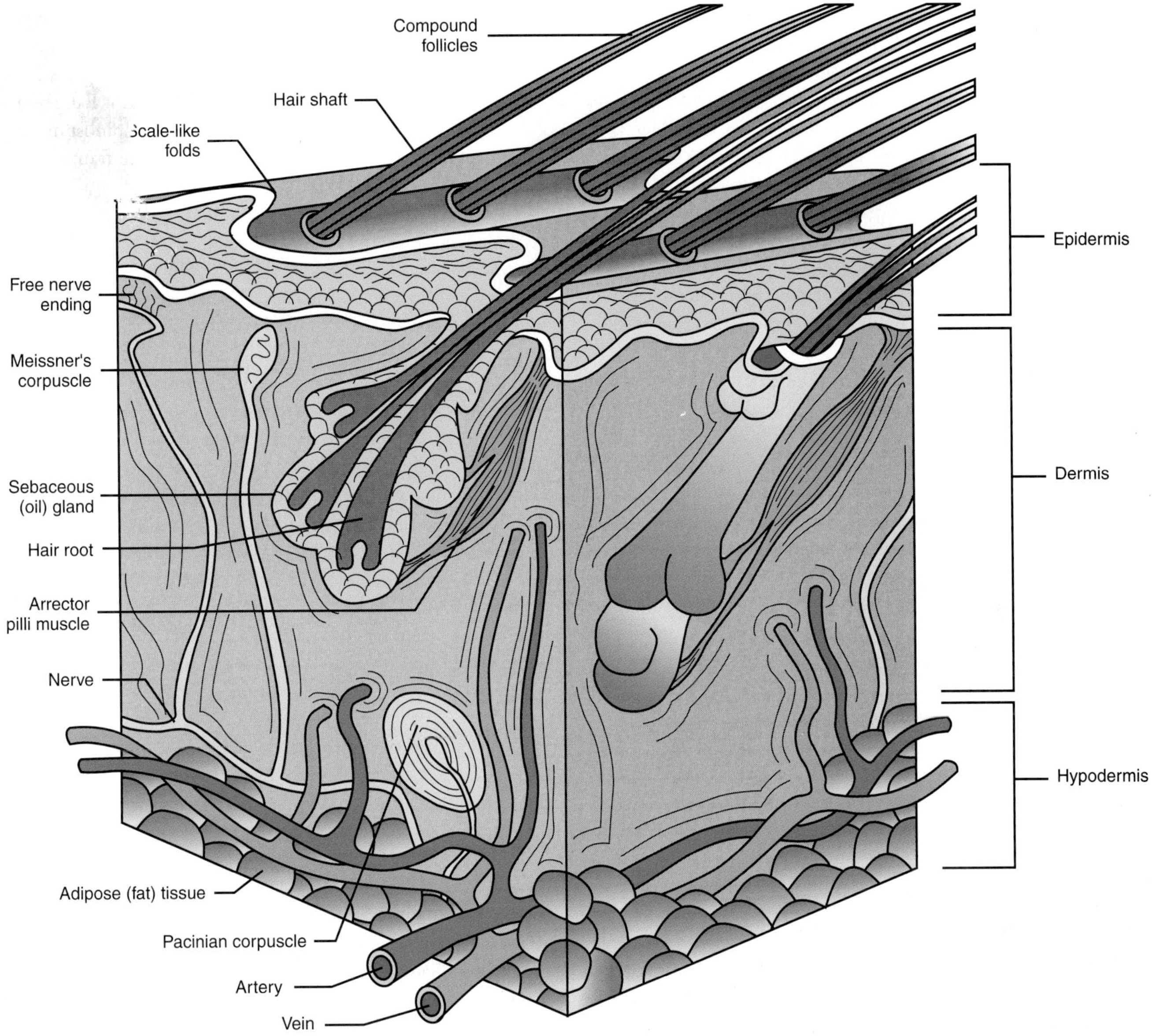

FIGURE **6-1** **Canine Skin.** Cubed section of canine skin and underlying subcutaneous tissue, as well as many structural details discussed in this chapter. Notice that epidermis of canine skin includes folds from which compound hairs arise.

The epidermis is composed of keratinized stratified squamous epithelium and forms an outer waterproof shield. The majority of skin, however, is composed of the underlying dermis, which is a tough, leathery layer composed of dense fibroelastic connective tissue. Only the dermis contains blood vessels. The epidermis is avascular but is provided nutrient molecules via interstitial fluid that diffuses up from the underlying dermis.

A third layer, the **hypodermis** or **subcutaneous layer,** is found below the dermis and is composed primarily of **adipose** tissue, which acts as a thermoinsulator and a mechanical shock absorber.

Figure 6-1 offers an overview of the structure of skin, which includes the dermis and epidermis, and of the hypodermis with its accessory structures. Let's examine these layers in greater detail.

EPIDERMIS

Cells of the Epidermis

Several different kinds of cells are found in the epidermis. The principal ones are **keratinocytes, melanocytes, Merkel cells,** and **Langerhans' cells.** The majority of these are keratinocytes. Keratinocytes, as their name implies, produce keratin, which is a tough, fibrous, waterproof protein that gives skin its resiliency and strength. Keratocytes located along the basement membrane are well nourished by the blood supply of the underlying dermis. Therefore these cells can grow and divide. As daughter cells are produced, they push older cells away from the life-sustaining nutrients of the dermis and toward the outer layers of the epidermis. As the older cells travel from the basal to the superficial layers, they undergo profound changes. They fill with keratohyaline granules; lose their nuclei, cytosol, and organelles; and ultimately become lifeless sheets of keratin. This process is called *keratinization,* and it enables millions of dead cells to rub off or exfoliate daily at no expense to the health of the animal. Remarkably, in humans, an entirely new epidermis forms every 7 to 8 weeks.

The pigment found in skin is produced by another type of cell, the *melanocyte,* which is found in the deepest **epidermal** layers. The melanocyte is octopus-like and possesses long projections that extend outward to all of the keratocytes in the basal layer. As its name implies, it produces **melanin,** a dark pigment, which it stores in membrane-bound granules called **melanosomes.** The melanosomes are transported to the tips of the cellular projections, where they are released into the intracellular space and ultimately absorbed by keratocytes. The keratocytes use the melanin to protect themselves from exposure to damaging ultraviolet rays.

The Langerhans' cell is a macrophage specific to the epidermis. Like other macrophages, it originates in bone marrow and subsequently migrates to the skin, where it phagocytizes microinvaders and where it plays an important role in helping to stimulate other aspects of the immune system.

At the epidermal-dermal junction, Merkel cells can be found in small numbers. They are always associated with a sensory nerve ending and are thought to aid in the sensation of touch. Merkel cells take on a half-dome shape, which perfectly complements the half-dome shape of the sensory nerve ending. Together, these components form what is called **Merkel disk.**

Layers of the Epidermis

Early histologists examined sections of human skin and found five distinct layers in the epidermis (Figure 6-2). These layers were given Latin names and are used to describe the epidermis in other mammalian species today. The deepest layer is the **stratum germinativum,** but it is also known as the **stratum basale** (basal layer). For the most part, this layer consists of a single row of keratocytes, which are firmly attached to the epithelial basement membrane and are actively engaged in cell division. The daughter cells move from the stratum basale to sequentially more superficial layers as they mature. In this way, they replace epithelial cells that have exfoliated at the skin's surface. Merkel's cells and melanocytes, as well as keratocytes, are found in this layer.

The next layer is the **stratum spinosum** (spiny layer), so named because when the cells of this epidermal layer are fixed for histological examination, they contract into spiculated masses that resemble sea urchins. These cells are sometimes called "prickle cells"; however, their cellular projections do not occur naturally, and the cells are normally smooth in situ. Unlike the stratum basale, the stratum spinosum contains several layers of cells that are held together by desmosomes. Although cell division is dramatic in the stratum basale, infrequent divisions are seen in the stratum spinosum. Langerhans' cells are found in greater abundance in the spinosum layer, where their slender projections form a weblike frame around the keratocytes.

The **stratum granulosum** (granular layer) is the middle layer of skin. It is composed of two to four layers of flattened, diamond-shaped keratocytes. The cytoplasm of these cells begins to fill with keratohyaline and lamellated granules, which in turn leads to the dramatic degeneration of the nucleus and other organelles. Without these vital parts, the cell quickly dies. The lamellated granules contain waterproofing glycolipids and are transported to the periphery of the cell, where their contents are discharged into the extracellular space. These glycolipids play an important role in helping the skin to be waterproof and in slowing water loss across the epidermis.

The **stratum lucidum** (clear layer) is only found in very thick skin. Most skin therefore lacks this layer. Microscopically, the stratum lucidum appears as a translucent layer composed of a few rows of flattened dead cells. In this and the outermost epidermal layer, the sticky contents of the keratogranules combine with intracellular tonofilaments to form keratin fibrils.

The **stratum corneum** (horny layer) is the outermost layer and dominates the epidermis. It constitutes up to three quarters of the total epidermal thickness and is composed of 20 to 30 rows of keratocytes. On sagittal section, the keratocytes have a paper-thin, almost two-dimensionality, yet when viewed from above, they appear hexagonal. Keep in mind that these are really only the remnants of keratocytes because the actual cell died in the stratum granulosum. They are sometimes called *horny* or *cornified cells,* but we commonly call them *dandruff* and recognize them as the flakes that occasionally drop on our shoulders.

Epidermis of Hairy Skin

Humans are unusual in their level of hairlessness because most mammals are covered with fur. Unlike the epidermis of people and other relatively hairless animals, skin covered with fur usually consists of three epidermal layers rather than five. These layers are the stratum basale, stratum spinosum, and stratum corneum. The stratum granulosum and stratum lucidum in general are missing. However, a few regions of five-layered epidermis are found in furry mammals, but these are usually seen in regions where the keratinization process has slowed and the skin is very thick.

The surface of "hairy skin" is covered in scalelike folds. Hair emerges from underneath the scales and is directed away from the opening. In dogs the hair is organized in clusters of three follicles per scale.

Periodically throughout the surface of the epidermis a knoblike elevation can be seen, which is called a **tactile elevation,** or epidermal papilla. Each tactile elevation is usually associated with a tactile hair. These special hairs are called

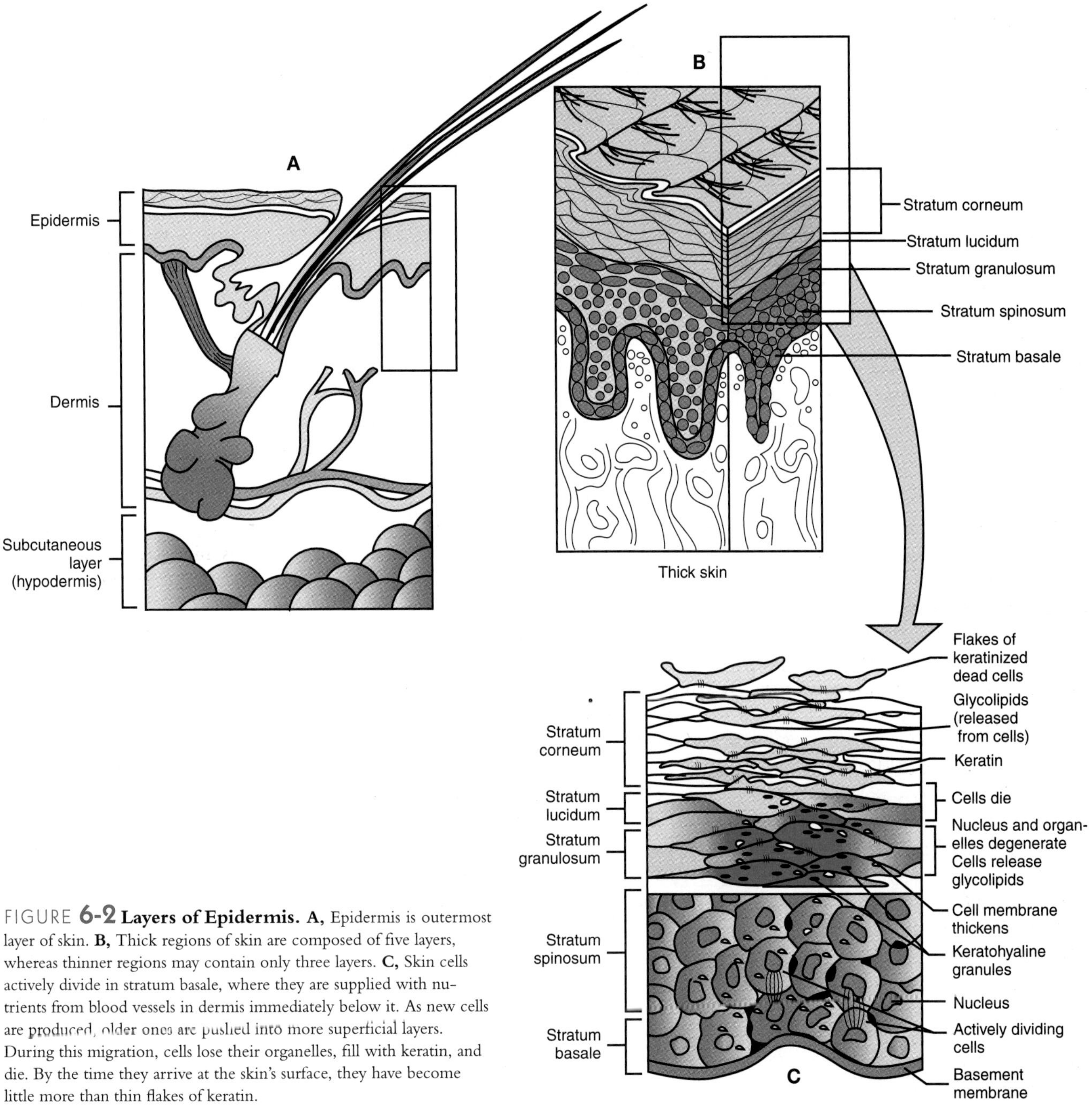

FIGURE **6-2** **Layers of Epidermis. A,** Epidermis is outermost layer of skin. **B,** Thick regions of skin are composed of five layers, whereas thinner regions may contain only three layers. **C,** Skin cells actively divide in stratum basale, where they are supplied with nutrients from blood vessels in dermis immediately below it. As new cells are produced, older ones are pushed into more superficial layers. During this migration, cells lose their organelles, fill with keratin, and die. By the time they arrive at the skin's surface, they have become little more than thin flakes of keratin.

tylotrich hairs, and they are important in the perception of touch (Figure 6-3).

DERMIS

The dermis makes up the greatest portion of the integument and is responsible for most of the structural strength of the skin. Unlike the epidermis, which is primarily cellular, the dermis is highly fibrous. It is composed of dense irregular connective tissue that contains collagen, elastic, and reticular fibers. Hair follicles, nerve endings, glands, smooth muscle, blood vessels, and lymphatics are all found in the dermis as well, creating a rich and interesting tissue community. Fibroblasts, adipocytes, and macrophages also are present and represent the most commonly found cellular elements.

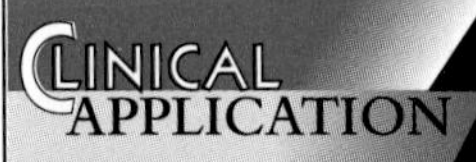

Why Don't the Tattoos on Cattle, Dogs, and Horses Slough Away?

When animals are tattooed, ink is injected into the dermis below the layer of the stratum germinativum. Here the cells of the dermis absorb the dye. Because cells of the dermis do not migrate to the skin's surface and slough the way epidermal cells do, the dye remains fixed in the dermal layer.

Author's note: Once I accidentally jabbed a graphite pencil tip into my ankle, and after the wound healed, it left a small circular gray mark. I know the pencil penetrated the dermis because I still have the mark today, 30 years later!

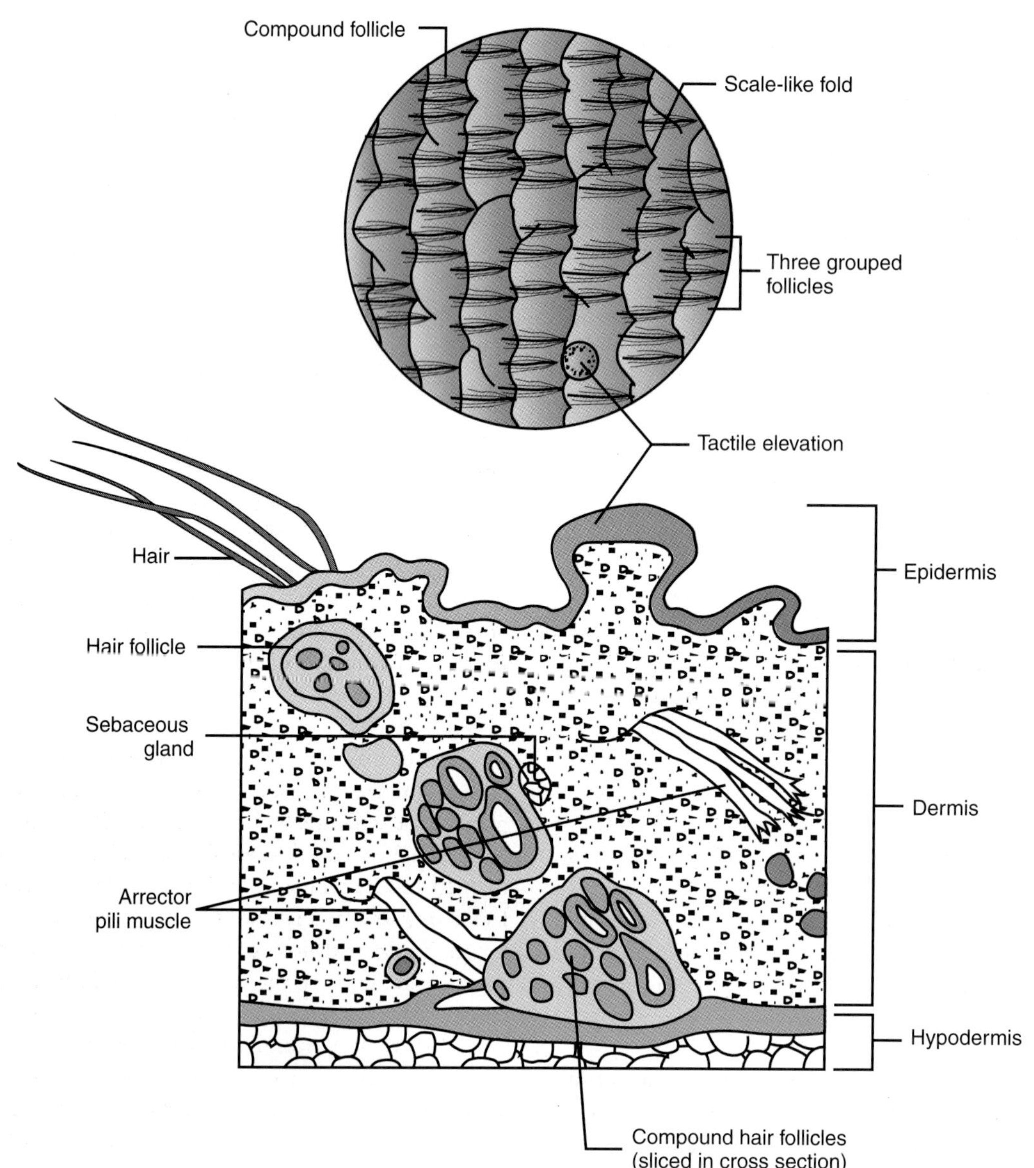

FIGURE **6-3** **Tactile Elevation and Tylotrich Hair.** Compound hairs, in the dog, are organized into groups of three. Interspersed among these groups are tactile elevations, which are prominent, knoblike extensions of epidermis. They are found in most mammalian species and often are associated with specialized sensory hairs called *tylotrich hairs.* Hair may be found medial, lateral, cranial, or caudal to tactile elevation. It is thought that this arrangement enables animals to detect subtle pressure, such as the light touch and movement of insects on skin.

The dermis is a tough layer that binds the superficial epidermis to the underlying tissues. It represents the "hide" of the animal and is used to make leather.

The dermis is composed of two layers: the thin and superficial **papillary layer** and the thick, deeper **reticular layer** (Figure 6-4). The papillary layer lies just underneath the epithelial layer of the epidermis and is composed of loose connective tissue with loosely woven fibers and ground substance. In most regions of the skin, the papillary layer of the dermis forms nipplelike projections, called *dermal papillae,* which rise up into the epidermis. These help to cement the epidermis and the dermis together. In addition, looping blood vessels are found in the papillary layer, which provide nourishment to the active cells of the stratum basale in the epidermis. The vessels also help to remove waste products and assist with temperature control of the body. Nerve endings or pain receptors and touch receptors called **Meissner's corpuscles** can also be found within the papillary layer. Receptors sensitive to temperature changes are present also.

The deeper reticular layer, which consists of dense irregular connective tissue, accounts for 80% of the dermis. The boundary between these two layers is indistinct because bundles of collagen fibers from the papillary layer blend into those of the reticular layer. The majority of fibrous bundles tend to run parallel to one another, and their orientation depends on the

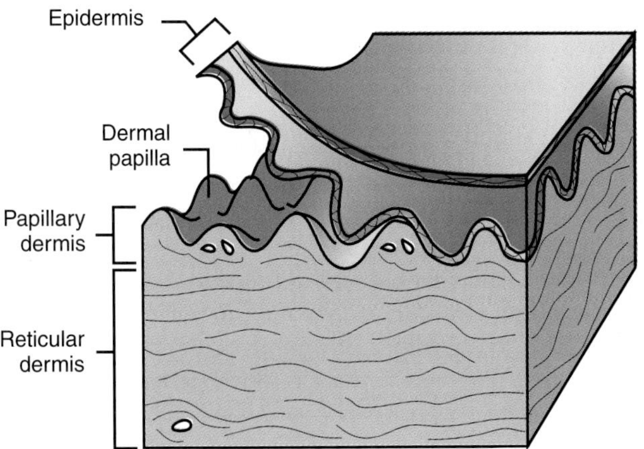

FIGURE **6-4** **Dermal Layers.** Dermis is composed of two layers: a papillary layer and a deeper reticular layer. Projections called *dermal papillae* help to cement the epidermis and dermis together. In addition, dermal papillae provide additional surface area for exchange of nutrients and waste and for temperature regulation.

direction of the stress placed on them. Separations between the bundles represent tension lines in the skin. Tension lines are important to surgeons because the healing of an incision occurs best if the incision is made parallel to the direction of the collagen bundles. In this way, fewer collagen fibers are disrupted, and less scar tissue is needed for healing. Wounds or incisions made perpendicular to the tension lines tend to gap open, particularly if that portion of the body bends or flexes. In regions where a great deal of bending occurs, such as around joints, dermal folds or flexure lines can be found. Here the dermis is tightly secured to underlying tissue.

Hypodermis or Subcutaneous Layer

The hypodermis is a thick layer that resides below the dermis. It is a loose layer of areolar tissue that is rich with adipose, blood and lymphatic vessels, and nerves. In addition, it contains a type of touch receptor called the **pacinian corpuscle.** Meissner's corpuscle in the dermis is sensitive to light touch, whereas the pacinian corpuscle in the hypodermis is sensitive to heavier pressure. The fibers of the hypodermis and those of the dermis are continuous with one another, blurring the distinction between these two layers. The hypodermis is important because it permits the skin to move freely over underlying bone and muscle without putting tension on the skin that would result in tearing.

TEST YOURSELF

1. Why is skin important? Can you think of five important functions of skin?
2. What is keratinization and why is it an important process?
3. Can you list all five layers of the epidermis? What is happening in each layer?
4. How is the skin of hairy animals different from that of humans?
5. How is the dermis different from the epidermis?

Special Features of the Integument

Pigmentation

Some regions of skin, mucous membranes, hooves, and claws are darkly pigmented, whereas other areas are not. **Pigmentation** is caused by the presence or absence of melanin granules in the armlike extensions of the melanocytes. Grossly, no pigmentation is apparent if the granules are concentrated around the nucleus in the cell body of the melanocyte. As the granules move into the cellular "arms" and into the surrounding tissue, however, pigmentation becomes grossly apparent. The more granules that exist in the "arms" of the melanocyte and surrounding tissue, the darker the pigmentation. The dispersion of the granules is controlled by the release of **melanocyte-stimulating hormone,** which in turn is controlled by the intermediate lobe of the **hypophysis.** The melanosomes are transported to the tips of the cellular projections, where they are released into the intracellular space and ultimately absorbed by keratocytes. The keratocytes arrange the melanin on the side of the cell that has the greatest amount of sun exposure. In this way, the pigment acts to protect the keratocytes from exposure to damaging **ultraviolet rays.**

Paw Pads

The foot of many animals is padded and quiet. Thick layers of fat and connective tissue form the foundation of the digital pads that bear the weight of the animal. The pad's outer surface is the toughest and thickest skin in the body. It is often pigmented and is composed of all five epidermal layers. Of these five layers, the outermost epidermal layer, the stratum corneum, is thicker than all of the others combined. The insulating fat together with the tough outer skin forms a protective barrier against abrasion and thermal variances, enabling the animal to walk on rough surfaces, hot roads, and cold snow. The surface of the pad feels rough, and an uneven surface is visible with the naked eye. On close inspection, minute conical papillae can be seen covering the entire pad (Figure 6-5). Sometimes the central surface of the pad may be worn smooth from walking on rough surfaces such as concrete. In this case, the central papillae are rounded or flattened rather than conical while the papillae on the periphery of the pad maintain their conical shape and therefore are more evident grossly.

Many species have multiple footpads. These include (1) the carpal pads, which reside on the caudal surfaces of the "wrist"; (2) the metacarpal and metatarsal pads, which are the central weight-bearing pads of the foot; and (3) the digital pads, which protect each of the digits.

In addition to thick adipose layers, the pad is composed of exocrine sweat glands and lamellar corpuscles. Histologically, the ducts from these sweat glands can be seen passing through the dermis to the stratum basale of the epidermis. Their glandular excretion is then expelled onto the surface of the pad.

Planum Nasale

It is not uncommon for people to judge their pet's health by the animal's nose. An alarmed client, for example, may telephone her veterinarian because her dog's nose is "too warm,"

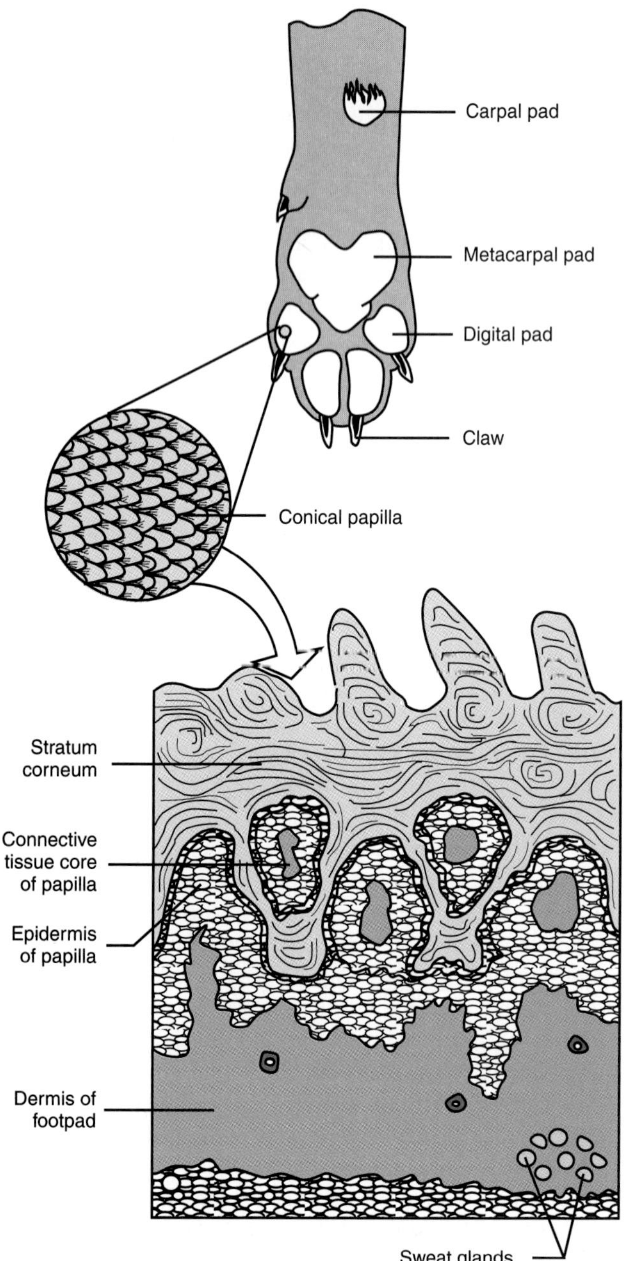

FIGURE **6-5** **Paw Pads.** Paw pads provide a tough, protective surface on which animals walk. Outer layer of pad is the thickest skin in the body and is composed of thousands of conical papillae. Papillae arise from stratum corneum, the outermost layer of epidermis.

"too wet," "too dry," or "just not right." The top of the nose in cats, pigs, and sheep, as well as in dogs, is called the **planum nasale** (Figure 6-6). In the cow and horse, the nose is commonly called the *muzzle* and is technically referred to as the **planum nasolabiale.** Like paw pads, the planum nasale represents an unusual form of skin. Although abnormalities in the appearance of the planum nasale can indicate certain illnesses, its wetness or dryness is usually not an indicator of the health status of the animal as a whole. Normal animals can have wet, dry, moist, hot, and cold noses. Let's take a look at the planum nasale in greater detail.

On close inspection, the nose of a dog appears to be composed of polygonal plates packed together. Although the planum nasale is usually pigmented and appears to be a tough, thick region of integument, histologically, the planum nasale in the dog is composed of only three epidermal layers. The stratum lucidum and stratum granulosum are not present. The outermost layer, the stratum corneum, is composed of only four to eight cell layers, which is surprisingly thin considering the exposed location of the nose and its heavy use, particularly in the dog. The epidermal surface is divided by deep surface grooves, which give it the appearance of being composed of multiple plaques. As with other regions of the skin, the dermis and epidermis interdigitate to form an irregular line of attachment that includes dermal papillae. Although often moist from nasal secretions and licking, the planum nasale in the dog contains no glands in the epidermis or dermis. However, in the sheep, pig, and cow, tubular glands are found.

Ergots and Chestnuts

Ergots and **chestnuts** are dark, horny structures found on the legs of horses, ponies, and other members of the equine family. Chestnuts are usually dark brown and are found on the inside of each leg between the knee and the elbow on the forearm and just below the hock on the hind leg (Figure 6-7). Ergots are similar but much smaller and are often overlooked because usually they are buried in the long caudal hairs of the fetlock. These structures are thought to be vestiges of the carpal and tarsal pads of the second and forth digits (now called "splint bones"), which regressed through evolution as the horse became an increasingly faster runner. Remnants of the fifth digit do not exist.

TEST YOURSELF

1. What causes pigmentation of skin?
2. How are paw pads and the planum nasale different from other regions of skin?

Cutaneous Pouches in Sheep

Cutaneous pouches are infoldings of skin found in sheep. Their three primary locations are in front of the eye, between the digits above the hooves, and in the groin (Figure 6-8). Respectively, these pouches are technically called the **infraorbital, interdigital,** and **inguinal pouches.** Each of the pouches contains fine hairs and numerous sebaceous and oil glands. The glands secrete a fatty, yellow substance, which covers and sticks to the skin when dry.

RELATED STRUCTURES OF THE INTEGUMENT

HAIR

For most animals, hair is essential for survival. By trapping insulating layers of air, hair plays an important role in maintaining body temperature. If dark in color, it can absorb light and, in this way, further assists in warming the animal. Coat

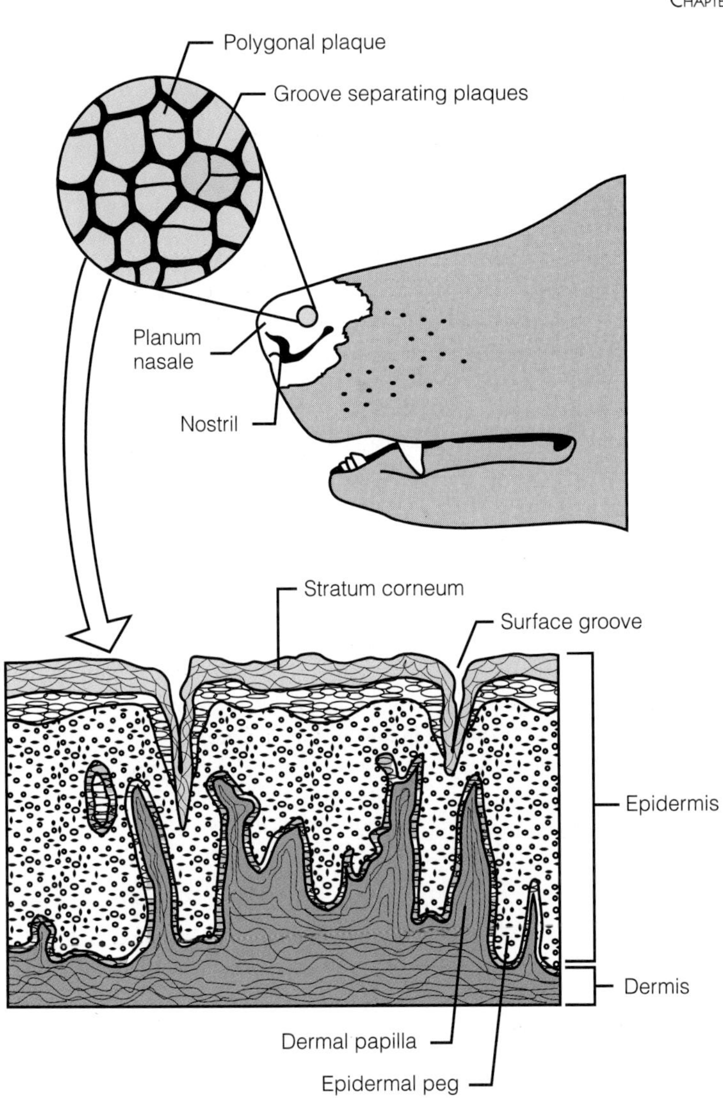

FIGURE **6-6 Planum Nasale.** Planum nasale is composed of polygonal plaques separated by epidermal grooves. Unlike footpads, the epidermis in the planum nasale is surprisingly thin and contains three rather than five layers.

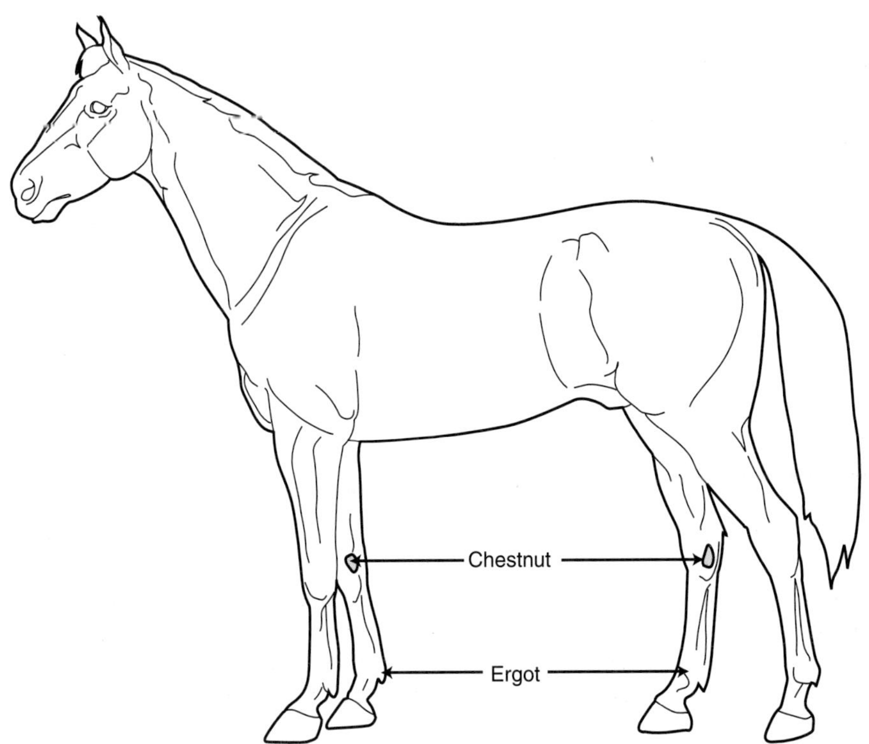

FIGURE **6-7 Location of Ergots and Chestnuts in the Horse.**

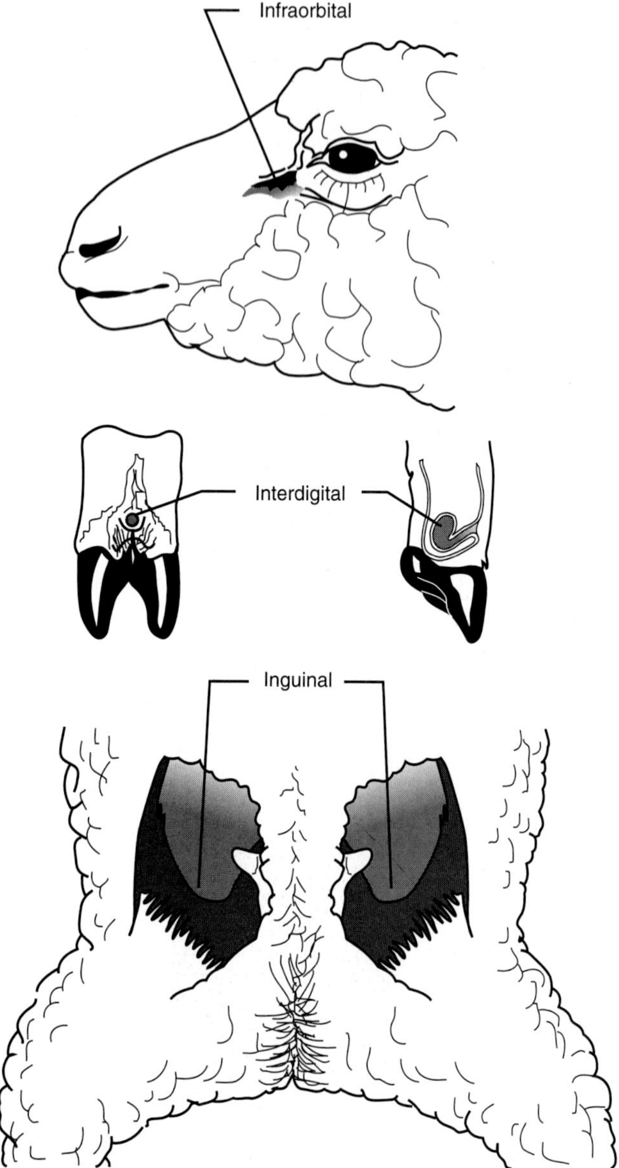

FIGURE **6-8** **Locations of Cutaneous Pouches in Sheep.**

CLINICAL APPLICATION **Skin Cancer**

With the increasing deterioration of the protective ozone layer that surrounds the earth, people are becoming more aware of the growing risk of skin cancer and the importance of protecting the skin from excessive exposure to the sun. However, we are less likely to consider skin cancer in animals, and cancer of the skin, particularly in certain species and breeds, is very common.

Because cancer is the aberrant growth of cells, skin cancer can stem from any of the cell types found in the epidermis or dermis. As you know, many different cell types make up these layers; however, three types of particular importance are the squamous cells, melanocytes, and **basal cells.**

Abnormal changes in the genetic programming of melanocytes, for example, can induce a deadly form of skin cancer called **malignant melanoma.** Malignant melanoma commonly occurs in aged, gray horses and initially appears as nodules under the tail base, in the perianal area, and in the scrotum. Later, these nodules will grow, ulcerate, and spread to multiple internal locations in the horse. Although they may appear on any area of the body in dogs and cats, they are most malignant in the oral cavity. In addition, although rare among pigs in general, malignant melanoma commonly occurs in the duroc-jersey breed.

Squamous cell carcinoma is another deadly form of skin cancer because it spreads rapidly to local lymph nodes and is aggressively invasive locally. It tends to form circular, ulcerated lesions that seem to "eat away" the surrounding tissue. Remarkably, squamous cell carcinoma commonly appears on the eyeball, nictitating membrane, and surrounding eyelids of cattle and horses. It is also seen on the planum nasale and on the earflaps of white cats and in the vulvar regions of merino ewes. It is one of the most common skin tumors in dogs over the age of 5. Areas of skin that receive prolonged sun exposure are most vulnerable to squamous cell carcinoma.

The **basal cell tumor** stems from the cells found in the basal layer of the epidermis, in hair follicles, and in sebaceous glands. They do not spread to other areas of the body and therefore are considered benign; however, they do recur after removal. Basal cell tumors grow slowly and are found on the head and neck in dogs. They are thought to be one of the most common tumors found in cats but account for only 6% of the neoplasms in dogs.

color may also play a critical role in protecting the animal via camouflage.

In most species of mammals, hair occurs as fur. Marine mammals such as whales, domestic pigs, human beings, and relatively few other species are exceptional in that the hair covering their bodies is sparse and thin. They have evolved to survive without fur. For the majority of animals, however, thick fur covers the greater surface of their bodies. Only the hooves, lips, paw pads, horns, nipples, inner folds of genitalia, and nasal regions may be devoid of hair. Hair coats tend to be thickest on the most exposed regions of the body, such as the back and sides, whereas the abdomen and inner sides of the proximal limbs are less densely covered.

Hair Strands and Their Follicles

The part of hair that is visible above the skin is called the **shaft,** and the portion buried within the skin is called the **root.** Hair is anchored by the **hair follicle.** The hair follicle is an invagination of the epidermis that extends from the skin surface to the dermis or, occasionally, the hypodermis. The deepest part of the hair follicle expands to form a **hair bulb.** At the base of the bulb is a mound of dermal cells called the **papilla.** The papilla is covered with rapidly dividing epithelial cells called the **matrix** (Figure 6-9, *A*). These cells are nourished by blood flow from vessels in the underlying papilla. Nourishment of the epithelial cells stimulates much cell division and growth. As the cells divide, older cells are pushed upward into the tunnel away from the papilla. These cells become keratinized, and as

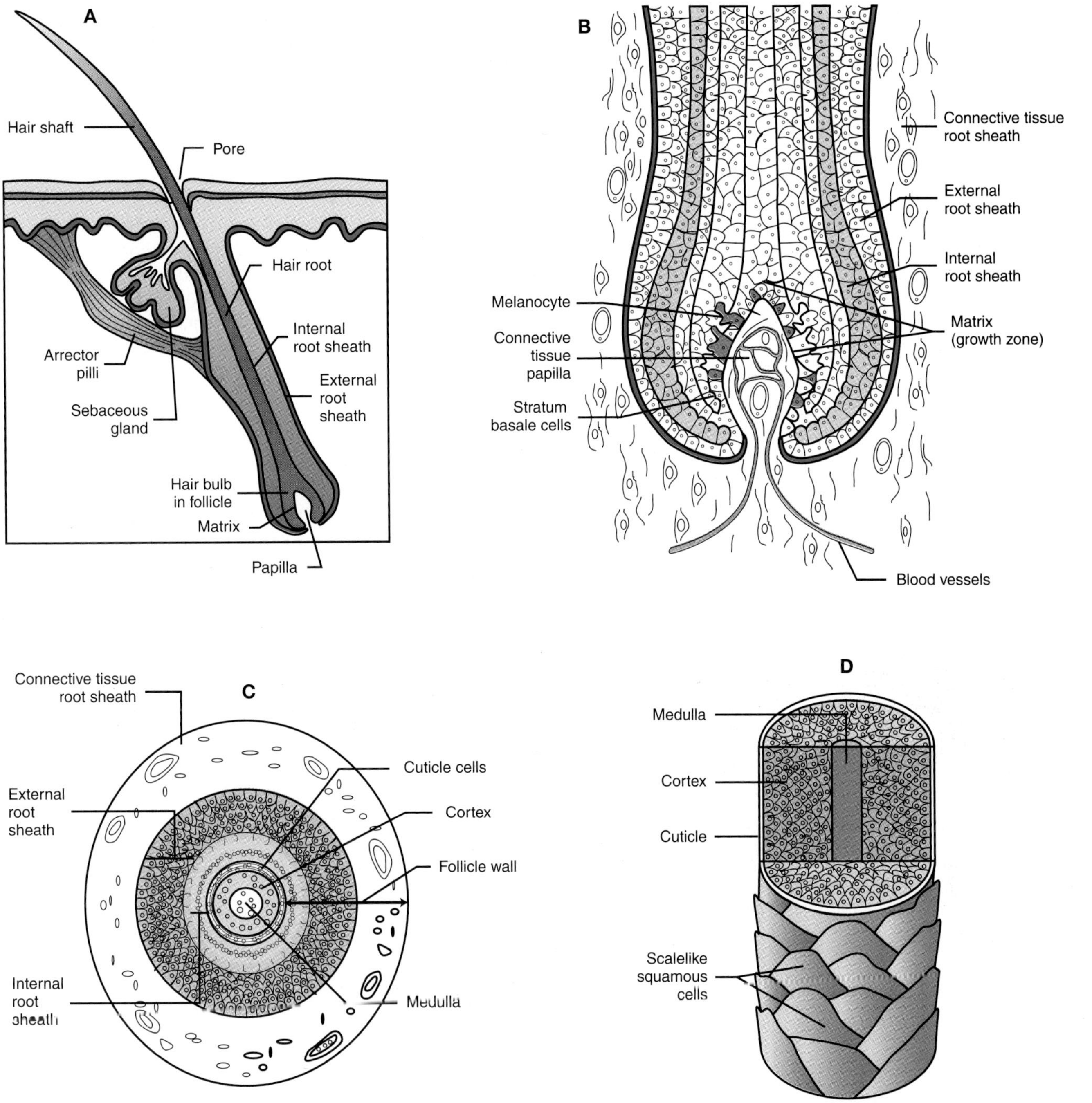

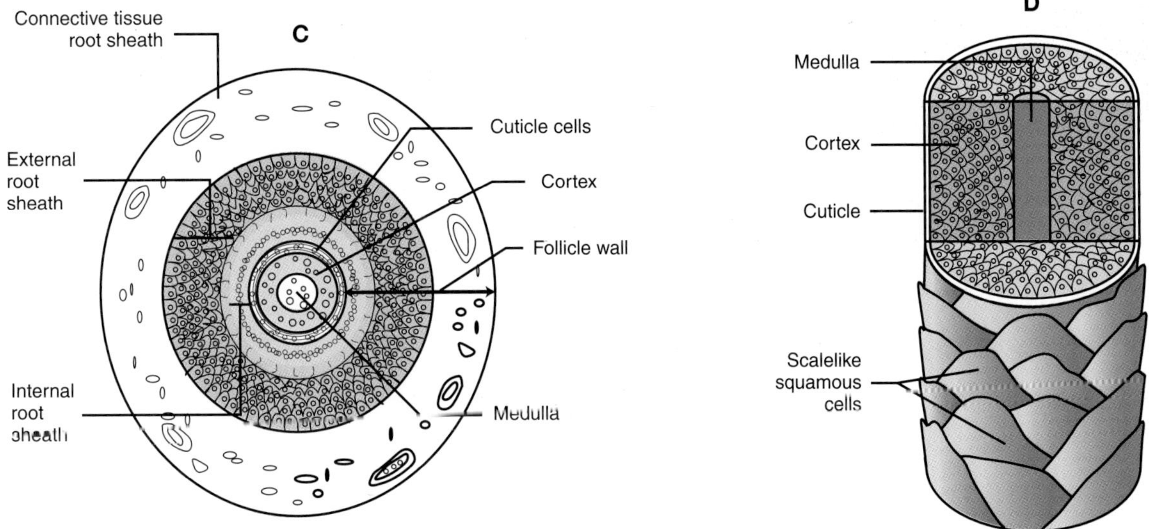

FIGURE **6-9 Hair Follicle. A,** Structures of a hair follicle. **B,** The matrix is composed of rapidly dividing epidermal cells that are supplied with important nutrients from the blood supply in the connective tissue papilla. A strand of hair is formed as daughter epithelial cells mature, fill with keratin, and move away from the papilla and its blood supply. Cells subsequently die and become part of the hair. **C,** The root sheath is composed of three layers: connective tissue root sheath, external root sheath, and internal root sheath. **D,** Dead epithelial cells make up hair. Each strand is organized into three layers: cuticle, cortex, and medulla.

they lose contact with the nutrition provided by the papilla, they die and become part of the developing hair. In this way, hair is constructed from dead epithelial cells.

A web of sensory nerve endings called the **root hair plexus** envelops the root, making it an important touch receptor when the hair is bent. The wall of the hair follicle is composed of three layers: an internal epithelial root sheath, an outer epithelial root sheath, and a dermal or connective tissue root sheath (see Figure 6-9, *B* and *C*).

Animals with fur often have compound follicles in which multiple hair strands emerge from a single **epidermal orifice,** or pore, although each strand has its own follicle and bulb. As many as 15 hairs may be associated with one pore. Usually in compound follicles, a single, long **primary hair** (also known as a *guard hair* or *cover hair*) is surrounded by shorter secondary hairs, or satellite hairs. In dogs, usually three compound follicles are grouped together to emerge from the same epidermal fold.

Hair is formed in three concentric layers (see Figure 6-9, *D*). The innermost layer (and central core) is called the **medulla.** It is composed of two to three layers of loosely arranged cells that are separated by spaces filled with liquid or air. The cells themselves contain flexible, *soft keratin* similar to that found in the stratum corneum of the epidermis. Surrounding the medulla is the **cortex.** Unlike the flexible medulla, the cortex is stiff and rigid because it is composed of *hard keratin* and is the thickest of the three layers. A single layer of cells arising from the edge of the papilla form the hair surface, which is called the **cuticle.** It is also composed of hard keratin. The cells of the cuticle are layered like shingles on a roof, which prevent the hairs from sticking together and forming mats. In some animals, such as sheep, however, the edges of the cells in the cuticle are raised, enabling them to "grab onto" the cuticle cells from other hair strands. In this way, wool threads can be created by twisting and pulling clumps of hair.

Growth Cycles of Hair

However unconsciously, we are all aware that hair undergoes a cycle of growing and falling out. When we remove a wad of hair from a clogged sink, when we vacuum up hair left behind by the dog on *his* favorite chair, and when we can cover the barn floor with a layer of hair from our horse after brushing, we know that it is normal for hair to fall out. Hair sheds to make room for the production of new strands. The volume of shedding is influenced by genetics and by the environment. For example, shedding is heaviest in the spring and fall for animals that live outside. Longhaired animals may shed more than shorthaired animals, and animals that are kept indoors may shed less than animals that are kept outdoors. In addition, hormonal changes may influence shedding. For example, many bitches after whelping lose a large percentage of their total hair volume at one time. Technically, this phenomenon is called **telogen effluvium,** but many breeders refer to it as "blowing the coat." Whether an animal is undergoing routine shedding or blowing its coat, hair is lost to make room in the follicles for the production of new hair strands. How does this happen?

When a hair is produced, dead keratinized epithelial cells push up and away from the dermal papilla and are organized into the layers that make up the hair shaft and root (Figure 6-10). As more cells are added at the base of the root, the hair lengthens. During this time of growth, the hair is said to be in the **anagen phase.** As one would expect, the maximum length achieved by the anagen hair is genetically predetermined. In

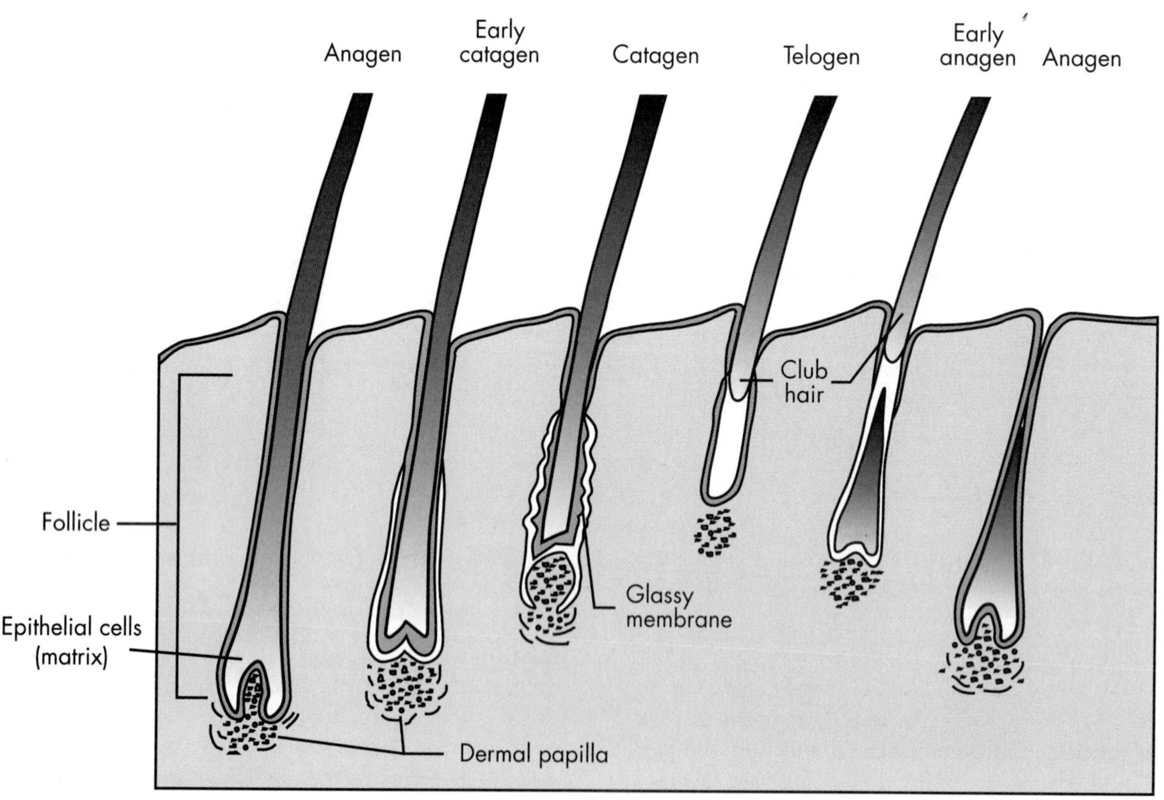

FIGURE **6-10** **Growth Cycles of Hair.** Three phases take place in the hair growth cycle. The *anagen* phase is a time of hair growth when the follicle is longest. The *catagen* phase occurs with the appearance of a thick glassy membrane and a shortening of the hair follicle. In addition, thickening of the basement membrane in the matrix separates epidermal cells from the dermal papilla. In the *telogen* phase, the hair follicle is very short, and the dermal papilla is separated from the bulb. The hair strand is rounded and resembles a club (therefore called *club hairs*).

this way, some species and breeds of animals have longhair coats, whereas others have short coats. When the maximum length of hair is achieved, the hair stops growing, the hair follicle shortens, and the hair is held in a resting phase. This quiescent period is called the **telogen phase** and can last from weeks to years depending on the location, type of hair, and species involved. The period of transition between the anagen and telogen phases is called the **catagen phase.**

Hair Color

Pigment in the cortex and medulla gives hair its color. Genetically programmed melanocytes, located at the base of the hair follicle, produce melanin, which is transferred to the cortical and medullary cells that form the hair strand. Different colors are achieved based on the quantity and type of melanin that is incorporated into the hair. Horses, for example, produce only one type of melanin, whereas the dog produces two. Yellow and reddish colors in the dog are achieved with **pheomelanin,** and the brown-black colors are formed by the presence of **tyrosine melanin.** In the horse, all colors are achieved by varying the amount and location of the melanin, not the type. Darker colors are generally achieved with greater quantities of melanin than lighter shades. In addition, pigmentation may occur uniformly throughout the hair to form a solid color, or it may be concentrated at just the base or just the tip of the strand to form agouti-type coloration.

As animals age, melanin production decreases, and the hair begins to turn gray. White hair is formed when the cortex loses its pigment entirely and the medulla becomes completely filled with air.

Types of Hair

Animals possess a variety of hair types. In general, hair has been categorized into three broad groups: primary or guard hairs, **secondary** or **wool-type hairs,** and tactile or sinus hairs. Primary hairs are generally straight or arched and are thicker and longer than secondary hairs. They are the dominant hairs in a complex hair follicle. As already mentioned, the complex hair follicle in the dog consists of one primary hair surrounded by numerous secondary hairs. Secondary hairs are softer and shorter than primary hairs. They are generally wavy or bristled in the dog and are the predominant hair type in species with wool-type coats. **Tactile hairs** are used as probes and feelers. They are well supplied with sensory endings that make them particularly sensitive to the slightest bending or touch. These hairs are commonly known as *whiskers* and can be found around the mouth and on the muzzle of many species, as well as mixed intermittently throughout the hair coat. The tactile hair is also called the *sinus hair* because of the presence of a large blood sinus, which is located in the connective tissue portion of the follicle.

Arrector Pili Muscles

In most animals, hair slopes from the nose to the tail. In some species or breeds of animal, the hair is more erect than in others. The degree of erection is called the **implantation angle.** The summer coats of horses, for example, are short and lie flat against the surface of the skin; therefore the implantation angle in these animals is relatively low. Dog breeds tend to have implantation angles that range from 30 to 40 degrees although the Chow, Airedale, and Scottish Terrier have angles as high as 45 degrees.

When frightened or cold, animals can make their hair stand up beyond the normal implantation angle. This is due to the presence of a small, smooth muscle called the **arrector pili muscle,** which is attached to each hair follicle and is innervated by the sympathetic nervous system. When the muscle contracts, it pulls the hair to an erect position. Perhaps you have seen a frightened cat "puffed up." This reaction is a defense mechanism designed to make the animal appear bigger and therefore less vulnerable to potential predators. In addition, hair that stands erect can better trap insulating layers of air than nonerect hair. So animals with erect hair coats stay warmer than animals with flat coats. In humans, contraction of the arrector pili muscles causes "goose bumps." The arrector pili muscle also is responsible for forcing sebum from the sebaceous gland, which helps keep the integument moist and supple.

TEST YOURSELF ✓

1. Can you draw and label the parts of a hair follicle?
2. How does hair form and grow?
3. What are the three cycles of hair growth?
4. Why does hair turn gray and then white as animals age?
5. What factors stimulate contraction of the arrector pili muscle? Why is this muscle important?

GLANDS OF THE SKIN

Sebaceous Glands

Sebaceous glands are generally found all over the body except in certain specialized regions, such as paw pads and the planum nasale. The glands are located in the dermis and may be simple or complex alveolar structures. Although most sebaceous glands have a single duct that empties into a hair follicle, others have ducts that empty directly onto the surface of the skin. This latter group of sebaceous glands is found at the mucocutaneous junctions of the lips, labia vulvae, penis, prepuce, anus, and eyelids. They are also found in the ear canal. In sheep, sebaceous glands empty directly onto the surface of the skin in the infraorbital pouches, interdigital pouches, and inguinal pouches. The sebaceous glands associated with hair follicles are found in the triangle formed by the surface of the skin, the hair follicle, and the arrector pili muscle.

Sebaceous gland alveoli are lined with epithelial cells that manufacture and store an oily, lipid substance composed primarily of glycerides and free fatty acids. Eventually, the cells become so full that they rupture and release their contents, together with cellular debris, into the center of the alveolus. The white, semiliquid mixture is called **sebum.** However, in sheep, sebaceous glands produce a substance that ultimately

CLINICAL APPLICATION Allergies: Itchy Business

When cats and dogs develop allergies, they do not usually develop congested sinuses and runny eyes and noses the way people do. Instead, dogs and cats develop itchy skin and ears. As in people, animals can develop an allergy to just about anything, including people dander! Imagine if your pet were allergic to you!

Allergies to inhalant particles, such as pollen, dust, and mold spores, are common. This type of allergy is called **atopy** and can cause seasonal itchiness (as in the case of ragweed pollen) or year-round itchiness (caused by house dust). Atopic dogs tend to rub their faces on the carpet, scratch in the axillae ("armpits") with their hind feet, and lick the tops of their paws. Food allergies and allergies to ectoparasites, such as fleas, are also very common. Dogs with flea allergies tend to "corncob chew" the base of their tail and the medial sides of their hind legs. Cats rarely chew but exhibit itchiness by excessive licking and grooming.

To some extent the veterinarian can distinguish between the various types of allergies by the pattern of **pruritus**, or itchiness, on the body. Areas that have been scratched or licked excessively will be excoriated, raw, and hairless. In chronic cases the skin may become **hyperpigmented** and turn black, or areas of white fur may exhibit "salivary staining" by turning the hairs yellow.

becomes **lanolin.** Because the epithelial cell is lost in the process of secretion, the sebaceous gland is classified as a holocrine structure.

When the arrector pili muscle contracts, it compresses the sebaceous gland, and the sebum is forced from the alveolus through the duct into the hair follicle. Here sebum coats the base of the hair and the surrounding skin and plays an important role in trapping moisture to prevent excessive drying. In this way, the skin and hair are kept soft, pliant, and somewhat waterproof. Sebum also possesses some antibacterial and antifungal properties, which reduce the skin's risk of infection.The sebaceous gland is sensitive to changes in levels of sex hormones and therefore is most productive during puberty in humans. Excessive amounts of sebum can clog the opening of the hair follicle, forming whiteheads. With time, the sebum turns black and forms blackheads which are also called **comedones.** If untreated, comedones may develop into pimples or **pustules.**

Sweat Glands

Sweat glands are also called *sudoriferous glands* and are found over the entire body of most domestic species, including pig, horse, cow, dog, and sheep. Not surprisingly, sweat glands produce sweat, a watery transparent liquid that helps cool the body through evaporation. Although sweat glands are numerous in most domestic species, only the horse produces a profuse sweat, which sometimes works itself into a white froth. The two types of sweat glands are eccrine and apocrine (Figure 6-11). Both are classified as merocrine glands because no cellular material is lost during their excretory function.

Eccrine Sweat Glands. The excretory portion of the **eccrine gland** consists of a simple coiled tube located in the dermis or hypodermis. It is connected to the surface of the skin by a long duct. In dogs, **eccrine sweat glands** are found only in the deep layers of the fat and connective tissue of footpads.

Apocrine Sweat Glands. Like eccrine sweat glands, **apocrine sweat glands** have a coiled excretory portion buried in the dermis or hypodermis with a single excretory duct. However, unlike eccrine sweat glands, apocrine glands empty into hair follicles rather than onto the surface of the skin. In the dog, apocrine glands are located in the external ear canal. Interestingly, dogs with long hair have more sebaceous and apocrine glands in their external ear canal than do dogs with short hair.

Tail Glands

Most felids (cats) and canids (dogs) possess an oval region at the dorsal base of their tails called the **tail gland** (Figure 6-12). This region may be grossly recognizable because of the presence of course, oily hairs. Apocrine and sebaceous glands are especially large in this region. Like sebaceous glands, apocrine glands are sensitive to changes in sex hormone levels, and therefore they become particularly active during puberty and estrus. The tail gland is thought to assist with the recognition and identification of individual animals.

Anal Sacs

Anal sacs and other related musk glands are famous for their powerful, foul-smelling secretions. Although skunks are shy and not often seen in the wild, it is not uncommon to catch the noxious odor of a skunk's spray from our car as we drive down a suburban or rural road. The odor can linger in the region for days. Cats and dogs have anal sacs, similar to musk glands that are located at the 5 and 7 o'clock positions relative to the anus. They are connected to the lateral margin of the anus by a small, single duct. The anal sac is lined with sebaceous and apocrine glands and acts as a reservoir for the secretions that are produced from these glands. When the animal defecates or becomes frightened, some or all of the anal sac contents are expressed. In this way, feces become coated with the secretions stored in the anal sac, and the unique smell of the animal is transferred to the environment. Thus defecation serves the dual purpose of elimination and of marking a territory or attracting a mate. Sometimes the small duct of the anal sac clogs and if untreated can lead to an infected anal sac. Clinically, animals with irritated or impacted anal sacs often drag their rumps along the ground to help alleviate the discomfort.

TEST YOURSELF

1. Name two types of sweat glands. How are they different from one another?
2. Where are anal sacs found and what is their importance to animals?

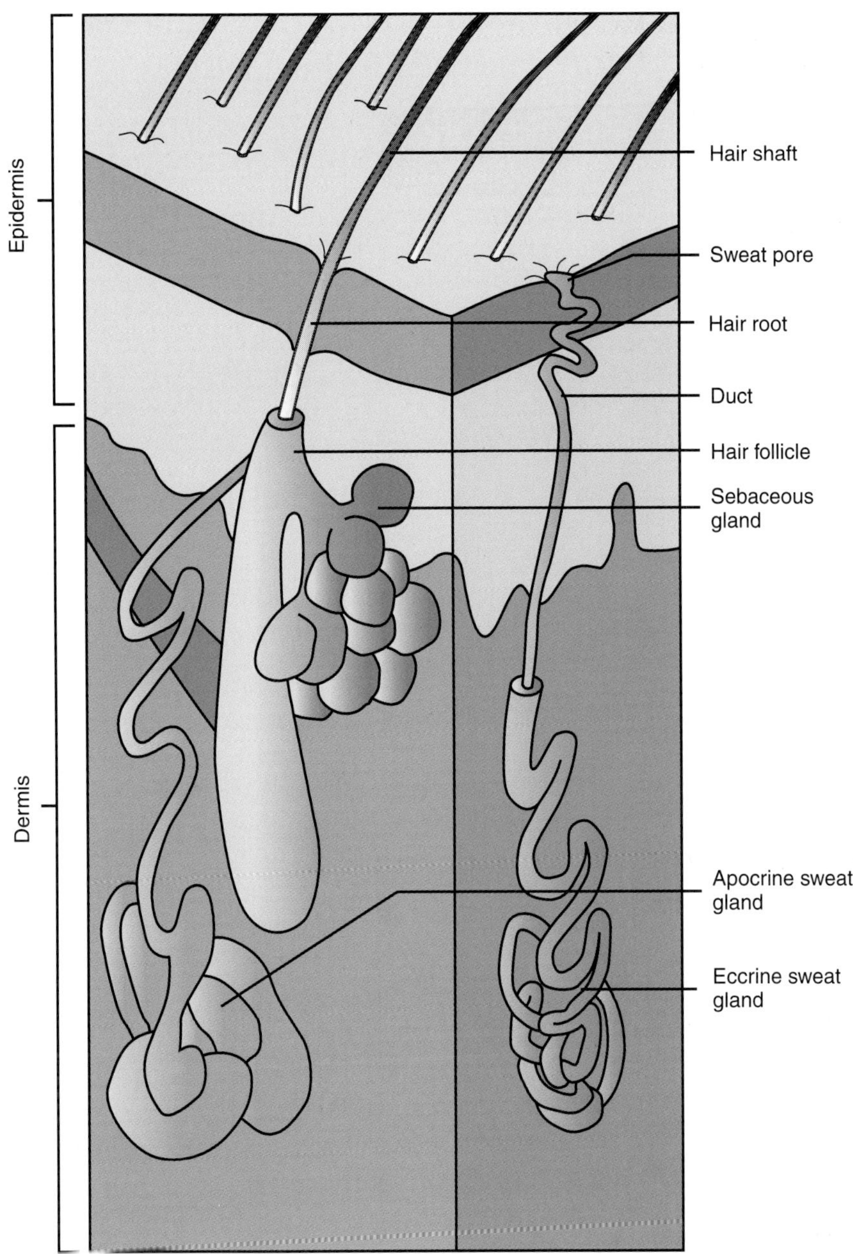

FIGURE **6-11** **Glands of Skin.** Two types of sweat glands are apocrine glands, with ducts that connect to hair follicles, and eccrine glands, which empty directly onto the skin surface. Sebaceous glands are also depicted.

Claws and Dewclaws

Many animals have **claws,** which are the hard, often pigmented outer coverings of the distal digits. Claws are important for maintaining good traction while running, walking, and climbing and serve as lifesaving tools for defense and for catching prey. In most animals, claws are nonretractable although, with the exception of the cheetah, cats can retract their claws (Figure 6-13). Interestingly, the claw of cats cannot be separated from the **distal phalanx bone.** A declaw procedure therefore necessitates amputation of the entire third phalanx. Fortunately, this procedure is usually limited to the front feet.

Dewclaws are the remains of digits that, in the course of evolution, are undergoing regression. In the dog, the dewclaw is the first digit, but actual bones are only found in the dewclaws of the forelimbs. In the cow, pig, and sheep, the medial and lateral dewclaws are the second and fifth digits, respectively. Of these three species, only the pig has dewclaws that contain bones. Both the **metacarpal bones** and **phalangeal bones** are present in the dewclaws of the pig, just as they are in the weight-bearing digits.

The Hoof

We all know what hooves are, but we might not know that another name for "hoof" is **ungula** and that hoofed animals are called **ungulates.** The horny outer covering is sometimes called a "claw," as well as a "hoof." Ruminants have four hooves per foot, with each one covering a digit. However,

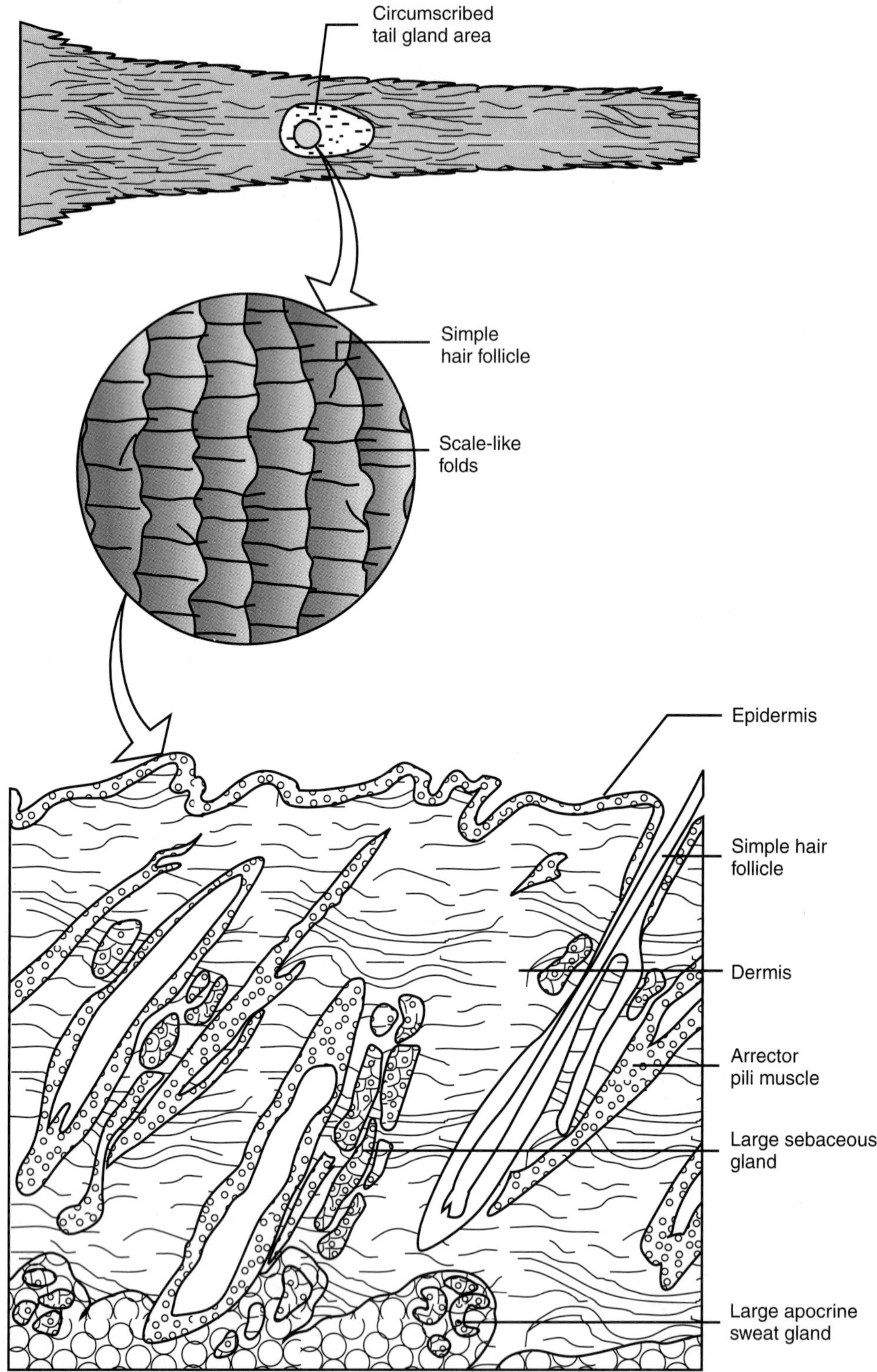

FIGURE **6-12** **Tail Gland Area.** Region of tail gland in dogs and cats is rich with apocrine and sebaceous glands, which become particularly productive when sex hormone levels are high. Simple, course hairs predominate, making the region look grossly different from surrounding areas.

weight is carried only on two of the four hooves in many ungulates, such as sheep, cow, and goat. The weight-bearing hooves represent the third and forth digits. Imagine walking only on your middle and ring fingers! In essence, that is what these species of farm animals are doing. Although their evolutionary ancestors had five toes, the "thumb" or first digit has disappeared, and the "index finger" and "pinky" (second and fifth digits) have regressed into what we call the dewclaws. These digits are found more proximally on the limb. Remarkably, the horse walks on only one digit, that being the third

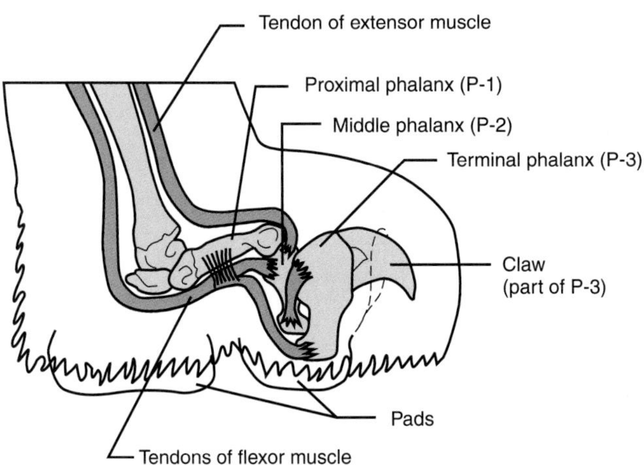

FIGURE **6-13** **Cat Claw.** The claw on a cat is an extension of the third phalanx. Declaw procedures involve complete amputation of this bone.

digit (equivalent to our middle finger or toe). As already mentioned, the splint bones, ergot, and chestnuts of equids (horses) are the only remaining vestiges of ancestral digits. See Figure 6-14 for an illustration of the equine foot.

Both claws and hooves rest on underlying sensitive tissue called the **corium.** The corium is firmly attached to the periosteum of the distal phalanx and is rich with blood vessels that provide nutrient molecules to the developing cells of the stratum basale in the hoof. In this way, the outer hoof is a modified epithelial layer, and the corium is modified dermis. The corium is well innervated and sensitive to pain, whereas the outer wall of the hoof has no sensation. In addition, the corium is divided into regions based on the anatomy of the overlying hoof. **Coronary corium,** for example, lies underneath the coronary band of the hoof, and **perioplic corium** underlies the periople (Figure 6-15).

The hoof grows from the corium of the coronary band downward. Growth of the hoof is continuous, and hooves that are not trimmed can become so long that they curl up like the shoes worn by elves. In wild horses the abrasion caused by running on rough surfaces is an important part of maintaining normal hoof length. Domestic horses, however, rely on a blacksmith to trim their feet. Horses are used for work to carry heavy riders, pull loads, and carry packs, often on hard roads and surfaces. This puts the equine hoof at greater risk for cracking or chipping, which in turn causes lameness and renders the horse unable to work. Long ago, it was discovered that nailing a rigid metal shoe to the plantar and palmar surface of the hoof increased the integrity of the wall and strengthened the foot. A horseshoe prevents excessive expansion of the hoof when the animal carries weight. It also improves traction and creates an additional barrier between the hoof and the ground. In this way, people could keep horses in a condition to work with greater regularity.

The skeletal foot of the horse includes the distal part of the second phalanx; the distal sesamoid bone, which is called the **navicular bone;** and the entire third phalanx, which is commonly known as the **coffin bone.** The coffin bone is cloaked in a layer of corium, which in turn is covered by the cornified hoof. The hoof and the corium form an elaborate array of interdigitations called **laminae.** The laminae consist of primary and secondary extensions, which increase the contact area between the corium and the **hoof wall.** These important interdigitations form the attachment between the hoof and the coffin bone.

The equine hoof is generally divided into three parts: the wall, the sole, and the frog. Let's examine each of these parts.

The Wall

The wall is the convex external portion of the hoof that is visible from the anterior, lateral, and medial views. It is divided into three regions: the toe, the quarters, and the heels (Figure 6-16). The **toe** is the front of the foot, and the **quarters** make up the lateral aspects. The **heel** is the portion of the wall that tapers downward and wraps around the back of the foot. The hooves of the front feet are angled at about 50 degrees, and those in the back are angled at about 55 degrees. Minute vertical lines representing **horn tubes** may be evident running from the coronary band to the ground. In addition, rings or ridges can be seen wrapping around the hoof. Like the rings in tree trunks, these lines or ridges represent periods of growth in the hoof.

The Sole

The **sole** is the plantar, or palmar, surface of the hoof. It is concave and fills the space bordered by the wall and the bars. The part of the sole that immediately surrounds the bars is called the **angle.** Like other external portions of the hoof, the outer layers of the sole are avascular and lack innervation. Deeper layers of the corium provide nutrient molecules and contain nervous input. The corium connects the sole to the underside of the coffin bone. A thin strip called the **white line** is formed at the junction of the sole and the hoof wall.

The Frog

The insensitive **frog** is a triangular, horny structure located between the heels on the underside of the hoof. The **point,** or apex, of the frog faces the toe, and the base runs across the caudal aspect of the foot between the heels. The frog is divided by a central depression known as the **central sulcus,** or cleft of frog. The frog is separated from the bars on the lateral and medial sides by a deep, concave region called the **collateral sulcus.** A thick pad of fat and fibrous tissue, called the *digital cushion,* lies beneath the sensitive frog.

Two large bands of cartilage, called the **lateral cartilages,** extend proximally from the distal phalanx and form an important structural support for the equine foot. These bands, together with the frog and digital cushion, work as a kind of circulatory pump to assist blood flow through the foot. As the horse bears weight, the frog is compressed against the bars, and the heel of the foot expands (Figure 6-17). In addition, the digital cushion is compressed against the lateral cartilages and the frog. This forces blood out of the corium, away from the

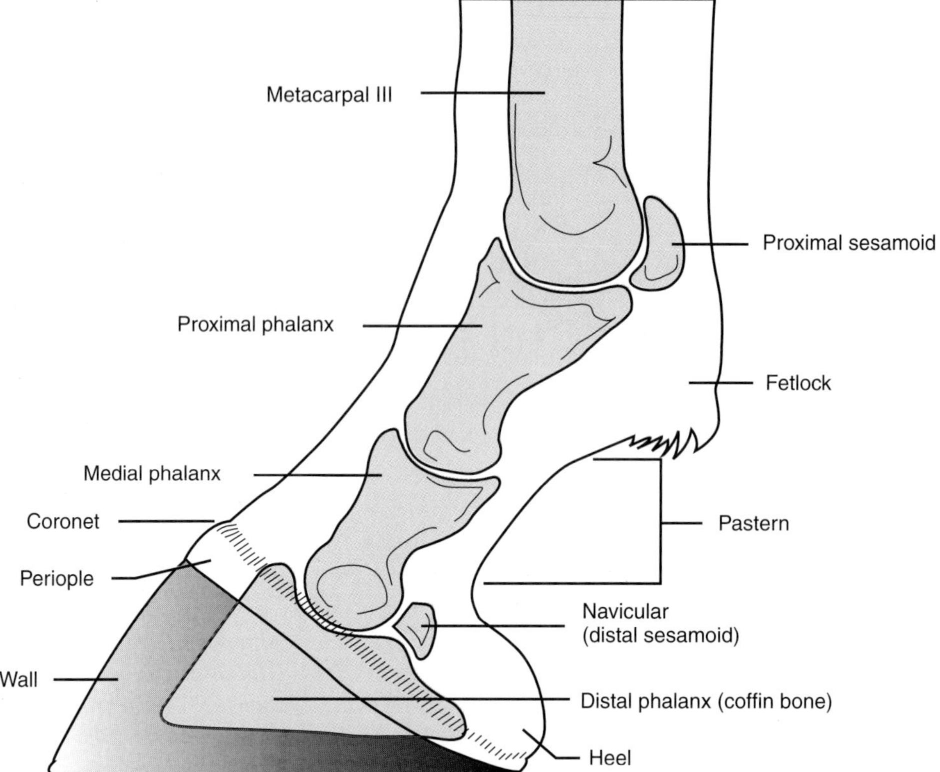

FIGURE **6-14** **Bones of Equine Foot.** The skeletal foot of the horse includes the distal part of the second phalanx; distal sesamoid bone, or *navicular bone;* and the entire third phalanx, commonly known as *coffin bone.*

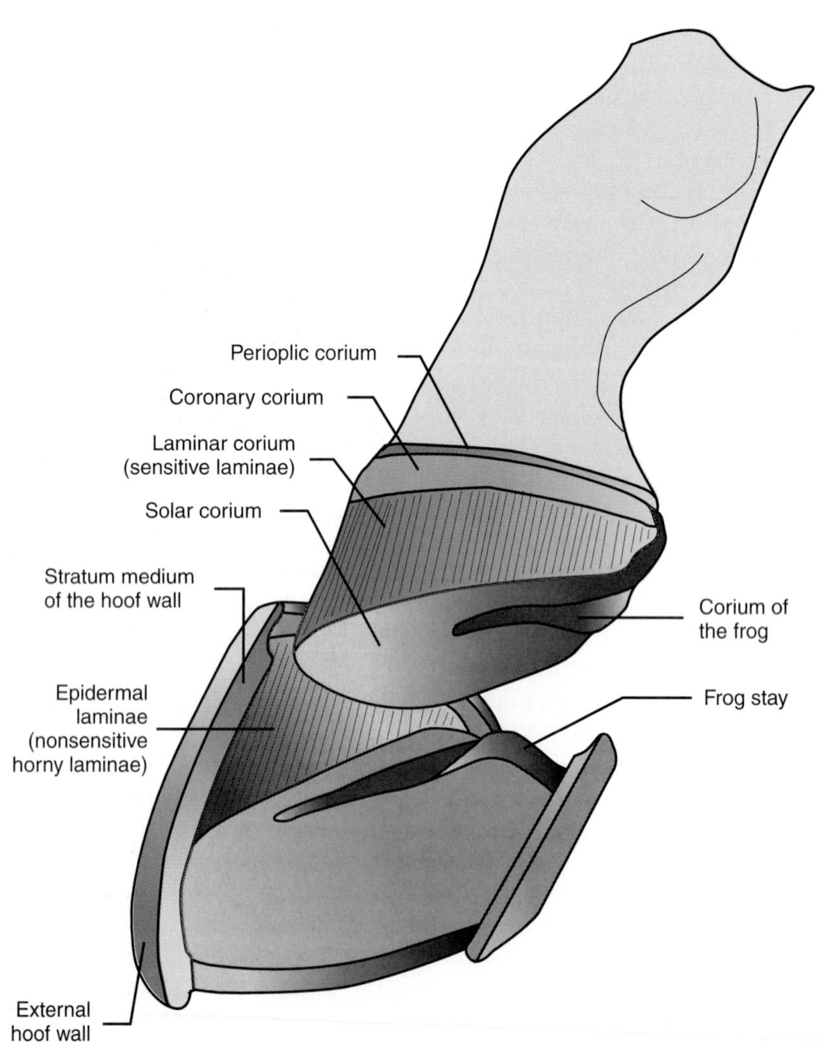

FIGURE **6-15** **Equine Laminae.** The hoof is held onto the coffin bone by delicate interdigitating laminae. When these laminae become inflamed, during a painful condition called *laminitis,* the connection between the hoof and the coffin bone is weakened. Consequently, the coffin bone may slip and rotate downward.

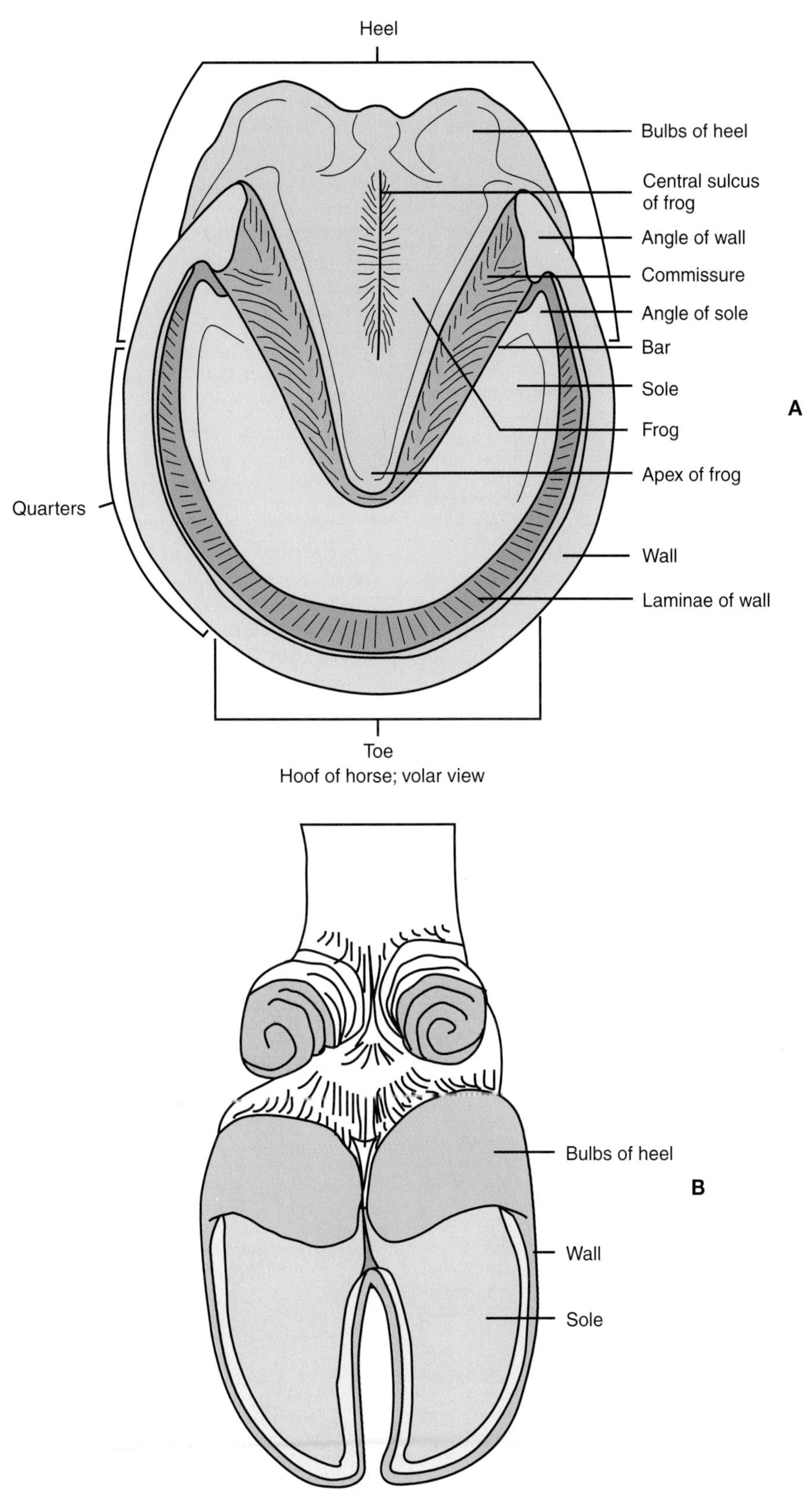

FIGURE **6-16** **Anatomy of Volar Region of Equine and Bovine Hoof. A,** Equine hoof. **B,** Bovine hoof.

CLINICAL APPLICATION Laminitis: A Painful Health Risk to Horses

Laminitis, or "founder" as it is commonly called, is an excruciatingly painful disorder that affects the feet (primarily the front feet) of horses and ponies. As its name implies, laminitis is inflammation of the delicate laminae that attach the hoof wall to the underlying corium. As with all inflammation, laminitis involves swelling. However, the outer wall of the hoof is rigid and cannot expand to accommodate the swelling of the inner foot. Therefore the laminae become compressed. Blood flow and circulation within the foot are inhibited, and the laminae degenerate. Because the laminae attach the coffin bone to the outer hoof, their degeneration may cause the distal phalanx or coffin bone to pull away from the hoof wall. Under the weight of the animal, the bone may rotate downward and push against the sole of the hoof. With very severe rotation, the distal phalanx can actually perforate the sole and, in this way, be fatal to the animal.

Because laminitis is acutely painful, affected animals are often recumbent for extended periods, standing only to urinate, defecate, and access water and feed. When standing, horses with laminitis tend to shift their weight away from the front feet to their hind legs to alleviate pressure in the toe. Their gait is slow and hesitant, and their heart rate and respiratory rate may be elevated because of the pain. A mild tap on the toe with hoof testers can elicit a strong pain response from the horse.

In cases of chronic laminitis, external changes to the hoof become evident. Circumferential rings in the outer hoof wall become pronounced, marking previous aberrations in hoof growth. The angle of the hoof is reduced, and the hoof consequently appears flattened. If rotation has occurred, the sole may appear "dropped." With corrective trimming of the hoof, change in diet, and good management techniques, some of these aberrant changes can be corrected.

Predisposing factors for laminitis include the following:

1. Engorgement of foods high in carbohydrates
2. Any systemic illness or condition that might lead to endotoxemia
3. Postoperative periods
4. Retained placentas in mares
5. Adverse reaction to drugs

Ponies, in particular, are prone to developing laminitis, particularly if they are permitted to graze on lush pasture or are fed diets rich in carbohydrates, such as corn, molasses, and grains. Treatment is designed to decrease swelling, relieve pain, and increase circulation in the feet. Prevention by adherence to a strict low-carbohydrate diet is essential in ponies and horses that are sensitive to carbohydrate levels.

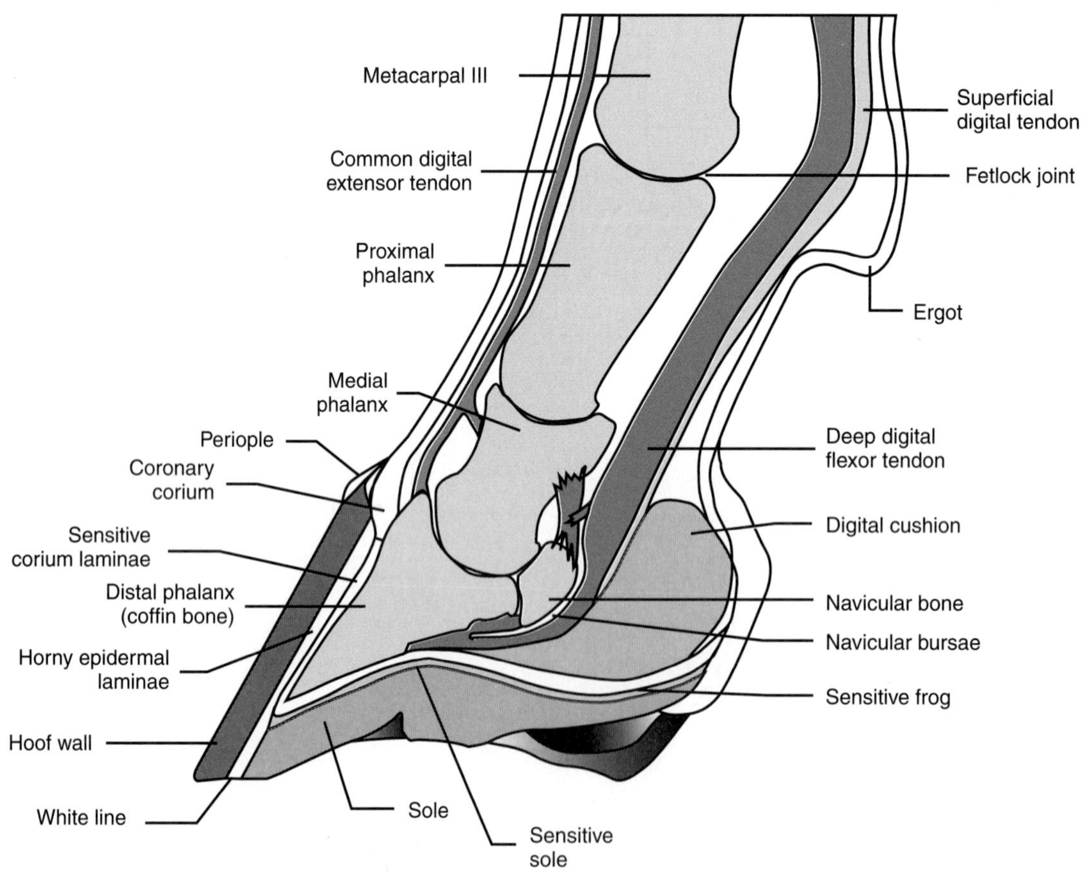

FIGURE **6-17** **Longitudinal Section of Equine Foot Showing Internal Anatomical Structures.**

foot, and into the digital veins. Shifting weight off of the foot releases the compressive force and enables blood to flow back into the corium via the digital arteries.

Horns

Like hooves, horns are epidermal in origin and are structurally similar to hair. They emerge from the horn processes of the frontal bones and take on diverse shapes and sizes in ruminating ungulate species, such as sheep, goats, cattle, buffalo, and antelope. In adults the horn is generally hollow and communicates directly with the frontal sinus. Like the hoof, it is a mass of horny keratin. The corium lies at the root of the horn and is bound to the horn process by periosteum. In addition, long, slender papillae of corium interdigitate with one another to form critical attachments that bind the outer horn to the underlying periosteum. The body of the horn is composed of tubules, which are packed close together to form a single mass. Although externally the diameter of the horn is larger at the base and forms a point at the apex, the wall of the horn is actually thinner at the base than at the apex. In fact, the apex of the horn is considerably stronger and denser than the horn base.

With the exception of the American Pronghorn, which sheds its horns annually, horns grow continuously throughout the life of the animal and can reach great lengths. Many domestic species of sheep, goats, and cattle are "dehorned" when young to facilitate their management by the farmer. Several different instruments and methods can be used to dehorn an animal, depending on the age and species involved. However, the standard procedure is to remove the horn or horn bud and to destroy (usually via cauterization) the corium to prevent further growth of the horn. Some species of domestic animals have been bred to be horn free. These breeds are called **polled breeds.** In nonpolled breeds, horns are found on both males and females. Unlike antlers, they are not sex specific.

In contrast to horns, antlers are found primarily on males, are dermal in origin, and arise as bony protuberances from the skull. They grow and are shed annually. Antlers lack a central core and internal blood supply but are nourished externally by a soft, velvetlike tissue. When the antler has completed its growth, a dense ring of connective tissue forms at the base of the antler, which restricts blood supply to the outer **velvet skin.** In this way, the velvet dies and subsequently is shed or scraped off by the animal. Loss of the velvet allows the antler to harden and become a formidable weapon, a status symbol, and an attractive male secondary sex characteristic. With time, the bony connection between the antler and the skull breaks down, the antlers fall off, and new growth begins.

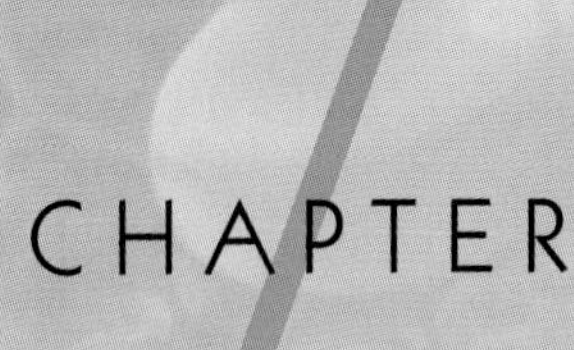

CHAPTER 7

THE NERVOUS SYSTEM

Robert L. Bill

The nervous system is a complex communication and regulatory system that is simultaneously sturdy yet very sensitive to alterations caused by disease, medications, or trauma. To better comprehend the changes occurring in an animal that is anesthetized, intoxicated with a neurotoxin (poison affecting the nervous system), or unable to properly move because of trauma (hit by car, intervertebral disk rupture, etc.), the veterinary technician must have a basic understanding of neurophysiology, that is, the physiology of the nervous system.

The nervous system has three basic functions: sensory functions, integrating functions, and motor functions. The nervous system *senses* changes from within the body or from outside of the body and conveys this information to the spinal cord and brain. In the brain and spinal cord, the sensory information is received, analyzed, stored, and *integrated* to produce a response. The response may be to command muscles to move or produce glandular secretions. This would be the *motor* function of the nervous system.

The branch of science that studies the nervous system is called **neurology** (*neuro-* refers to the nervous system, and *logos* means "study of").

BASIC STRUCTURAL UNIT: THE NEURON

Several cell types are located within the nervous system. The **neuroglia,** or **glial cells** (from the Greek *glia,* meaning "glue"), constitute a group of cells that structurally and functionally support and protect the nervous system. However, although glial cells may make up half of the cells found in the nervous system, they are not the cells directly involved in transmission of the information or "impulses" through the nervous system. This function is the responsibility of another group of cells called the **neurons.**

Although neurons in different parts of the nervous system vary in their physical appearance, their basic structure is the same (Figure 7-1). The structure of the neuron can be divided roughly into the central cell body (also called the **soma** or **perikaryon)** and the two different types of extensions from the cell body called **dendrites** and **axons.**

The dendrites *receive stimuli,* or "impulses," from other neurons and convey this stimulation to the cell body. Dendrites also may be modified into sensory receptors that receive, or "sense," stimuli such as heat, cold, touch, pressure, stretch, or other physical changes from inside or outside of the body. Dendrites tend to be short, multibranched projections extending from the soma. (The word *dendro* is derived from the Greek word for "branch," and under microscopic examination, the dendrites resemble the branches of a tree.)

The axon is the other type of extension from the soma and conducts the nervous impulse away from the soma toward another neuron or other type of cell. In contrast to the short, branched dendrites, the axon is a single process that can be very long. For example, a single axon in the horse may extend several feet from the spinal cord all the way to the lower leg.

Axons often are covered by a fatty substance called **myelin.** Myelin, when chemically prepared for examination under the microscope, appears white. For that reason, nervous tissue containing many myelinated axons is often referred to as **white**

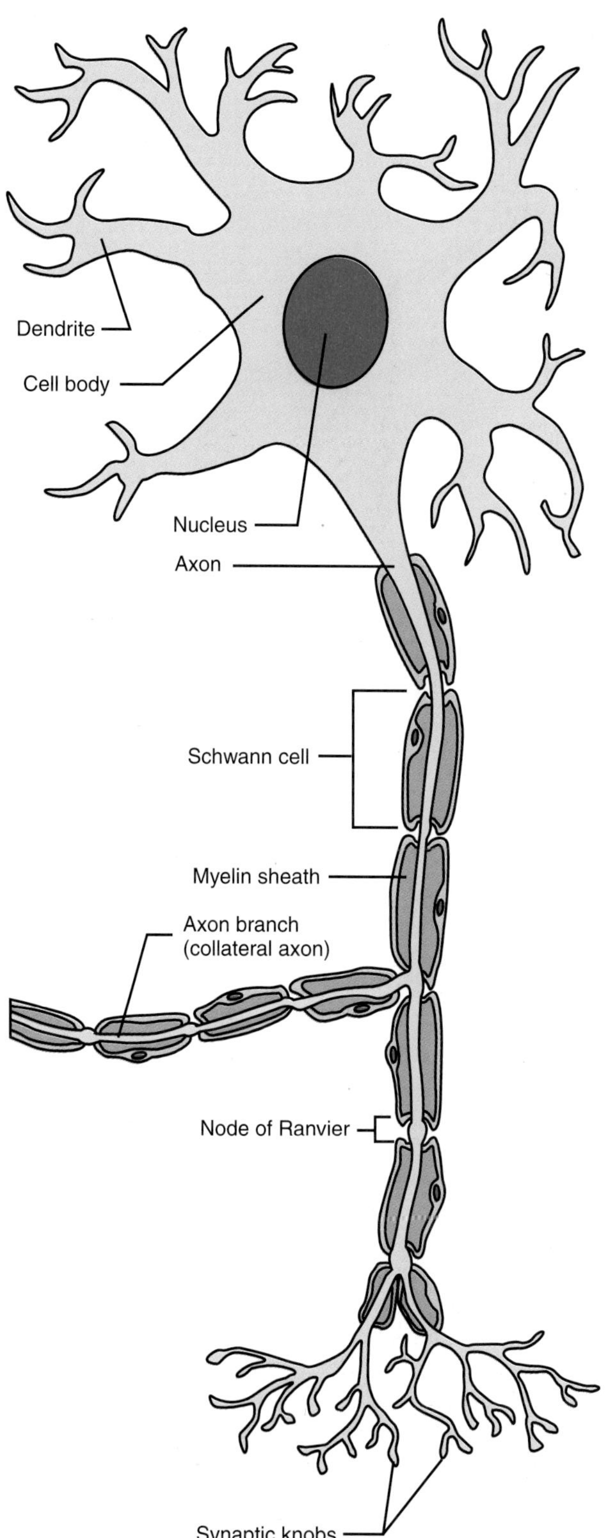

FIGURE **7-1** **Structure of Neuron.**

matter. Conversely, nervous tissue that does not have myelin stains dark and is called **gray matter.** The **myelin sheath** is actually the cell membrane of specialized glial cells called **oligodendrocytes** in the brain and spinal cord and **Schwann cells** in the nerves outside of the brain and spinal cord. These special glial cells are wrapped around the axon like a thin pancake might be tightly wrapped around a pencil or wooden rod. Because the axon of most neurons is fairly long, it takes multiple Schwann cells or oligodendrocytes lying end-to-end to cover the entire length of the axon. Between adjacent glial cells are small gaps in the myelin sheath called **nodes of Ranvier.** The myelin sheath and nodes of Ranvier work together to enhance the speed of conduction of the nervous impulses along the axon. Hence, myelinated axons conduct nerve impulses faster than unmyelinated axons (Figures 7-2 and 7-3).

TEST YOURSELF ✓

1. How are the functions of neurons and neuroglia different from each other?
2. Name the parts of a typical neuron.
3. How are the dendrites and axons different in structure and function?
4. What is the difference between gray matter and white matter?
5. What is the relationship between the myelin sheath and the nodes of Ranvier?

ORGANIZATION OF THE NERVOUS SYSTEM

Many schemes are used to describe the anatomical or functional organization of the nervous system. Because the organizational terminology sets the foundation of any discussion on the nervous system, we first discuss how this terminology is used.

Anatomical Location: CNS vs. PNS

A simple way to organize the nervous system anatomically is to think of it as being divided into two components: the **central nervous system** and the **peripheral nervous system.** As the name implies, the central nervous system (CNS) is anatomically composed of the brain and the spinal cord, which are found associated within the "central" or cranial-caudal axis of the animal's body. *Peripheral* means "to the side" or "away from the center"; therefore the peripheral nervous system (PNS), comprises those components of the nervous system that extend away from the central axis outward toward the periphery of the body. The **cranial nerves** are those nerves of the PNS that originate from the brain, and **spinal nerves** are those PNS nerves that emerge from the spinal cord.

Direction of Impulses: Afferent vs. Efferent

Some nerves conduct electrical impulses from the periphery toward the CNS, and other nerves conduct impulses in the opposite direction from the CNS toward the periphery. These two functional types of nerves are called **afferent nerves** and **efferent nerves.** Afferent nerves conduct nervous impulses *toward* the CNS (*ad-*, "toward"; *ferre,* "to carry"), whereas

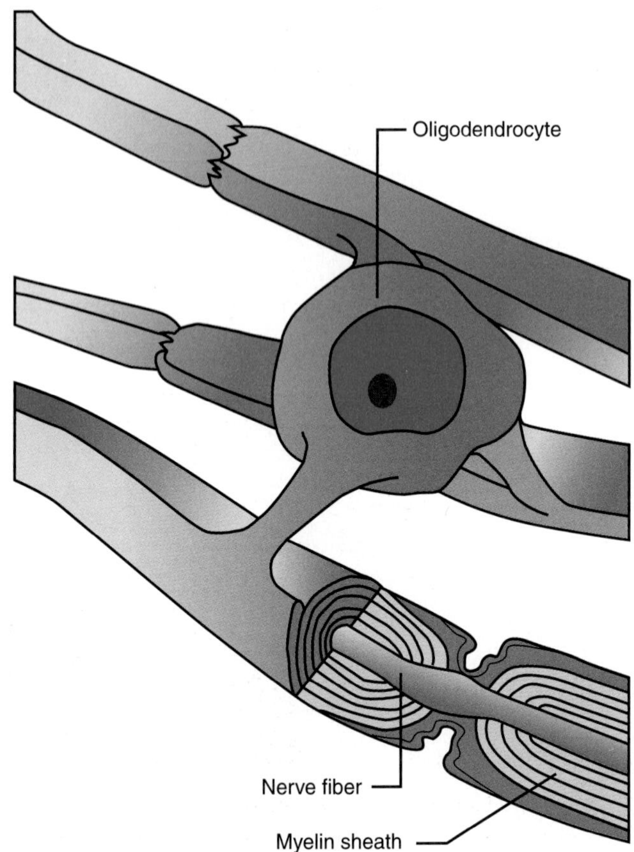

FIGURE **7-2** **Oligodendrocyte, Nerve Fiber, and Myelin Sheath.** Oligodendrocyte wraps around nerve fibers in central nervous system to form myelin sheaths.

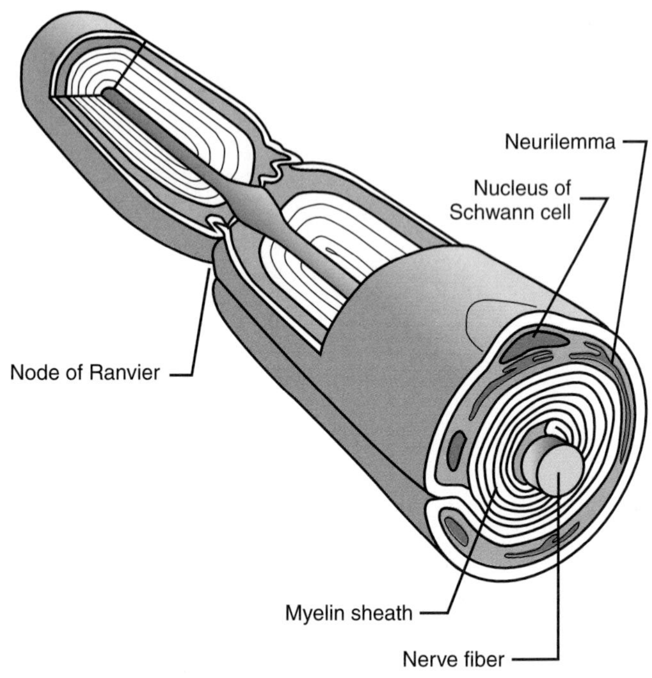

FIGURE **7-3** **Schwann Cell Wraps Around Peripheral Nerve Fiber to Form Thick Myelin Sheath.**

efferent nerves conduct nervous impulses *away* from the CNS (*ex-*, "away"; *ferre,* "to carry").

Because afferent nerves conduct sensations from the sensory receptors in the skin and other locations in the body, afferent nerves are also called **sensory nerves.** In contrast, efferent nerves conduct impulses from the CNS toward muscles and other organs. Because the efferent impulses are the ones that, among other things, cause skeletal muscle contraction and movement, efferent nerves are often called **motor nerves.** Thus cranial nerves and spinal nerves in the PNS and nerve tracts in the CNS may carry nerve fibers that are sensory, motor, or both.

FUNCTION: AUTONOMIC VS. SOMATIC

When an animal turns its head in response to its name being called by its owner, efferent (outgoing) motor impulses from the brain are consciously sent to the muscles in the neck to turn the head toward the sound. This conscious, or voluntary, control of skeletal muscles is referred to as a **somatic nervous system** function. Because the action of the animal turning its head was caused by voluntary initiation of efferent impulses, this function would be classified as a somatic motor function. Impulses being sent to the CNS from receptors in the muscle, skin, eye, or ear would be classified as somatic sensory function because they are consciously perceived by the brain.

In contrast to the voluntary movement of the somatic nervous system function, animals do not have to consciously think to contract their intestines, to increase their heart rate in response to a threat, or to stimulate release of digestive juices in response to ingestion of a meal. The animal also does not have to be consciously aware of blood pressure receptors informing the body that the blood pressure is too low or of stretch receptors indicating that the lungs have inflated. The part of the nervous system that controls and coordinates these automatic functions is called the **autonomic nervous system.** (*Auto-* means "self," and *nomos* means "law"; so the autonomic nervous system is the self-regulating system.)

Like the somatic (voluntary) system, the autonomic system also has motor nerves and sensory nerves. However, instead of these motor nerves going to skeletal muscle to cause voluntary limb or body movement, these autonomic motor nerves send impulses to smooth muscle, cardiac muscle, and endocrine glands to regulate a wide variety of automatic body functions. Autonomic sensory nerves receive the afferent sensory impulses from sensory receptors that are used to automatically regulate these body functions.

TEST YOURSELF

1. What are the anatomical differences between the CNS and the PNS?
2. Which are afferent nerves: motor nerves or sensory nerves? Which are efferent?
3. Identify each of the following as being controlled by the autonomic or the somatic nervous system and as being either sensory or motor:
   - Conscious movement of the forelimb
   - Slowing of the heart rate in response to an increased blood pressure
   - Constriction of blood vessels in the skin in response to cold temperatures
   - Perception of pain from an injection of antibiotics
   - Perception of amount of acidity present in the duodenum

NEURON FUNCTION: DEPOLARIZATION AND REPOLARIZATION

It is often said that a nerve "fires" or that an impulse is conducted from one end of a neuron to the other. What actually is occurring in the neuron when a nerve "fires"? Understanding the concepts of depolarization and repolarization is important for understanding how drugs like local anesthetics can prevent nerves from firing or how imbalances of sodium or potassium in the body can adversely affect nerve function.

RESTING STATE, POLARIZATION, AND RESTING MEMBRANE POTENTIAL

When a neuron is not being stimulated, it is said to be in a **resting state.** However, even when the neuron is "resting" it is still working to maintain its resting state. Specialized molecules located on the neuron's cell membrane pump sodium ions (Na^+) from the inside of the neuron to the outside and pump potassium ions (K^+) from the outside to the inside. This specialized molecule is called the **sodium-potassium pump** (Figure 7-4).

Sodium (Na^+) cannot readily diffuse or leak through the cell membrane on its own. Because sodium cannot diffuse across the membrane, the action of the sodium-potassium pump causes a higher concentration of sodium to accumulate *outside* the cell. The action of the sodium-potassium pump and the negative charges inside the cell cause a higher concentration of potassium to accumulate *inside* the cell. By separating the sodium on one side of the membrane (outside) and the potassium on the other (inside), the cellular membrane separating the two is said to be polarized (it has two distinct "poles" of ions on either side of the membrane).

The distribution of positive and negative charges from sodium, potassium, proteins, and other charged ions on either side of the neuronal membrane creates a difference in electrical charge across the membrane, with the inside of the neuron being more negatively charged than the outside. This electrical

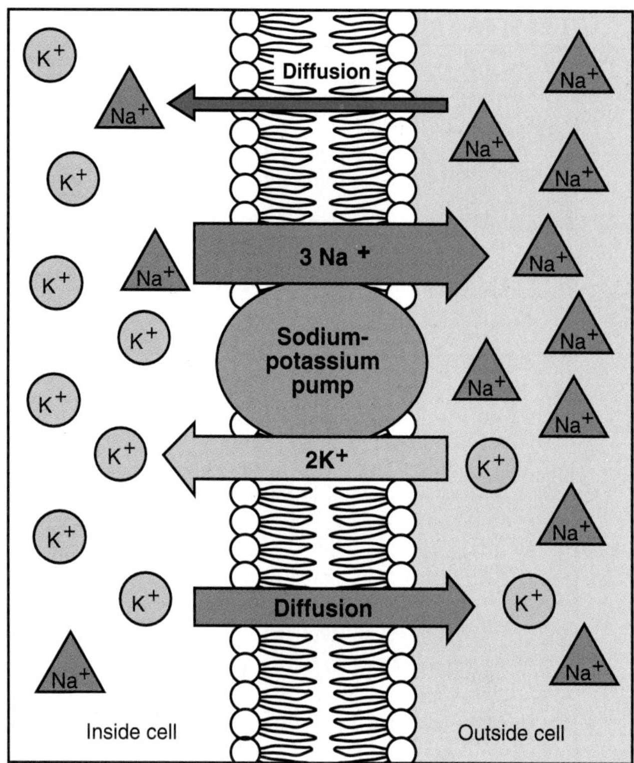

FIGURE **7-4** **Sodium-Potassium Pump.** This cellular mechanism is located in the plasma membrane and actively pumps sodium ions (Na^+) out of the neuron and potassium ions (K^+) into the neuron.

difference in charges across the membrane is called the **resting membrane potential.** The net negative resting membrane potential usually is stated as a certain negative number of millivolts (e.g., -70 mV) indicating the net negative charge within the cell. By selectively pumping sodium out and potassium in, the sodium-potassium pump maintains this negatively charged resting membrane potential.

DEPOLARIZATION

When an impulse from an adjoining neuron or from a specific type of external stimulus (heat, touch, taste, etc.) stimulates a neuron, a set of specific steps occurs, resulting in the nerve "firing" or depolarizing. At the point where the stimulus occurs on the neuron, a specialized molecular structure on the neuron cell membrane called a *sodium channel* opens. This sodium channel allows *only* sodium ions (Na^+) to pass through it. Because a higher concentration of sodium ions exists outside the cell than inside the cell, the sodium ions readily flow through the open sodium channels from the outside to the inside by passive diffusion. Not only is the sodium "driven" into the cell by the concentration gradient (the differences in concentration between the outside and inside), but the positive sodium (Na^+) ions are attracted into the cell by the net negative charge inside the cell. Remember, opposite charges attract each other, and therefore the positive Na^+ ion is attracted toward the relatively negative charge within the cell.

Depolarization refers to this opening of the sodium chan-

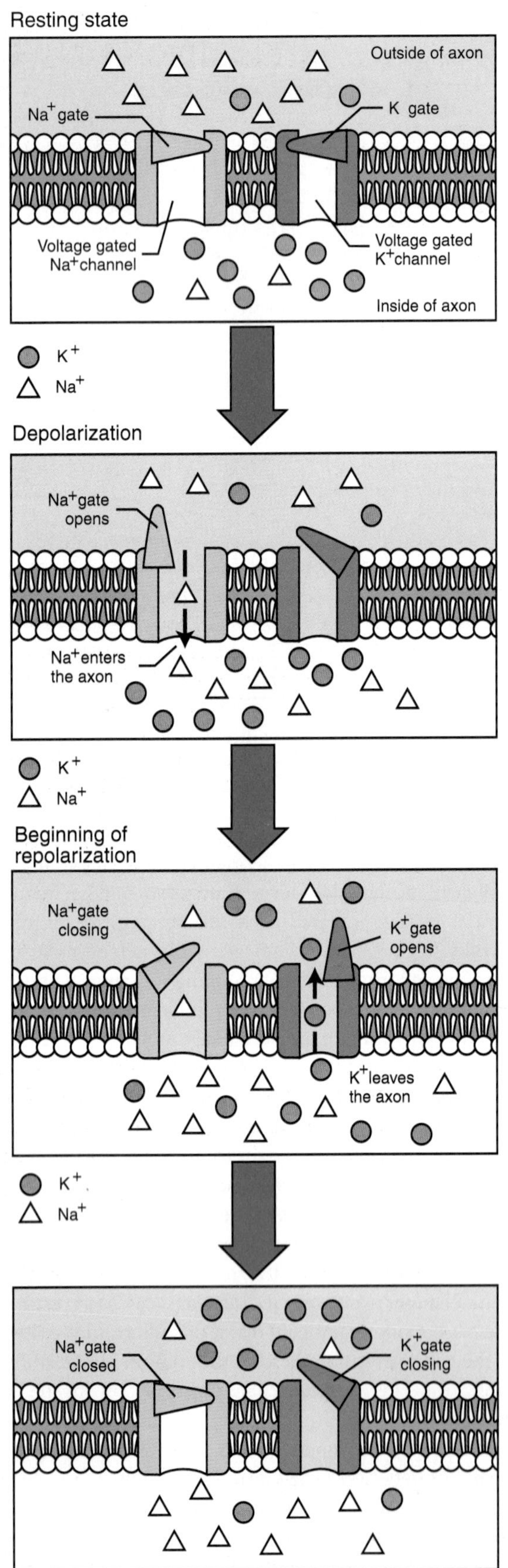

FIGURE **7-5 Depolarization and Repolarization.** Sodium gates open during depolarization and close during repolarization. Potassium gates open during repolarization phase but are closed during depolarization.

nels and the sudden influx of many sodium ions into the cell. It is called *de*polarization because the sodium influx results in the loss of two distinct poles of sodium and potassium on either side of the membrane. If we hooked an electrical meter to the neuron, we would see the inside of the neuron go from a negatively charged resting membrane potential to a net positive charge during depolarization (Figure 7-5). This shift inside the cell from negative to positive makes sense when we consider the positive sodium ions flooding into the neuron. This large change in electrical charge from negative to positive is called the **action potential** and signals the depolarization of the neuron.

REPOLARIZATION

Within a fraction of a second after sodium begins to flood into the cell during depolarization, the sodium channels snap shut, halting the influx. Almost simultaneously, specialized potassium channels open up in the cellular membrane. Like the sodium channels, the potassium channels only allow potassium ions to pass through them.

With the potassium channels open, the potassium ions (K^+) passively diffuse out of the cell, propelled by both the potassium's concentration gradient (high concentration inside, lower concentration outside) and the strong positive charge brought into the cell by the influx of sodium ions. Remember, "like" charges repel; therefore the positive potassium ions are repelled by the relatively positive charge inside of the neuron caused by the sodium influx. This outflow of potassium ions continues until these specialized potassium channels snap shut a split second after they have opened. Because the potassium ions (K^+) are positive, the exodus of potassium ions out of the neuron causes the charge inside the cell to swing back in the negative direction.

This change of the cell's charge back toward the net negative resting membrane potential is called **repolarization.** The cell is said to be *re*polarized because the sodium and potassium ions are once again on opposite sides (opposite poles) of the cell membrane. The only difference between the end of the repolarization phase and the resting state is that the sodium and potassium ions are on the opposite sides from where they began. To restore the sodium and potassium to their original locations on either side of the membrane, the sodium-potassium pump quickly moves the "misplaced" sodium and potassium ions back to their original sides.

Students often think of the acts of depolarization and repolarization as involving a molecular tidal wave of ions moving back and forth. The truth is that relatively few sodium and potassium ions move at each point of the depolarization-repolarization cycle, which explains why the cycle is completed rapidly and why even minor imbalances in sodium or potassium can greatly affect normal neuron function.

DEPOLARIZATION THRESHOLD, CONDUCTION, AND ALL-OR-NONE PRINCIPLE

Not every depolarization stimulus results in the complete depolarization-repolarization cycle. The initial stimulus must be sufficient to make the neuron respond. When the stimulus is strong enough to cause complete depolarization, it is said to have reached **threshold,** causing the cell to depolarize or "fire."

To understand how this works, let's use an example in which a neuron with sensory receptors on its dendrites receives a very weak stimulus. The weak stimulus results in only a few sodium channels opening and therefore only a small influx of sodium ions into the neuronal cell. Because of this, we would only see a slight positive change in neuron charge from the resting membrane potential. Because the charge was not very significant, the cell did not reach threshold and the few sodium channels that opened would close without causing further effect on other sodium channels. The sodium-potassium pump would quickly move the few displaced sodium ions from inside back to outside, and the neuron would go back to its resting state. In this case, the stimulus failed to depolarize the neuron, and the information from the sensory receptors in the dendrites was not transmitted to the brain.

If, however, the stimulus on these dendritic sensory receptors had been larger, more sodium channels would have opened and a greater number of sodium ions would have entered the neuronal cell. This would have produced a significant positive change in the membrane potential in that immediate area of the cellular membrane. If the change was sufficient to reach the threshold, sodium channels adjacent to this area would also open. This would allow sufficient sodium influx into these adjacent areas to reach threshold, causing further adjacent sodium channels to open. In other words, the initial stimulus causes a spreading wave of sodium channels to open over the entire neuron. This wave of sodium channels opening to allow sodium influx is called the **wave of depolarization.** As you recall, the strong influx of sodium ions during depolarization was called the *action potential;* therefore this wave of depolarization is also called the *conduction of the action potential.* Thus, when someone speaks of a "nerve impulse," they are speaking of the wave of depolarization or conduction of the action potential.

Regardless of how strong the initial stimulus was, if it was sufficient to achieve threshold, the action potential would be conducted along the entire neuron with a uniform strength. This phenomenon is called the **all-or-none principle** because either the complete neuron depolarizes to its maximum strength or it does not depolarize at all.

CLINICAL APPLICATION: Local Anesthetics

Local anesthetics are drugs that are injected into superficial areas of the body to block the conduction of sensations from that area of the body. You have experienced this form of anesthesia when your dentist administered a local anesthetic to numb an area of your mouth. Local anesthetic drugs like *lidocaine* prevent sensory nerves from depolarizing despite stimulation from the dental or surgical procedure. If these sensory nerves do not depolarize, the brain is "unaware" of any sensations from that area of the body, and therefore you do not feel pain. Lidocaine prevents the sensory neuron from depolarizing by blocking the sodium channels through which sodium ions usually flood into the neuronal cell. If the sodium channels are "plugged" by the local anesthetic molecule, no sodium can flood into the cell despite the channels being stimulated to open. No sodium influx means the internal positive charge change does not occur in the neuron, threshold is not attained, and the stimulus is not turned into a depolarization wave.

Anesthesia means "without sensitivity." If a sensory nerve does not depolarize, the animal's brain does not perceive sensations from that area of the body. Local anesthetics are used not only to anesthetize areas of the body for minor surgical procedures but also to aid in identifying sources of pain that cause lameness in horses. In a lame horse, a local anesthetic is injected into selected sensory nerves to prevent them from responding to stimulation. The veterinarian determines if injection into that particular nerve improves the horse's movement or lessens the lameness. If it does, the veterinarian knows that the source of the problem is in the area of the leg or hoof whose sensations are supplied by the "blocked" nerve. If the injection of the nerve does not improve the lameness, the veterinarian injects another specific sensory nerve and repeats the process until the horse appears to have less pain.

REFRACTORY PERIOD

If a second stimulus arrives at the dendrites or on the neuron's soma while the sodium channels are all open or while the potassium molecules are moving rapidly through their open channels, the stimulus would be incapable of causing a second depolarization. Because cells in the depolarization and early repolarization phases are already in the process of executing the depolarization-repolarization cycle, they can't depolarize again until the cycle is completed. Thus any stimulus arriving at that point in the depolarization-repolarization cycle would die out. The neuron is said to be in a **refractory period** because it is refractory or "insensitive" to new stimulations. The period of sodium influx and early potassium outflow is a part of the refractory period during which no stimulus of any size can cause the cell to depolarize again. This period is called the *absolute refractory period* because the cell "absolutely" cannot respond. However, if a very large stimulus comes during the tail end of the repolarization period, it may be possible to stimulate another depolarization. Therefore, during this part of the refractory period, the cell may depolarize again if the stimulus is much larger than normal. This period is called the *relative refractory period* because the cell is still refractory to stimuli of normal intensity but may respond to "relatively" larger stimuli.

HOW MYELINATED AXONS CONDUCT ACTION POTENTIALS QUICKER: SALTATORY CONDUCTION

If all neurons sent their wave of depolarization or their conduction of action potentials from one sodium channel to the next in a series of tiny steps, the transmission of the nerve impulse would be relatively slow from one end of a neuron to

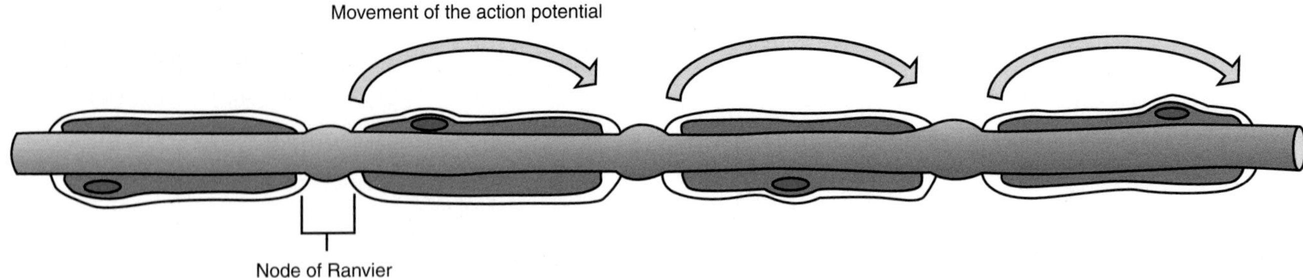

FIGURE **7-6** **Saltatory Conduction.** A nerve impulse moves from one node of Ranvier to the next, producing rapid conduction of the nerve impulse.

the other. Think of the sodium channels as a set of tiny dominos set up in a line several feet long. When we tip over the first domino, we know that it is going to take some time for the last domino to fall. The same thing happens if each sodium channel opening stimulates only the next adjacent channel to open.

If, however, our domino line only required every tenth or hundredth domino to tip over, the speed at which we would reach the end of the domino line would be greatly accelerated. In neurons with axons wrapped in a myelin sheath, a similar effect happens with the depolarization wave. Like a rubber coating on an electrical wire that prevents electrical shorts, the myelin sheath prevents sodium ions from flowing across the neuronal cell membrane. Therefore depolarization in myelinated axons only can take place at the gaps in the myelin sheath that occur at the nodes of Ranvier. Thus, when the sodium influx at one node is sufficient to open adjacent sodium channels, the next available sodium channel is at the next node of Ranvier. The depolarization wave in the myelinated axon "skips" from one node of Ranvier to the next, greatly accelerating the rate at which the depolarization wave moves from the soma to the other end of the axon. This rapid means of conducting an action potential is called **saltatory conduction** (the word *saltatory* is derived from the Latin *saltare,* which means "to leap"; Figure 7-6).

The rapid conduction of impulses through myelinated neurons by saltatory conduction makes processes such as vision and fine motor control possible in "large" animals, such as the domestic animal species and ourselves. An example of how important the myelin sheath and saltatory conduction is to normal function can be illustrated in people with *multiple sclerosis (MS).* In persons with MS, the myelin sheath is damaged, resulting in the inability to see properly, the loss of normal muscle control, and an inability to make coordinated movements. With a damaged myelin sheath, the nerves may still conduct impulses, but their conduction is much slower, resulting in loss of rapid communication needed for complex, integrated functions of the nervous system.

TEST YOURSELF

1. During depolarization, what ion channels open and what ion moves? Where does it move?
2. During repolarization, what ion channels open and what ion moves? Where does it move?
3. What normally maintains the resting membrane potential of a neuron during the resting state?
4. What is threshold? What role does threshold play in the all-or-none principle?
5. What is the difference between the absolute and the relative refractory period?
6. Explain why waves of depolarization are conducted faster in myelinated axons than in unmyelinated ones?

HOW NEURONS COMMUNICATE: THE SYNAPSE

Once the depolarization wave, or action potential, has been successfully conducted to the end of the axon, the nerve impulse must be transmitted to the next neuron or to the cells of the target organ or tissue. Because two adjacent neurons do not physically touch each other, this process cannot be accomplished by continuing the depolarization wave. Instead, the neuron must release a chemical that stimulates the next neuron or cell. This perpetuation of the nerve impulse from one neuron to the next cell is called **synaptic transmission.**

The **synapse** is the junction between two neurons or a neuron and a target cell. The synapse consists of a physical gap between the two cells called the **synaptic cleft.** The neuron bringing the depolarization wave to the synapse and releasing the chemical to stimulate the next cell is called the **presynaptic neuron.** The chemical released by the presynaptic neuron is called the **neurotransmitter,** and the neuron that contains the receptors that receive the neurotransmitter is the **postsynaptic neuron** (Figure 7-7).

If we look closely at the end of the axon on the presynaptic neuron, we see a slightly enlarged bulb called the **terminal bouton** (*bouton,* meaning "button"), **synaptic end bulb,** or

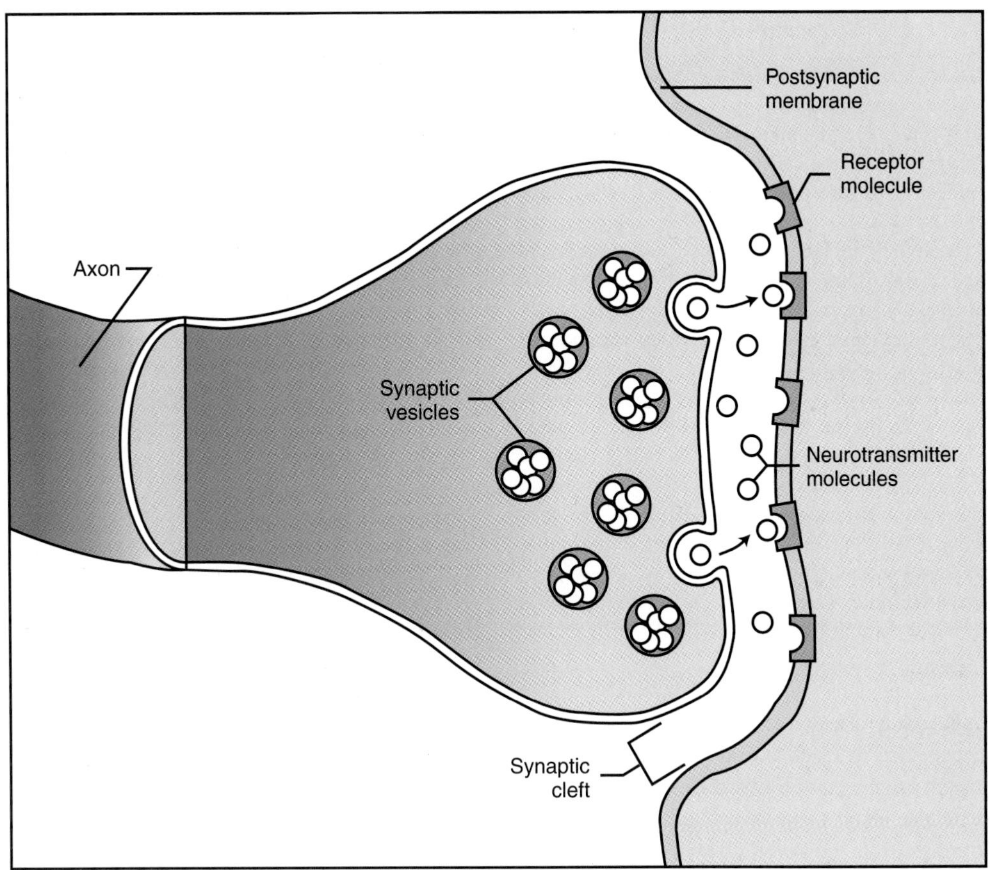

FIGURE **7-7** **Chemical Synapse.** Neurotransmitters are released into the synapse, where they combine with receptors on the postsynaptic membrane.

synaptic knob. The synaptic knob contains many mitochondria that provide energy for the processes that occur here. Multiple vesicles (small sacs) also contain the neurotransmitter. When the axon's wave of depolarization reaches the synaptic knob, calcium channels open in the knob's cellular membrane, resulting in an influx of calcium into the synaptic knob. This influx of calcium causes the vesicles containing neurotransmitter to fuse with the knob's cellular membrane and dump their contents into the synaptic cleft. These neurotransmitters diffuse rapidly across the synaptic cleft toward the postsynaptic membrane.

On the postsynaptic membrane are specialized proteins called **receptors.** The neurotransmitter released by the synaptic knob combines with these receptors and triggers a change in the postsynaptic cell. However, the postsynaptic membrane receptors are very specific about which neurotransmitters they will bind. If the neurotransmitter and receptor are not matched, they will not bind to each other and no change will be triggered in the postsynaptic cell. An analogy that illustrates this concept is that of a lock and key. Only certain keys (types of neurotransmitters) will fit in a lock (the receptor) and cause the lock to open (the receptor to trigger cellular changes). Thus synaptic transmission is only effective if receptors to the neurotransmitter exist on the postsynaptic cell's membrane.

Types of Neurotransmitters and Their Effect on Postsynaptic Membrane

Many different types of neurotransmitters are associated with synapses in both the CNS and PNS. Generally, we can classify these neurotransmitters into two categories: **excitatory neurotransmitters** or **inhibitory neurotransmitters.** As their name implies, excitatory neurotransmitters have an "excitatory" effect on the postsynaptic membrane when they combine with their specific receptors. Specifically, excitatory neurotransmitters usually cause an influx of sodium so that the postsynaptic membrane moves toward threshold. If the postsynaptic membrane is stimulated sufficiently by enough excitatory neurotransmitters, then threshold will be attained and depolarization of the postsynaptic membrane will occur.

In contrast to excitatory neurotransmitters, inhibitory neurotransmitters tend to "hyperpolarize" the postsynaptic membrane, making the inside of the cell more negative instead of positive and moving the charge within the postsynaptic cell farther away from threshold. When inhibitory neurotransmitters combine with their specific receptors on the postsynaptic side, they may cause chloride channels or potassium channels to open up on the postsynaptic membrane. This allows the negatively charged chloride ions (Cl^-) to enter the postsynaptic cell and potassium (K^+) ions to leave the cell, making the inside

Clinical Application: Poisons That Affect the Nervous System

Every year animals are injured or killed by nervous system poisons in the form of insecticides (flea products, bug sprays, agricultural chemicals), rodenticides (mice and rat killers), poisonous plants, or other chemical poisons that disrupt the function of the synapse. Many of these poisons act by combining with or blocking the neurotransmitter receptors on the postsynaptic membranes. To combine with the receptors, these poisons must have a similar molecular structure to the natural neurotransmitters in the body.

Many of these poisons bind with the receptors just like the natural neurotransmitters do, thereby stimulating the postsynaptic cell or neuron. In these cases of poisoning, we see an overstimulation of some aspect of the nervous system or the tissues innervated (supplied with nerves) by that part of the nervous system. Animals may show signs of seizures or muscular tremors, indicating stimulation of the somatic motor system, or overstimulation of the autonomic nervous system, resulting in vomiting or changes in respiration, heart rate, or other autonomic functions.

In some cases the poison can combine with the receptor, but it does *not* produce an effect. In this case the poison would *prevent* the natural neurotransmitter from combining with the receptor to produce its normal effect. Because the poison acts as a blocker of that receptor, we would see a suppression of that part of the nervous system. A classic example of this effect is curare, the nerve poison found on the skin of the brightly colored poison dart frogs in South America. Curare combines with the receptors on skeletal muscles and prevents the presynaptic neuron's neurotransmitter from stimulating the muscle to contract. Therefore curare paralyzes the animal's muscles. South American natives use this toxin to coat the tips of their hunting arrows or spears to paralyze animals hit with the arrow or spear. In this way, the animals are easily captured even if the arrow itself was not fatal.

We use a similar effect medically to paralyze the normal respiratory movements of animals during open chest surgery. By paralyzing the respiratory muscles, we can more easily ventilate (breathe for the animal) with a machine without fighting the body's own contraction of the diaphragm and rib cage muscles.

of the cell more negatively charged (a change in charge that is opposite from that needed to reach threshold).

Neurotransmitters usually can be classified as excitatory or inhibitory based on the effect they have on the postsynaptic cell. Some neurotransmitters, however, can have an excitatory effect on some cells and an inhibitory effect on others, so it is difficult in most cases to make sweeping statements about whether a given neurotransmitter is one or the other.

Acetylcholine is one of the most commonly studied neurotransmitters in the body. It can be either an excitatory or inhibitory neurotransmitter depending on its location in the body. At the junction between somatic motor neurons and the muscles they supply, acetylcholine is an excitatory neurotransmitter that causes muscular contraction. However, at the site where nerves synapse with the heart, acetylcholine has an inhibitory effect that slows the heart rate.

Norepinephrine, dopamine, and **epinephrine** are all neurotransmitters that belong to a group called **catecholamines.** Norepinephrine is associated with arousal and "fight or flight" reactions of the sympathetic nervous system. Epinephrine is released primarily from the adrenal medulla (center of the adrenal gland) and therefore plays more of a role as a hormone in the fight or flight reactions of the sympathetic nervous system. Dopamine is found within the brain where it is involved with autonomic functions and muscle control. Humans with a decreased number of functioning dopamine neurons show the muscle tremors and shaky gait associated with Parkinson's disease.

Gamma-aminobutyric acid (GABA) and **glycine** are two neurotransmitters that are inhibitory. GABA is found in the brain, and glycine is found in the spinal cord. Some groups of tranquilizers, such as diazepam (Valium), work by increasing the GABA effect on the brain, thus inhibiting activity in the brain and producing tranquilization with sedation.

One postsynaptic membrane may have multiple types of presynaptic neurons across the synaptic cleft. For example, a postsynaptic motor neuron in the brain may have some presynaptic neurons that release the excitatory neurotransmitter acetylcholine into the synaptic cleft and other presynaptic neurons that release the inhibitory neurotransmitter GABA into that same synaptic cleft. Depending on which set of neurons is more active—the excitatory acetylcholine-releasing neuron or the neurons releasing the GABA inhibitory neurotransmitter—the postsynaptic motor neuron may either be stimulated or inhibited.

By having both inhibitory and excitatory neurotransmitters, the nervous system can selectively increase or decrease activity of specific parts of the brain or spinal cord. Drugs or poisons that imitate inhibitory or excitatory neurotransmitters will cause CNS depression or CNS-increased activity, respectively. For example, ivermectin, a commonly used antiparasitic drug (kills parasites), causes an increased inhibitory neurotransmitter effect. In animals receiving an overdose of ivermectin, the main clinical signs are severe depression, loss of normal control of voluntary movements, and coma, all of which reflect inhibition of the neuronal activity in the brain.

Stopping and Recycling the Neurotransmitter

If the neurotransmitter were released, combined with its corresponding receptor, and remained in the synapse or on the postsynaptic receptor, the postsynaptic cell would either continue to be excited or continue to be inhibited, depending on the type of receptor being stimulated. Therefore the body must have a way of stopping the effect of the neurotransmitter quickly so that this does not occur.

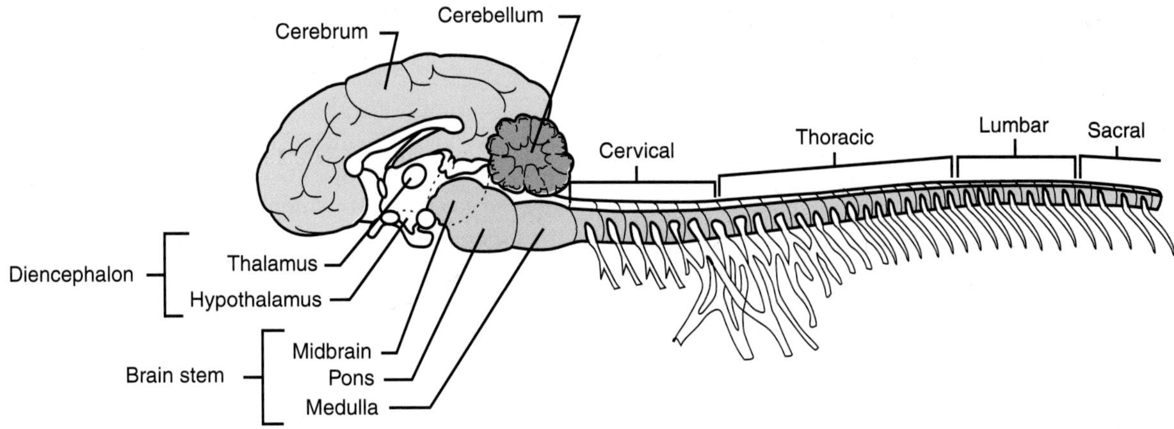

FIGURE **7-8** **Anatomy of Central Nervous System.**

In the case of acetylcholine, the neurotransmitter is broken down quickly by an enzyme found on the postsynaptic membrane called **acetylcholinesterase.** The *-ase* on the end of the word tells us that this compound is an enzyme that acts on acetylcholine. The broken down components of acetylcholine are reabsorbed by the synaptic knob, reassembled into new acetylcholine molecules, and repackaged into vesicles for release with the next wave of depolarization. If acetylcholinesterase is prevented from working, acetylcholine will not be broken down and acetylcholine receptors will continue to be stimulated. This is what happens when animals are exposed to poisonous levels of flea products containing organophosphate insecticides. In organophosphate poisoning the insecticide combines with the acetylcholinesterase and inactivates it. The small amount of acetylcholine normally released by presynaptic neurons causes overstimulation of acetylcholine receptors, resulting in diarrhea, vomiting, difficult breathing, and constricted pupils.

After the release of norepinephrine from the presynaptic neuron, the norepinephrine is rapidly taken back into the synaptic knob, where it is broken down into its components by the enzyme monoamine oxidase (MAO). Any norepinephrine not reabsorbed by the synaptic knob is degraded by another enzyme called *catechol-O-methyl transferase* (COMT). Compared with acetylcholinesterase, the activity of MAO and COMT is relatively slow, which helps to explain why effects of these excitatory neurotransmitters can linger for awhile after their release. One of the mechanisms by which human antidepression medications work is by blocking MAO or COMT, which allows norepinephrine to prolong its excitatory effect on the brain.

Because drugs and poisons encountered in veterinary medicine often produce their effects by increasing or decreasing excitatory or inhibitory neurotransmitter effects or by affecting the enzymes that terminate these effects, it's important that the veterinary technician understand the concepts of synaptic function and neurotransmitter release and termination.

TEST YOURSELF ✓

1. What role do the synaptic cleft, presynaptic neuron, neurotransmitter, and postsynaptic neuron play in the continuation of a depolarization wave from one nerve to another?
2. What is the functional relationship between a neurotransmitter and a receptor? Will any neurotransmitter stimulate any receptor?
3. What is the difference between an excitatory and an inhibitory neurotransmitter?
4. How is acetylcholine different from acetylcholinesterase?
5. What are catecholamines?
6. What is GABA and glycine?

THE BRAIN: GENERAL STRUCTURE AND FUNCTION

Neurological disease or disorders affecting the brain produce clinical signs that sometimes can be identified as belonging to specific areas of the brain. Although knowing all the centers or nuclei (clusters of neurons within the CNS) of the brain is not essential, the veterinary technician should be familiar with what the various areas of the brain do to better understand the effect of neurological disease and medications that affect the CNS (Figure 7-8).

In general, we can think of the brain as being divided into four different sections: the **cerebrum,** the **cerebellum,** the **diencephalon** (meaning "between brains"), and the **brain stem.** Each section of the brain has its own particular function, with the brain stem and diencephalon being the more "primitive" parts of the brain, the cerebellum coordinating motor control, and the "highest centers" of function being found in the cerebrum. Therefore disease in each part of the brain would produce different clinical signs.

CEREBRUM

The cerebrum is made up of the gray matter **cerebral cortex** (outer layer of the brain) and white matter fibers beneath the cortex, including the **corpus callosum** (set of fibers that connect the two halves of the cerebral cortex). It is the largest part of the mammalian brain in domestic animals and constitutes the area of the brain responsible for those functions most commonly associated with "higher-order" behaviors (learning, intelligence, awareness, etc.). The cerebrum receives and interprets sensory information; initiates conscious (voluntary) nerve impulses to skeletal muscles; and integrates neuron activity that is normally associated with communication, expression of emotional responses, learning, memory and recall, and other behaviors associated with conscious activity.

The wrinkled appearance of the surface of the lobes of the cerebral hemispheres is due to the folds called **gyri** (plural of **gyrus**) separated by deep grooves called **fissures** and more shallow grooves called **sulci** (plural of **sulcus**). The most prominent groove is the **longitudinal fissure,** which divides the cerebrum into right and left **cerebral hemispheres** (Figure 7-9). Each hemisphere is divided by sulci into **lobes.** Different lobes of the cerebral hemispheres specialize in certain functions. For example, a section of lobes in the front half of the brain contains the organized areas that initiate voluntary motor functions, whereas the lobe immediately posterior to this section contains the area that identifies the locations of sensations in or on the body.

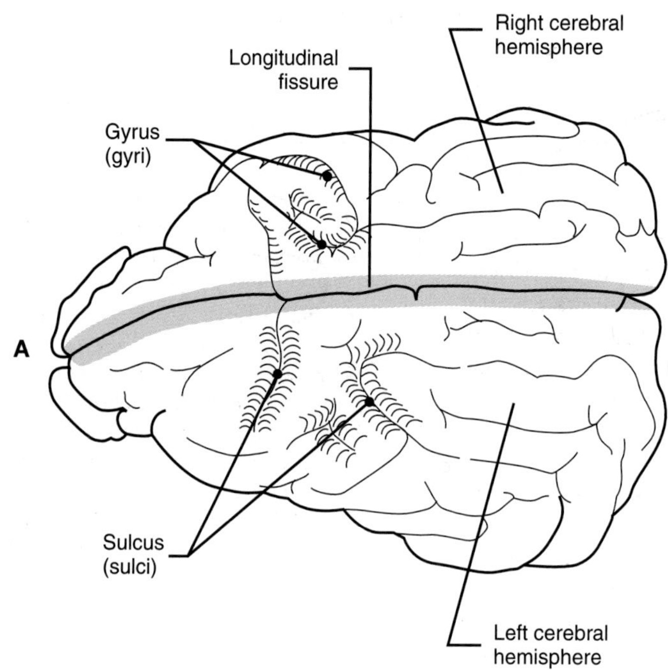

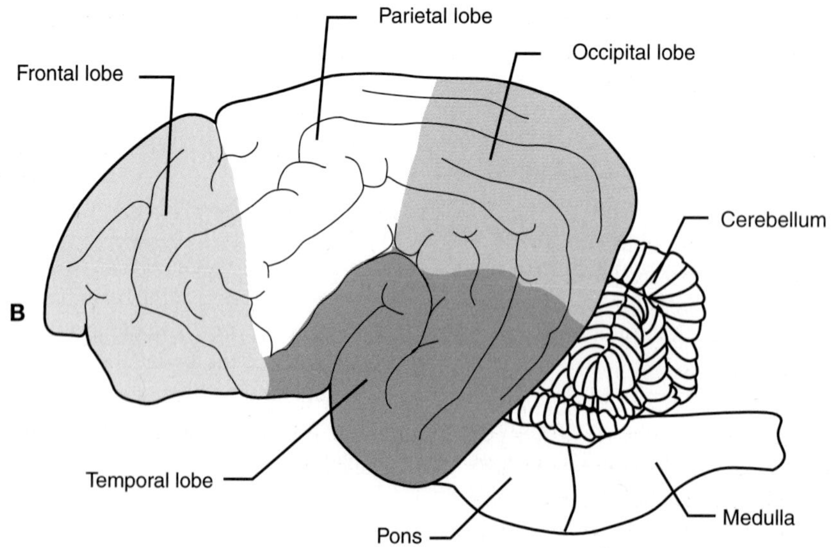

FIGURE **7-9** **Sulci and Gyri of Cerebrum. A,** Top view. **B,** Side view.

If certain lobes of the cerebrum contain neurons that begin to fire spontaneously as a result of drugs, cellular damage, or neurotransmitter imbalance, the animal can exhibit spontaneous movements, seizure activity, abnormal behaviors, or hallucinations, depending on which lobes are affected. If parts of the cerebrum become damaged and nonfunctional from lack of oxygen, poisonous substances, or blood clots (strokes), the animal may lose the perception of specific sensations, may experience loss of voluntary movement, or may be unable to retain or recall information (unable to learn).

CEREBELLUM

The cerebellum is the second largest component of the brain and allows the body to have coordinated movement, balance, posture, and complex reflexes. Essentially, the cerebellum compares the movement the body intends to do with the actual position of muscles and joints to determine if the intentions of the cerebral cortex are actually being carried out. If the movements are not being carried out, the cerebellum will stimulate or inhibit muscles to fine-tune the movements.

For example, if you flex your arm, you can feel your biceps muscle contract while the opposing triceps muscle relaxes. When your arm begins to flex, stretch receptors associated with the muscles send feedback to the cerebellum to keep it informed of the position of the arm. The cerebellum then sends impulses to both the cerebral cortex and the muscles involved in the arm movement so that adjustments in the contraction can be made.

In addition to making the voluntary body movements smooth and accurate, the cerebellum also uses this same afferent sensory feedback from the muscles to maintain posture and balance.

Damage or disease involving the cerebellum results in hypermetria, a condition in which voluntary movements become jerky and exaggerated. A condition like this occurs in pigs with cerebellar disease and causes the affected animals to exhibit a "goose-step" gait in which the lifting and placing of the foot becomes exaggerated. Similar abnormal gaits can be seen in the young of other species born with an incompletely developed cerebellum or in animals with viral or bacterial disease that affects the cerebellum.

DIENCEPHALON

The diencephalon serves as a nervous system passageway between the primitive brain stem and the cerebrum. Although many structures are associated with the diencephalon, veterinary technicians need to be familiar with the following three major ones: (1) the **thalamus,** which acts as a relay station for regulating sensory impulses to the cerebrum; (2) the **hypothalamus,** which essentially is an interface between the nervous system and the endocrine system; and (3) the **pituitary,** which is the endocrine "master gland" that regulates hormone regulation throughout the body. The hypothalamus region also plays major roles in temperature regulation, hunger, thirst, and components of rage and anger responses. Disease or drugs that result in fever (hyperthermia) or compulsive eating or drinking often involve centers within the hypothalamus.

BRAIN STEM

The brain stem is the connection between the brain and the spinal cord. It is composed of the **medulla oblongata,** the **pons,** and the **midbrain.** This section of the brain is heavily involved in autonomic control functions related to the heart, respiration (including coughing, sneezing, and hiccupping), blood vessel diameter (vasomotor control), swallowing, and vomiting. Many of the cranial nerves (see later text) originate from this area of the brain. Because the functions related to the heart, blood vessel diameter, and respiration are critical to life, damage to the brain stem can result in the animal dying from respiratory failure or cardiovascular collapse.

TEST YOURSELF

1. What part of the brain is responsible for conscious thought and perception of sensations?
2. What are the correct names for the "bumps" and "fissures" that make the cerebral cortex appear wrinkled?
3. What part of the brain is critical for coordination, posture, and fine motor control? How does this part of the brain accomplish these responsibilities?
4. What part of the brain serves as a relay station for impulses going to and from the cerebrum?
5. Which part of the brain controls many autonomic functions related to cardiovascular function, respiration, and gastrointestinal tract functions?

OTHER CLINICALLY IMPORTANT STRUCTURES OF THE BRAIN

Other structures in the brain are important for the veterinary technician to be aware of because of their role in how drugs or disease affect the brain or their role in diagnostic procedures used in veterinary medicine.

Meninges

The **meninges** are a set of connective tissues that surround the brain and spinal cord. The three layers of the meninges, from outside to innermost layer, are the **dura mater,** the **arachnoid,** and the **pia mater.** These connective tissue layers of the meninges contain a rich network of blood vessels that supply nutrients and oxygen to the superficial tissues of the brain and spinal cord. The fluid, fat, and connective tissue found between the layers of the meninges also provide some cushion and distribution of nutrients for the CNS. Inflammation of these meningeal membranes from virus or bacterial infections is called *meningitis.*

Cerebrospinal Fluid

The brain and spinal cord are bathed and protected from the hard surface of the skull by a fluid called the **cerebrospinal**

Clinical Application: Epidural Anesthesia and Radiographic Contrast Materials

We sometimes inject anesthetic agents into the spaces between the spinal cord meninges to produce spinal cord anesthesia. Anesthetic drugs introduced in this way block depolarization waves from moving up and down the spinal cord and thus remove the perception of pain from the caudal part of the body. This is called **epidural anesthesia** because the anesthetic is injected into a space between one layer of meninges called the *dura* and the surrounding bone. "Epidurals" have the advantage of decreasing the perception of pain without having to anesthetize the brain. By not anesthetizing the brain stem and diencephalon, the body can more readily maintain its normal autonomic function during the anesthesia.

Another example of the spaces between the meninges being used in veterinary medicine occurs when an animal is suspected of having spinal trauma. For example, dachshunds often suffer from a rupture of intervertebral disks (so-called slipped disk) between the lumbar vertebrae or caudal thoracic vertebrae. The rupture of an intervertebral disk forces the gelatinous material inside the disk through the fibrous ring of the disk and dorsally into the spinal cord. The pressure exerted by the gelatinous material compresses, or completely closes off, the space between the meninges on the ventral side (the underside) of the spinal cord at the point of disk rupture. To identify the existence of this material pushing up against the spinal cord, we can inject a radiopaque dye (a dye that shows up on radiographs or x-ray films) into the spinal cord meningeal space, take a radiograph, and look for places along the spinal cord where the dye did not flow. These areas where the dye is not found would indicate where the ruptured gelatinous intervertebral disk material is pressing against the spinal cord and causing damage. This procedure is called **contrast radiography** or **myelography.**

fluid (CSF). This clear, slippery CSF circulates between layers of the meninges and through cavities (canals and ventricles) inside of the brain and spinal cord. In addition to its cushioning function, the CSF's chemical composition may be involved in regulation of certain autonomic functions, such as respiration and vomiting. For example, if the pH of the CSF becomes more acidic, the respiratory center in the brain stem will increase the respiratory rate. Because the CSF circulates throughout the CNS, infection, inflammation, or cancer in the brain or spinal cord can cause the CSF to change in the amount of protein or cells (white blood cells, cancer cells) it contains. Veterinarians can diagnose certain nervous system diseases or cancer by taking a sample of CSF ("CSF tap") and examining it for particular types of cells or specific changes in the CSF composition.

Blood-Brain Barrier

The **blood-brain barrier** is a functional barrier separating the capillaries in the brain from the nervous tissue itself. Unlike other capillaries in the body that have small openings between the cells of the capillary walls, the capillary wall cells in the brain are aligned tightly together without these openings, or *fenestrations.* In addition, the capillaries in the brain are covered by the cell membranes of glial cells. Thus the tightly constructed capillary wall and the additional glial cell membranes result in a cellular barrier that prevents many drugs, proteins, ions, and other molecules from readily passing from the blood into the brain. In this way the blood-brain barrier protects the brain from many poisons circulating in the bloodstream. For example, the heartworm preventative drug ivermectin is poisonous to insects and parasites but does not adversely affect the dogs and cats that receive it. The reason for this "selective toxicity" of ivermectin is that mammals have a blood-brain barrier that prevents ivermectin from reaching target receptors on cells within the brain; however, insects or parasites do not have a blood-brain barrier and thus the ivermectin can readily reach target receptors throughout the nervous system.

Cranial Nerves

Cranial nerves are a special set of 12 pairs of nerves in the peripheral nervous system that originate from the brain. Each pair of cranial nerves is conventionally numbered in Roman numerals from I through XII (1 through 12). The cranial nerve itself may contain axons of motor neurons, axons of sensory neurons, or combinations of both. Cranial nerve I (CN I, olfactory nerve) and cranial nerve II (CN II, optic nerve) are both examples of a pure sensory cranial nerve. The olfactory nerve is responsible for conveying sensory impulses from receptors in the nose to the brain for the sense of smell, and the optic nerve is responsible for perception of light and vision. Unlike CN I and II, CN III is the oculomotor nerve and, as the name implies, is a motor cranial nerve that controls eye movement. Other cranial nerves, like CN V (trigeminal nerve), control muscles of the jaw for chewing and also convey sensations from the nose, mouth, and part of the throat. Thus CN V is an example of a cranial nerve that serves both sensory and motor functions. See Table 7-1 for a list of the different functions of the twelve cranial nerves.

Two mnemonic devices (memory aids) can be used for remembering the names of the cranial nerves and their functions (sensory, motor, or both). In the first one, each word of the saying begins with the same letter as the corresponding cranial nerve. Of course, you have to remember which "O" represents which cranial nerve in the first three cranial nerves, but the saying still helps students remember their names more readily (Table 7-2).

The next mnemonic device tells you whether the cranial nerve in question is a sensory nerve, a motor nerve, or both sensory and motor (see Table 7-2). In the saying, the words beginning with "S" indicate that the corresponding nerve is primarily sensory. If the word begins with "M" the corresponding nerve is primarily a motor nerve, and if the word begins with "B" the nerve is both sensory and motor.

Table 7-1 Functions of 12 Cranial Nerves

Number	Name	Type	Key Functions
I	Olfactory	Sensory	Smell
II	Optic	Sensory	Vision
III	Oculomotor	Motor	Eye movement, pupil size, focusing lens
IV	Trochlear	Motor	Eye movement
V	Trigeminal	Both sensory and motor	Sensations from the head and teeth, chewing
VI	Abducent	Motor	Eye movement
VII	Facial	Both sensory and motor	Face and scalp movement, salivation, tears, taste
VIII	Vestibulocochlear	Sensory	Balance, hearing
IX	Glossopharyngeal	Both sensory and motor	Tongue movement, swallowing, salivation, taste
X	Vagus ("wanderer")	Both sensory and motor	Sensory from gastrointestinal tract and respiratory tree, motor to the larynx, pharynx, parasympathetic motor to the abdominal and thoracic organs
XI	Accessory	Motor	Head movement, accessory motor with vagus
XII	Hypoglossal	Motor	Tongue movement

Table 7-2 Mnemonic Devices for Cranial Nerve Names and Functions

Cranial Nerve	Nerve Name	Word of the Saying	Type of Nerve	Word of the Saying
I	Olfactory	On	Sensory	Six
II	Optic	old	Sensory	sailors
III	Oculomotor	Olympus'	Motor	made
IV	Trochlear	towering	Motor	merry,
V	Trigeminal	top,	Both sensory and motor	but
VI	Abducent	a	Motor	my
VII	Facial	fine,	Both sensory and motor	brother
VIII	Vestibulocochlear	vocal	Sensory	said,
IX	Glossopharyngeal	German	Both sensory and motor	"Bad
X	Vagus	viewed	Both sensory and motor	business,
XI	Spinal accessory	some	Motor	my
XII	Hypoglossal	hops.	Motor	man."

TEST YOURSELF

1. What are the protective membranes that surround, support, and protect the CNS?
2. What is the fluid called that bathes, cushions, and aids in transport of materials to and from the CNS?
3. What helps keep dangerous poisons or certain drugs from leaving the blood and entering the brain? What is the structural makeup of this?
4. What are the 12 cranial nerves? Which nerves are motor, which are sensory, and which are both?

THE PARASYMPATHETIC AND SYMPATHETIC NERVOUS SYSTEMS

As mentioned previously, the autonomic nervous system controls many functions of the body at a subconscious level. These automatic functions are performed by two divisions of the autonomic nervous system: the **sympathetic nervous system** and the **parasympathetic nervous system.** These two systems generally have opposite effects on organs or tissues, and whichever system dominates at any given moment determines the state of the organ systems.

STRUCTURE

The first anatomical difference between these two systems is where the peripheral nerves of each system emerges from the CNS. The nerves for the sympathetic nervous system emerge from the thoracic and lumbar vertebral regions in the back. Thus the sympathetic system is often referred to as the **thoracolumbar system.** In contrast, the parasympathetic system emerges from the brain and the sacral vertebral regions and therefore is called the **cranial sacral system.**

The efferent motor nerves of both the sympathetic and parasympathetic nervous systems are composed of a sequence of two neurons. The first neuron has its cell body in the brain or spinal cord and extends its axon out from the CNS to a cluster of neuronal cell bodies outside of the CNS called an autonomic **ganglion.** Here the first neuron synapses with one or more second neuron(s), which then connect to the target organ (e.g., endocrine gland, smooth muscle). The first neu-

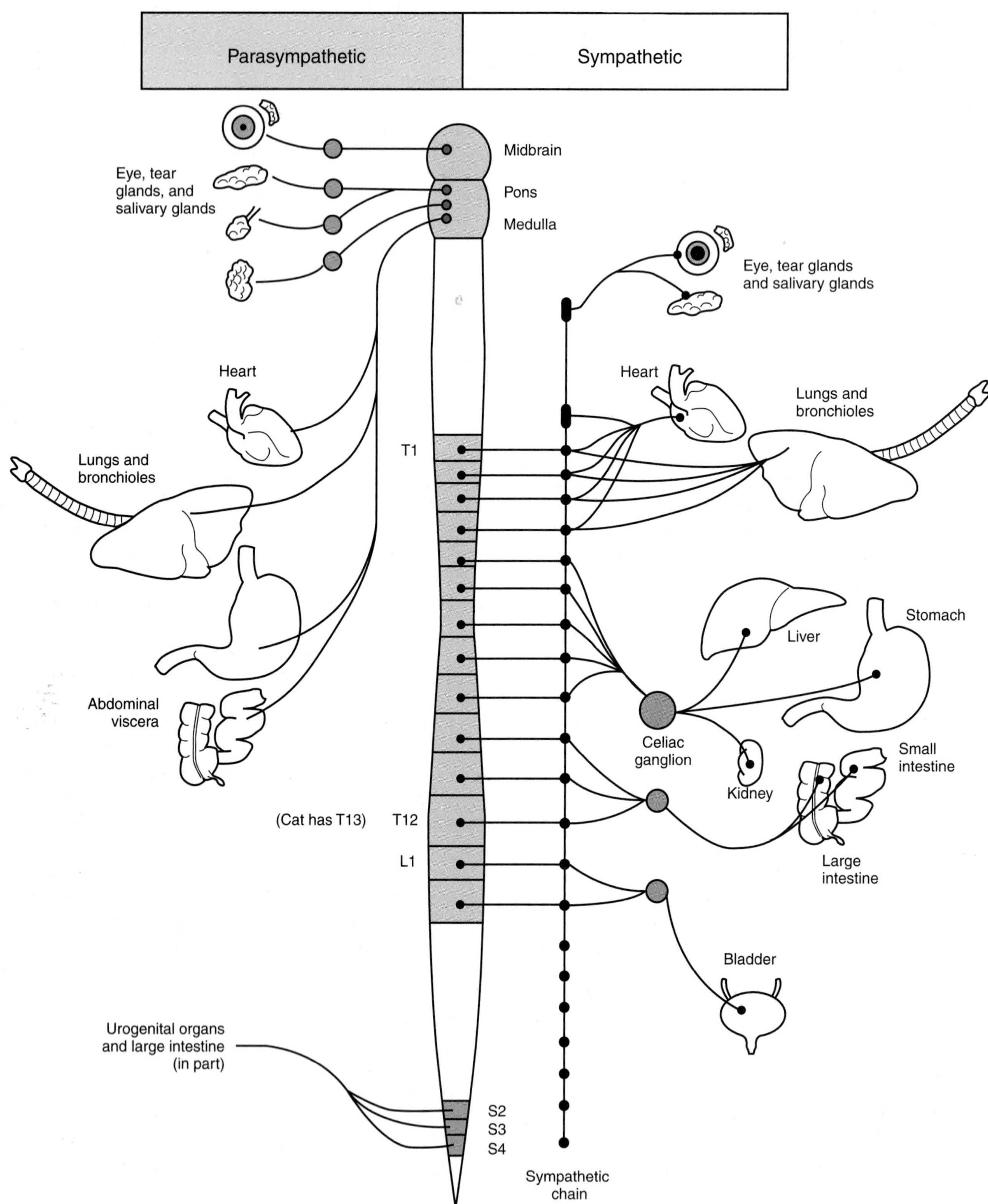

FIGURE **7-10** **Structure of Parasympathetic and Sympathetic Nervous System.**

ron is called the **preganglionic neuron** because it is "before" the ganglia. The second neuron is the **postganglionic neuron,** so named because it carries the impulse from the ganglia onto the target organ.

The sympathetic and parasympathetic systems also differ anatomically in the length of the preganglionic and postganglionic neurons (Figure 7-10). The sympathetic preganglionic neuron originates in the thoracic and lumbar segments of the spinal column. Outside the thoracolumbar area of the spinal column are a series of autonomic ganglia (many ganglion) that

Table 7-3 Effects of Sympathetic and Parasympathetic Nervous System

	Sympathetic System Effect	Parasympathetic System Effect
Heart rate	Increases	Decreases
Force of heart contraction	Increases	No significant effect
Diameter of bronchioles	Increases (dilates)	Decreases (constricts)
Diameter of pupil	Increases (dilates)	Decreases (constricts)
Gastrointestinal motility, secretions, and blood flow	Decreases	Increases
Diameter of skin blood vessels	Decreases	No significant effect
Diameter of muscle blood vessels	Increases	No significant effect
Diameter of blood vessels to kidney	Decreases	No significant effect

form a chain called the **sympathetic ganglion chain.** The sympathetic preganglionic neuron extends out from the spinal cord and either synapses with a neuron within the ganglion chain or passes through the ganglionic chain and synapses with a neuron located beyond the sympathetic chain. Each sympathetic preganglionic neuron usually synapses with many postganglionic neurons in a wide variety of locations in the sympathetic chain or in ganglions outside the sympathetic chain. This helps explain why the sympathetic nervous system responses are usually spread throughout the body and involve several organs simultaneously.

The sympathetic postganglionic neuron extends the remaining distance to the target organ. Thus the sympathetic postganglionic neuron is much longer than its corresponding preganglionic neuron.

Unlike the short preganglionic neuron, the parasympathetic preganglionic neuron is quite long and originates from the **nuclei** (clusters of neurons in the brain) of several cranial nerves and from the sacral region of the spinal cord. Thus the parasympathetic system is called the *craniosacral division* of the autonomic nervous system.

In contrast to the sympathetic preganglionic neuron, which terminates close to the spinal cord, the parasympathetic preganglionic neuron travels directly from the CNS to its target organ, where it synapses with a short postganglionic neuron in the target organ. Thus the parasympathetic preganglionic neuron is relatively long compared with the very short postganglionic neuron.

General Functions

The sympathetic nervous system is often called the "fight or flight system," meaning this is the system that helps the body cope with emergency situations in which an animal might have to defend itself (fight) or escape (flee or take flight). In contrast, the parasympathetic nervous system could be called the "rest and restore system" because of its ability to decrease the strong excitatory effects of the fight or flight system (bring the body back to resting state) and its ability to facilitate all the processes that will replace those body stores used up during the emergency (restore).

Using this simple model of fight or flight or rest and restore, we can make sense of the clinical signs observed with stimulation of either part of the autonomic nervous system. Table 7-3 summarizes these effects. In a fight or flight situation, the animal needs to move rapidly; therefore the muscles are going to be working vigorously. To meet the needs of the muscles, the bronchioles (airway passages) increase in diameter (bronchodilation) to allow a greater exchange of oxygen and carbon dioxide. Once the oxygen leaves the lungs and enters the blood, it must be delivered rapidly. Therefore the heart rate and force of the cardiac contractions both increase, which increases the rate at which blood is moved around the body. Finally, to deliver more blood into the working muscles, the small blood vessels (arterioles) supplying the muscles dilate (vasodilation).

In contrast to the dilation of skeletal muscle blood vessels under sympathetic stimulation, the small blood vessels supplying the skin, gastrointestinal tract (GI tract), and the kidney constrict, thereby reducing blood flow to these areas so that the blood can be more readily redirected toward the muscles. During this time when blood is redirected away from these organs, the digestive and absorptive function of the GI tract and the filtering function of the kidney are temporarily suspended or decreased until the crisis passes. The decreased blood supply to the skin also means that superficial wounds will bleed less.

Why would eye pupil dilation be of benefit to an animal in a fight or flight situation? Obviously, opening up the pupil admits more light, but an additional benefit may be an increase in peripheral vision (can see "out of the corner of the eye"). Thus the sympathetic nervous system may allow the animal to take in a wider field of vision and see better under dim light conditions.

It's pretty easy to see how the parasympathetic nervous system antagonizes (works against) many but not all of the sympathetic nervous system effects. The parasympathetic system causes the GI tract to increase its activity, thus digesting and absorbing nutrients that are needed to replenish the body energy stores used during the fight or flight situation. The parasympathetic system also reduces the heart rate and reduces the sympathetic system's dilation of the bronchioles. The parasympathetic system has little effect on the blood vessels in most parts of the body other than the GI tract; thus the return to normal diameter is from other regulatory mechanisms other than parasympathetic innervation.

Drugs or diseases that imitate, stimulate, or inhibit either the parasympathetic or sympathetic nervous system produce physiological changes that mimic one of these branches of the

CLINICAL APPLICATION

Sympathetic Nervous System Produces Many of the Signs Associated With Shock or Blood Loss

One of the key roles of the sympathetic nervous system is to maintain arterial blood pressure. In situations involving a loss of blood volume (e.g., bleeding), a loss of fluid in the blood (e.g., dehydration), or a large amount of dilation of blood vessels throughout the body (e.g., shock), the arterial blood pressure can drop to a point at which the brain may not continue to receive adequate blood flow. The body responds to this loss of arterial blood pressure by causing massive stimulation of the sympathetic nervous system. The heart pounds rapidly and fiercely in the chest to increase the output of blood into the arteries while simultaneously the small blood vessels (arterioles) in the skin, GI tract, kidney, and other areas constrict. The effect of this increased cardiac output and the arteriole vasoconstriction results in an increased arterial blood pressure and more blood directed to the brain. The increase in blood arterial pressure from the increased cardiac output and vasoconstriction would be like the increase in air pressure within a rubber tube if you blew forcefully into the tube while simultaneously pinching the far end. The vasoconstriction (narrowing of blood vessels) of the small blood vessels supplying the skin also explains why the skin and mucous membranes of people or animals with a sudden decrease in blood pressure appear quite pale.

autonomic system. Therefore the veterinary professional should know how and why the sympathetic and parasympathetic nervous systems affect the body.

NEUROTRANSMITTERS AND RECEPTORS

The sympathetic nervous system primarily uses norepinephrine as its key neurotransmitter. As stated previously, norepinephrine, epinephrine, and dopamine are all part of a group of neurotransmitters and hormones called *catecholamines.* Because epinephrine and norepinephrine used to be called *adrenalin* and *noradrenalin,* respectively, the neurons that release norepinephrine are said to be **adrenergic neurons.** In addition to the release of norepinephrine from postganglionic adrenergic neurons, the body's sympathetic response also comes from release of epinephrine and norepinephrine from the medulla (inner part) of the adrenal gland. The adrenal medulla acts like a cluster of adrenergic neurons releasing the epinephrine and norepinephrine into the bloodstream, where they are quickly distributed to many receptors throughout the body.

Neurotransmitters can only work on cells that contain specific receptors capable of binding with the particular neurotransmitter molecules. Thus blood vessels in the skin, the GI tract, and the skeletal muscle must have adrenergic or catecholamine receptors to epinephrine or norepinephrine. What we find is that there are actually different types of sympathetic receptors on the tissues or organs affected by the sympathetic nervous system. **Alpha$_1$-adrenergic receptors** typically are found on blood vessels and cause the vasoconstriction of the skin, GI tract, and kidney associated with sympathetic stimulation. The increase in heart rate and force of contraction are the result of stimulation of **beta$_1$-adrenergic receptors** by catecholamines, and the bronchodilation associated with sympathetic stimulation results from **beta$_2$-adrenergic receptor** stimulation.

Sympathetic nervous system drug effects and side effects can be explained by the specificity (selectiveness) of the drug molecule for alpha$_1$-, beta$_1$-, or beta$_2$-receptors. Therefore it is important for the veterinary professional to remember the different adrenergic receptors and the organs or tissues with which they are associated.

The neurons associated with the parasympathetic nervous system secrete acetylcholine. Therefore these neurons often are referred to as **cholinergic neurons.** Although norepinephrine is the neurotransmitter associated with sympathetic nervous system effects, the preganglionic neuron (the neuron that emerges from the CNS and synapses with the postganglionic neuron) in both the sympathetic and parasympathetic nervous system is a cholinergic neuron releasing acetylcholine.

Like the adrenergic receptors of the sympathetic nervous system, the **cholinergic receptors** for acetylcholine also come in different types. The two types of acetylcholine receptors are called **muscarinic** and **nicotinic.** The nicotinic acetylcholine receptors are found primarily on the postganglionic neurons of both the sympathetic and parasympathetic nervous system, as well as between motor neurons and muscle in the somatic (voluntary) motor system. The muscarinic cholinergic receptors are found on the target organs and tissues supplied by the postganglionic neuron of the parasympathetic nervous system.

Certain toxins (like nicotine or plants containing nicotine-like compounds) may selectively stimulate the nicotinic cholinergic receptors more than the muscarinic cholinergic receptors, whereas others may selectively affect the muscarinic receptors. Therefore the veterinary professional should understand the differences between the two receptors for acetylcholine, where they are located in the body, and the potential effects that stimulation or inhibition might produce (Figure 7-11).

TEST YOURSELF

1. Which system is responsible for "fight or flight" and which is responsible for "rest and restore"?
2. Compare and contrast the sympathetic and parasympathetic nervous systems as far as their preganglionic neurons; their postganglionic neurons; where the preganglionic neurons emerge from the CNS; their neurotransmitters; and their impact on the heart, GI tract, blood vessels, bronchiole diameters, and size of the pupil.
3. With which branch of the autonomic nervous system are the alpha$_1$-, beta$_1$-, and beta$_2$-receptors associated? What happens to the body when these particular receptors are stimulated?
4. With which branch of the autonomic nervous system are muscarinic and nicotinic receptors associated?

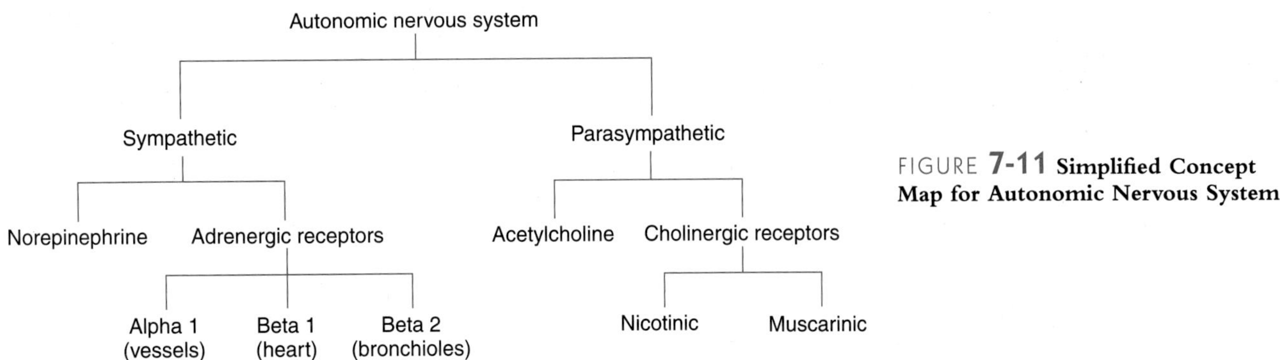

FIGURE **7-11** **Simplified Concept Map for Autonomic Nervous System.**

REFLEXES AND THE REFLEX ARC

Reflexes are rapid, automatic responses designed to protect the body and maintain homeostasis. Reflexes can be **somatic reflexes,** which involve contraction of skeletal muscles, or **autonomic reflexes,** which regulate smooth muscle, cardiac muscle, and endocrine glands.

Regardless of whether the reflex is somatic or autonomic, all reflexes have the same basic structure called the **reflex arc.** The reflex arc originates from a sensory receptor, which detects a change either in the environment or within the body itself. Once stimulated to threshold, the sensory receptor sends an action potential along the sensory neuron and terminates in the gray matter of the spinal cord or brain stem. In the CNS gray matter, the sensory neuron synapses with other interneurons, which serve to integrate the incoming sensory impulse with other impulses from other sensory neurons. Finally, the integrated response of the reflex is sent out from the spinal cord or brain stem by the **motor neuron,** which ends at the target organ (muscle or endocrine gland). If the motor neuron is a somatic neuron, the reflex arc ends in contraction or inhibition of skeletal muscle. If it is an autonomic neuron, the reflex arc ends in smooth muscle within an organ or blood vessel, cardiac muscle, or endocrine glands.

Stimulation of skeletal muscle (somatic) reflex arcs are commonly used in veterinary medicine to aid in the diagnosis of spinal cord trauma, peripheral nerve damage, or muscle disease. Various types of somatic reflexes are evaluated by the veterinarian, including the stretch reflex, the withdrawal reflex, and the extensor reflex. Understanding how these somatic reflex arcs function and are regulated is important for comprehending how normal and abnormal reflexes can indicate disease or damage in the nervous system or musculoskeletal system.

STRETCH REFLEX

The **stretch reflex** is considered a simple "two neuron" or "monosynaptic" reflex arc because it involves only the afferent sensory neuron and an efferent motor neuron (with only one synapse between them) without any interneurons (Figure 7-12). The sensory receptor in the stretch reflex arc is a specialized structure within the muscle called the **muscle spindle.** If a muscle is stretched, the muscle spindle also stretches and sends impulses via the afferent somatic sensory neuron to the spinal cord. At the spinal cord, the sensory neuron synapses with the efferent motor neuron that innervates the *same* muscle. Stimulation of the motor neuron causes that muscle to contract in response to the stretching of the muscle. In this way, the body can maintain the tension or tone of a muscle to meet an increased force applied to stretch the muscle or prevent an overstretching of a muscle caused by contraction of opposing muscles.

You may have had this reflex tested in your own doctor's office, whereby your patellar ligament (located just below your kneecap) was tapped. In this situation, the force against the ligament slightly stretched the large quadriceps femoris muscle on your thigh, stimulating a reflex arc that resulted in contraction of the quadriceps and the subsequent extension of the lower leg (a slight kick).

When stimulated by the stretch receptor, the afferent somatic sensory neuron from the muscle spindle does more than just cause the stretched muscle to contract. Branches off the sensory neuron will synapse with another reflex arc to cause the opposing muscles to relax. Therefore, when the stretch receptor in your quadriceps femoris muscle initiated the stretch reflex arc, a branch off the sensory neuron also synapsed with an *inhibitory* interneuron in the spinal cord. This inhibitory interneuron released inhibitory neurotransmitters at a synapse with the motor neuron to the semimembranosus and semitendinosus muscles, the muscles which normally oppose the quadriceps femoris muscle. By inhibiting stimulation of these opposing muscles, the quadriceps femoris muscle could contract without antagonism.

Finally, another branch off of the stretch receptor's sensory neuron enters the spinal cord and goes up to the brain so that the cerebellum can coordinate the movement and the conscious sensory centers in the cerebral cortex can be "informed" of the stimulation and the subsequent limb movement.

WITHDRAWAL REFLEX

The **withdrawal reflex,** also called the *flexor reflex,* happens when you rapidly withdraw the limb, or flex the joints, after accidentally touching a hot stove or stepping on a sharp object with your bare foot (Figure 7-13). In both of these situations a strong stimulus to a receptor causes the sensory somatic neuron

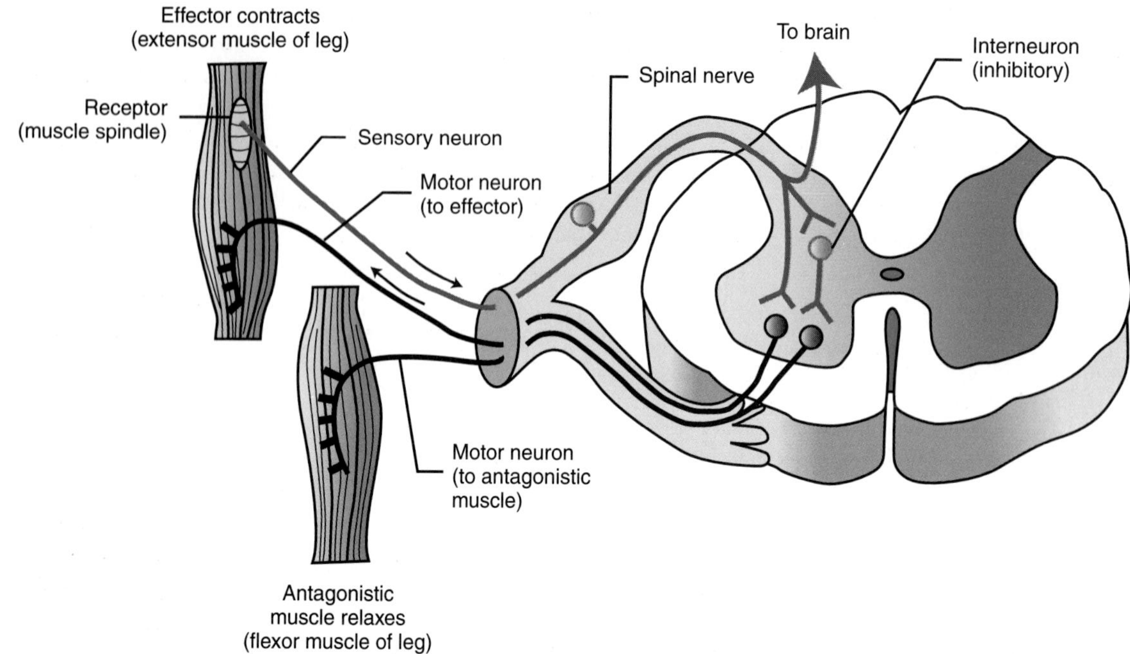

FIGURE **7-12** **Basic Reflex Arc as Illustrated by Simple Stretch Reflex.**

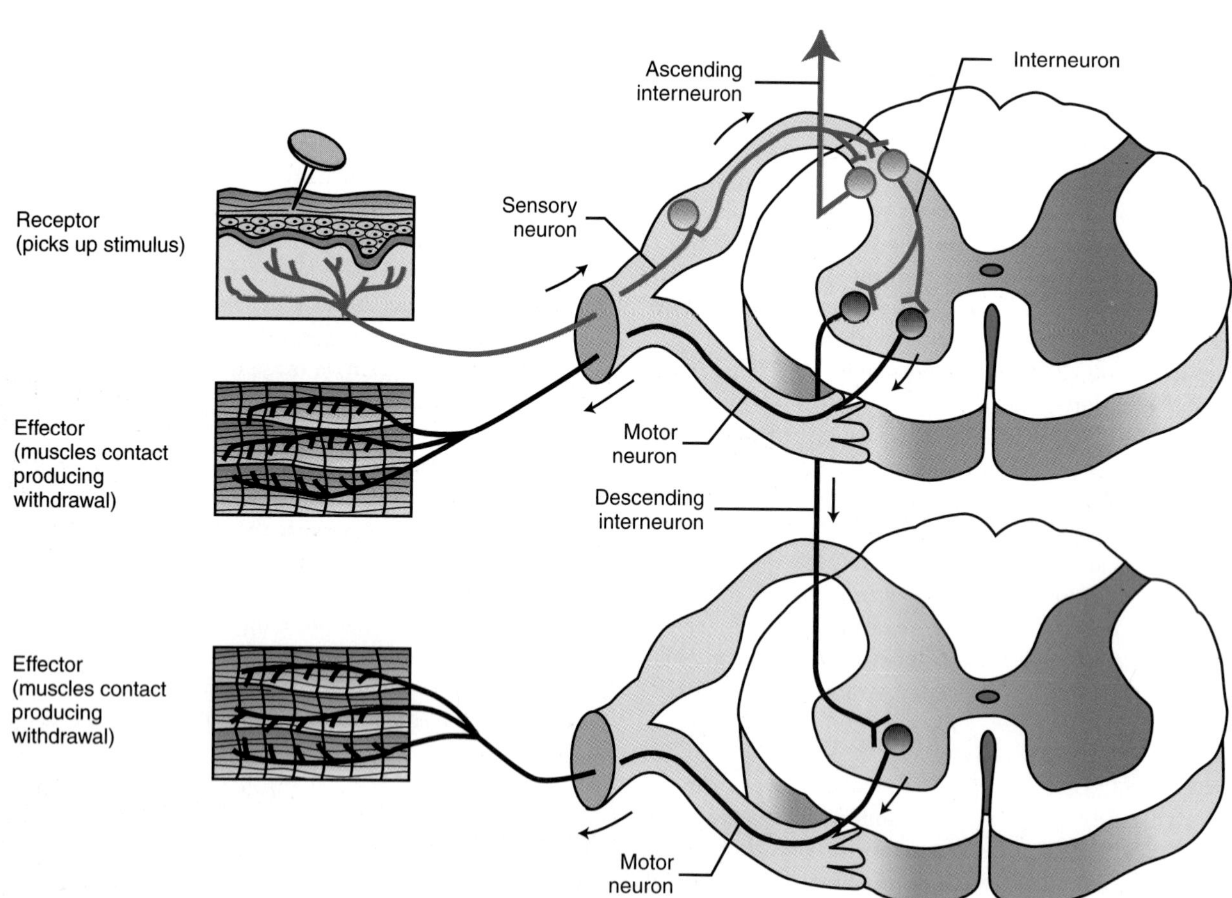

FIGURE **7-13** **Flexor (Withdrawal) Reflex.** Reflex arc involves several spinal segments. Some branches of spinal reflex arc extend to motor nerves in other spinal segments, resulting in relatively complex reflex movement.

to send impulses to the spinal cord. Unlike the simpler stretch reflex, the withdrawal reflex involves synapsing with several interneurons. Some of these interneurons will synapse with motor neurons that will cause contraction of a specific set of muscles responsible for pulling the limb away from the painful stimulus. Other interneurons will inhibit those opposing muscle groups so that the withdrawal of the limb is rapid and complete. This reflex can be complicated because many different muscles may be involved in the withdrawal from the painful stimulus.

Even though the reflex arc may involve several interneurons, several motor neurons, and several different segments of the spinal cord, the reflex still occurs without the brain being "aware." In other words, the limb has been withdrawn from the painful stimulus before the brain becomes consciously aware of the stimulus itself.

Cross Extensor Reflex

If you step on a sharp tack, resulting in the leg being withdrawn rapidly before the brain is aware of what is going on, you should fall over. The reason you don't is that when the withdrawal reflex arc is stimulated, the afferent somatic sensory neuron also synapses with another set of interneurons, causing extensor muscles in the opposite leg to contract and thus support the weight of your body when the other leg flexes. This reflex is called the **cross extensor reflex** because the afferent sensory impulse "crosses" to the other side of the spinal cord and stimulates the muscles that extend the opposite limb (Figure 7-14). Reflexes that start on one side and travel to the opposite side of the body are said to be **contralateral reflexes.** Reflexes, like the stretch reflex, are called **ipsilateral reflexes** because the stimulus and response are on the same side of the body. The veterinary technician needs to be familiar with the terms *contralateral* and *ipsilateral* because they are used for a variety of applications in veterinary medicine other than reflexes.

Role of Upper CNS in Moderating Reflexes

An animal with severe spinal cord damage in the area of the first or second lumbar vertebrae (L1, L2) can still have reflexes in the hind limb. Even though the sensory impulses from the hind limbs are blocked from reaching the brain or the conscious motor impulses from the brain to the hind limbs cannot travel through the damaged section of the spinal cord, the reflex arcs in the lumbar spinal cord segments L3 to L5 caudal

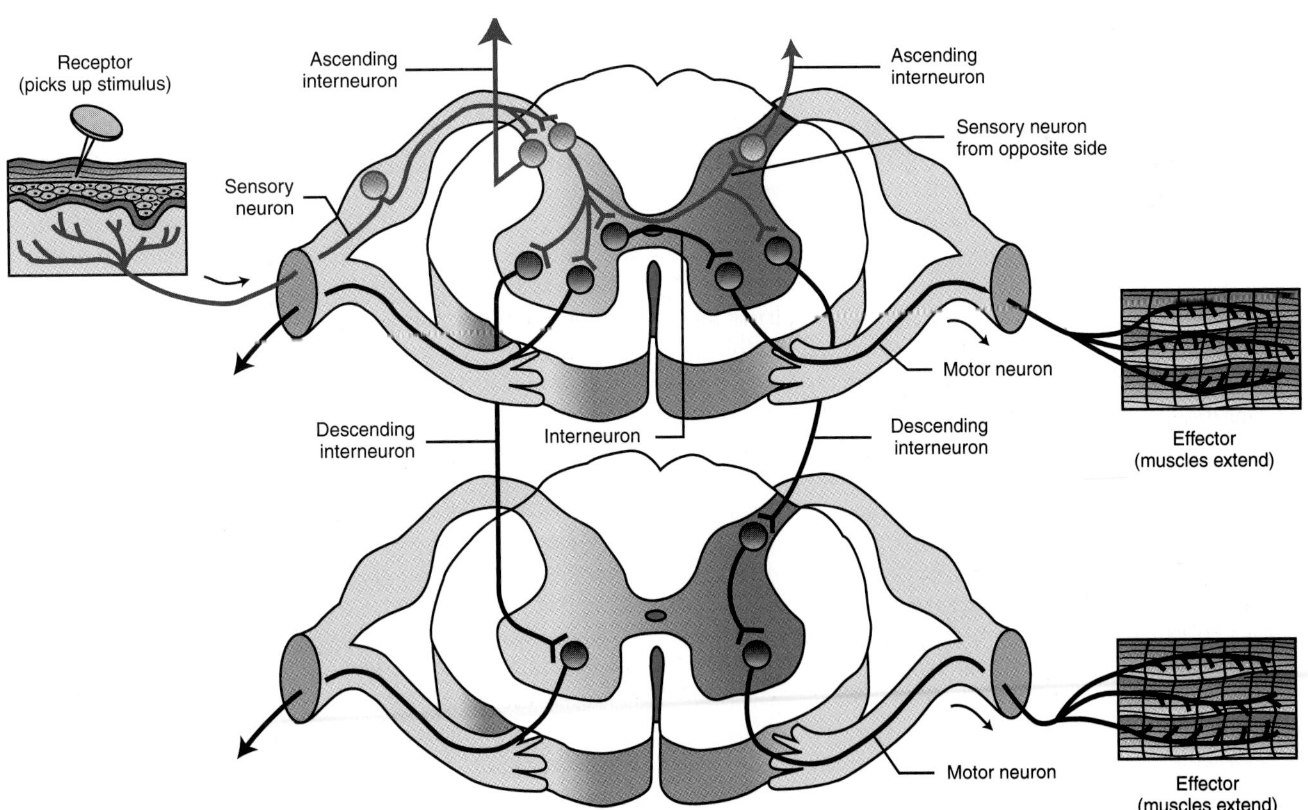

FIGURE **7-14** **Crossed Extensor Reflex.**

CLINICAL APPLICATION Dachshund With Intervertebral Disk Disease

Gretchen is an 8-year-old, spayed, female miniature dachshund presented as suddenly being unable to move her hind legs. On examination the veterinarian observes that Gretchen cannot stand on her rear legs and does not yelp when the skin on her rear toes is pinched. She does, however, react to firm squeezing of the toes themselves. The veterinarian concludes that a spinal cord trauma is interfering with the sensory impulses reaching the brain and with conscious motor impulses from the brain reaching the muscles of the hind limb.

With the history and Gretchen's breed, spinal trauma from the rupture of an intervertebral disk is the most likely cause. In these situations the material from the disk between vertebrae can rupture forcibly against the adjacent spinal cord, producing severe trauma and swelling that renders the spinal cord at that segment nonfunctional.

Before ordering radiographs, the veterinarian must localize the area of the spinal cord where the trauma is most likely to have occurred. In this way the radiograph will be focused directly over the suspected site with the vertebrae lined up to better see the presence of disk material in the spinal canal and to see a narrowing of the affected disk space.

The veterinarian tests several somatic reflexes (withdrawal, crossed extensor) in the hind limb and determines that the reflexes that travel through segments of spinal cord caudal (toward the tail) to L3 (lumbar vertebral segment 3) are all hyperreflexive. This means that these reflex arcs are functional but are not being dampened by the upper CNS. Therefore these spinal cord segments must be caudal to the spinal cord trauma. The reflex arcs that travel through L1, L2, and L3 are all hyporeflexive or nonexistent. The reflex arcs at these spinal cord segments have been broken because of the trauma to these spinal cord segments. The reflexes that involve spinal cord segments cranial (toward the head) to T13 (thoracic vertebral segment 13) are normal. These spinal cord segments are unaffected and still have communication with the upper CNS.

The veterinarian orders the radiographs centered over L2 on Gretchen. The radiographs indicate narrowed disk space between vertebrae L1 and L2. Because Gretchen's owner rushed her in quickly, the veterinarian could arrange emergency surgery to decompress the pressure on the spinal cord by removing part of the vertebral bone over the affected areas. Gretchen slowly recovered over several days until she could walk with 90% of her normal strength and control.

to (below) the trauma are still intact and can still function. The animal, however, is unaware that the hind limbs are moving because it cannot receive any sensory information as a result of the spinal cord damage at L1 to L2.

Not only are the reflex arcs functioning in the hind limb despite the damage to the spinal cord at L1 to L2, but the reflex responses are **hyperreflexive.** This means when the veterinarian taps on the patellar ligament, the quadriceps muscles contract with more force and produce more limb movement than normal. This illustrates an important concept used by veterinarians to diagnose location of spinal cord injuries. The upper CNS normally produces a dampening or inhibitory effect on the reflex arcs. Thus, under normal conditions, the patellar stretching usually only produces a relatively small "kick" because of the dampening effect of the upper CNS. With spinal cord trauma, this dampening effect from the upper CNS is blocked, and any intact reflex arcs caudal to the spinal cord trauma are now exaggerated or hyperreflexive.

If spinal cord trauma occurs where the reflex arc enters or leaves the spinal cord or if the afferent sensory nerve or efferent motor nerve of the reflex arc are damaged, the reflex will be less than normal, or **hyporeflexive.** In other words, if the arc is broken anywhere, the reflex will not function.

By stimulating different somatic reflex arcs, knowing through which spinal cord segments the reflex arc travels, and observing whether the response is normal, hyperreflexive, or hyporeflexive, the veterinarian can localize the area of the spinal cord in which trauma or disease has occurred.

OTHER REFLEXES OF CLINICALLY SIGNIFICANT IMPORTANCE

Many reflexes are used to assess the clinical condition of patients in veterinary medicine. Most are complex reflexes relating to posture, gait, the animal's ability to right itself, and the placement of limbs. Two other reflexes that the veterinary technician should understand are the **corneal reflex** and the **pupillary light reflex (PLR)**. These two reflexes are routinely used when assessing an animal for depth of anesthesia and when performing a physical examination.

The **corneal reflex** arc originates from receptors on the epithelium of the cornea (the clear surface of the eye), travels via sensory neurons in CN V to the pons (brain stem), synapses with neurons in the pons, then travels via CN VII to the muscles that blink the eye. When an animal is anesthetized, the neurons in the pons become less responsive. Therefore, as anesthesia deepens, the corneal reflex (also called the "corneal blink reflex") becomes less responsive and provides the veterinary technician with an idea of the animal's depth of anesthesia.

The PLR is a test for a reflex arc that includes the retina (light-sensing layer of the eye), the optic nerve (CN II), neuron clusters in the diencephalon of the brain, and motor neurons of CN III (which supplies the muscle of the iris that constrict the size of the pupil). A normal response to shining the light in the eye of an animal is for the iris in both eyes to constrict, thus making the pupil smaller. Normally this pupillary constriction would reduce the amount of light entering the eye and protect the retina against bright light. Because shining the light in one eye causes a constriction in both eyes, the reflex arc must cross over to the other side of the body. By examining the PLRs in both eyes, a veterinarian can evaluate each reflex arc and identify whether an animal has a visual problem in the retina, optic nerve, or the motor nerve. Note that the PLR does *not* assess vision. An animal with damage to the visual centers in the cerebral cortex can be blind but have normal PLRs in both eyes.

TEST YOURSELF

1. What are the differences between an autonomic reflex and a somatic reflex?
2. What role do the sensory receptor, sensory neuron, interneuron, and motor neuron play in the reflex arc?
3. What is the sensory receptor in the stretch reflex? What results from the stretch reflex arc stimulation? Is this an ipsilateral or contralateral reflex?
4. What happens in a withdrawal reflex? Is this reflex more or less complex than the stretch reflex?
5. How is the cross extensor reflex tied in with the withdrawal reflex? Is the cross extensor reflex an ipsilateral or contralateral reflex?
6. What is the role of the upper CNS on the reflex arc? If the CNS influence is removed or blocked, do reflexes become hyporeflexive or hyperreflexive?
7. If trauma occurs in the segment of the spinal cord through which a particular reflex arc passes, will the reflex arc be hyperreflexive or hyporeflexive?
8. What is the corneal reflex? How is it used in veterinary medicine?
9. What is the result of a normal PLR?

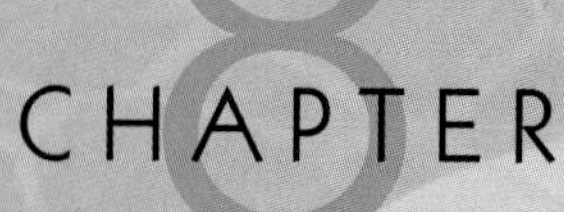

THE CARDIOVASCULAR SYSTEM

Keith Nelson Strickland

In this chapter we provide a basic description of the cardiovascular anatomy and physiology of domestic animals, such as dogs, cats, horses, and ruminants.

CARDIOVASCULAR ANATOMY

LOCATION, SHAPE, AND SIZE OF THE HEART

The heart lies within the thorax within the **mediastinum.** The mediastinum is the central space that separates the left and right pleural cavities. The mediastinum is divided into cranial, medial, and caudal sections. The trachea and mainstem bronchi, the esophagus, lymph nodes, and vascular structures lie within the medial mediastinum on top of the heart, and the sternum lies below the heart. The location of the heart in the thorax is important to appreciate and is more easily done by relating the parts of the heart to external landmarks, such as the intercostal spaces, the costochondral junctions, the elbow, and so on. The carnivore heart is ovoid, and in dogs, it extends from approximately the third to the sixth intercostal space. The long axis of the heart normally forms a 45-degree angle with the sternum. The base is directed craniodorsally, and the apex lies to the left of midline at the junction of the diaphragm and the sternum. The angle can vary with the conformation of the thorax; deep-chested breeds have a larger angle, and barrel-chested breeds have a lower angle. The projection of the base of the heart intersects the middle of the fourth rib, and the most dorsal part of the heart reaches to the line connecting the acromion with the ventral end of the last rib. The apex beat of the heart can be palpated from both sides of the chest but is normally slightly more pronounced on the left side. The heart is almost completely surrounded in the thorax by the lungs, except where the heart makes contact with the right ventrolateral thoracic wall in an area known as the *cardiac notch.* Puncture of the right ventricle is possible through the right fourth and fifth intercostal spaces at the level of the costochondral junction.

The heart is ausculted more easily in dogs and cats because the heart is less covered by the forelimbs than it is in horses and ruminants. The areas for optimal perception of the sounds made at the levels of the valves may be summarized as follows: (1) **pulmonic valve,** low in the left third intercostal space; (2) aortic valve, high in the left fourth intercostal space; (3) left atrioventricular valve (mitral valve), at the costochondral junction in the left fifth intercostal space; and (4) right atrioventricular valve (tricuspid valve), low in the right third or fourth intercostal space (Figure 8-1).

In cats the heart extends from the third and fourth to the sixth and seventh ribs. The long axis of the heart forms a more acute angle with the sternum, therefore resulting in more sternal contact, especially in cats in their second decade of life. The areas for optimal perception of the sounds made at the

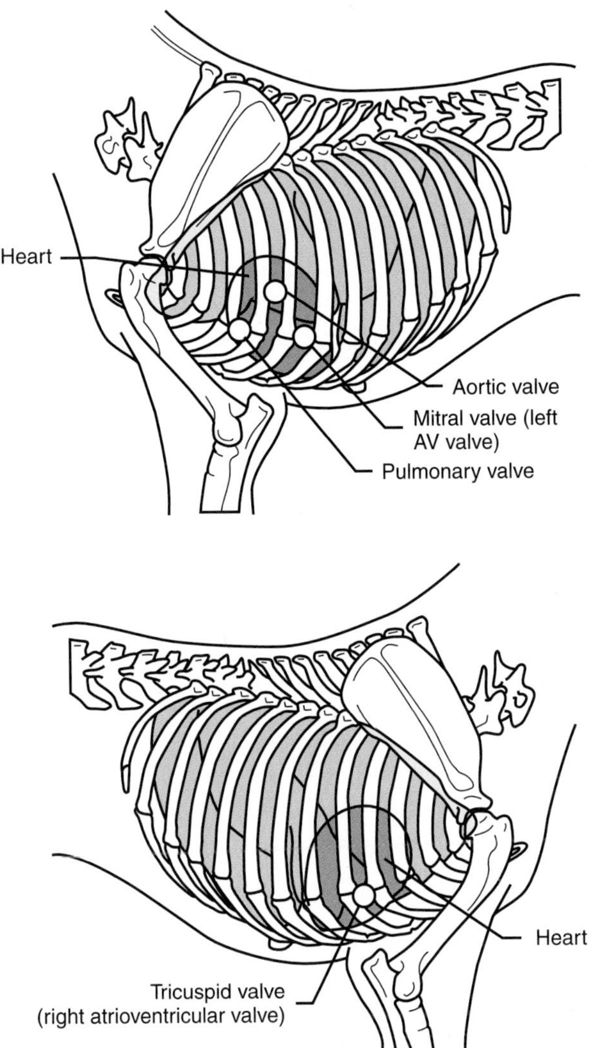

FIGURE **8-1** **Position of Canine Heart in Thoracic Cavity.** When listening to the heart with a stethoscope, you can remember positions of the valves by remembering *PAM: P* is pulmonary valve; *A* is aortic valve; and *M* is mitral, or left atrioventricular, valve.

levels of the valves in cats may be summarized as follows: (1) left atrioventricular valve (mitral valve), at the costochondral junction in the left sixth intercostal space; (2) aortic and pulmonic valves, high in the left fourth intercostal space; and (3) right atrioventricular valve (tricuspid valve), low in the right fifth intercostal space. Puncture of the heart is possible by inserting a needle from the right at the level of the costochondral junction on either side of the fifth rib, although it is difficult because the organ is small.

The equine heart lies primarily on the left side of the thorax and forms an irregular and laterally compressed cone. It lies in the mediastinum just cranial to the diaphragm. Significant variation in heart size is seen among the various types of horses. It typically lies between the second and sixth intercostal space, with the apex at the level of the point of the elbow.

The ruminant heart is also placed asymmetrically in the thorax; about 60% of the heart on the left side extends from the second intercostal space to the fifth space. The size of the heart of sheep and goats is quite variable among different breeds. The bovine heart is unique in that the skeleton of connective tissue (fibrous base) that surrounds the atrioventricular and arterial openings contains two ossicles (ossa cordis).

The heart of a normal dog is about 0.7% to 0.8% of its body weight. However, variations are associated with gender, age, breed, and level of activity. The heart of a normal cat is about 0.33% of its body weight. Cats have smaller hearts than dogs relative to their body size.

CLINICAL APPLICATION: Pericardial Effusion

Pericardial effusion (fluid in the pericardial sac) can cause a serious clinical syndrome called *cardiac tamponade.* Accumulation of fluid in the pericardial sac can impair cardiac filling, cause signs of congestive heart failure, and reduce cardiac output. Symptomatic pericardial effusion is treated by performing a pericardiocentesis. A needle or catheter is placed into the pericardial space, and the effusion is drained. Neoplasia is a common cause of hemorrhagic pericardial effusion.

PERICARDIUM, EPICARDIUM, MYOCARDIUM, AND ENDOCARDIUM

The heart is surrounded by a fibroserous covering called the **pericardium.** The pericardium is thin and is divided into the fibrous and serous pericardia. The fibrous pericardium is the outer covering, and it attaches to the great vessels as they leave and enter the heart base. The fibrous pericardium extends to the diaphragm to form the sternopericardiac ligament at the apex of the heart. This connection anchors the heart in position in the thorax. The serous pericardium lines the fibrous pericardium and covers the heart, forming the **epicardium.** The space between the two layers of the serous pericardium is called the *pericardial cavity,* and it normally contains a small volume of fluid. This fluid lubricates the heart as it moves during contraction and relaxation within the pericardial sac. The portion of the serous pericardium that lines the fibrous pericardium is called the *parietal layer,* and the portion that overlies the heart is called the *visceral layer.*

The left and right phrenic nerves course from cranial to caudal across each side of the heart. The ventral vagal trunk also courses from cranial to caudal, paralleling the phrenic nerves more dorsally at the level of the aorta on the left side of the thorax.

The **myocardium** is the muscular layer between the epicardium and the **endocardium,** which is the thin membrane that covers the whole internal surface of the heart. The myocardium makes up the majority of the heart's mass (Figure 8-2). The cardiac muscle cells (myocytes) are connected by structures called *intercalated disks* that contain gap junctions and desmosomes. The myocytes are anchored to each other by desmosomes and gap junctions allow the transfer of ions from cell to cell. This transfer of ions from cell to cell directly transmits the depolarizing current across the heart, making the

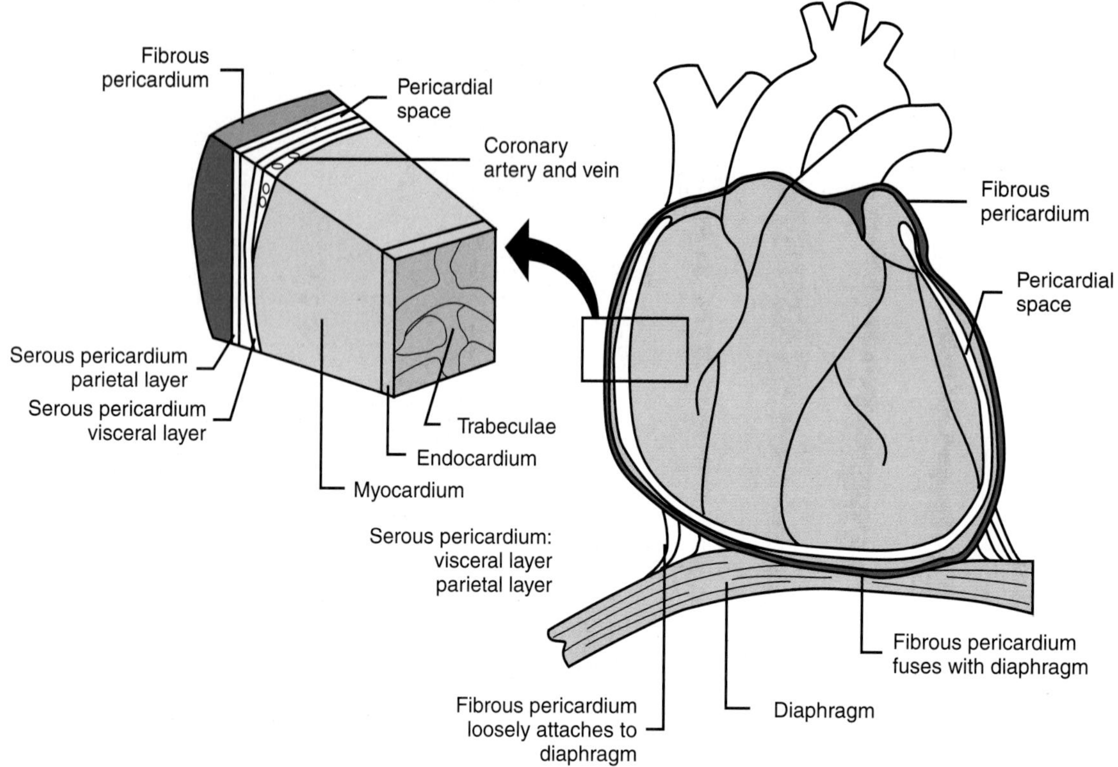

FIGURE **8-2** **Layers of Pericardium.**

myocardial tissue a functional syncytium. A fibrous skeleton (also referred to as the *base*) separates the heart into an atrial syncytium and a ventricular syncytium. Because this fibrous tissue does not conduct electrical impulses, it shields the electrical activity in the atria from the ventricles. This fibrous skeleton base also serves as an anchor for the atrioventricular valves. When stimulated by an electrical impulse, the cardiac muscle cells contract. Because the myocardium functions as a syncytium, this contraction occurs throughout the myocardium virtually at the same time so as to squeeze the blood out of the atrium or ventricle. The contraction increases the pressures inside the chambers of the heart and forces valves to open and blood to flow.

Heart Chambers, Valves, and Associated Vessels

The heart has four chambers: two atria and two ventricles. The heart is divided into left and right sides by partitions known as the *interatrial* and *interventricular septum*. The interatrial septum separates the left and right atria, and the interventricular septum separates the left and right ventricles. The atria receive and hold venous blood (blood coming to the heart), and the ventricles pump the blood away from the heart (arterial blood). The **aorta** is the major artery associated with the left ventricle, and the **pulmonary artery** is the major artery associated with the right ventricle (Figure 8-3).

Vena Cavae, Azygos Vein, and Thoracic Duct

In general, venous blood enters the heart through two large vessels called the *cranial* and *caudal vena cava*. Venous blood also enters the heart from the coronary circulation (to be discussed elsewhere). Three major vessels contribute to blood flow entering the cranial vena cava: (1) the brachiocephalic veins, (2) the azygos vein, and (3) the thoracic duct. The axillary veins join with the external and internal jugular veins to form the brachiocephalic veins, which join to form the cranial vena cava. The cranial vena cava receives blood from the head, neck, chest wall, and thoracic limbs. As the azygos vein courses forward from the region of the third lumbar vertebra, it collects blood from the lumbar, subcostal, dorsal intercostals, esophageal, and bronchoesophageal veins. The azygos vein enters the cranial vena cava adjacent to where the cava enters the right atrium. The thoracic duct drains all of the lymph from the body, except the right thoracic limb and the right side of the head and neck, which are drained by the right lymphatic duct. The thoracic duct originates in the cranial portion of the sublumbar region and courses through the thorax between the aorta and the azygos vein (right dorsal border of the aorta and the ventral border of the azygos vein).

A species variation exists with regard to the formation of the cranial vena cava. In dogs and pigs, the left external jugular

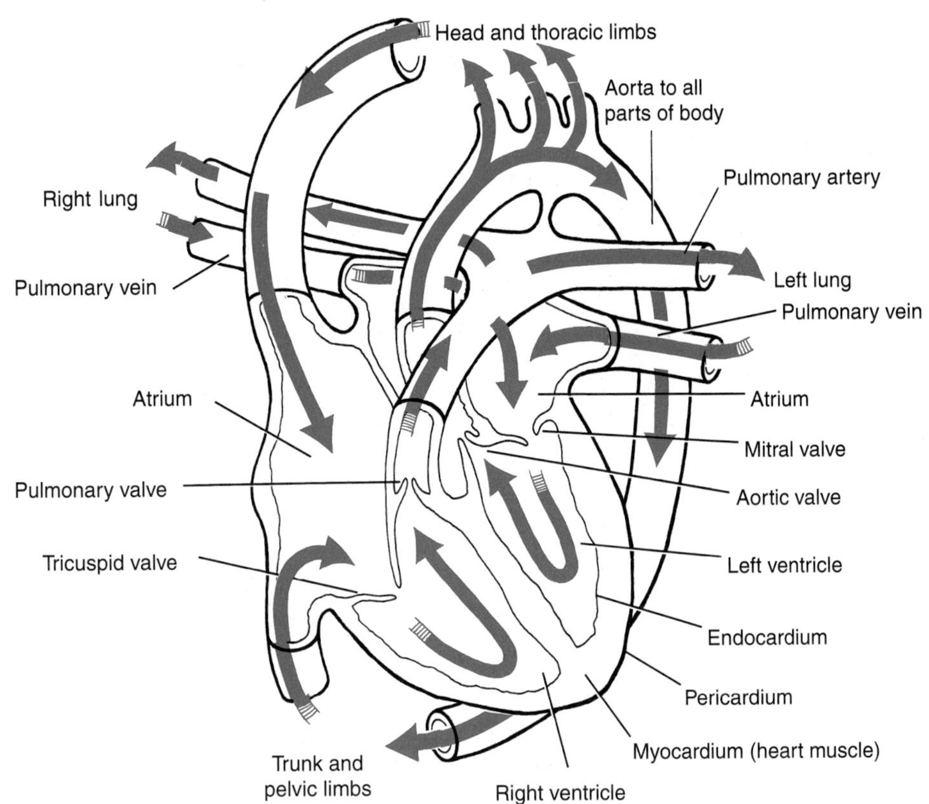

FIGURE **8-3** **Basic Chamber Arrangement of Mammalian Heart.** Arrows indicate direction of blood flow. (From McBride DF: *Learning veterinary terminology,* ed 2, St Louis, 2002, Mosby.)

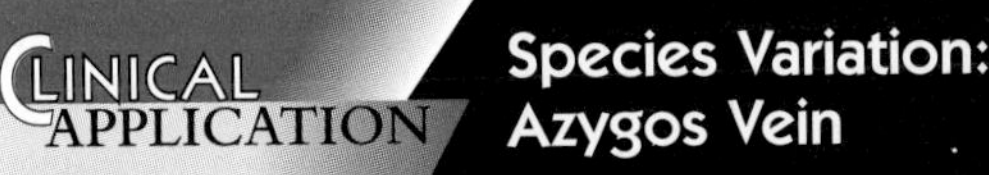

The equine heart may be distinguished from the bovine heart by the presence of a single right azygos vein.

vein combines with the left subclavian vein and the right external jugular vein combines with the right subclavian vein to form the left and right brachiocephalic veins, which come together to form the cranial vena cava. In horses and ruminants, on the other hand, the left and right external jugular veins combine to form a bijugular trunk, which joins with the left and right subclavian veins to form the cranial vena cava.

The common iliac veins converge ventral to the seventh lumbar vertebra to form the caudal vena cava. In the abdomen, the caudal vena cava ascends to the right of the aorta in the retroperitoneal space between the left and right psoas muscles. Many vessels join with the caudal vena cava as it courses cranially through the abdomen. These vessels include the deep circumflex iliac, renal, testicular or ovarian, phrenicoabdominal, and hepatic veins. At the level of the liver, the caudal vena cava courses ventrally and somewhat to the right to pass through the caudate lobe of the liver. From there it courses through the right crus of the diaphragm into the thorax, where it eventually enters the caudal border of the right atrium. The right phrenic nerve is closely associated with the caudal vena cava at this level.

TEST YOURSELF

1. Describe the general location of the heart in a canine and compare it with the location of the heart in a horse.
2. Describe the general structure of the heart.
3. List the layers of the heart wall.

THE RIGHT ATRIUM

The **right atrium** receives deoxygenated blood from the cranial and caudal vena cava and the coronary sinus (the opening of the great coronary vein of the coronary circulation) (Figure 8-4). It acts as a holding chamber of venous blood destined to be pumped into the lungs by the right ventricle. The right atrium also serves as a conduit for venous blood flow into the right ventricle. The right atrium is divided into a right atrial body and an auricle. The right auricle is a blind sac that extends cranially from the right atrial body, which lies dorsal to the right ventricle. The inner surface of the medial wall of the *right* atrial body is smooth, whereas the surface of the lateral wall of the right atrial body and the right auricle is lined with pectinate muscles. These muscles form a network of hills

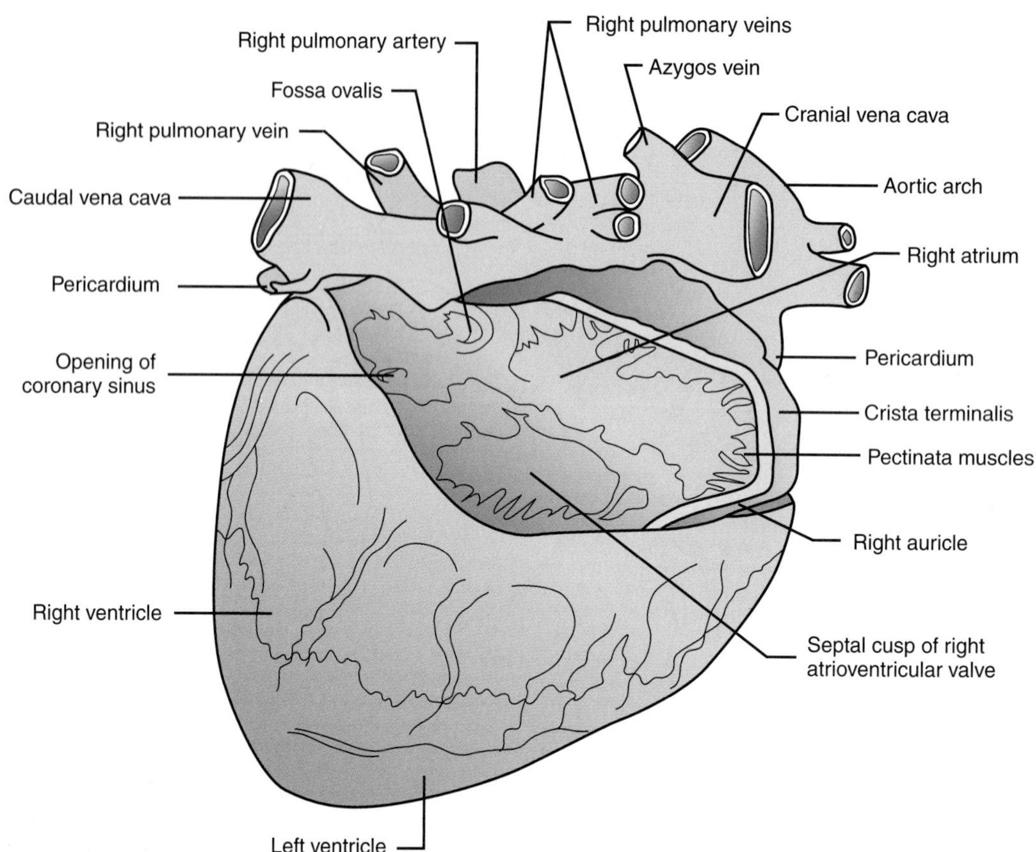

FIGURE **8-4** **View of Heart With Right Atrium Exposed.**

and furrows that give it an uneven, or trabeculated, surface. In the fetus, the *foramen ovale* is an opening between the right and left atria where blood is shunted from the right side to the left side of the heart, bypassing the lungs. Normally the foramen ovale closes at birth and forms a remnant called the *fossa ovalis* (see Figure 8-6). The coronary venous blood flow enters the right atrium through an ostium, or opening, in the floor of the right atrial body called the *coronary sinus.* The coronary sinus lies ventral to the opening of the caudal vena cava. The dorsomedial wall of the right atrial body is called the *interatrial septum* because it is the wall that separates the left and right atria. The crista terminalis is a smooth-surfaced, thick-walled section of the heart muscle. It is shaped like a half-moon and resides at the entrance to the auricle. Pectinate muscles radiate from this semilunar structure into the auricle.

Right Atrioventricular Valve (Tricuspid Valve)

The right atrioventricular (AV) valve, also called the **tricuspid valve,** separates the right atrium and auricle from the right ventricle (Figure 8-5). It is a one-way valve that opens during ventricular relaxation, or diastole, allowing the passage of blood from the right atrium to the right ventricle. During ventricular contraction, or systole, the valve closes, thereby preventing blood from flowing backward from the right ventricle to the right atrium.

The valve apparatus is composed of valve leaflets, a valve annulus (ringed structure), chordae tendineae, papillary muscles, an atrial wall, and a ventricular wall.

Valve leaflets are attached to the fibrous base that supports the AV junction. The free ends of the valve leaflets are attached to the papillary muscles by fibrous strands called *chordae tendineae.* The papillary muscles arise from the apical portion of the right ventricle. In humans the valve has three leaflets; in dogs and cats, it has two major leaflets (septal and parietal). The parietal or ventral leaflet is larger and more mobile than the septal or dorsal leaflet. The junctions between the two valve leaflets are called the *cranial* and *caudal commissures.* The atrial surface of the leaflets is smooth, and the ventricular surface is divided into a rough zone (along the edges of the leaflets, where the chordae tendineae attach) and a clear zone that extends from the rough zone to the attachment of the leaflets to the annulus.

The function of the chordae tendineae and the papillary muscles are to prevent the valve leaflets from prolapsing back into the atrium during ventricular contraction. Chordae tendineae are strong, fibrous strands that extend from the fibrous layer of the valve leaflets. These fibrous strands extend to the papillary muscles located on the interventricular septum. Branching of the chordae tendineae is variable, producing both primary and secondary attachments to the ventricular surface and papillary muscles.

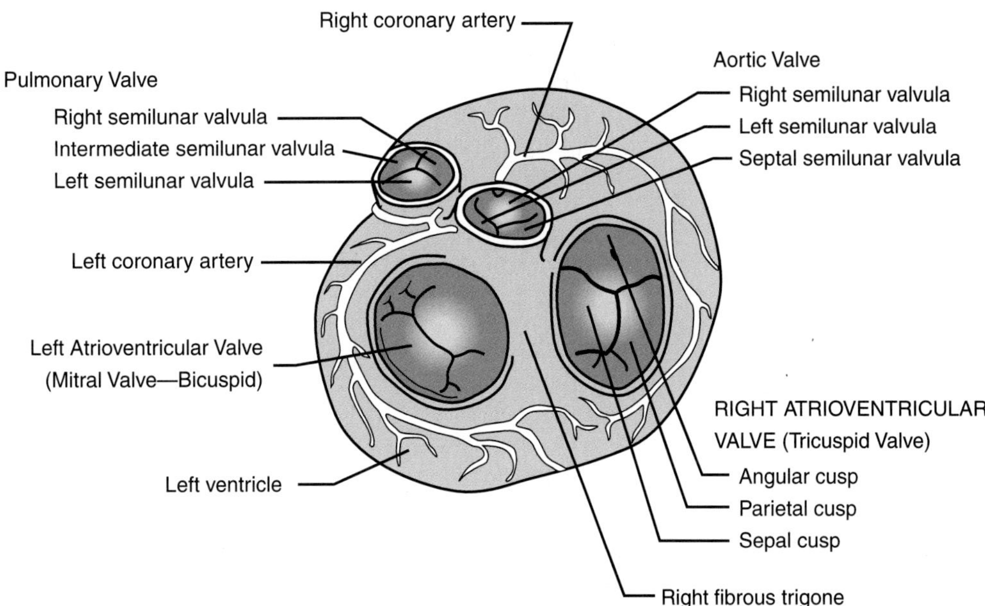

FIGURE **8-5** **Valves of Heart.**

Usually three main papillary muscles in the right ventricle and a small papillary muscle of the conus all attach to the parietal cusp via chordae tendineae. The septal cusp chordae tendineae attach to small muscular ridges or papillae dorsal to the papillary muscles. The main papillary muscles arise from the apical third of the interventricular septum, and the papillary muscle of the conus is the most cranial of the papillary muscles. The papillary muscle of the conus arises along the dorsal region of the crista supraventricularis, which is a small ridge of tissue on the interventricular septum that lies between the body of the right ventricle and the right ventricular outflow tract.

THE RIGHT VENTRICLE

The right ventricle pumps deoxygenated venous blood into the low-pressure **pulmonary circulation.** The walls of the right ventricle are considerably thinner than the walls of the left ventricle because it is required to generate less force to get the blood to flow into the low-resistance pulmonary circulation. The left ventricular walls are much thicker because it must generate approximately five times more force to eject blood into the high-pressure **systemic circulation.** The right ventricle partially wraps around the cranial aspect of the left ventricle. When the right ventricle contracts, its motion is like a bellows.

The right ventricle is divided into two sections: (1) the caudal or inflow area just below the tricuspid valve and (2) the outflow tract (or infundibulum), which ascends cranially and to the left toward the pulmonic valve. The body of the right ventricle (free wall and the apical interventricular septum) is trabeculated, and the areas dorsal to the papillary muscles and the outflow tract are smooth. The body of the right ventricle contains several large papillary muscles arising from the apical portion of the interventricular septum. The body and the outflow tract are separated by an indistinct ridge of tissue (crista supraventricularis), which is located along the interventricular septum. The papillary muscle of the conus arises from this ridge. A thin, muscular strand of tissue called the *trabecula septomarginalis* (or moderator band) runs from the interventricular septum to the free wall of the right ventricle and contains the right bundle branch (a part of the conduction system that conducts electrical impulses to the right ventricular free wall during ventricular excitation).

THE PULMONIC VALVE

The pulmonic valve is a semilunar valve that prevents blood from flowing from the pulmonary artery back into the right ventricle when the ventricle is filling with blood from the right atrium. The pulmonic valve is cranial and to the left of the tricuspid valve. Remember that the right ventricle wraps around the left ventricle so that the tricuspid valve is on the right side of the left ventricle and the pulmonary outflow tract (infundibulum) and the pulmonic valve are on the cranial aspect of the left side of the left ventricle. This is why the sounds associated with the closure of the pulmonic valve are best appreciated from the left side of the thorax. The pulmonic valve consists of an annulus and three cusps.

PULMONARY ARTERIES

The pulmonary artery delivers deoxygenated blood from the right ventricle to the lungs. The main pulmonary artery begins at the level of the pulmonic valve and arches dorsocaudally to the left of the aorta and dorsal to the body of the left atrium. The main pulmonary artery branches to form divergent left and right pulmonary arteries, which deliver blood to their respective lung lobes. The left and right pulmonary arteries course along the lateral aspect of the corresponding bronchi. The **ligamentum arteriosum** connects the pulmonary artery to the descending aorta. In a fetus, the descending aorta is connected to the proximal portion of the left branch of the pulmonary artery via the ductus arteriosus. After birth, the ductus arteriosus normally constricts and over time fibroses to form the ligamentum arteriosum (Figure 8-6).

PULMONARY VEINS

The pulmonary veins deliver oxygenated blood from the lungs to the left atrium. The pulmonary veins course along the ventromedial aspect of their respective bronchi, and three pulmonary veins from each side of the lungs enter the dorsal aspect of the left atrium. The pulmonary veins often merge to form four to six veins before entering the left atrium; consequently four to six vein orifices, or ostia, are found in the dorsal aspect of the left atrial body.

CLINICAL APPLICATION — Valvular Stenosis

Congenital **stenosis** of the pulmonic valve is the third most common congenital cardiac defect in dogs. It results when the valve annulus is hypoplastic or if the valve cusps are fused, or both, thus effectively narrowing the passageway for blood to travel into the pulmonary artery. Stenosis of the pulmonic valve results in a **murmur,** which is heard best during systole on the left third to fourth intercostal spaces on the left side of the thorax at the heart base.

THE LEFT ATRIUM

The left atrium receives and holds oxygenated blood from the pulmonary veins. The left atrium is divided into a left atrial body and a left auricle. The left atrium is on the left dorsocaudal aspect of the heart base above the left ventricle. The left auricle extends cranially on the left side of the heart. The carinae of the trachea and the mainstem bronchi are dorsal to the body of the left atrial body, and the left ventricle is ventral. The branching of the main pulmonary artery occurs just cranial to the left atrial body.

CLINICAL APPLICATION — Patent Ductus Arteriosus

A **patent ductus arteriosus** is the most common congenital cardiac defect in dogs. In this scenario, the ductus remains open and allows shunting of blood from the aorta to the pulmonary artery—a potential cause of left-sided congestive heart failure.

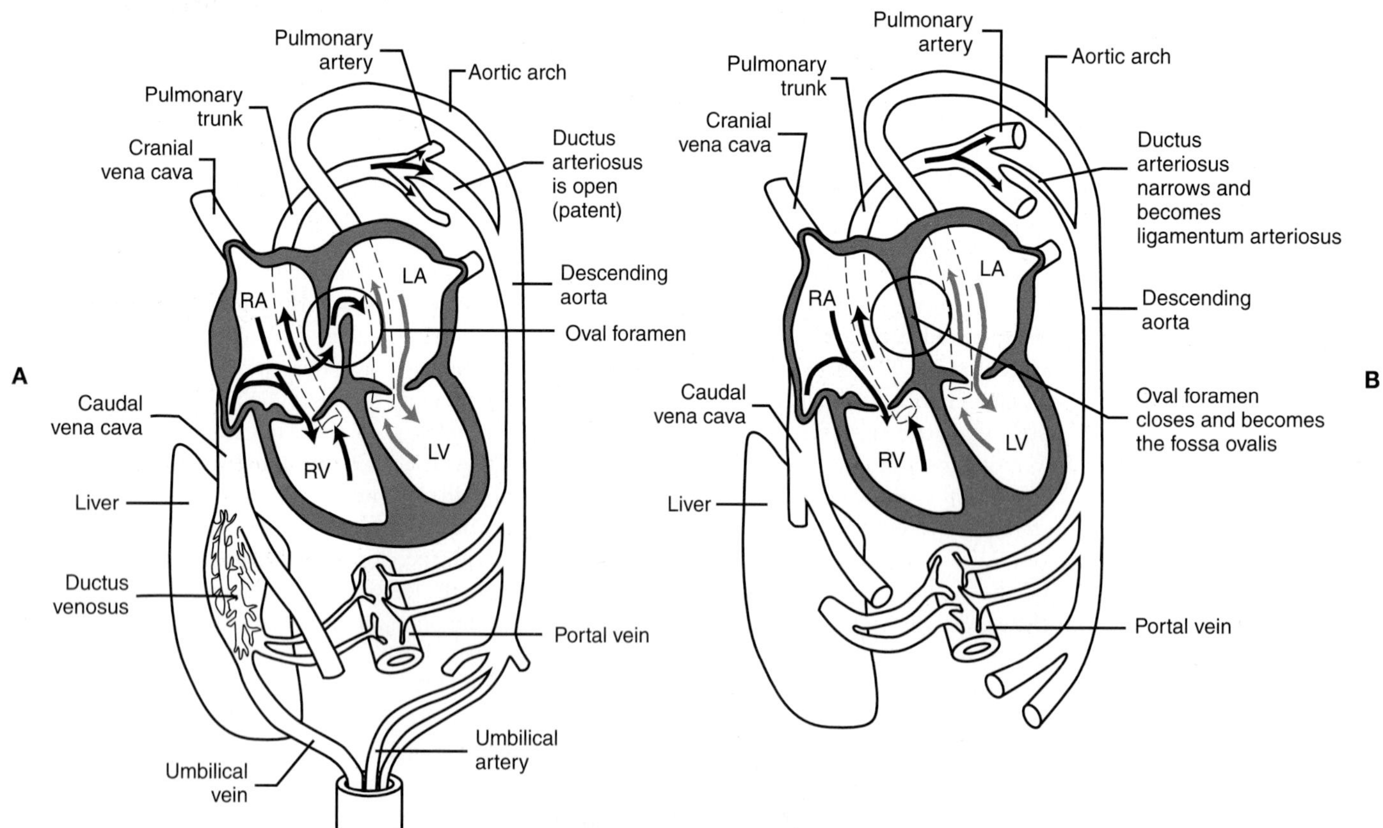

FIGURE **8-6** **Circulatory Patterns in Fetus and in Newborn. A,** Fetal circulation. **B,** Circulation after birth. *LA,* Left atrium; *LV,* left ventricle; *RA,* right atrium; *RV,* right ventricle.

LEFT ATRIOVENTRICULAR VALVE (MITRAL VALVE)

The left AV valve **(mitral valve)** lies between the left atrium and the left ventricle and prevents the backflow of blood from the left ventricle into the atrium during ventricular contraction. During diastole, the left AV valve is open because the pressures in the left ventricle are lower than in the left atrium. When the valve is open, oxygenated blood can flow from the left atrium and pulmonary veins into the left ventricle. When the ventricle is stimulated to contract, ventricular pressures increase and the left AV valve closes. The mitral valve consists of two leaflets: a septal (or anterior) leaflet and a parietal (or posterior) leaflet. The septal leaflet is the larger of the two (the opposite is true regarding the tricuspid valve leaflets). The aortic root is continuous with the base of the septal leaflet. Like the right AV valve, the left AV valves have a smooth atrial surface and a ventricular surface with rough and clear zones. In addition to the two larger cusps, small cusps may be present in the commissures. Large papillary muscles (a cranial or subauricular papillary muscle and a caudal or subatrial one) are located within the left ventricle ventral to each commissure. Chordae tendineae extend from the tips of the valve leaflets to the papillary muscles; typically each leaflet receives chordae from each papillary muscle. The chordae extend from each papillary muscle as a single strand, and secondary and tertiary branches are common.

Clinically, malfunction of the left AV valve is the most common cause of congestive heart failure in adult dogs. When this valve malfunctions, it leaks and allows blood to flow backward into the left atrium instead of out of the left ventricle into the aorta. The valve leaks when the heart is pumping blood, and this causes a systolic heart murmur heard best over the left fifth intercostal space at the apex of the heart.

THE LEFT VENTRICLE

The left ventricle is the thick-walled pumping chamber that ejects oxygenated blood into the systemic circulation. The left ventricle is the largest structure of the heart (Figure 8-7). The ventricle is conical in shape, and the walls are two to three times the thickness of the right ventricular walls. The left

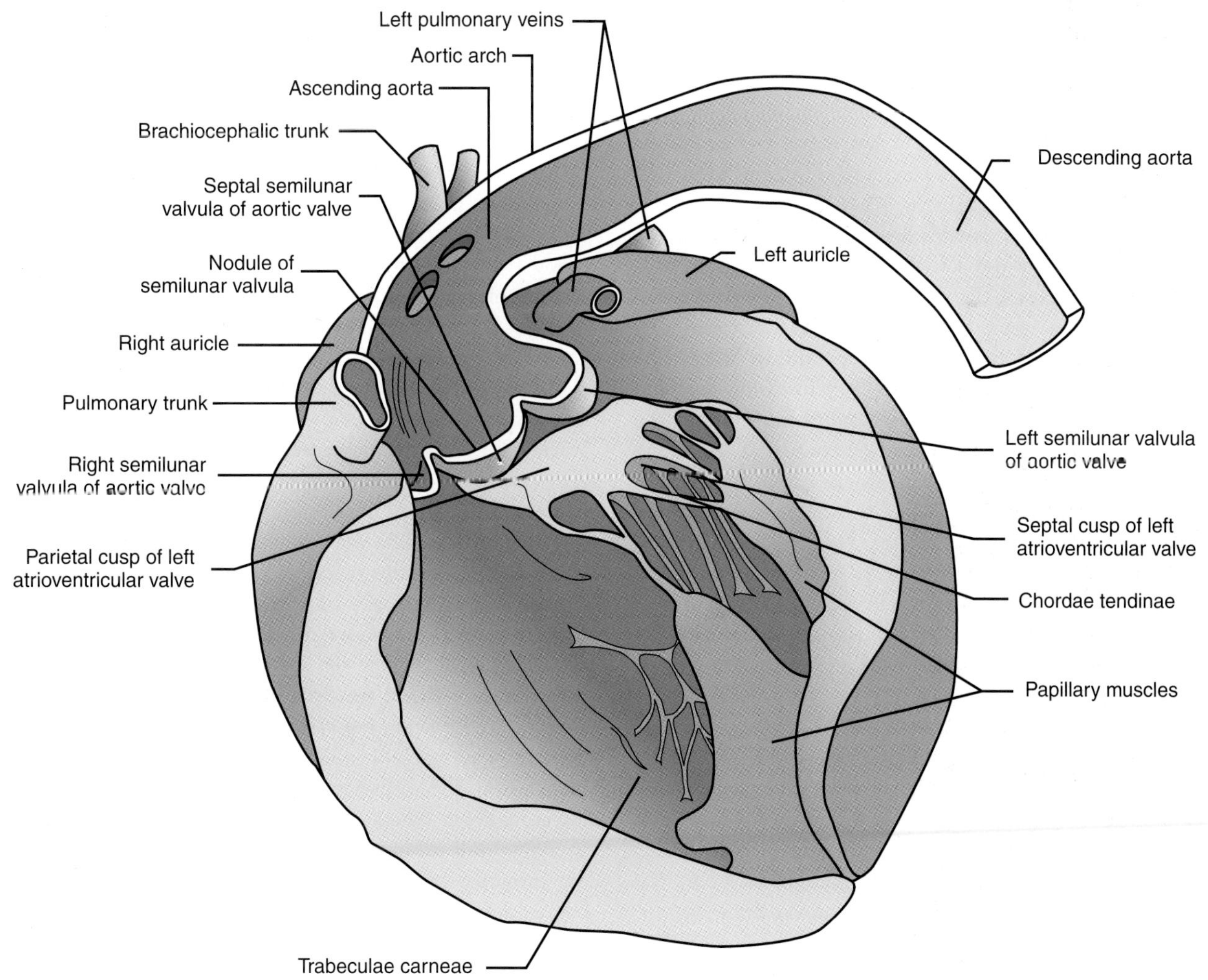

FIGURE **8-7** **Interior of Left Ventricle.**

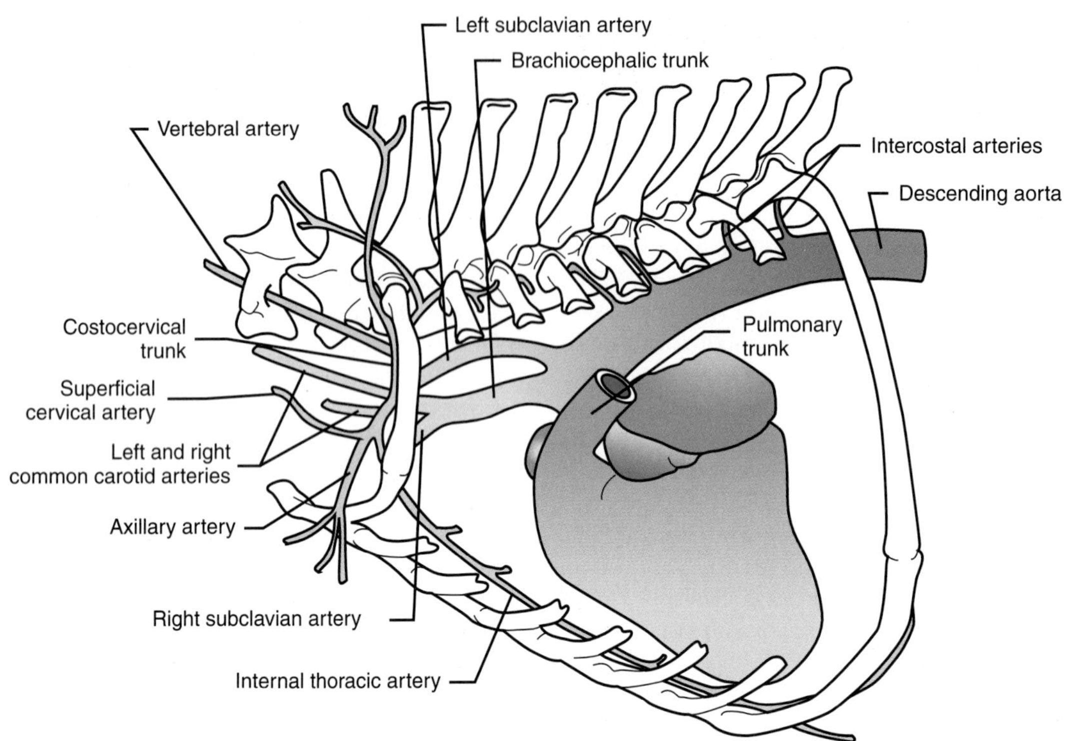

FIGURE **8-8** **Aortic Arch and Its Branches.**

ventricle occupies the caudal and left regions of the heart ventral to the left atrial body. There are two regions of the left ventricle, defined during diastole, when the left AV valve is open. The inflow tract extends from the tips of the left AV valve to the apex of the left ventricle. The outflow tract extends from the apex to the **aortic valve,** which is just cranial to the septal leaflet of the left AV valve. The interventricular septum is the medial boundary of the outflow tract. The interventricular septum has two parts: a membranous part and a muscular part. The membranous septum lies beneath the junction of the noncoronary and the left coronary cusps of the aortic valve. The muscular septum extends from the apex of the heart to a crest just below the area of the membranous septum, below the noncoronary cusp. The left ventricle is less trabeculated than the right ventricle. In addition, no moderator bands reach across the ventricle's lumen as on the right side. Two papillary muscles in the left ventricle are a cranial and a caudal papillary muscle.

The Aortic Valve

The aortic valve is similar to the pulmonic valve. Both have three semilunar cusps. The aortic cusps are designated as left, right, and noncoronary. Nodules are found in the middle of the free borders that, when the valve is closed, resemble a peace sign or the symbol for Mercedes Benz. Behind each cusp the aorta is slightly dilated into the sinuses of Valsalva—one for each valve cusp.

In veterinary medicine, the aortic valve can cause a problem if stenosis is present or if the valve is infected. If the valve is stenotic, blood flows quickly through the stenosis and creates a systolic murmur that is most audible over the third to fourth left intercostal spaces at the level of the left base. Aortic stenosis is the second most common congenital heart defect in dogs. If the valve is infected, it leaks blood back into the ventricle from the aorta at the time when the ventricle is normally receiving blood from the left atrium. A leaky aortic valve causes the diastolic murmur of aortic **valvular regurgitation.** Infection of valves is rare but can be catastrophic when it happens.

The Aorta and Major Arteries

The aorta consists of three segments: the ascending aorta, the aortic arch, and the descending aorta. The ascending aorta arises from the cranial aspect of the heart directly behind the tissue at the junction of the right ventricular outflow tract and the right auricle. The ascending aorta angles dorsocranially as it accommodates the blood ejected from the left ventricle (Figure 8-8). The proximal portion of the ascending aorta or the aortic root, just above the aortic valves, contains sinuses associated with each of the aortic valve leaflets. The left and right sinuses contain the ostia of the right and left coronary arteries. These sinuses are also called the *sinuses of Valsalva* in humans. The brachiocephalic trunk and left subclavian artery branch from the aortic arch, or transverse aorta. The descending aorta begins when the aorta has completely turned, and it is divided into thoracic and abdominal sections. The ventral, left proximal portion of the descending aorta contains the connection of the ligamentum arteriosum. The ligamentum arteriosum courses cranioventrally to connect with the proximal portion of the left branch of the pulmonary artery. The descending aorta courses caudally just beneath the spine within the dorsal mediastinum, initially on the left side but on midline as it crosses the diaphragm. During its course, it sends off

Clinical Application: Feline Aortic Thromboembolism

Cats with cardiomyopathy may develop an intracardiac thrombus that embolizes and becomes lodged in aortic trifurcation (also called a "saddle thrombus"). This condition is associated with a poor prognosis and short survival times.

branches to the spine and vertebrae. The abdominal aorta courses caudally within the retroperitoneal space. Several major arterial branches of the abdominal aorta supply the liver, gastrointestinal tract, spleen, kidneys, and genital organs. The aorta branches into the two external iliac and the common iliac arteries just under the sixth or seventh vertebrae (see Figure 8-8).

Test Yourself

Identify and describe the cardiac chambers and the valves that are associated with each chamber.

Surface of the Heart

The surface of the heart contains grooves in which the coronary arteries and veins are located. The coronary groove lies between the atria and the ventricles and contains coronary vessels and fat. The interventricular grooves are the superficial separations of the right and left ventricles. The paraconal interventricular groove obliquely transverses the auricular side of the heart and contains the paraconal (left anterior descending) branch of the left coronary artery. The subsinuosal interventricular groove on the atrial surface of the heart marks the position of the interventricular septum and contains the terminal portion of the left coronary artery, the subsinuosal interventricular branch.

The Coronary System

Left and right coronary arteries arise from the root of the aorta. The opening of each coronary artery is called an *ostium* (orifice), and the right and left ostia lie within each corresponding sinus. In the canine, the left coronary artery emerges beneath the pulmonary trunk and quickly divides into the left circumflex and paraconal interventricular (left anterior descending coronary artery in humans) coronary arteries. An interventricular septal branch most commonly arises from the left anterior descending coronary artery, but it occasionally arises from the short, left main coronary artery. The paraconal interventricular coronary artery supplies the craniolateral free wall of the left ventricle and part of the caudal interventricular septum, as well as the right ventricular outflow tract. The left circumflex coronary artery can be found in the coronary groove between the left atrium and ventricle. The left circumflex coronary artery supplies the caudolateral left ventricular free wall and much of the left atrium.

The right coronary artery is smaller than the left coronary artery. It originates from the right coronary ostium in the right sinus and courses within the coronary groove on the right side, much like the left circumflex coronary artery does on the left side. The right coronary artery supplies the majority of the right ventricular free wall, as well as much of the right atrium and portions of the proximal pulmonary artery and aorta. The atrial branch of the right coronary artery supplies the sinoatrial (SA) node.

Some species variations exist with regard to the dominance of the right and left coronary arteries. In the canine the left coronary artery supplies a larger portion of the heart than does the right coronary artery. However, in the horse the coronary arteries share the supply of the heart more equally, compared with other species. In ruminants the left coronary artery is larger than the right (limited to a circumflex course) (Figure 8-9).

The great cardiac vein ascends from the apex of the heart adjacent to the left anterior descending coronary artery and then courses within the coronary groove adjacent to the left circumflex coronary artery. The great cardiac vein empties blood in the caudal aspect of the right atrium via the opening called the *coronary sinus.*

Blood Vessels

The vessels directly associated with the heart are discussed in the preceding text. The following series of drawings illustrates portions of the systemic arteries and veins (Figures 8-10 through 8-16). We cannot describe every blood vessel in several species; however, a basic description seems appropriate. The dog is used as the model here. See Box 8-1, pp. 182-183, for an outline of these arteries and veins.

The arterial wall is composed of three layers, or tunics: (1) the innermost lining (tunica interna) is called the *endothelium,* (2) a middle tunic (tunica media) is composed of smooth muscle tissue and elastic connective tissue, and (3) the tunica adventitia is the outer fibrous layer. Arteries are characterized by the structure of the media and are grouped in three major classes: (1) the media of the largest arteries (e.g., the aorta and the pulmonary trunk) predominantly have elastic fibers so that the arteries can expand and recoil so as to propel the blood forward; (2) the smaller arteries have a media that is primarily composed of smooth muscles, and the diameter of the lumen of these arteries is carefully controlled by the autonomic nervous system; (3) the smallest arteries (resistance arterioles) regulate the resistance to blood flow and blood pressure. Vasoconstriction and vasodilation of the arterioles are also very carefully controlled by the autonomic nervous system.

Capillaries

The capillaries are small vessels that are reduced to a layer of endothelium and supported by a thin layer of connective tissue. The capillaries are the sites of exchange between the blood and the tissues; hence they are called *exchange vessels.* They are distinguished from the small arterioles in that arterioles have some layers of smooth muscle that capillaries lack. Sinusoids are a special type of capillary found in the liver, spleen, and bone marrow.

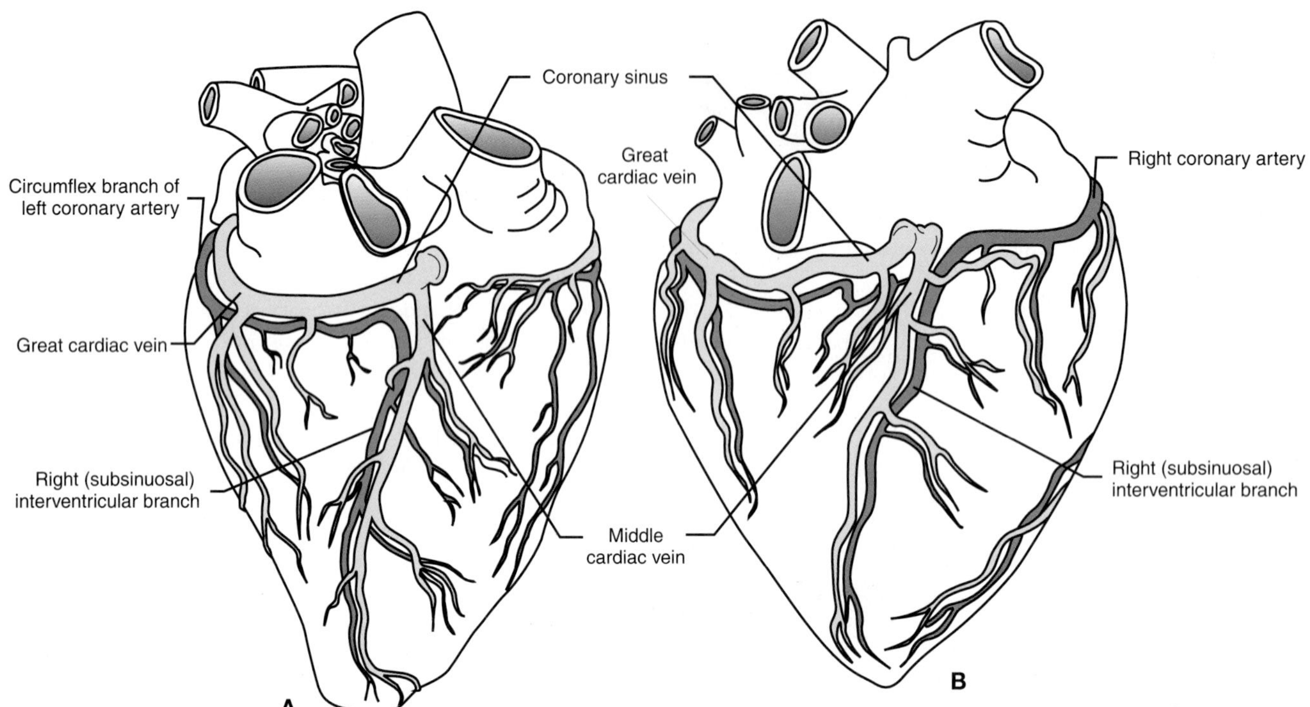

FIGURE **8-9** **Various Patterns of Coronary Circulation on Heart Viewed From the Right.** **A,** Carnivores and ruminants: right (subsinuosal) interventricular branch is continuation of left coronary artery. **B,** Horse and pig: right (subsinuosal) interventricular branch is continuation of right coronary artery.

Veins

Veins are constructed like arteries with thinner walls. The smallest veins, called *venules,* do not contain smooth muscle in the media. The larger veins contain some smooth muscle that allows venoconstriction or venodilation to control the amount of blood returning to the heart.

CLINICAL APPLICATION — Venipuncture Sites

The most common sites for venipuncture in small animals are the cephalic vein on the dorsal aspect of the antebrachium, the external jugular veins in the superficial cervical region, and the lateral saphenous vein on the lateral aspect of the hock.

TEST YOURSELF

1. Describe the differences between the types of blood vessels.
2. On a diagram, locate and identify the major arteries that supply the abdominal viscera.
3. On a diagram, locate and identify the major arteries of the forelimb.
4. On a diagram, locate and identify the major arterial branches of the abdominal aorta.
5. On a diagram, locate and identify the major venous systems of the body.

CARDIOVASCULAR PHYSIOLOGY

THE CIRCULATORY SYSTEMS

The cardiovascular system is divided into two separate circulations: the systemic circulation and the pulmonary circulation. Each circulatory system is divided into a venous and arterial system. Beginning in the systemic venous system, deoxygenated blood flows toward the heart in veins to the right atrium. From there it travels into the right ventricle, from which it is pumped into the pulmonary circulation, specifically the pulmonary artery. Vessels that carry blood toward the heart are called *veins,* and vessels that carry blood away from the heart are called *arteries.* The pulmonary arteries are the only arteries that carry deoxygenated blood. The pulmonary veins are the only veins that carry oxygenated blood. Blood in the pulmonary arteries travels to the pulmonary capillary beds, where carbon dioxide is lost and oxygen is picked up. The oxygenated blood then travels through the pulmonary veins to the left atrium and the left ventricle, from which it is pumped into the systemic arterial circulation so that it can deliver oxygen and nutrients to the tissues. The larger arteries branch into smaller arteries, called *arterioles,* that provide the majority of the resistance to blood flow, thus protecting the capillary beds from the high pressures of the systemic arterial system and maintaining blood pressure and steady tissue perfusion. Once the blood reaches the capillary beds, oxygen and other nutrients are lost to the tissues and waste products, such as carbon dioxide, are picked

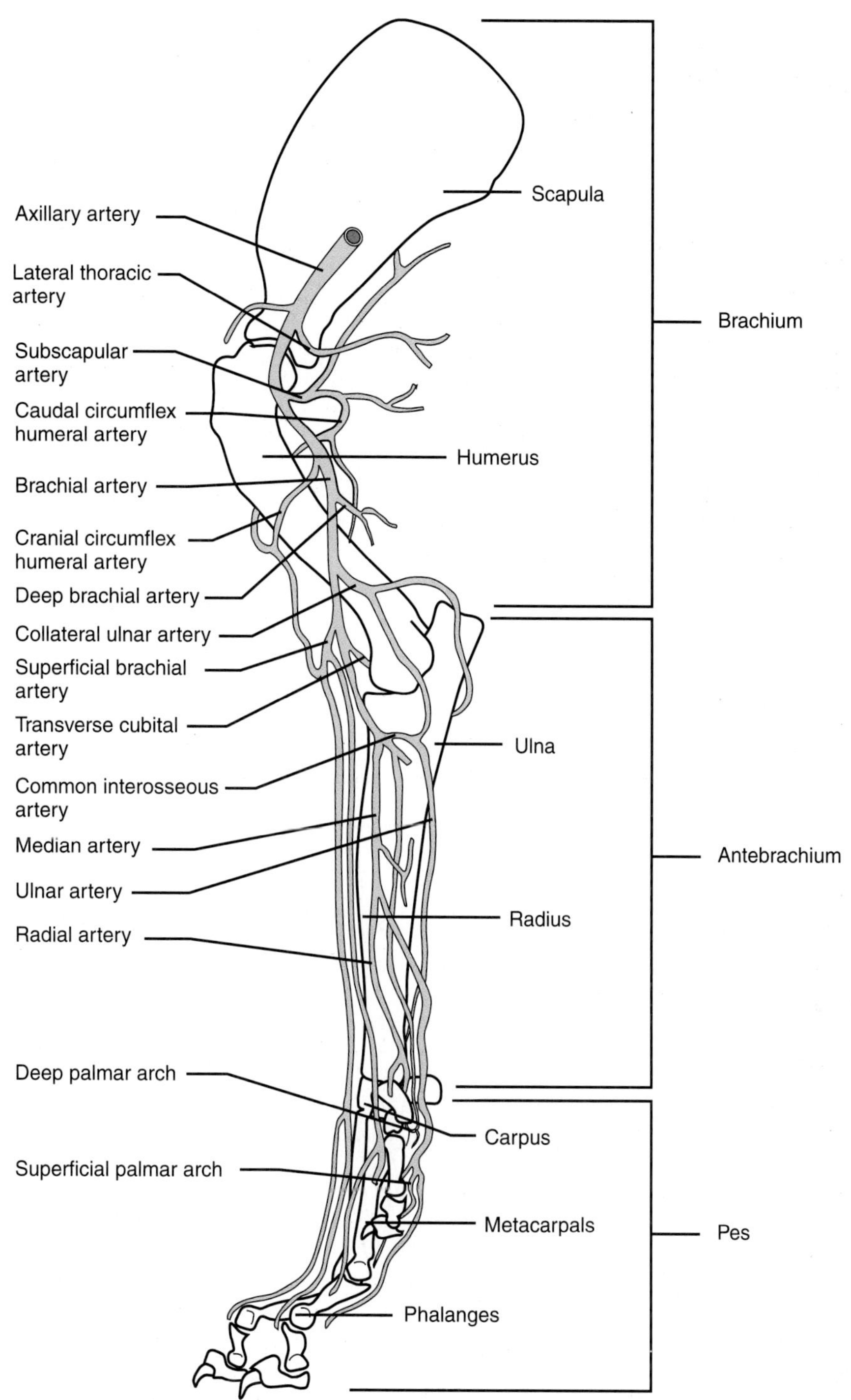

FIGURE **8-10** **Arteries of Canine Forelimb (Medial Aspect).**

up to be delivered away from the tissues via systemic veins (Figure 8-17, p. 183).

The systemic arterial circulation is regarded as a high-pressure system, and the pulmonary and systemic venous circulations are regarded as low-pressure systems. High hydrostatic pressure is required to perfuse tissues with a high resistance to blood flow (such as the brain, heart, and kidney), as well as to overcome gravitational forces to perfuse tissues above the heart. The pulmonary circulation is regarded as a low-pressure system because the pulmonary system has a low resistance to blood flow. High blood pressures in venous systems may cause fluid to leak from the vessels and to accumulate as edema (e.g., with congestive heart failure). The average blood flow (given in millimeters per minute [ml/min])

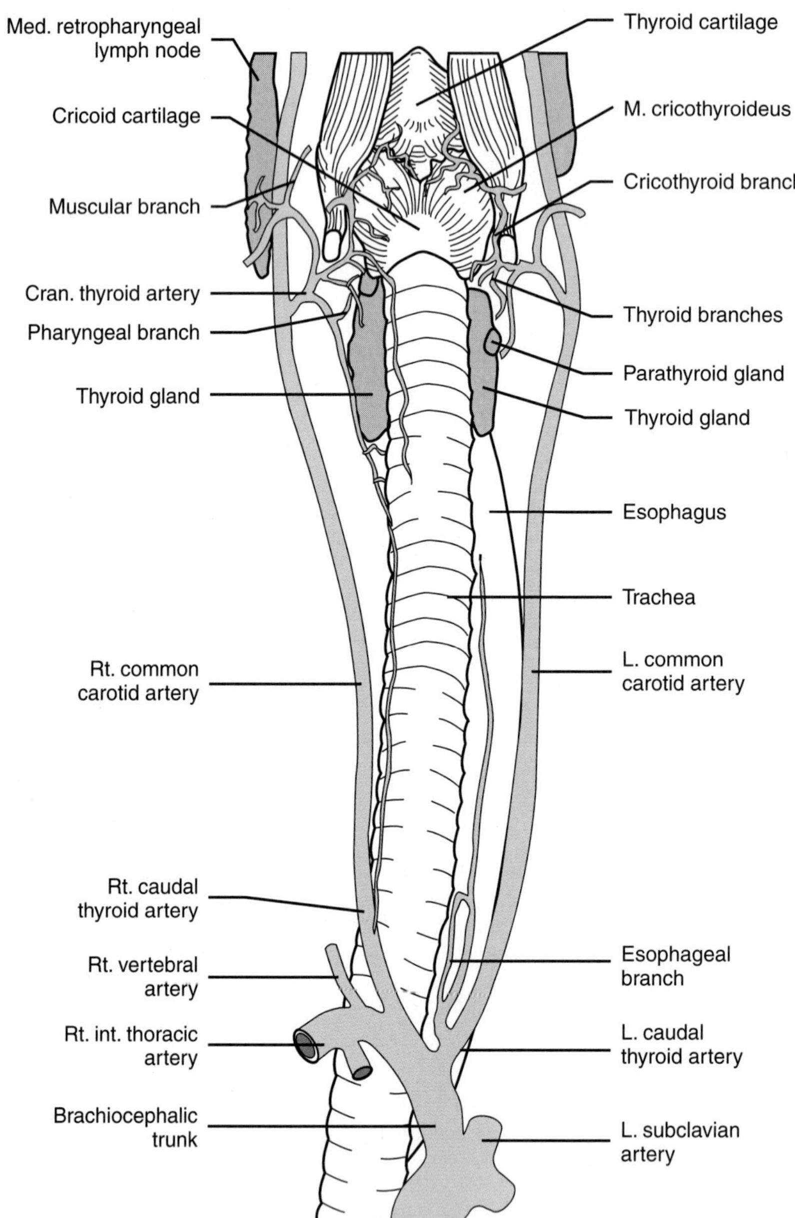

FIGURE **8-11** **Common Carotid Arteries and Their Relation to Larynx, Trachea, and Other Structures.**

is about the same in the pulmonary and systemic systems. However, the systemic system contains a much larger percentage of the total blood volume. Of the total blood volume, the pulmonary circulation contains about 15%; the systemic system, about 80%; and the heart, about 5%. Within the systemic circulation, the systemic veins contain the majority of the blood volume (65%). The systemic arteries and arterioles contain about 10%, and the systemic capillary beds contain about 5% of the total blood volume.

Functions of the Cardiovascular System

The cardiovascular system functions to maintain normal blood pressure within the arteries, to maintain blood flow to the tissues, and to maintain normal blood pressures within the capillaries and veins. The cardiovascular system must be able to carry out these functions during rest and during exercise. Maintenance of normal blood pressures allows proper tissue perfusion. Tissue perfusion is important because it allows (1) the delivery of oxygen and other nutrients (such as glucose)

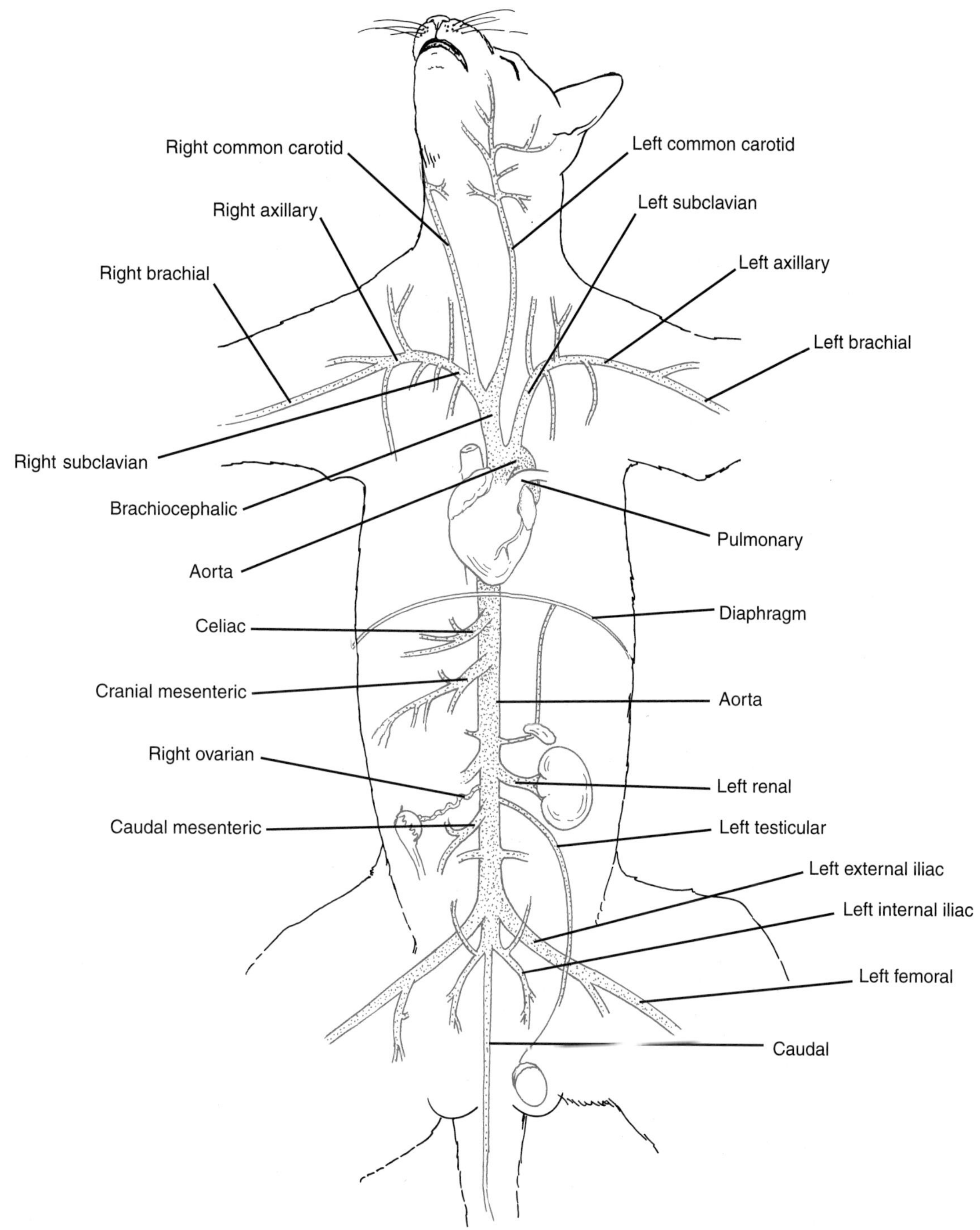

FIGURE **8-12** **Branches of Abdominal Aorta in Cat.** (From McBride DF: *Learning veterinary terminology,* ed 2, St Louis, 2002, Mosby.)

to the tissues, (2) the removal of waste products (such as carbon dioxide) from the tissues, and (3) the transport of hormonal messages from one part of the body to another. Maintenance of normal blood pressures within the capillary and veins is important in the prevention of edema formation.

Blood pressure is the force exerted by the blood against the inner walls of the blood vessels. All vessels in the cardiovascular system have this force within them, but typically the term *blood pressure* refers to systemic arterial blood pressure. The systemic arterial blood pressure rises and falls in coordination with the cardiac cycle (rises with systole and falls with diastole) (Figure 8-18, p. 184). The maximum pressure achieved during ventricular contraction is called the *systolic blood pressure.* The *diastolic blood pressure* is the lowest pressure that remains in the arteries when the ventricles are relaxing. When the ventricles contract, the blood is ejected into the large arteries, whose walls stretch and recoil as the pressures increase and decrease, respectively. This expanding and recoiling of the arterial wall

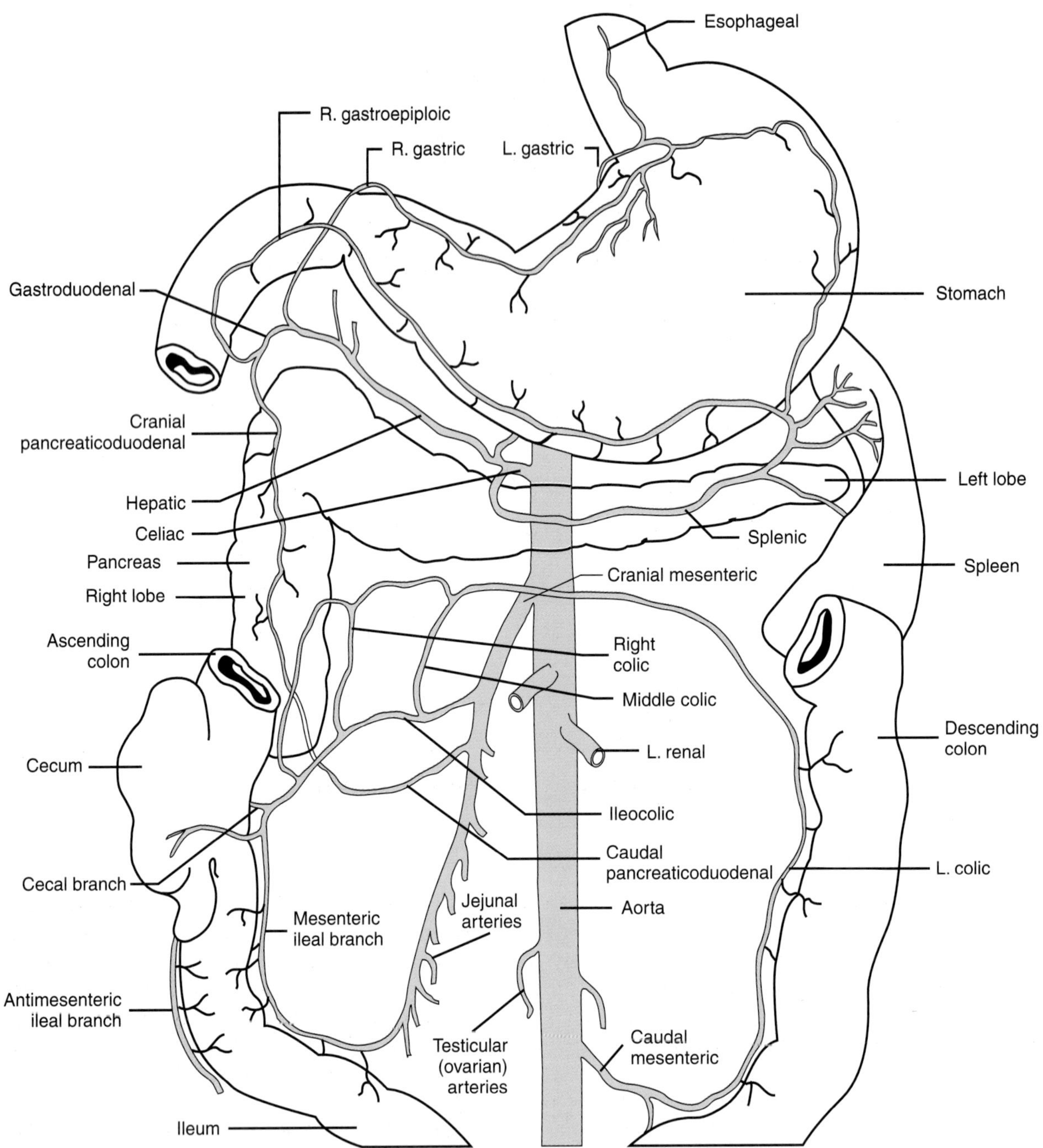

FIGURE **8-13** **Visceral Branches of Abdominal Aorta (Ventral Aspect).**

can be felt as a pulse. The pulse pressure is the difference between the systolic and diastolic pressures, and the greater the pulse pressure, the stronger the palpated pulse.

The friction created between the blood and the arterial vessel wall limits the flow of blood; this force is called *peripheral* or *systemic resistance.* For blood to flow forward, the blood pressure must be greater than the peripheral resistance. Peripheral resistance and blood pressure can be changed by many things. For example, **sympathetic nervous system** input to the arterioles will cause vasoconstriction and a subsequent increase in the blood pressure. Conversely, increases in parasympathetic activity cause vasodilation and a decrease in blood pressure. Furthermore, local mediators of vascular tone affect the resistance to blood flow independent of the **autonomic nervous system.** The ability to change the resistance to blood flow allows the autonomic system to select the organ systems that it wants to perfuse. For example, at rest the **parasympathetic nervous system** predominates, and blood flow is directed toward the digestive system; however, during exercise, the sympathetic nervous system is dominant, and blood flow goes preferentially to the muscles rather than the gastrointestinal tract. The vital organs (brain, heart, and kidney) are

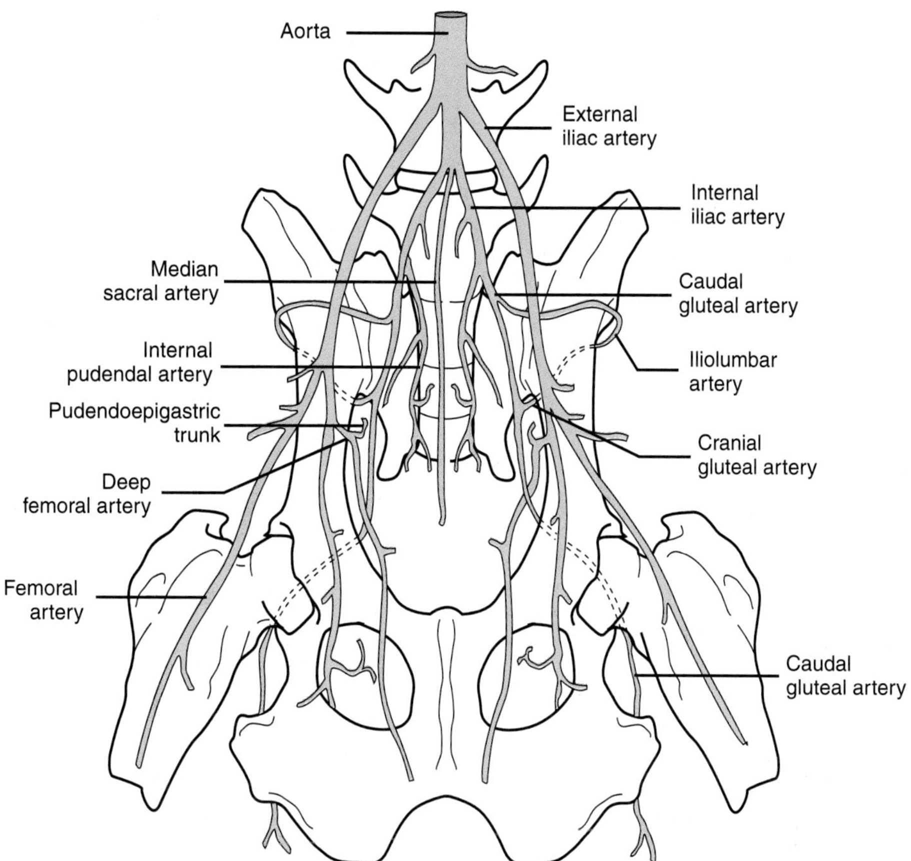

FIGURE **8-14** **Termination of Abdominal Aorta.**

preferentially perfused above all other tissues. Control of vasoconstriction and vasodilation by the vasomotor center is especially important in the arterioles of the splanchnic region (abdominal viscera). When fully dilated (as in the case with hypotensive shock), these vessels can accommodate nearly all of the blood volume in the body, and the arterial blood pressure becomes very low.

The function of the heart is dictated by a balance among the level of **contractility** (inotropic state), the forces opposing the pumping action of the heart (afterload), and the forces that are associated with filling the heart during diastole (preload). Many factors influence the performance of the heart (heart rate, autonomic input, hormonal input, drugs, metabolic products, synchrony of the atria and ventricles, etc.).

The level of contractility is determined, at the molecular level, by the interaction of calcium ions and the contractile proteins (actin and myosin). However, many mechanisms affect the concentration of calcium ions in the myocytes. The level of autonomic nervous system activity, specifically, the sympathetic nervous system, greatly impacts the level of contractility. Stimulation of cardiac beta-adrenergic receptors by norepinephrine (neurotransmitter of the sympathetic nervous system) increases the rate and extent of myocardial contraction by increasing the amount of calcium available to the contractile apparatus. Furthermore, Starling's law describes an increase in contractility associated with stretching of sarcomeres (which happens when venous return is increased). In addition, a limited positive relationship exists between the force generated by the myocardium and the frequency at which it is stimulated (i.e., within limits, the faster the heart beats, the stronger it contracts).

The **afterload** is the sum of the forces that the ventricle must contract against to make blood flow forward. Among other things, blood pressure plays an important part in determining the afterload. In states in which the blood pressure is high (e.g., systemic hypertension), the afterload is also high and the function of the heart is impaired. If the afterload is low, the heart can eject blood easily into the arterial system. In the case of sustained elevated afterload, the heart muscle compensates by becoming thicker, therefore allowing the heart to generate the forces necessary to move blood forward.

The **preload** essentially is the amount of blood in the heart just before it contracts (also called the *end-diastolic volume* [EDV]). Preload is determined by the amount of venous return and, in some disease states, the amount of blood that has been regurgitated into the atrium by a leaky AV valve or the amount

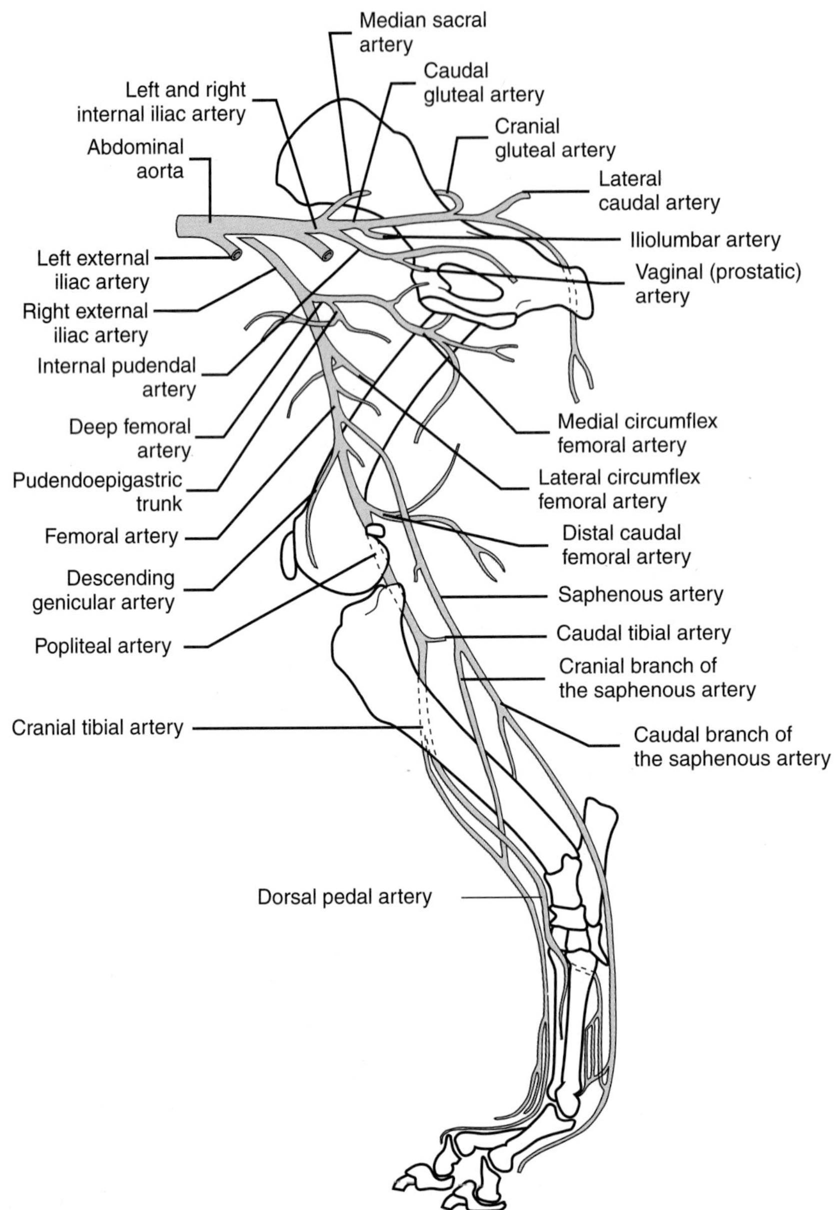

FIGURE **8-15** **Arteries of Canine Hindlimb (Medial Aspect).**

of blood left in the heart after a weak systolic contraction (as with myocardial failure). Increases in preload stretches the heart muscle, which contracts more strongly, (Starling's principle) and the cardiac output is increased. Conversely, if the preload is reduced, cardiac output may decrease.

TEST YOURSELF

1. Trace the pathway of blood flow through the heart.
2. Describe the pressure changes that occur in the heart throughout the cardiac cycle.
3. Explain the concepts of preload and afterload.

THE CARDIAC CYCLE

For the heart to function as a pump, it must contract and relax in a cyclical pattern. The heart contracts and relaxes in response to electrical stimuli generated from specific parts of the heart known as *pacemakers.* The cardiac cycle is divided into two parts: systole and diastole. **Systole** is the period in which the heart is contracting and generating pressure within the heart so that blood can be ejected into the systemic and pulmonary circulations. The period when the heart is relaxed and is filling with blood is called **diastole.** In general, reference to systole or diastole is made with regard to the ventricles (even though the atria also undergo systole and diastole).

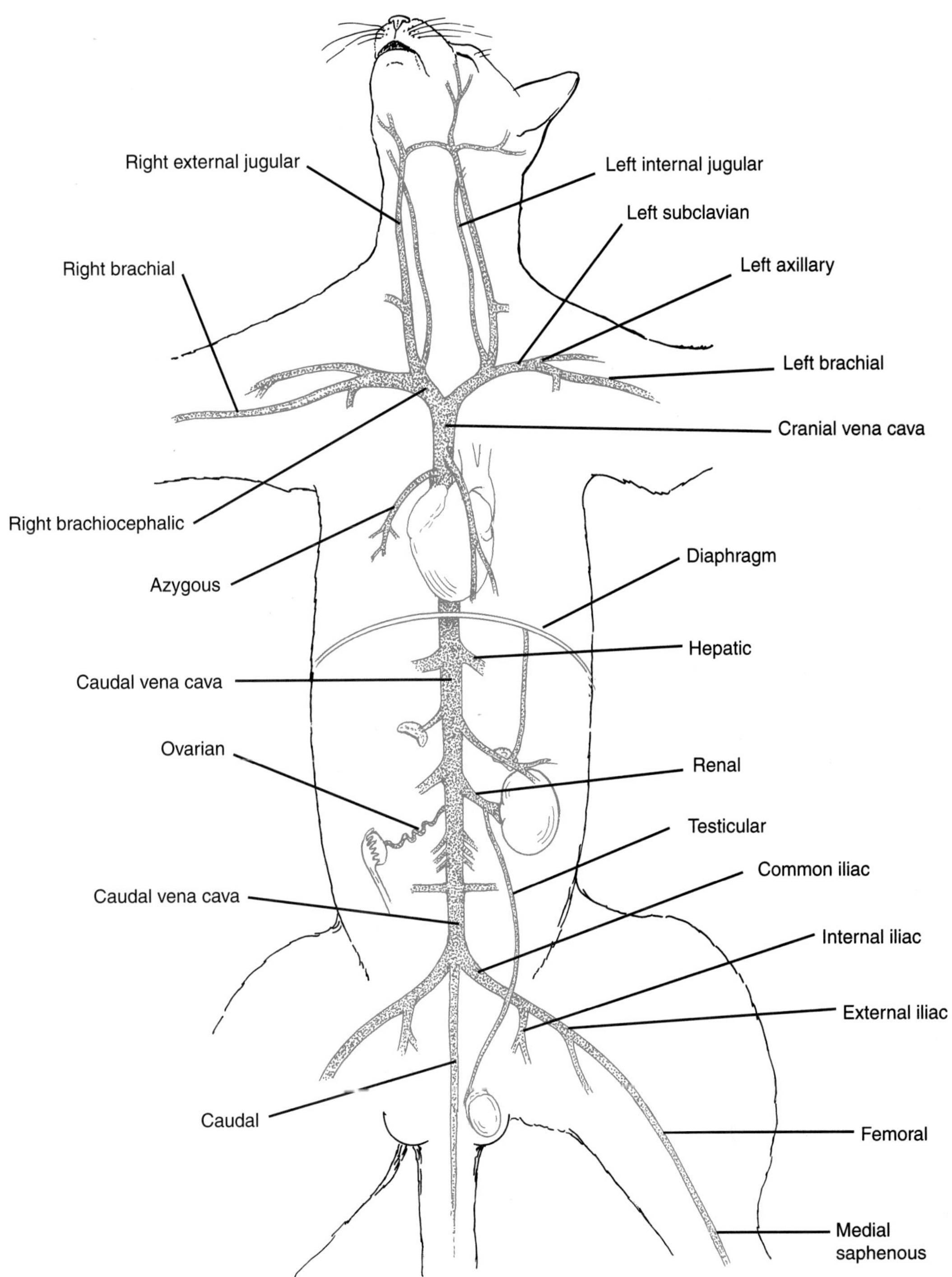

FIGURE **8-16** **Venous System in Cat.** (From McBride DF: *Learning veterinary terminology,* ed 2, St Louis, 2002, Mosby.)

At the end of diastole, the ventricle has filled to a maximum volume (EDV). Electrical systole precedes mechanical systole. When the electrical stimulus reaches the ventricles, the myocardium begins to contract and pressure begins to increase within the ventricle. Once the pressure in the ventricle is higher than that of the atrium, the AV valves close. The myocardium continues to tense, and pressure continues to increase. This period is known as the *isovolumetric contraction period* because the AV valves and the semilunar valves are closed and the volume in the ventricle is unchanged (provided that the AV valves are not insufficient). The first heart sound occurs when the AV valves close. The semilunar valves open when the pressure in the ventricle equals or exceeds the pressure in the aorta or pulmonary artery (depending on which side is being described). Ventricular ejection occurs when the semilunar valves open and ends

Box 8-1 The Systemic Arteries

AORTIC ARCH

- Aortic arch
  - Coronary arteries (aa.)
  - Brachiocephalic trunk
    - Right subclavian artery (a.)
      - Vertebral a.
      - Costocervical trunk
        - Deep cervical a.
      - Internal thoracic a.
        - Ventral intercostal a.
        - Cranial epigastric a.
        - Musculophrenic a.
      - Superficial cervical a.
      - Common carotid a.
  - Left subclavian a. (same branches as right subclavian a.)

AXILLARY ARTERY (SEE FIGURE 8-10)

- Axillary a.
  - External thoracic a.
  - Lateral thoracic a.
  - Subscapular
- Brachial a.
  - Deep brachial a.
  - Collateral ulnar a.
  - Superficial brachial a.
    - Cranial superficial antebrachial a.
      - Dorsal common digital aa.
  - Transverse cubital a.
  - Common interosseous a.
    - Ulnar a.
    - Cranial interosseous a.
    - Caudal interosseous a.
      - Superficial palmar arch
        - Palmar common digital aa.
      - Deep palmar arch
        - Palmar metacarpal aa.
- Median a.
  - Radial a.

COMMON CAROTID ARTERY (SEE FIGURE 8-11)

- Common carotid a.
  - Caudal thyroid a.
  - Cranial thyroid a.
  - External carotid a.
    - Occipital a.
    - Cranial laryngeal a.
    - Ascending pharyngeal a.
    - Lingual a.
    - Facial a.
    - Caudal auricular a.
    - Parotid a.
    - Superficial temporal a.
    - Maxillary a.
      - Inferior alveolar a.
      - External ophthalmic a.
      - Ethmoidal a.
      - Palatine aa.
      - Infraorbital a.
  - Internal carotid a.

THORACIC AORTA

- Thoracic aorta
  - Dorsal intercostals aa.
- Bronchoesophageal a.
  - Bronchial branches
  - Esophageal branches
  - Dorsal costoabdominal a.

ABDOMINAL AORTA (SEE FIGURES 8-12 AND 8-13)

- Abdominal aorta
  - Phrenicoabdominal aa.
  - Lumbar aa.
  - Celiac a.
    - Left gastric a.
    - Hepatic a.
      - Hepatic branches
      - Right gastric a.
    - Gastroduodenal a.
    - Cranial pancreaticoduodenal a.
    - Right gastroepiploic a.
  - Splenic a.
    - Pancreatic branches
    - Short gastric aa.
    - Left gastroepiploic a.
  - Cranial mesenteric a.
    - Caudal pancreaticoduodenal a.
    - Jejunal aa.
    - Ileal aa.
    - Ileocolic a.
      - Middle colic a.
      - Right colic a.
      - Cecal aa.
  - Renal aa.
  - Testicular (ovarian) aa.
  - Caudal mesenteric a.
    - Left colic a.
    - Cranial rectal a.
  - Deep circumflex iliac aa.
  - External iliac aa.
  - Internal iliac aa.
  - Median sacral a.
    - Lumbar a. VI
  - Median caudal a.

EXTERNAL ILIAC ARTERY (SEE FIGURES 8-14 AND 8-15)

- External iliac artery
  - Deep femoral a.
    - Pudendoepigastric trunk
      - Caudal epigastric a.
      - External pudendal a.
  - Femoral a.
    - Lateral circumflex femoral a.
    - Proximal, middle, and distal caudal femoral aa.
    - Saphenous a.
      - Cranial branch
        - Dorsal common digital aa.
      - Caudal branch
        - Plantar common digital aa.

Box 8-1 The Systemic Arteries—cont'd

EXTERNAL ILIAC ARTERY—CONT'D
- Popliteal a.
  - Cranial tibial a.
    - Dorsal pedal a.
    - Plantar metatarsal aa.
  - Caudal tibial a.

INTERNAL ILIAC ARTERY
- Internal iliac artery
  - Umbilical a.
  - Caudal gluteal a.
    - Iliolumbar a.
    - Cranial gluteal a.
- Internal pudendal a.
  - Prostatic (vaginal) a.
    - Artery of the ductus deferens (uterine a.)
    - Caudal vesical a.
  - Middle rectal a.
  - Urethral artery
  - Ventral perineal a.
  - Artery of the penis (clitoris)
    - Artery of the bulb
    - Deep artery
    - Dorsal artery

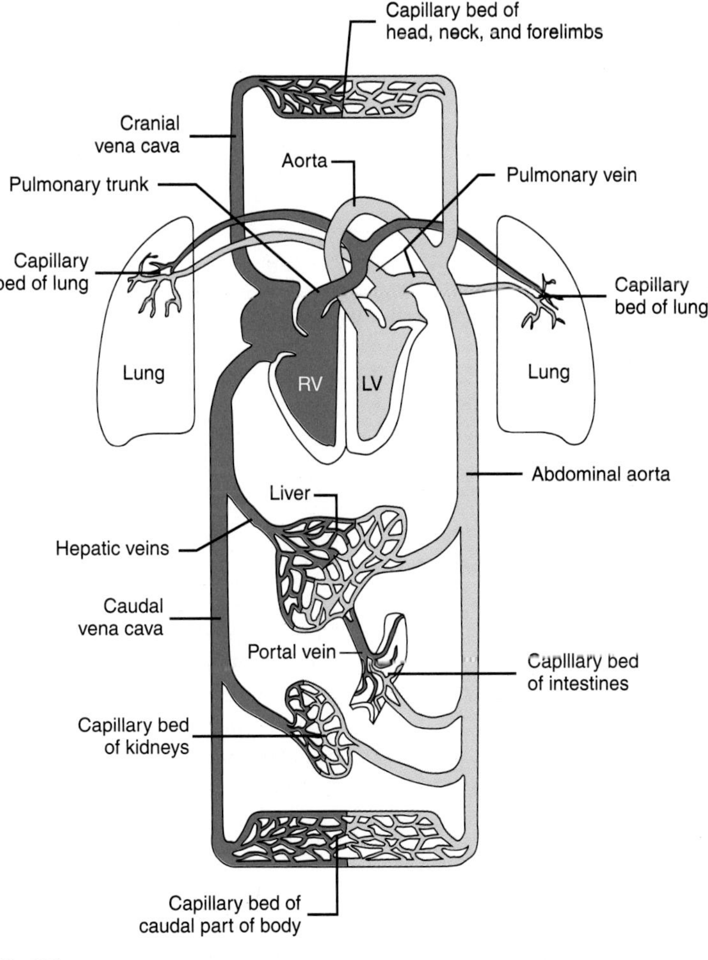

FIGURE **8-17** **Systemic and Pulmonary Circulatory Systems.** *LV,* Left ventricle; *RV,* right ventricle.

when they close. The amount of blood left in the heart at the end of systole is called the *end-systolic volume* (ESV). The amount of blood that is ejected from the ventricle during each systole is called the *stroke volume* (EDV - ESV = SV). The end of systole coincides with the closure of the semilunar valves (the second heart sound).

The first part of diastole, also called the *isovolumetric relaxation time,* occurs when the semilunar valves and the AV valves are closed. During this time, the ventricle relaxes, and the pressure inside the ventricle decreases even though the volume of blood in the ventricle does not change. Once the pressure has become less than that within the atrium, the AV valves open and the ventricle begins to fill with blood. This early filling period is passive and may be accompanied with the third

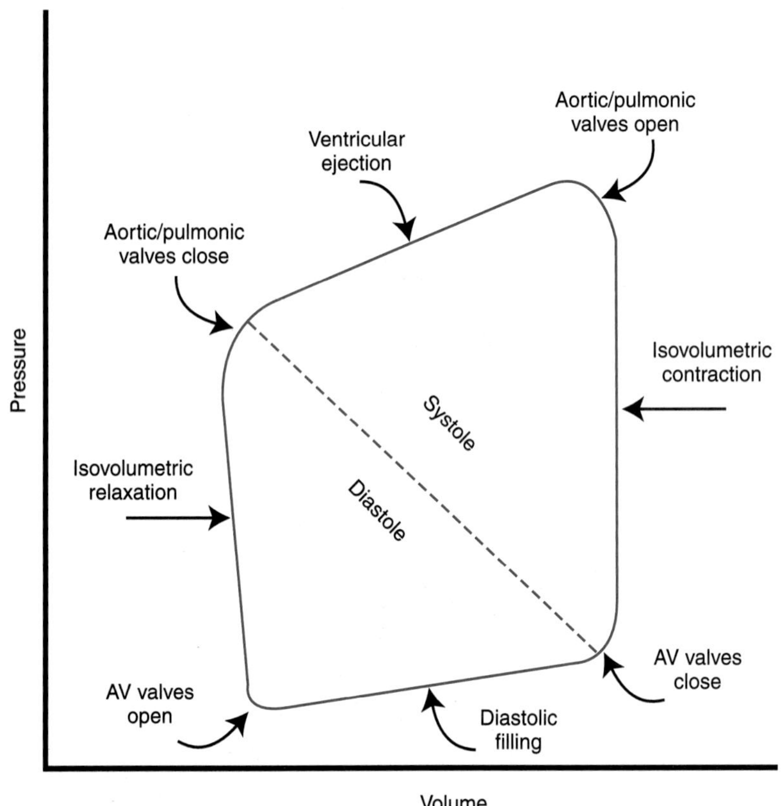

FIGURE **8-18** **Cardiac Cycle Represented by Pressure-Volume Loop.** *AV,* atrioventricular.

heart sound (normal in horses and ruminants but abnormal in carnivores). About 60% of the diastolic filling occurs during this initial, rapid-filling phase. The slow-filling phase follows the rapid-filling phase. The atria contract and augment the ventricular filling just before the next systole. Atrial contraction contributes approximately 20% to 30% of the filling volume in a normal animal. A fourth heart sound may accompany atrial contraction. This fourth heart sound can be normal in ruminants or equine but is usually associated with cardiac disease in carnivores. The phases of diastole occur almost simultaneously in animals with rapid heart rates.

Properties of Cardiac Muscle Fibers

Cardiac muscle is similar to skeletal muscle in that both are striated muscles. However, some important differences should be noted. In contrast to skeletal muscle, impulses travel from cell to cell in cardiac muscle tissues. Because the impulses travel from cell to cell across the myocardial tissue, the heart contracts as a unit or it does not contract at all. In addition, cardiac tissues have automaticity and may initiate a wave of depolarization independently, whereas skeletal muscle tissue must be stimulated by a nerve ending. Automaticity is a unique characteristic of cardiac tissue that allows parts of the heart to take on pacemaker activities by being self-excitable. These automatic tissues (such as the SA node) initiate their own depolarizations that initiate the depolarization of the rest of the heart so that the heart beats in a rhythmic fashion. The majority of the heart is composed of contractile muscle tissue, and only a small portion is automatic. Another difference between cardiac muscle and skeletal muscle is that cardiac muscle tissues have a long refractory period (the inexcitable period) compared with skeletal muscle tissue. The refractory period in cardiac tissues is about 200 times as long as that of skeletal tissues.

Like skeletal muscle tissue, depolarization of cardiac muscle tissue is associated with the influx of sodium through voltage-regulated, time-dependent, fast sodium channels. This wave of depolarization (created by the influx of sodium ions) travels across the myocardial tissue down T tubules to activate L-type calcium channels, which allow calcium into the myocyte to stimulate calcium release from the sarcoplasmic reticulum. Excitation-contraction coupling links the wave of depolarization with the sliding and cross-linking of the myofilaments.

Cardiac Impulse Propagation

The heart is required to pump a tremendous amount of blood throughout the life of an animal. The rhythmic pumping action of the heart is a result of the heart's intrinsic ability to spontaneously depolarize. Specific areas of the heart are normally responsible for the generation of the **action potentials** that stimulate the heart muscle to contract. These areas are called *automatic tissues* because they can depolarize spontaneously. Impulses are conducted across specific pathways so that parts of the heart are activated at the appropriate time in the cardiac cycle. In other words, the myocardial tissue is excited in a specific pattern that facilitates the pumping function of the heart. The sequence of activation is as follows: (1) the SA node

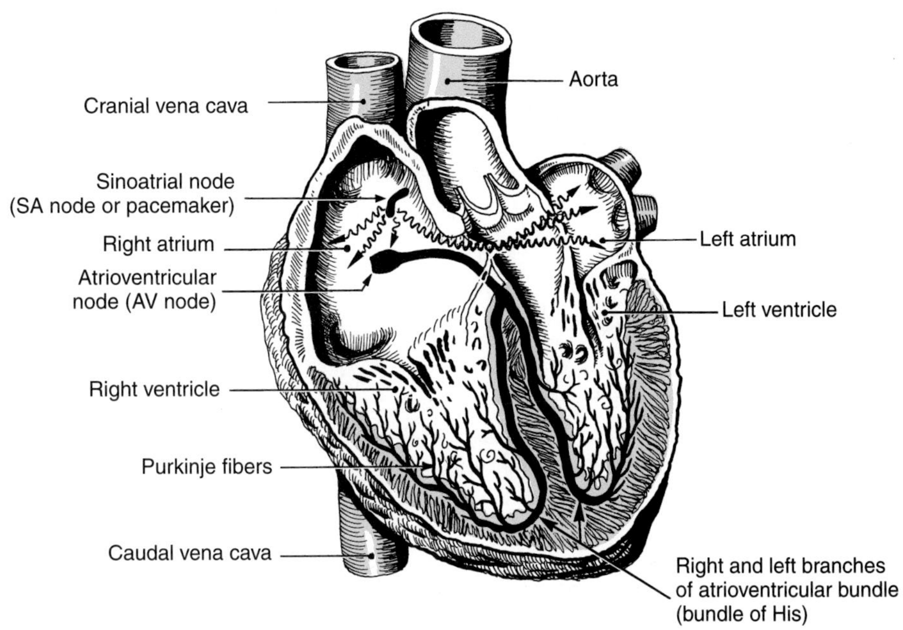

FIGURE **8-19** **Conduction System of Heart.** Sinoatrial node (pacemaker), located in wall of right atrium, sets basic heart rhythm. (From McBride DF: *Learning veterinary terminology,* ed 2, St Louis, 2002, Mosby.)

spontaneously depolarizes; (2) the wave of depolarization takes two routes, first to the AV node via specialized conduction fibers and, second, across the atrial myocardium to stimulate atrial contraction; (3) the impulse travels through the AV node into the bundle of His in the AV junction; (4) the impulse travels within the left and right bundle branches toward the ventricular apex; and (5) from the bundle branches the impulse travels through the Purkinje fibers to the myocardium (Figure 8-19). This sequence of activation allows the contraction to be coordinated and efficient. While the impulse is depolarizing the atria, it is traveling slowly through the AV node so that the atria have enough time to contract and empty blood into the ventricles just before the ventricles are excited and contract. Once the impulse reaches the ventricular myocardium, it excites the septum, papillary muscles, apex, and heart base (in that order) to facilitate ejection of blood out of the ventricle.

Action potentials (depolarization wave) in cardiac tissue are associated with the influx and efflux of ions across the cell membrane. The action potential of an automatic tissue, such as the SA node, is characterized by a spontaneous influx of positive ions (sodium, potassium, or calcium) that causes the membrane potential to become more positive. Once the cell membrane potential reaches a threshold voltage, calcium channels open and calcium flows into the cell, causing it to depolarize. Once the cell has depolarized, the calcium channels become inactive and potassium begins to flow out of the cell again, making the cell negative and polarized. The cycle repeats in adjacent tissues, thereby effectively pacing the adjacent myocardium. The action potential of nonautomatic tissue is characterized by a negative resting membrane potential that is brought to threshold by the wave of depolarization from adjacent cells. When the tissue reaches the threshold potential, voltage-regulated, fast sodium channels open and allow sodium to enter the cell, thereby depolarizing the cell. At less negative voltages, the calcium channels are activated and allow calcium to enter the cell. The flow of calcium ions maintains the cell in a depolarized state for a specific amount of time, after which the calcium channels become inactive and potassium ions flow out of the cell to repolarize the cell. The cell is not depolarized again until another wave of depolarization arrives.

Although cells in most parts of the heart have intrinsic pacemaker ability, the normal heart rhythm is determined by the SA node. The SA node has the fastest rate of spontaneous depolarization. The dominant pacemaker suppresses all other pacing sites (such as the AV node, Purkinje system, etc.). If the SA node did not fire, then one of the other subsidiary pacemakers would rescue the cardiac rhythm, only at a slower rate. The intrinsic pacing rate of the AV node is approximately 40 to 60 beats/min, and the intrinsic pacing rate of the Purkinje fibers is between 20 to 40 beats/min in the canine. The pacing rate of automatic tissues is variable among species. Note that the function of the conduction system is to allow for faster activation of the myocardium. If the myocardium had to rely on cell-to-cell transmission of the impulse, it would take much longer to depolarize the heart.

The heart rate is determined by several factors, such as body temperature; however, the most important factor is the autonomic nervous system. The balance between the sympathetic and parasympathetic nervous system determines the rate of spontaneous depolarization of the SA node and the other subsidiary pacemakers. When the sympathetic nervous system is stimulated, the rate of spontaneous depolarization is faster and the heart rate increases; when the parasympathetic nervous system is activated, the heart rate slows (Figure 8-20). The cardioregulatory centers are located in the medulla oblongata.

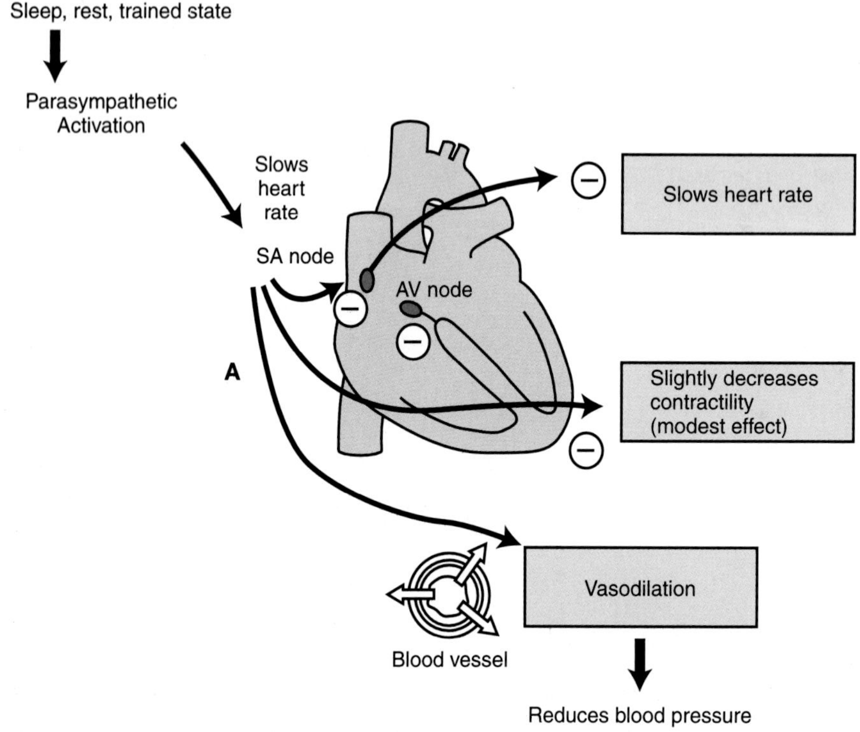

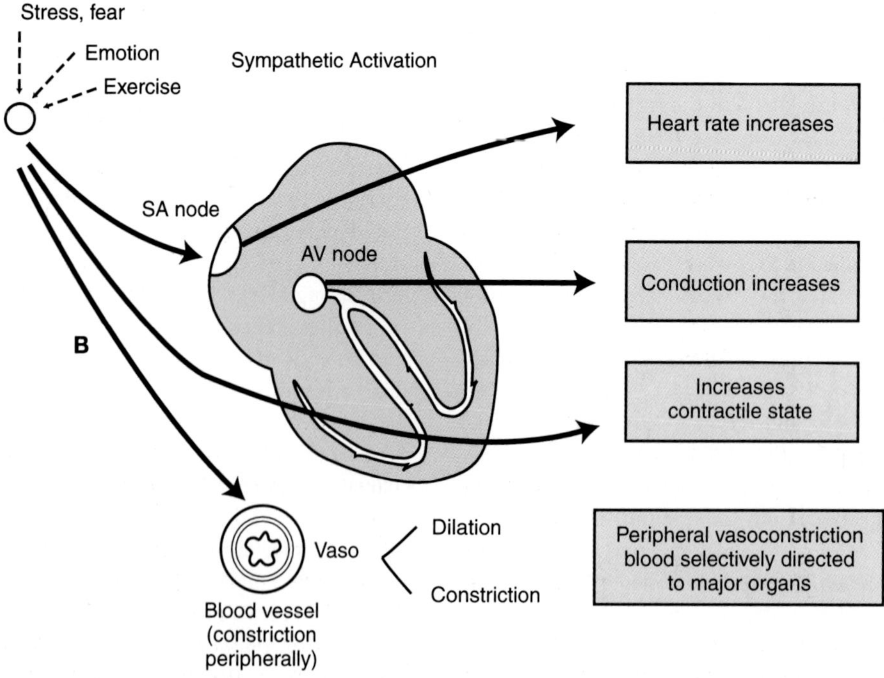

FIGURE **8-20** **Regulation of Heart Rate and Blood Pressure.** Balance between sympathetic and parasympathetic nervous system determines rate at which SA node "fires," or depolarizes. **A,** Parasympathetic activation. **B,** Sympathetic activation.

These regulatory centers reflexively increase and decrease sympathetic and parasympathetic tone based on input from structures called *baroreceptors* in the vessels and heart chambers. Baroreceptors detect changes in blood pressure. If blood pressure decreases, baroreceptors send a message to the cardioregulatory center to increase sympathetic tone, which increases heart rate and causes vasoconstriction to bring the blood pressure back to normal. If the baroreceptors detect high blood pressure, the message is transmitted to the cardioregulatory center to decrease sympathetic tone and to increase parasympathetic tone, which decreases the heart rate and causes vasodilation to bring blood pressure back to normal.

TEST YOURSELF

1. Describe the cardiac cycle.
2. Explain the origin of the heart sounds.
3. Describe the difference between automatic and nonautomatic cardiac tissues.
4. Describe the role of the SA node.

EXCITATION-CONTRACTION COUPLING

For the heart to be an effective pump, the contraction of the myocardium must be coupled with the electrical activity that determines when the heart muscle should contract. This process is called *excitation-contraction coupling.* You'll need an understanding of the ultrastructure of the myocytes to grasp the concept of excitation-contraction. The ultrastructure of cardiac muscle is arranged so that the tissue can contract. Cardiac tissue is composed of connective tissue and myocytes. Cardiac myocytes are arranged as a syncytium. This means that all of the cells are connected via structures called *intercalated disks.* The atrial syncytium is separated from the ventricular syncytium by a fibrous ring so that the electrical activity in the atria is insulated from the electrical activity in the ventricular syncytium. Each myocyte consists of numerous structures, called *myofibrils,* and a cell membrane (also called the *sarcolemma*). Myofibrils contain longitudinally arranged sarcomeres, which are the fundamental contractile units of the myofibril. The end of each sarcomere is marked by a structure called the *Z line.* The sarcomere contains thin filaments (known as *actin*) that project from the Z lines toward the center of the sarcomere. The thick filaments (known as *myosin*) project from the middle of the sarcomere and are parallel to the actin filaments. The region where actin and myosin overlap is called the *A band,* and the region where only the thin filaments are located is called the *I band.* The *H band* is the region where only the myosin filaments are located. A transverse tubule system (T tubules), which is part of the sarcolemma, is in close association with the sarcoplasmic reticulum at the level of the Z lines (Figure 8-21).

The process of excitation-contraction is complex and not completely understood. It involves the movement of calcium ions into and within the myocytes. Normally, the calcium concentration inside the cell is much smaller than outside the cell. Therefore a large chemical gradient exists from outside to inside the cell. The cell membrane (or sarcolemma) is relatively impermeable to calcium; so calcium must enter the cell through channels. These calcium channels are called *L-type calcium channels,* and they are located in the region of the Z line where the T tubules are in close association with the sarcoplasmic reticulum. As the electrical impulse (wave of depolarization) travels across the myocardial tissue, voltage-regulated, L-type calcium channels become activated and allow calcium to enter the cell. The calcium that enters the cell stimulates the release of calcium from the sarcoplasmic reticulum. The sarcoplasmic reticulum is a membrane-limited structure that surrounds the myofibrils within the myocardial cell. The basic function of the sarcoplasmic reticulum is to store calcium during diastole and to release calcium during systole. Calcium ions that are released from the sarcoplasmic reticulum interact with regulatory proteins that cause conformational changes that allow the contractile structures to interact and cause contraction of the myocytes. Specifically, calcium binds to troponin C, creating a conformational change in the tropomyosin molecule, thus allowing actin and myosin to interact and contract. When repolarization of the myocytes occurs, the calcium channels close and calcium is pumped back into the sarcoplasmic reticulum, where it is stored during diastole. Excess calcium also may leave the myocytes by way of an exchange mechanism known as the *sodium-calcium exchanger.* During diastole, the calcium no longer interacts with troponin, and tropomyosin conforms to prevent the interaction between actin and myosin. The myocytes relax as the calcium is removed from the contractile apparatus and is pumped into the sarcoplasmic reticulum by an energy-dependent process.

TEST YOURSELF

1. Discuss excitation-contraction coupling. What are the roles of actin, myosin, and calcium?
2. Discuss the concept of spontaneous depolarization.
3. Describe an action potential from automatic tissue. Describe an action potential from nonautomatic tissue.
4. Describe the role of the fast sodium channels.
5. Describe ventricular repolarization.

THE ELECTROCARDIOGRAM

Because body fluids can conduct electrical currents, the electrical activity of the heart can be detected on the surface of the body and may be monitored with an instrument called an **electrocardiograph.** The electrocardiograph creates a graphic recording called an **electrocardiogram (ECG).** An ECG is recorded by placing metal electrodes in specific locations on the skin. The electrical activity of the heart follows a specific pattern that is reflected on the ECG as either positive or negative deflections, depending on the direction the impulses are traveling. These deflections

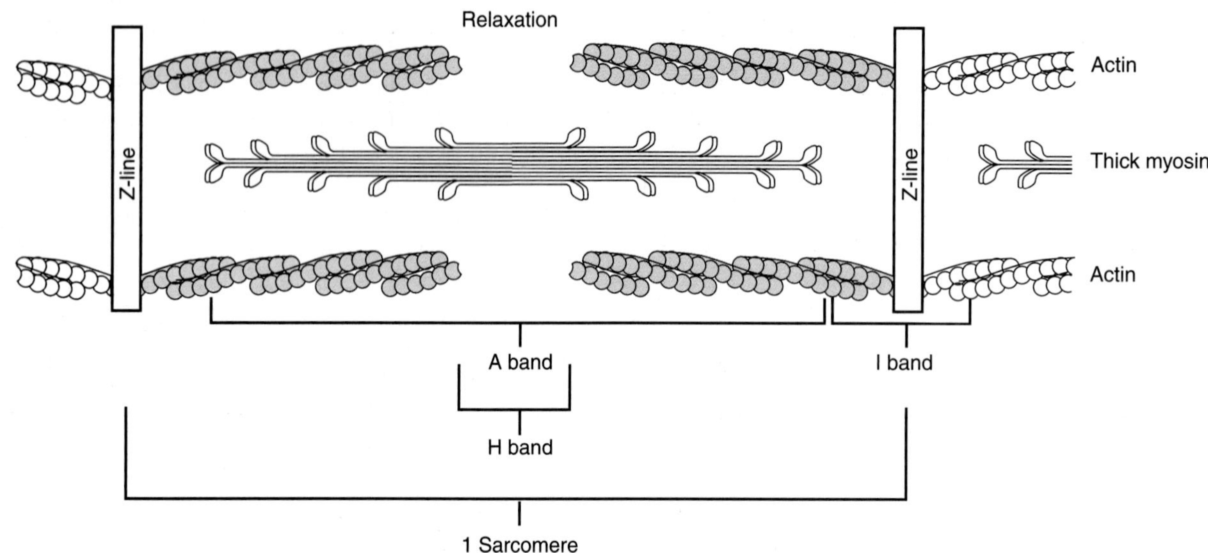

FIGURE **8-21** **Schematic Concept of Myocardial Contractile Proteins.**

FIGURE **8-22** **Normal P-QRS-T Complex.**

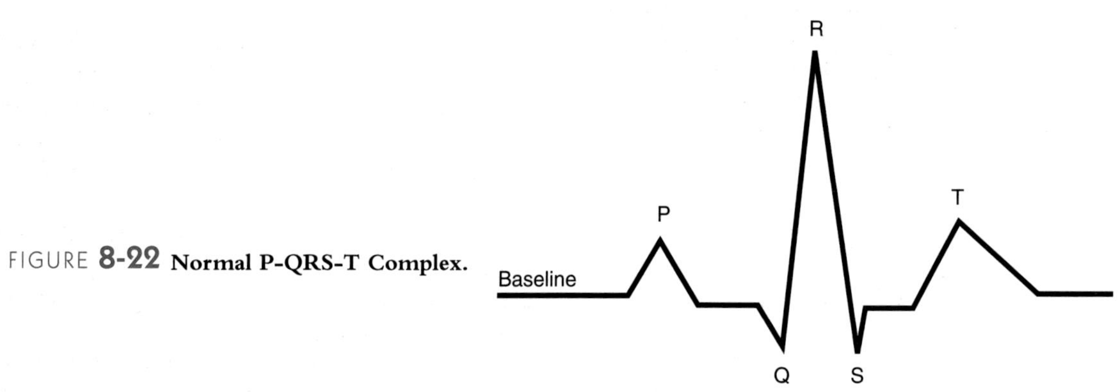

are also referred to as *waves*. Between electrical events, the myocardium stays polarized and the ECG does not record anything. When the SA node fires and the atria depolarize, the ECG detects this change and a wave is created. The wave associated with atrial depolarization is called the *P wave*. When the ventricles depolarize, another set of waves is created. The group of waves associated with ventricular depolarization is called the *QRS complex*. After depolarization, the ventricles have to repolarize, and this event is recorded as the *T wave*.

To summarize: the P wave is caused by atrial depolarization, the QRS complex is caused by ventricular depolarization, and the T wave is caused by ventricular repolarization (Figure 8-22).

Clinically, three reasons are given to evaluate an ECG. First, the heart rate can be calculated. Second, the cardiac rhythm can be determined. Third, the P-QRS-T complexes can be evaluated for conduction abnormalities or cardiac chamber enlargement.

HEART RATE

Two methods can be used to calculate the heart rate on an ECG. The first method is determining the average

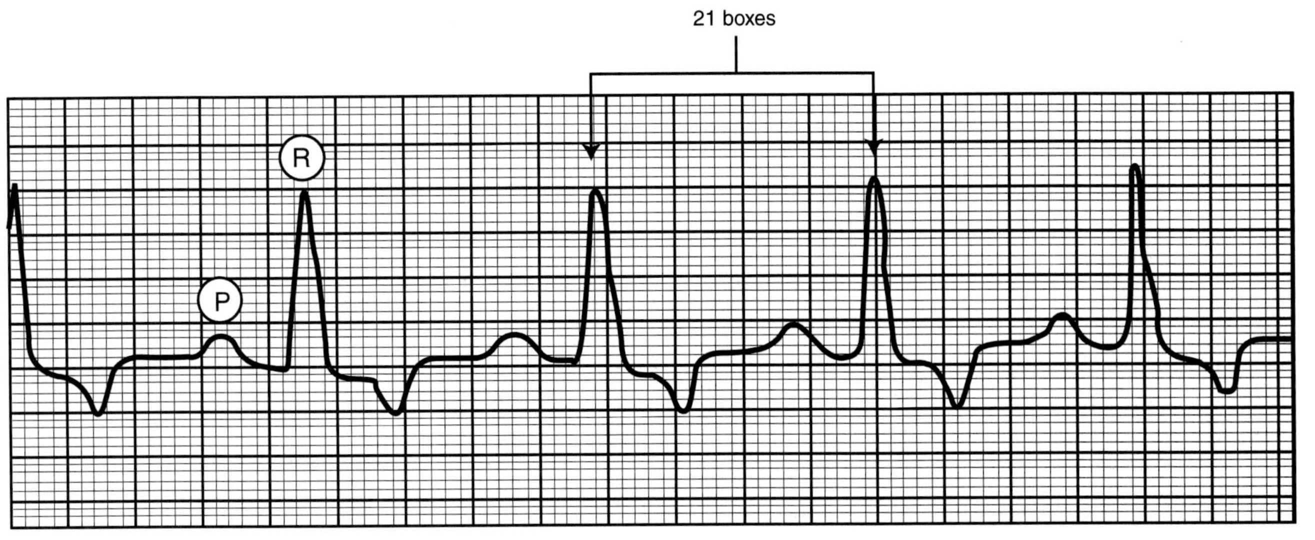
21 boxes
R
P
A
21 boxes => 3000 divided by 21 = approx. 150 beats/min
Number of small boxes between R waves divided into 3000
(if the paper speed is 50 mm/sec)

FIGURE **8-23** **A,** Calculating heart rate by instantaneous method. *Continued*

> **CLINICAL APPLICATION — ECG Patterns**
>
> ECG patterns are important because they allow the assessment of the heart's ability to conduct impulses and therefore allow us to judge its condition. For example, the period between the beginning of the P wave and the beginning of the QRS complex (PR interval) indicates how long it takes the impulse to travel through the AV node. In some disease states, the impulse takes too long to get through the AV node and sometimes does not reach the ventricles. This condition is called *AV* or *heart block.*

heart rate. First, the paper speed is determined. At 25 mm/sec, 1 mm equals 20 milliseconds (ms) and 1 cm equals 200 ms. Once the paper speed has been established, count the number of QRS complexes within a specific time interval (3 seconds, or 7.5 cm). Next, multiply the number of complexes by 20. If the paper speed is 50 mm/sec, then multiply the number of complexes within 7.5 cm by 40 (7.5 cm equals 1.5 seconds at a paper speed of 50 mm/sec). The second method of calculating the heart rate is determining the instantaneous heart rate. Count the number of small boxes (1 mm) between QRS complexes and divide that number into 3000, if the paper speed is 50 mm/sec, or into 1500, if the paper speed is 25 mm/sec. This method gives you the heart rate at that moment. This method is particularly useful for short periods of very high heart rates (Figure 8-23).

CARDIAC RHYTHM

The normal cardiac rhythm is a sinus rhythm (Figure 8-24, *A*). A sinus rhythm is a rhythm that is determined by the SA node within the right atrium. A sinus rhythm is characterized by a series of P waves that are associated with QRS-T complexes. In other words, a P wave exists for every QRS-T, and those P waves are related to a QRS-T complex.

Rhythms that are too slow or too fast are called *arrhythmias.* If the heart rate is too slow, the heart cannot pump an adequate amount of blood to meet the body's needs. Conversely, if the heart rate is too fast, the heart cannot fill with blood adequately and the pumping function of the heart will be abnormal. Bradyarrhythmias are abnormal heart rhythms characterized by a slow heart rate (see Figure 8-24, *B*). Specific bradyarrhythmias include the following: sinus bradycardia, sinus arrest, and AV block. Tachyarrhythmias are abnormal heart rhythms characterized by fast heart rates (see Figure 8-24, *C*). Tachyarrhythmias are further characterized as being supraventricular (from above the AV junction) or ventricular (from below the AV junction). Premature complexes are complexes that occur early and are either supraventricular or ventricular in origin. Many premature complexes constitute a tachycardia. For example, 10 premature ventricular complexes (PVCs) in a row would be called *ventricular tachycardia*; 10 premature atrial complexes (PACs) in a row would be called a *supraventricular tachycardia.* Arrhythmias are most commonly associated with heart disease but also can be associated with drugs, such as sedatives, narcotics, and general anesthesia. Clinically, a tachycardia is characterized as being either a wide-complex or a narrow-complex tachycardia. Wide-complex tachycardias are usually ventricular tachycardias, and

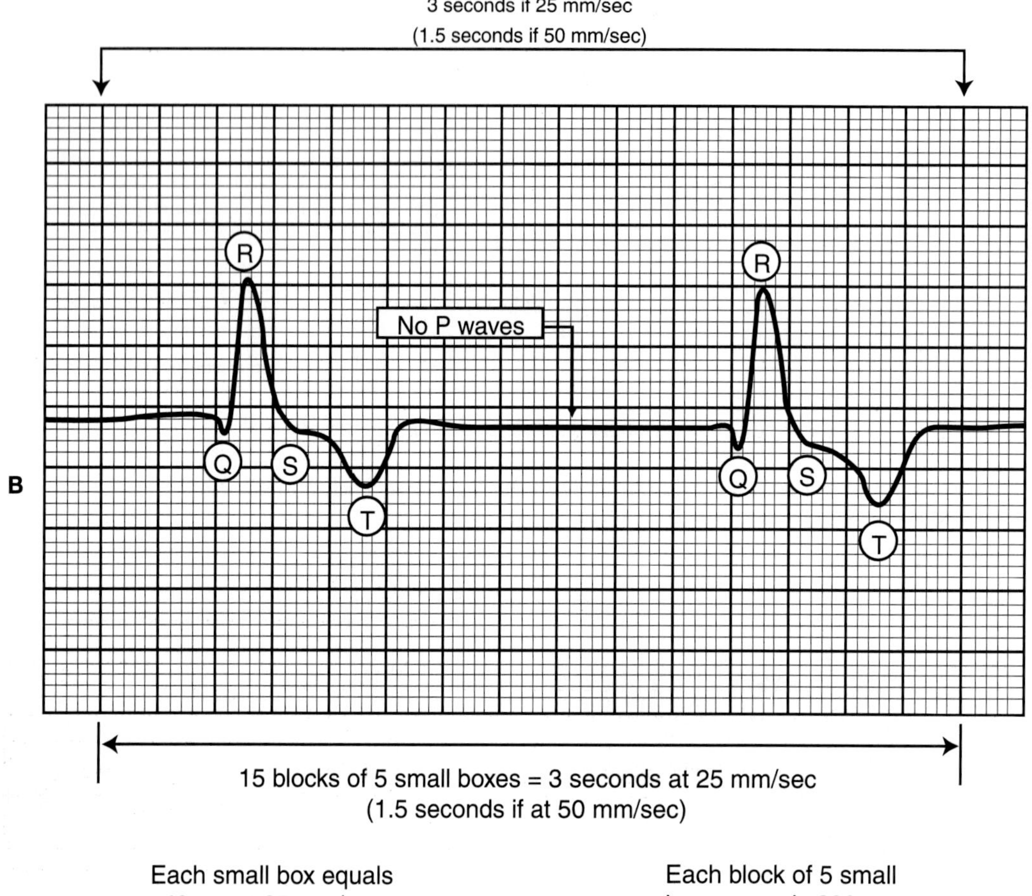
Find 3 seconds and multiply number of
QRS-T complexes by 20
3 seconds if 25 mm/sec
(1.5 seconds if 50 mm/sec)
R
No P waves
R
Q
S
T
Q
S
T
B
15 blocks of 5 small boxes = 3 seconds at 25 mm/sec
(1.5 seconds if at 50 mm/sec)
Each small box equals
40 ms at 25 mm/sec
or 20 ms at 50 mm/sec
Each block of 5 small
boxes equals 200 ms
at 25 mm/s or
100 ms at 50 mm/s
therefore... 2 complexes times 20 = 40 beats/min
(if the paper speed is 25 mm/sec)

FIGURE **8-23, cont'd** **B,** Calculating average heart rate.

narrow-complex tachycardias are usually supraventricular tachycardias. A terminal cardiac rhythm is ventricular fibrillation. Ventricular fibrillation is characterized electrocardiographically by coarse or fine unorganized deflections (see Figure 8-24, *D*). This rhythm is a life-threatening event and must be stopped by a process called *defibrillation,* whereby an electrical shock is applied to the heart.

Chamber Enlargement or Conduction Abnormalities

The ECG may show evidence that the heart is enlarged. Chamber enlargement may be present if a part of the P-QRS-T complex is of greater amplitude or has a longer duration than normal. For example, a tall P wave is suggestive of right atrial enlargement (p-pulmonale). A P wave that is wide (longer duration) may suggest left atrial enlargement (p-mitrale). A tall R wave or a widened QRS may suggest left ventricular enlargement, and a deep S wave may suggest right ventricular enlargement. In addition, conduction abnormalities may mimic chamber enlargement patterns. If the right bundle branch is blocked, right ventricular enlargement is mimicked. Furthermore, if the left bundle branch is blocked, the pattern is suggestive of left ventricular enlargement. In the cases of chamber enlargement or conduction abnormalities, the mean electrical axis may need to be determined. The mean electrical axis is the sum direction in which the ventricles are depolarizing. The mean electrical axis is determined by evaluating the heart's depolarization from the infor-

Cardiac Rhythm

What is normal?

The normal cardiac rhythm for dogs and cats is a sinus rhythm (NSR).

How do I recognize an NSR?

There are P waves associated with the QRS complexes.

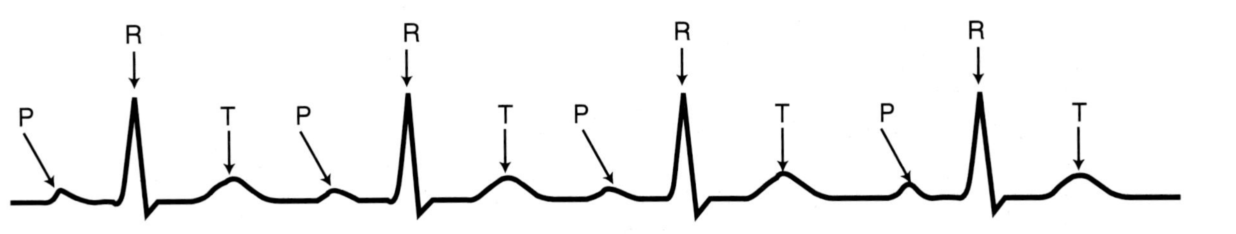

Rhythms with slow heart rates = Bradycardias

Abnormal sinus rhythms ⟶ Sinus bradycardia
Sinus arrest

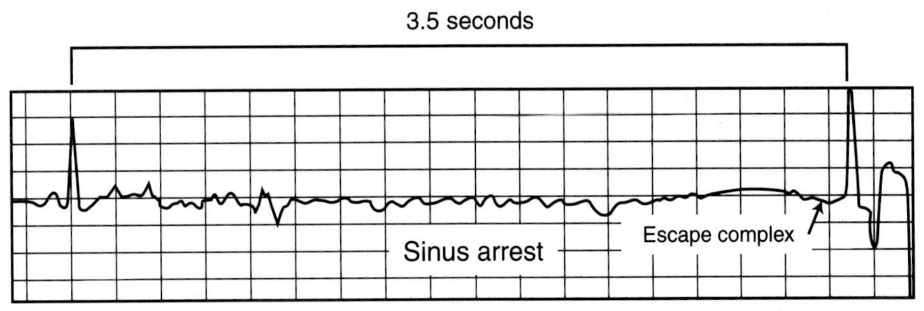

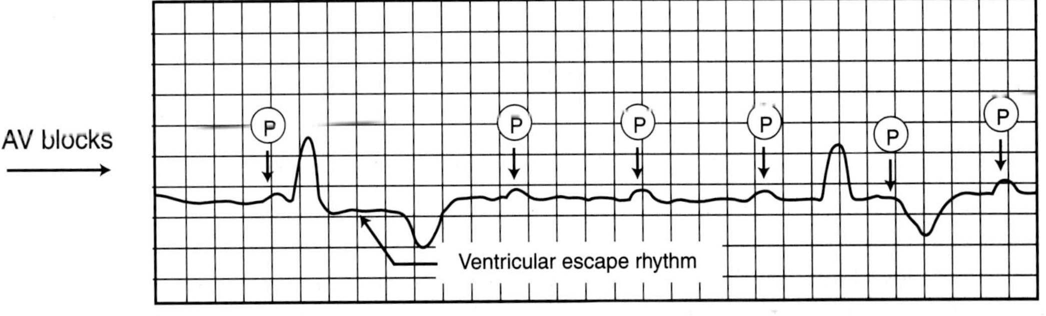

FIGURE **8-24** **A,** Normal sinus rhythm in dog. **B,** Bradycardias. *Continued*

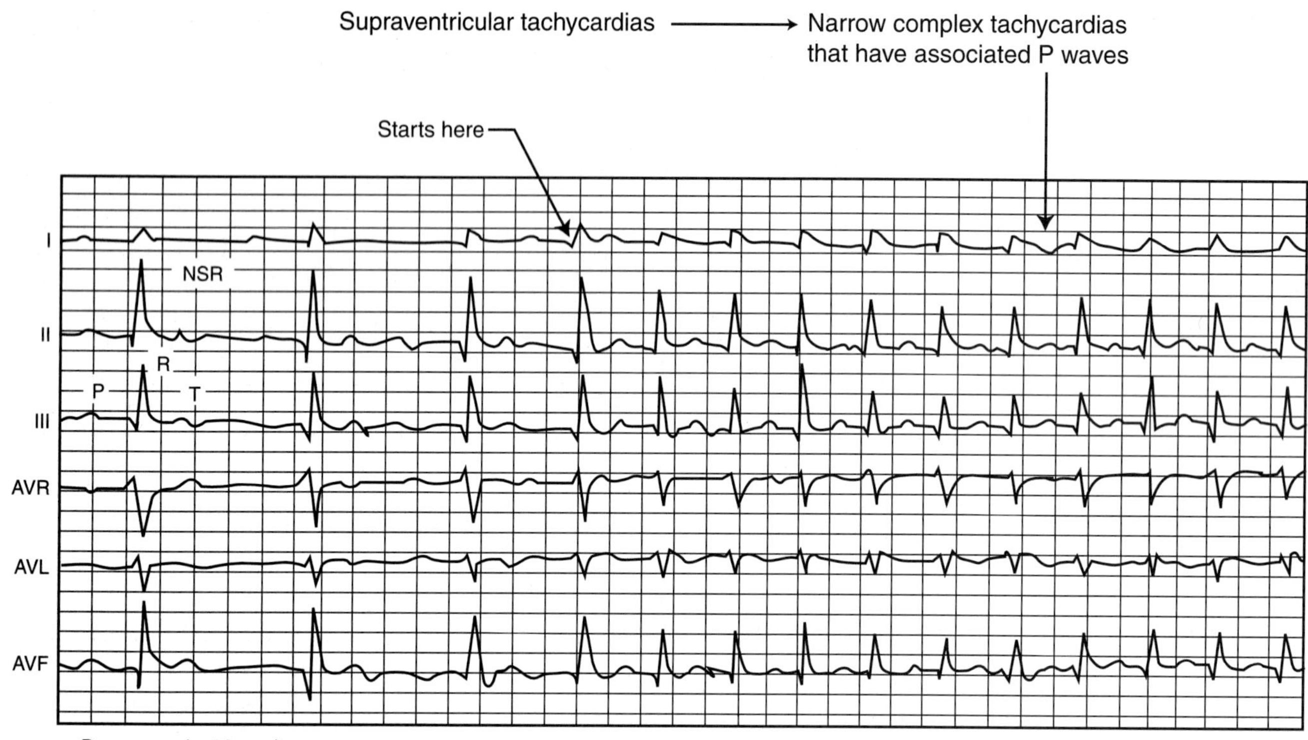

C

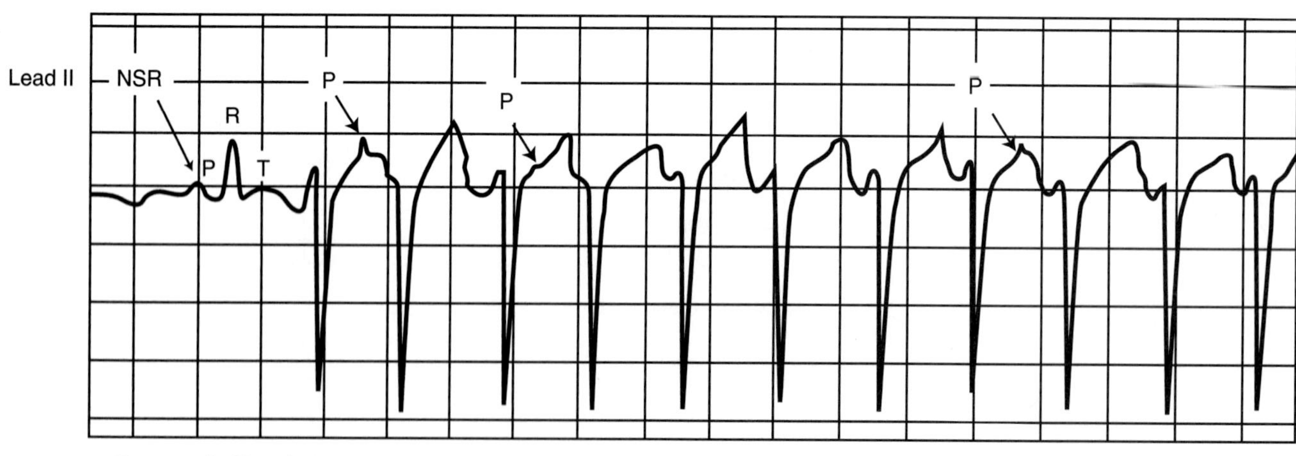

FIGURE **8-24, cont'd C,** Supraventricular tachycardia (SVT) (leads I, II, III, AVR, AVL, AVF—paper speed 50 mm/sec at standard sensitivity) and ventricular tachycardia (VT) (lead II—paper speed 25 mm/sec at standard sensitivity).

Continued

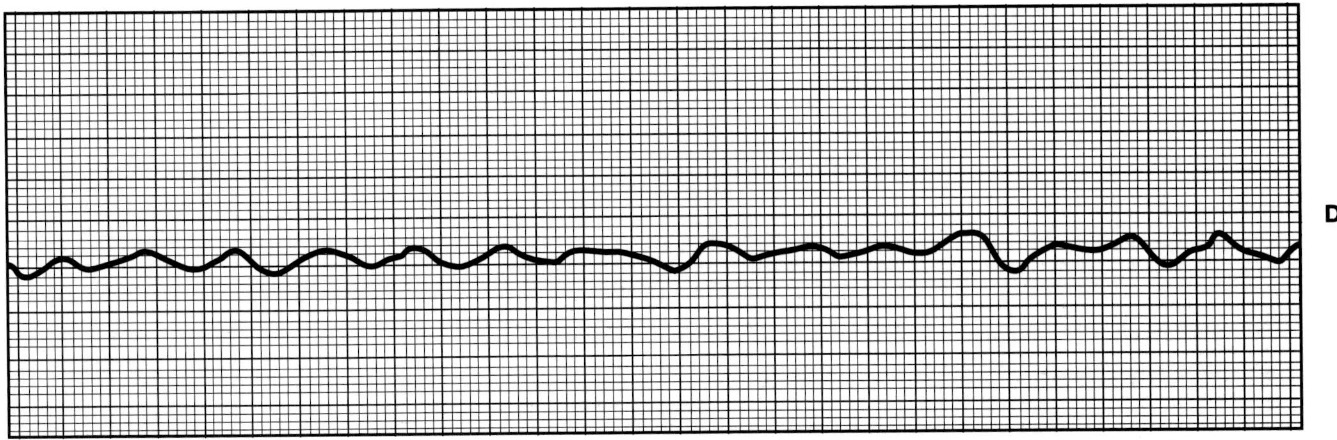

FIGURE **8-24, cont'd** **D,** Ventricular fibrillation (VF) (paper speed 50 mm/sec at standard sensitivity).

mation given by multiple leads. The standard limb leads are leads I, II, and III; the augmented limb leads are leads aVR, aVL, and aVF. These different leads "look" at the heart's electrical activity from different vantage points. If the sum direction is to the right, right ventricular enlargement or right bundle branch block is possible. If the sum direction is to the left, left ventricular enlargement or left bundle branch block is possible.

TEST YOURSELF

1. Describe the normal waves of the ECG.
2. Explain the importance of the various patterns seen on an ECG.
3. Describe how the autonomic nervous system controls the heart rate.
4. Describe how the autonomic nervous system controls blood pressure.
5. In a diagram, describe the aortic arch and its major branches.

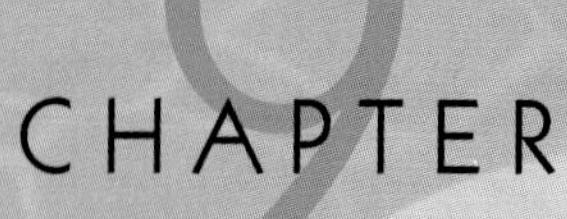

CHAPTER 9

Blood, Lymph, and Immunity

Joann Colville

BLOOD

Blood—say the word and some people cringe, others faint, and, if you believe Anne Rice (author of vampire books), others drool. But no matter what you think about blood, all common domestic animals need it. In this section of the chapter we'll explore the red, sticky, salty fluid and find out how it keeps animals alive and healthy.

Blood is actually classified as a connective tissue. It is the fluid connective tissue that flows all over the body in the vessels of the cardiovascular system. Its three main functions are transportation, regulation, and defense.

1. Blood is a transport system.
   - It carries oxygen, nutrients, and other essential compounds to every living cell in the body. Oxygen is carried by **hemoglobin** in the red blood cells. Nutrients and other essential compounds are dissolved in the blood plasma.
   - It carries the waste products of cellular metabolism, primarily carbon dioxide, away from the cells to the waste disposal organs that excrete them from the body, which are most often the lungs and the kidneys.
   - It transports hormones from endocrine glands to target organs.
   - It transports white blood cells from the bone marrow, where they are produced, to the tissues, where they will do their work.
   - It transports **platelets** to the site of damage to a vessel wall. Once there, the platelets will form a clump to prevent blood from escaping out of the vessel.
2. Blood is a regulatory system.
   - It aids in regulation of body temperature. Body temperature regulators are located in the brain and are partially influenced by the temperature of the blood that passes through or over them.
   - It aids in tissue fluid content. The normal state of the body **(homeostasis)** is one in which, within very narrow limits, the composition of body tissue fluid is maintained as constant as possible. If an animal is low in tissue fluid (dehydration) because of vomiting, diarrhea, profuse sweating, or a pathological condition that causes it to lose fluid, some of the plasma (not the cells and larger protein molecules) will leave the bloodstream and enter the body tissues in an effort to compensate for the fluid loss. This leaves less plasma in the bloodstream, and the cells become more concentrated **(hemoconcentration).** If an animal has too much body fluid, for instance, after subcutaneous fluids are administered, the excess fluid will enter the bloodstream. This extra fluid in the plasma dilutes the cells **(hemodilution)**.

- It aids in regulation of blood pH (acid-base balance). Normal blood pH falls in a range of 7.35 to 7.45, with the ideal being 7.4, which is slightly alkaline (see Chapter 10 for a more detailed description of blood pH). Blood must be maintained within this narrow range for the animal to remain in a state of homeostasis. Therefore the pH must remain slightly alkaline in an effort to buffer the acidic waste products of cellular metabolism that it carries. The pH of arterial blood is slightly more alkaline than that of venous blood (blood that has picked up the waste products).

3. Blood is a defense system.
   - White blood cells provide defense against foreign invaders entering the body through **phagocytosis** (ingesting the invaders) or their involvement in immunity.
   - In addition to the platelets that exist in blood, 13 clotting factors are found in blood that are necessary for blood to clot. These factors are activated when a blood vessel wall is damaged. The clotting process is complex, and if a clotting factor is missing, blood will not clot. The clotting factors are listed in Table 9-1.

Table 9-1 Clotting Factors

Factor Number	Common Name
I	Fibrinogen
II	Prothrombin
III	Tissue factor
IV	Calcium
V	Proaccelerin
(VI	No longer considered a clotting factor)
VII	Proconvertin
VIII	Antihemophilic factor A
IX	Christmas factor, antihemophilic factor B
X	Stuart-Prower factor
XI	Plasma thromboplastin antecedent
XII	Hageman factor
XIII	Fibrin stabilizing factor

COMPOSITION

Blood is a fluid in which cells and cell fragments are suspended and compounds such as oxygen, electrolytes, hormones, nutrients, and drugs are either dissolved or suspended. The liquid portion of blood is plasma. The cellular portion of blood is composed of red blood cells **(erythrocytes)**, white blood cells **(leukocytes)**, and platelets **(thrombocytes)** (Figure 9-1).

The term **whole blood** is used to denote blood contained

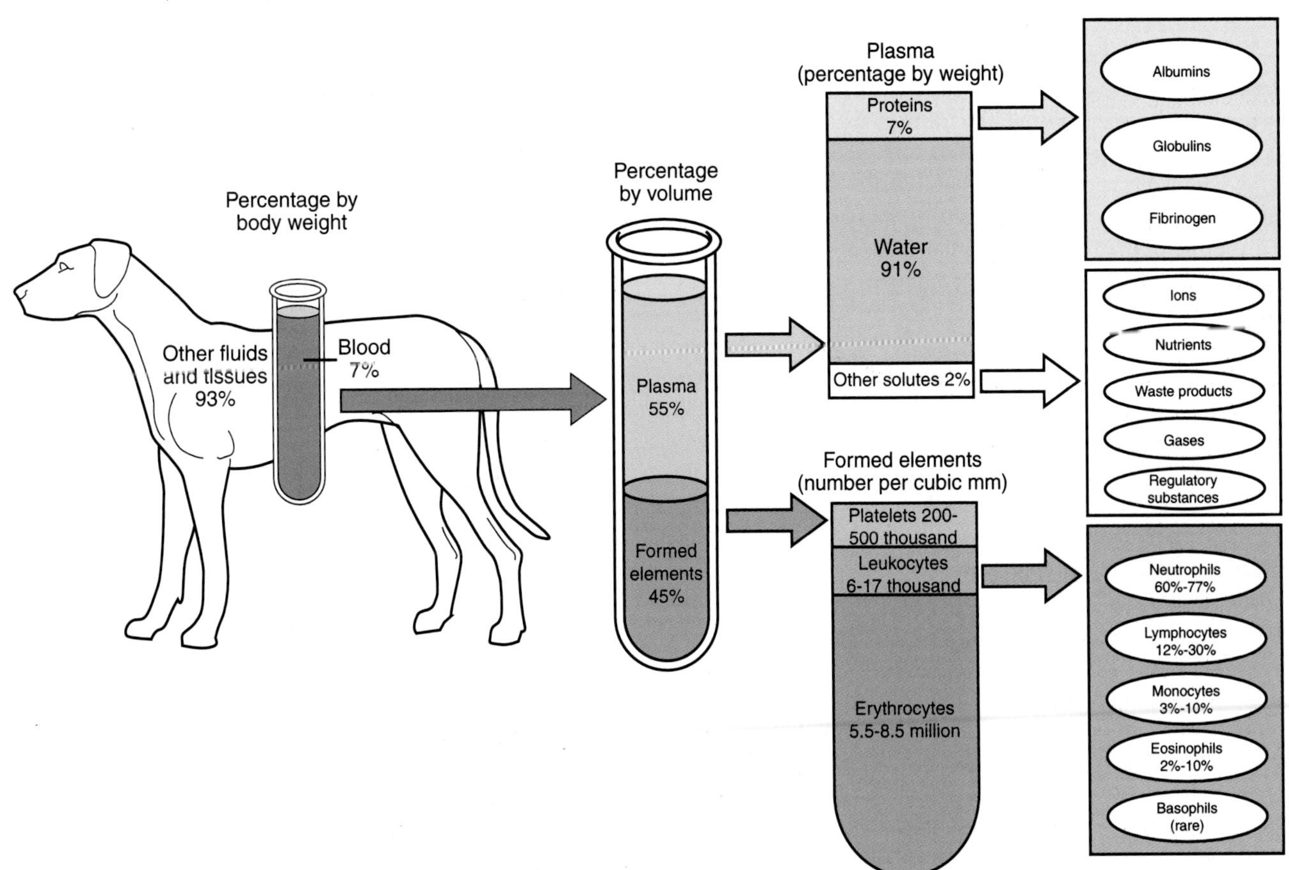

FIGURE 9-1 **Composition of Whole Blood.** Values are approximate for blood components in normal adult dog.

CLINICAL APPLICATION Postprandial Lipemia

If an animal has eaten just before a blood sample is drawn, the plasma may appear cloudy because fat from the digested food is still being suspended in the plasma. This condition is called **postprandial lipemia** (*postprandial* means after eating, and *lipemia* means fat in the blood) and can make the plasma or serum unsuitable for laboratory analysis, depending on the analytical method used. For this reason, blood samples for laboratory analysis should be drawn before an animal is fed or a couple of hours after feeding.

in the cardiovascular system or a sample that contains plasma and all its cellular components. **Peripheral blood** is whole blood that is flowing through the blood vessels that carry blood to and from the heart and lungs. Peripheral blood is drawn into a syringe or tube for laboratory analysis.

PLASMA

Plasma is the fluid portion of blood. It makes up from 45% to 78% of a blood sample volume, depending on the species of the animal and the size of its red blood cells. In species with small red blood cells (e.g., goat and cat), plasma makes up a larger percent of the blood sample. In species with larger red blood cells (e.g., dog), plasma makes up a relatively smaller portion of the blood sample. Imagine if you were to take two identical glasses and put 100 BBs in one and 100 marbles in the other. If you fill the glasses the rest of the way with water, you can put more water in the glass with the BBs. This would be like an animal with small red blood cells. Red blood cells make up the next largest component of blood after the plasma. The white blood cells and platelets make up a small portion of the total volume of the blood sample.

Plasma is about 93% water. It contains many substances dissolved or suspended in it. Plasma proteins such as albumins, globulins, and fibrinogen make up the majority of these substances. The gases most abundant in plasma are oxygen, carbon dioxide, and nitrogen. Lipids, amino acids, metabolic wastes, and electrolytes (such as sodium, potassium, calcium, magnesium, chloride, and bicarbonate ions) are also found in plasma. When systemic drugs are administered to an animal, they are carried to their site of action by plasma. Frequently these drugs have to attach themselves to a transport plasma protein, such as albumin, to make themselves soluble in the plasma.

A whole blood sample appears red because of the many red blood cells suspended in the plasma. The blood cells in the sample make it impossible to see through the sample. If the blood cells are removed from the sample, the remaining plasma appears transparent and clear to varying degrees of yellow. The intensity of the yellow color of plasma is determined by the concentration of hemoglobin breakdown products in the plasma. Hemoglobin is the protein in red blood cells that makes them red and enables them to carry large amounts of oxygen. When worn out, red blood cells are removed from circulation and the hemoglobin is broken down and released. The breakdown products of hemoglobin include **bilirubin,** which is yellow (this topic will be discussed further with hemoglobin). The hydration of the patient can also play a factor in plasma color. In a dehydrated patient, all the constituents of plasma, including bilirubin, are more concentrated. This could result in a deeper yellow plasma.

CLINICAL APPLICATION Anticoagulants, Plasma, and Serum

Remember the blood clotting factors that were mentioned earlier? These factors must be present in sufficient quantities for blood to clot. If we want to prevent blood from clotting, we can add something to it that ties up one of the clotting factors. Substances that tie up clotting factors and prevent blood from clotting are called **anticoagulants.** (*Coagulation* is another word for clotting.) If an anticoagulant is added to a blood sample in a tube or syringe, it will not clot. One of the most common anticoagulants is ethylenediaminetetraacetic acid (EDTA). EDTA prevents clotting by tying up calcium, clotting factor number IV (no calcium, no clot).

If anticoagulant is added to a blood sample as it is drawn from an animal, the sample will not clot because all the clotting factors are not present. If the blood sample is then centrifuged (spun at a high speed), the fluid that rises to the top of the tube is plasma.

If no anticoagulant is added to a blood sample as it is drawn from an animal, the blood will clot. If the clotted blood is centrifuged, the fluid that rises to the top of the tube is called **serum.** When blood clots, one of the dissolved plasma proteins, fibrinogen, is converted to insoluble fibrin, which precipitates out of solution as a meshwork of tiny fibers (hence its name) and helps make up the framework of the clot. Removing fibrinogen from plasma by allowing it to clot converts plasma to serum.

Many of the diagnostic clinical chemistry tests performed on a patient are run on either plasma or serum. After the sample has been centrifuged, the plasma or serum can be drawn off and analyzed or frozen for analysis at a later date. (Whole blood cannot be frozen because blood cells rupture easily during the freezing and thawing processes.)

CELLULAR COMPONENTS OF BLOOD

The cells suspended in plasma fall into the following three categories: (Figure 9-2):

- Red blood cells (erythrocytes) that carry oxygen from the lungs to the cells and tissues of the body
- Platelets (thrombocytes) that help prevent leaks from damaged blood vessels
- White blood cells (leukocytes). Five types of white blood cells can be differentiated on a stained blood smear. Three of these have granules in their cytoplasm and are named by how these granules stain using standard hematology stains. These cells are called **granulocytes**. They are **eosinophils** (red granules),

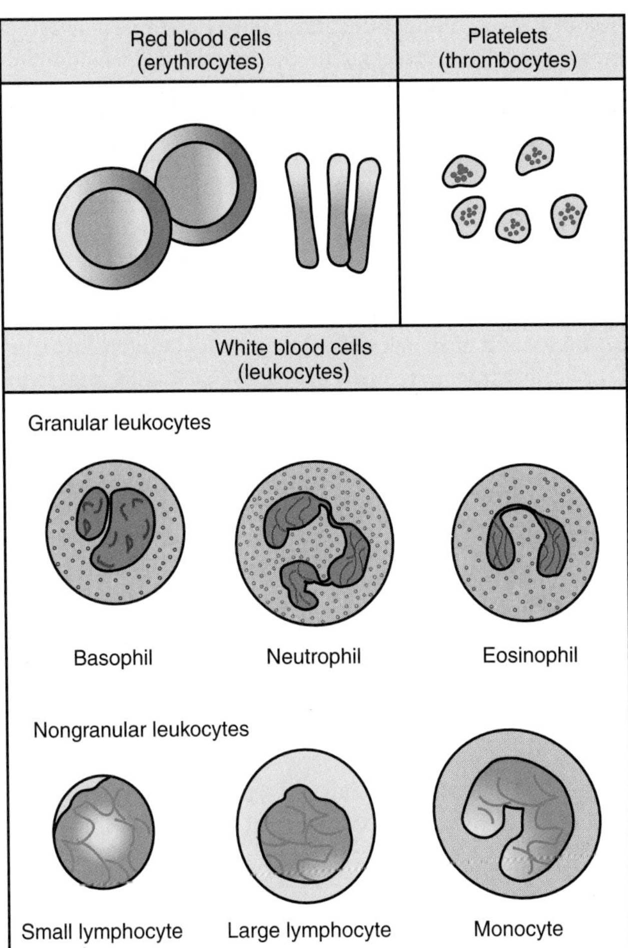

FIGURE **9-2 Cellular Components of Blood.** Red blood cells (erythrocytes), platelets (thrombocytes), and white blood cells (leukocytes).

basophils (blue granules), and **neutrophils** (granules that stain neither blue nor red). The other two types of white blood cells do not have granules in their cytoplasm; so they are called **agranulocytes** (or *nongranular leukocytes*). The agranulocytes are the **monocytes** and the **lymphocytes.** Each cell type has specific functions within the body. We'll discuss each of them in more detail shortly.

A Word About Stains

Throughout this chapter, you'll read about cells and structures that stain specific colors. These colors are based on the use of common hematology (blood) stains. There are many hematology stains with many different names, but they all have similar staining characteristics. Many of these are Romanosky-type stains that combine basic blue and acidic red dyes dissolved in methyl alcohol. Cellular structures that are basic (alkaline) will stain blue, and structures that are acidic will stain red. These stains are called *polychromatic stains* because they stain more than one color.

Wright's stain is the most widely used hematology stain. The basic part of a Wright's stain is methylene blue. The acidic part is eosin. Other Romanovsky-type stains that are available but used less often are Giemsa, Leishman's, Wright-Giemsa, and May-Grünwald stains. Modified Wright's stains are also available. They offer faster staining times but do not stain some cellular structures as well as Wright's stain.

Hematopoiesis

Hematopoiesis is a general term for the production of all blood cells. Blood cells are not immortal, and so they are constantly being produced. They function for a specific time and then die of old age. Some blood cells, especially leukocytes, leave the circulation to fight off foreign invaders in the tissues, where they can be killed in action. For an animal to remain healthy, it needs a sufficient number of all its blood cells all the time. As blood cells die or are destroyed, they need to be replaced. For this reason, hematopoiesis is a continuous process.

In an early fetus, most hematopoiesis takes place in the liver and spleen. As the fetus develops the bone marrow gradually takes over production of the blood cells. In a newborn animal, most of the blood cell production is occurring in the active bone marrow. This is called the **red bone marrow** based on its gross appearance. At this young age the red bone marrow is found in nearly all bones because of the great demand for blood cells as the animal grows and matures. The older the animal becomes, the less it requires a high blood cell production rate; therefore some of the red bone marrow is converted to inactive **yellow bone marrow,** again named for its gross appearance. Yellow bone marrow is composed of yellow fat cells that have replaced some of the active red marrow. In a mature animal, most of the red bone marrow is found at the ends of long bones (e.g., femur, tibia, humerus, and ulna) and flat bones (e.g. hip bones, sternum, and ribs). The rest is all yellow bone marrow. If the need arises, the liver and spleen have a limited capacity to participate in hematopoiesis but not to a life-sustaining capacity.

All blood cells have a common ancestor. Scattered about the bone marrow is a population of cells called the **pluripotent stem cells** (PPSCs). This name, although complicated, simply means that these cells are primitive cells (stem cells) that have lots of potential (pluripotent). One PPSC has the potential to develop into any one of the blood cells. The type it becomes is determined by the chemical or physiological stimulus that acts on the stem cell. Each blood cell type has its own set of stimuli that is required to activate a PPSC to start down the path of development of that specific blood cell. Once a PPSC has been stimulated to produce a specific blood cell, it is an irreversible process; that is, it can't partially develop into a red blood cell and then "change its mind" and become a neutrophil. Hematopoiesis is a one-way street. For example, one of the stimuli for red blood cell production is produced in the kidney. When these specialized kidney cells detect decreased oxygen levels in the blood **(hypoxia),** they perceive this as the need for more red blood cells to carry oxygen. In response to this need, they produce a hormone called **erythropoietin,** which is carried to the bone marrow by blood. There it will stimulate some of the PPSC cells to begin their development into red blood cells. Other stimuli are necessary to complete the production of red blood cells. The production of red blood cells along with production of all the other blood cells involves numerous cell divisions so that one PPSC eventually becomes many cells. For example, one PPSC eventually becomes many red blood cells when stimulated properly. Similarly, different stimuli are required for the production of platelets and for each white blood cell. Without these specific stimuli, the PPSCs will not develop into any mature blood cells.

With the exception of some lymphocytes, the complete development of the blood cells takes place in the red bone marrow. If you were to look at the bone marrow under a microscope, you would see all blood cell lines with cells in all stages of development, from very immature to fully functional and mature. Under normal conditions the bone marrow has reserve pools of mature blood cells and doesn't release the cells into circulation until they are needed. The size of the pool varies with the cell type, and some stimulus from the body is necessary to release the cells. However, hematopoiesis is a continuous process; so constant stimulation and release of cells is occurring to replace those that die or are killed.

Certain pathological conditions may stimulate a massive release of cells. For example, an invading microorganism can result in a large number of neutrophils being released from the bone marrow and traveling to the site of the infection to control the infection by killing the microorganisms. If the infection is severe enough the bone marrow may deplete its reserve of mature neutrophils and have to start sending out immature neutrophils. This is like sending a child to do an adult's work. It is just not as effective.

Another neat aspect about PPSCs is that they are self-perpetuating. When a PPSC is stimulated to begin production down a cell line, it undergoes a mitotic division. The result of that division is that one cell continues to develop into the blood cell while the other cell goes back into the stem cell pool.

Blood Storage

An animal's body can control its circulating volume of blood at any given time. When an animal is at rest, it does not need as much oxygen going to its muscles; so in a way, it has extra blood. The spleen is a spongelike organ in the abdomen that can hold a lot of blood. When the body does not need all of its blood circulating, the spleen will swell up and store blood until it is needed (think of a sponge that can sop up a lot of water). When the animal is physically active the spleen contracts and puts the stored blood back into circulation so that more oxygen is going to the muscles (think of squeezing the sponge). More details on the important functions of the spleen are discussed later.

CLINICAL APPLICATION Blood Volume

How do you know if you can draw 200 ml of blood from an animal without causing serious problems? Our limit is 25% of the total blood volume. This is more blood than you'd routinely draw from an animal, but let's look at a worse case scenario. An animal that loses 25% of its total blood volume has about a 50:50 chance of survival.

First, you need to know how much blood an animal has. The total blood volume for any animal can be estimated using the animal's *lean* body weight. *Lean* is the operative word here. A 13.5-kg (30-lb) house cat is not lean. So, if you want to figure the total blood volume on this cat, think of it as a 3.5- to 4.5-kg (8- to 12-lb) cat. As a broad rule of thumb, figure 50 to 100 (average, 75) ml of blood/kg lean body weight. High-strung animals tend to have a higher volume because they are always pacing, bouncing, running, or otherwise being active and therefore require more oxygen in their muscles.

Using these guidelines, we figure that a 454-kg (1000-lb) horse has a total blood volume of about 34,000 ml, or 34 L (454 kg × 75 ml of blood/kg = 34,050 total blood volume). Taking 200 ml of blood from this horse would result in a blood loss of 0.5% of the total blood volume (200 ml divided by 34,000 ml and multiplied by 100 to get a percent), which is not a problem.

Now let's consider a 16-kg (35-lb) dog with a total blood volume of 1193 ml. Drawing 200 ml from this dog would result in a blood loss of 16%. This is still not a problem, but we'd be getting closer to trouble.

A Pint's a Pound the World Around

Another way to determine the total blood volume is to figure that blood makes up 6% to 8% (average, 7%) of an animal's lean body weight. Of course, this would give you the *weight* of total blood volume, so you need to convert that amount to a liquid measure. A pint of water weighs a pound. So, because blood is mostly water, we can use that conversion rate. From here we need to convert it into metric measure because that is how syringes are calibrated. There are 2 pints in a quart, and a quart is approximately equivalent to a liter. There are 1000 ml in a liter. So now it becomes a simple math problem.

Using these guidelines, we figure that a dog weighing 75 lb (34kg) has a total blood volume of approximately 5.25 lb (75 lb × 7%), which is 5.25 pints of blood. If 2 pints is 1 quart, 5.25 pints are 2.625 quarts, or approximately 2.625 L. Move the decimal point to the right three places, and the total blood volume of this dog is 2625 ml. A 200-ml blood loss for this animal would amount to about a 10% loss of total blood volume. This would not be a significant loss for the dog.

On the other hand, a cat weighing 10 lb (4.5 kg) has a blood volume of 0.7 lb, or 0.7 pints. This converts to 350 ml. A blood loss of 200 ml would result in a loss of 57% of its total blood volume. The cat would probably die of shock before you draw that much blood from it.

TEST YOURSELF

1. What are the main functions of blood?
2. What is one of the most common causes of hemoconcentration and how can it affect blood cell counts in peripheral blood?
3. What is the most abundant component of plasma?
4. What are the three cellular components of blood?
5. What is the difference between red bone marrow and yellow bone marrow?
6. What is the difference between plasma and serum?
7. How does one cell population, the PPSCs, give rise to all the different blood cells?
8. What is the total blood volume of a 675-lb (lean body weight) animal? How about a 3-lb animal?

RED BLOOD CELLS

Red blood cells (RBCs) are also known as *erythrocytes.* An older term for them was *red corpuscles,* but this name is not used any more.

Formation

The process of red cell production is called **erythropoiesis.** RBCs start out as PPSCs in red bone marrow. Erythropoietin, a hormone produced by the kidney, is just one of the many stimuli necessary for complete RBC development. Erythropoietin is released when the kidney cells detect hypoxia in the blood. With this stimulation a PPSC starts to undergo mitotic divisions as it develops into several immature RBCs. Each step toward maturation requires a specific stimulus, and many stimuli have not yet been identified.

An immature RBC is a large cell with lots of dark blue cytoplasm and a large, round nucleus with a loose chromatin pattern. As the cell matures the nucleus becomes more condensed and smaller **(pyknotic)** until finally it is completely pushed out of the cell. The cytoplasm stains blue at this early stage because of the metabolic processes that are occurring. Some of the processes keep the cell alive; others result in protein synthesis, which is important for hemoglobin production. At some point during the maturation process, hemoglobin production begins in the cytoplasm. Hemoglobin stains red. When you add the red hemoglobin to the already blue cytoplasm, you get a lavender cytoplasm. This is called **polychromasia,** and its presence in circulating RBCs indicates that the cells are not yet fully mature but that hemoglobin production is happening. As the cell approaches maturity, its amount of cytoplasm decreases and it is filled with hemoglobin. When all the hemoglobin is produced the metabolic activities of the cell shut down. This leaves just hemoglobin to stain the cytoplasm; so we have a red cytoplasm, which is the mark of a mature RBC.

Characteristics

A mature RBC is a membranous sac that contains about 65% water and 35% solids (mainly proteins), with hemoglobin making up about 95% of the solids. With few exceptions, mature mammalian RBCs are round, biconcave (both sides are pushed in) disks that have no nucleus and stain red because of the presence of hemoglobin (see Figure 9-2). Immature RBCs keep their nuclei until their last stage of development before maturity. These nucleated RBCs normally stay in the bone marrow until they have matured and are not found in peripheral blood. The immature nucleated RBCs are metabolically active and busy producing the hemoglobin that will eventually allow them to carry oxygen to all the cells in the body.

Different species have different-sized RBCs with varying degrees of paleness in the center, when viewed on a stained blood smear. This paleness is called *central pallor* and is a result of that area being thinner (remember the biconcave shape?) and therefore containing less hemoglobin to stain red. Of the common domesticated animals, dogs have the largest RBCs (7 μm in diameter) and the greatest degree of central pallor. In decreasing order the cat, horse, cow, sheep, and goat (3 to 4 μm in diameter) have smaller RBCs. A micrometer is one millionth of a meter; therefore even the largest RBCs are pretty small.

Llamas and deer have elliptical or oval RBCs, and deer have sickle-shaped (like a crescent moon) RBCs. Birds, fishes, amphibians, and reptiles have elliptical RBCs that are nucleated even when they are mature.

The biconcave disk shape of RBCs serves the following three important functions.

1. Because the RBC membrane is deformable (can change shape) but not elastic, the RBC can take in water and swell (which results in the RBC forming a

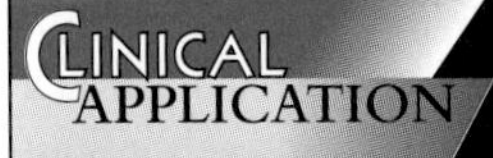

Polychromasia and Nucleated Red Blood Cells (nRBCs)

Under normal conditions, all but about 1% of the RBCs in circulation are mature.

If the animal has a sudden loss or destruction of RBCs, the bone marrow attempts to compensate by producing more RBCs in a shorter time. In its hurry to get RBCs into circulation, the red bone marrow frequently sends out cells that are not quite mature. These cells still have some metabolic activity going on in their cytoplasm; therefore they will pick up some blue stain. There is some hemoglobin present that will stain red. The result is lavender cytoplasm, or polychromasia.

Hemoglobin production begins before the cell loses its nucleus. If the bone marrow perceives a great need for oxygen-carrying hemoglobin, it may send out all its polychromatophilic (lavender) nonnucleated cells and then also start sending nucleated RBCs. In both cases these are immature cells that do not have their full complement of hemoglobin yet, and so they cannot carry a full load of oxygen. They can carry some oxygen, which is better than nothing when more RBCs are needed.

The presence of polychromasia and nucleated RBCs indicates that the bone marrow is responding to a need for more oxygen-carrying capacity of blood. This is a good thing.

sphere) without rupturing the membrane. Look at it this way. Take a small plastic bag and fill it about two-thirds full of water. Now you have a bag with a deformable membrane (you can readily change its shape). To a certain limit you can add more water, but when the bag is full of water, it is not as deformable. Eventually you will burst the membrane of the bag if you try to add too much water. Likewise, if a RBC becomes too full of water, the membrane will burst, causing destruction of the cell (hemolysis; Figure 9-3).

2. The biconcave shape provides more membrane surface area for diffusion of oxygen and carbon dioxide to take place.
3. The disk shape results in a shorter diffusion distance in and out of the cell compared with a sphere. Animals that have a less pronounced biconcave shape (sheep and goats) tend to have a higher number of RBCs, thereby providing a large surface area through increased numbers of cells rather than increased amount of membrane per cell.

Function

The function of a mature RBC is to carry oxygen to all the tissues of the body. It does this through the production of the protein *hemoglobin* that binds with the oxygen. The mature RBC is a sac of hemoglobin, water, and structural components that help maintain the biconcave shape.

Hemoglobin

Hemoglobin is a protein composed of two components—heme and globin. These two components are produced by the RBC as it matures. Heme is the pigment portion and is produced in the mitochondria; globin is the protein portion and is produced by ribosomes. Every heme group can carry a molecule of oxygen. Four heme groups attach to each globin molecule. Therefore each hemoglobin molecule can carry four molecules of oxygen. The oxygen attaches to iron atoms (Fe^{++}) that are part of each heme group.

Normal Hemoglobin Types

- **Embryonic hemoglobin** is found early in developing fetuses.
- **Fetal hemoglobin** is present in fetal blood during mid to late gestation and up to a couple months after birth. It has its highest concentration at birth and is gradually replaced by adult hemoglobin. Fetal hemoglobin functions very well in the low oxygen environment in the uterus because its affinity for oxygen is higher than normal adult hemoglobin.
- **Adult hemoglobin** is found in the RBCs of all animals, beginning a couple of weeks to a couple of months after birth. It gradually replaces the fetal hemoglobin as the primary type of hemoglobin being produced.

Function of Hemoglobin. The major function of hemoglobin is to transport oxygen to the tissues. It exists in the following two normal physiological states:

1. **Oxyhemoglobin:** hemoglobin that is carrying oxygen. One oxygen molecule is associated with each iron (Fe^{++}) molecule.
2. **Deoxyhemoglobin:** hemoglobin that has given up its oxygen. This is also known as *empty hemoglobin*.

Factors such as pH, temperature, and oxygen and carbon dioxide levels influence the ability of the hemoglobin molecule to carry oxygen. (See Chapter 10 for a good description of oxygen transfer at the cellular level.)

Carbon Dioxide Transport. Carbon dioxide is transported directly and indirectly in the RBCs and is dissolved in the plasma. Three fourths of the carbon dioxide is transported by indirect RBC transport: Carbon dioxide (CO_2) diffuses into the RBCs, where it is transformed into carbonic acid, then ionizes into hydrogen ions and bicarbonate ions ($H_2O + CO_2 = H_2CO_3 = H^+ + HCO_3^-$). Deoxyhemoglobin accepts the hydrogen ion, and the bicarbonate diffuses back into the

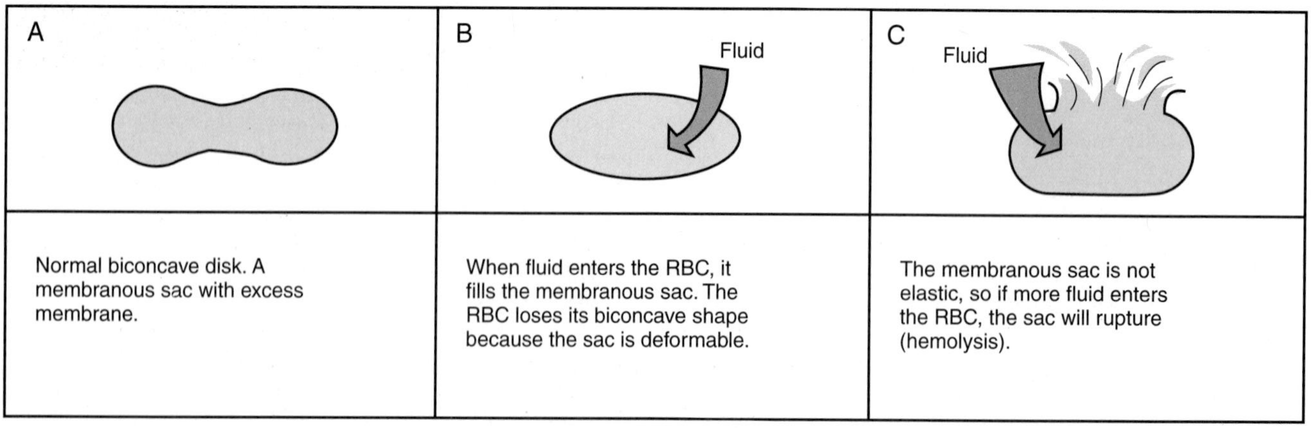

A	B	C
	Fluid	Fluid
Normal biconcave disk. A membranous sac with excess membrane.	When fluid enters the RBC, it fills the membranous sac. The RBC loses its biconcave shape because the sac is deformable.	The membranous sac is not elastic, so if more fluid enters the RBC, the sac will rupture (hemolysis).

FIGURE 9-3 **Hemolysis: Rupturing of Red Blood Cells (RBCs). A,** Normal biconcave disk. Membranous sac with excess membrane. **B,** When fluid enters RBC, it fills membranous sac. RBC loses its biconcave shape because sac is deformable. **C,** Membranous sac is not elastic, so if more fluid enters RBC, sac will rupture (hemolysis).

plasma. In the lungs, bicarbonate converts back to CO_2 and H_2O and is eliminated via respiration.

Even though the RBCs don't use metabolic energy to bind, transport, and release oxygen, they need energy to maintain their biconcave shape and membrane deformability. After hemoglobin has been produced, the mitochondria shut down, and the RBC must look elsewhere for a source of energy. Because the RBC is pretty much only a sack of hemoglobin, it must look in the plasma outside the cell for its source of energy. One of the best sources of energy is glucose; therefore mature RBCs depend on plasma glucose for energy.

RBC Life Span and Destruction

The normal life span of a RBC varies with the species. In dogs the average life span is 110 days. In cats it is about 68 days. RBCs in horses and sheep live up to 150 days, and RBCs in cows can live as long as 160 days. On the other end of the scale are mice, whose RBCs live only 20 to 30 days. Human RBCs live 120 days, on average. As RBCs wear out, they are replaced by young RBCs from the bone marrow in the never-ending erythropoietic cycle.

The process of aging is called **senescence.** As the RBC becomes senescent, enzyme activity decreases (especially glycolytic enzyme, the enzyme that helps break down glucose), and the cell loses its deformability. It becomes rounder, and its volume decreases. Ninety percent of the destruction of senescent RBCs occurs by **extravascular hemolysis,** that is, RBCs are destroyed outside the cardiovascular system by macrophages (large phagocytic cells) found all over the body. Macrophages remove senescent RBCs from circulation and break them down into components that can be recycled in the body or eliminated as waste material. Macrophages of the spleen are especially active in removing aging, dead, and abnormal RBCs.

Extravascular Hemolysis

Once inside a macrophage the membrane of the RBC is destroyed. Iron from the heme plus the amino acids from globin molecules are recovered from the macrophages. Iron is transported to the red bone marrow. The amino acids are returned to the liver, where they are used to build more proteins. The heme is disassembled and eliminated from the body. To do this it is first converted to bilirubin, which is then carried to the liver by the plasma protein *albumin*. It has to attach itself to albumin because bilirubin at this stage is not water soluble. At this point the bilirubin is classified as unconjugated or free bilirubin. In the liver bilirubin is joined or conjugated to a compound called *glucuronic acid*. The combined bilirubin and glucuronic acid molecule is water soluble and excreted as a bile pigment into the intestines. The bilirubin is now classified as conjugated bilirubin. In the intestines, conjugated bilirubin is converted into urobilinogen by bacteria. Some of this urobilinogen is reabsorbed and eliminated in the urine as urobilin. Some is converted to another compound, stercobilinogen, and excreted in the stool as stercobilin. Urobilin and stercobilin are two pigments normally present in urine and feces and help give them their normal color.

Intravascular Hemolysis

About 10% of normal RBC destruction takes place by intravascular hemolysis, that is, the destruction takes place within blood vessels. While in circulation the RBC is subjected to many metabolic and mechanical stresses. These can result in RBC fragmentation or destruction. When the RBC membrane ruptures within a vessel, hemoglobin is released directly into the blood. The free hemoglobin is picked up by **haptoglobin,** a transport plasma protein, and carried to the macrophages of the mononuclear phagocyte system in the liver for further breakdown. Once in the liver the process proceeds as in extravascular hemolysis.

When haptoglobin is filled with free hemoglobin, excess free hemoglobin appears in the plasma **(hemoglobinemia).**

CLINICAL APPLICATION — Blood Glucose and Red Blood Cell (RBC) Metabolism

Blood is living tissue even after it has been taken from an animal. A fresh blood sample in a tube still contains living RBCs that use plasma glucose for energy. The problem is that the glucose cannot be replenished after the RBCs use it. Diagnostic laboratory analysis of a blood sample often involves measuring blood glucose levels to look for or monitor diseases, such as diabetes mellitus. A patient with uncontrolled diabetes will have an elevated blood glucose level. If RBCs are not removed from the blood sample quickly enough, they could eat up enough glucose to bring an elevated blood glucose level down into the normal range. This could lead to a misdiagnosis and possibly inappropriate treatment. RBCs could even use enough glucose to take a normal blood glucose level down below normal. Samples that sit around long enough before the RBCs are removed can have a blood glucose level of zero. Therefore when the blood glucose level is to be measured, we must centrifuge the sample and remove the RBCs soon after the sample is drawn to achieve an accurate result.

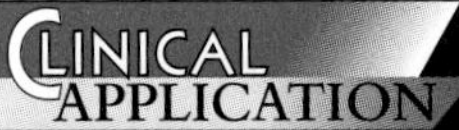

Jaundice (Icterus)

Excess RBC breakdown results in an excess amount of unconjugated bilirubin in plasma **(hyperbilirubinemia).** If the amount of bilirubin exceeds the ability of the liver to conjugate it, the excess bilirubin is deposited in tissues. This causes the tissues to turn yellow, and the condition is called **jaundice,** or *icterus.* The two terms are used interchangeably. Clinically, jaundice is most readily seen as a yellowish color of the mucous membranes and the white (sclera) of the eye.

Jaundice can also be associated with a liver disease that prevents the liver from conjugating even the normal amount of bilirubin presented to it. This causes the bilirubin from normal RBC breakdown to build up in the blood and eventually be deposited in tissues. If the bile ducts are obstructed the conjugated bilirubin cannot be passed with bile into the intestines; therefore it backs up into the bloodstream and into tissues. Jaundice again will occur.

This free hemoglobin is carried to the kidney, where it is eliminated in the urine (hemoglobinuria).

Intravascular hemolysis results in pink, red, or brown plasma (hemoglobinemia). If excess hemoglobin is being eliminated in the urine, the urine may also be red **(hemoglobinuria).**

Anemia and Polycythemia

Anemia is a pathological condition that results in decreased oxygen-carrying capacity of the blood. It can be caused by the following:

- A low number of circulating mature RBCs, caused by blood loss, blood destruction, or decreased RBC production. Hemorrhage, RBC parasites, and radiation therapy for cancer are just some of the conditions that can cause this type of anemia.
- Too little hemoglobin being produced for the normal number of RBCs. Even though the bone marrow is producing the proper number of RBCs, not enough hemoglobin is available to fill each RBC. This is often the result of a deficiency of one of the substances needed to synthesize heme or globin. Iron deficiency is a common cause of this type of anemia.

Polycythemia is an increase above normal in the number of RBCs. Three types of polycythemia are as follows:

1. Relative polycythemia is seen with is a loss of fluid from blood (hemoconcentration). This commonly occurs in animals that are dehydrated because of vomiting, diarrhea, profuse sweating, or not drinking enough water.
2. Compensatory polycythemia is a result of hypoxia. The bone marrow is stimulated to make more RBCs because the tissues are not getting enough oxygen. Animals living in high altitudes develop compensatory polycythemia. A patient with congestive heart failure may become polycythemic because the heart is not pumping enough blood to the tissues, and so a hypoxic condition results. This causes the kidney to produce more erythropoietin that will stimulate the PPSCs to develop into more RBCs.
3. Polycythemia rubra vera is a rare bone marrow disorder characterized by increased production of RBCs for an unknown reason.

TEST YOURSELF

1. What is the physiological state of blood that acts as the stimulus for erythropoiesis?
2. What causes polychromasia in developing red blood cell (RBC) cytoplasm?
3. How does having a deformable but not elastic membrane affect a RBC when fluid enters the cell?
4. How does a RBC carry oxygen to tissues?
5. Where does bilirubin come from? How is it eliminated from the body?
6. What is the difference between polycythemia and anemia?
7. How can you use the hematocrit to evaluate a patient for anemia?
8. What is the buffy coat?

CLINICAL APPLICATION: Hematocrit and Packed Cell Volume

One of the most important diagnostic screening tests performed on blood is the **packed cell volume (PCV)** (also called the **hematocrit**). An anticoagulated blood sample is placed in a small tube and centrifuged at a high speed. This causes the cells with a higher specific gravity to settle in the bottom of the tube, while the plasma, with a lower specific gravity, stays on top of the cells. The RBCs settle on the bottom and make up 28% to 55% of the sample volume, depending on the species. The height of the column of RBCs is measured in proportion to the height of the entire sample, allowing the percentage of RBCs to be determined. This value is called the *PCV* and is expressed as a percentage (Figure 9-4). The PCV is a useful test to screen a patient for anemia. The percentage of RBCs will be smaller if the animal has a low RBC count or if the RBCs are smaller than normal (two of the causes of anemia). The PCV also can be used to screen for patient dehydration that causes relative polycythemia and hemoconcentration.

Even though most people use the terms *PCV* and *hematocrit* interchangeably, technically the terms are different. The hematocrit is determined by automated hematology instruments that actually count the number of RBCs per specific volume of whole blood sample. The hematocrit is also expressed as a percentage of RBCs in a blood sample, but it is considered more accurate because the RBCs were counted directly by the instrument. When a centrifuge is used, we must rely on the efficiency of the centrifuge to pack the cells tightly enough to squeeze all the plasma out from between the cells but not so tightly that some of the cells rupture. Because of this difference in procedure, sometimes a discrepancy exists between the PCV reported from a centrifuged blood sample and the hematocrit reported from an automated hematology instrument.

The white blood cells and platelets lie on top of the RBC column in what is called the *buffy coat* because grossly it appears cream or buff colored. The thickness of the buffy coat can be used as an indicator of the total number of leukocytes and platelets in the sample. The thicker the buffy coat, the more white blood cells and platelets present. Most often a thicker buffy coat is caused by an increased number of white blood cells (leukocytosis).

The plasma from the hematocrit tube can be placed on an instrument called a *refractometer* to determine the total plasma protein. This value is a useful screening test for the hydration of an animal. A dehydrated animal will have less water in its plasma, resulting in an elevated total protein concentration.

PLATELETS

Platelets are also known as *thrombocytes.* They are not complete cells but are pieces of cytoplasm that have been isolated and released from giant, multinucleated cells **(megakaryocytes)** in the bone marrow. Even though they are not complete cells, platelets often are listed as one of the blood cell types in peripheral blood.

Formation

Production of platelets is called **thrombopoiesis.** The parent cell of platelets is the megakaryocyte that is produced from the PPSC in bone marrow. As it develops it undergoes incomplete mitosis, whereby the nuclei divide but the cytoplasm does not. This results in a cell that has many nuclei and lots of cytoplasm. The megakaryocyte does not leave the bone marrow. Instead, it breaks off small chunks of cytoplasm and sends them into circulation as platelets.

Characteristics

Platelets in circulation are round and have numerous small, purple granules scattered throughout the cytoplasm (see Figure 9-2). The granules contain, among other things, some of the clotting factors that are necessary for blood to clot. Platelets are usually smaller than RBCs, but occasionally giant platelets are seen. Giant platelets are considered more physiologically active than smaller platelets.

Function

Platelets are an essential part of **hemostasis,** the process by which blood is prevented from leaking from damaged blood vessels. Platelets have specific roles in the clotting process. These roles depend on adequate numbers of platelets being present and normal platelet function. The three specific platelet functions are as follows:

1. **Maintenance of vascular integrity.** Platelets help nurture the endothelial cells lining the vascular system. The platelets attach to the endothelium and release endothelial growth factor into the endothelial cells. If platelets are not present in adequate numbers, numerous RBCs can migrate through the endothelial wall and produce **petechiae** (small hemorrhages) around the body.
2. **Platelet plug formation.** If the lining of a blood vessel is damaged, the exposed connective tissue attracts platelets, which adhere irreversibly to it (platelet adhesion). The platelets adhere to the exposed connective tissue and to each other in an effort to stop the hemorrhage. Absence of platelet adhesion can result in bleeding disorders. Once the platelets have adhered to the site of injury, they change shape and develop pseudopods that allow them to intertwine with each other (platelet aggregation). As the platelets squeeze together, they release platelet factors, which are necessary to complete the clotting process.
3. **Stabilization of the hemostatic plug by contributing to the process of fibrin formation.** Blood clots when the soluble plasma protein *fibrinogen* is converted to insoluble strands of fibrin. For this to happen, various clotting factors and enzymes found in blood and tissue work together in a series of complex reactions. Thirteen different factors have been identified as necessary for clotting to take place. In most cases, each of these factors has to be activated by another factor. Once the factor is activated, it causes the activation of another factor. Sounds complicated, doesn't it? It is. Think of this process as a row of dominos set about an inch apart. If you knock over the first domino, it will fall against the second domino, knocking it over. Then the second domino knocks over the third domino, and so on. This is similar to the clotting process. One reaction leads to another reaction in a cascade effect that will eventually lead to the generation of large quantities of a substance called *thrombin* on the aggregated platelets' surfaces.

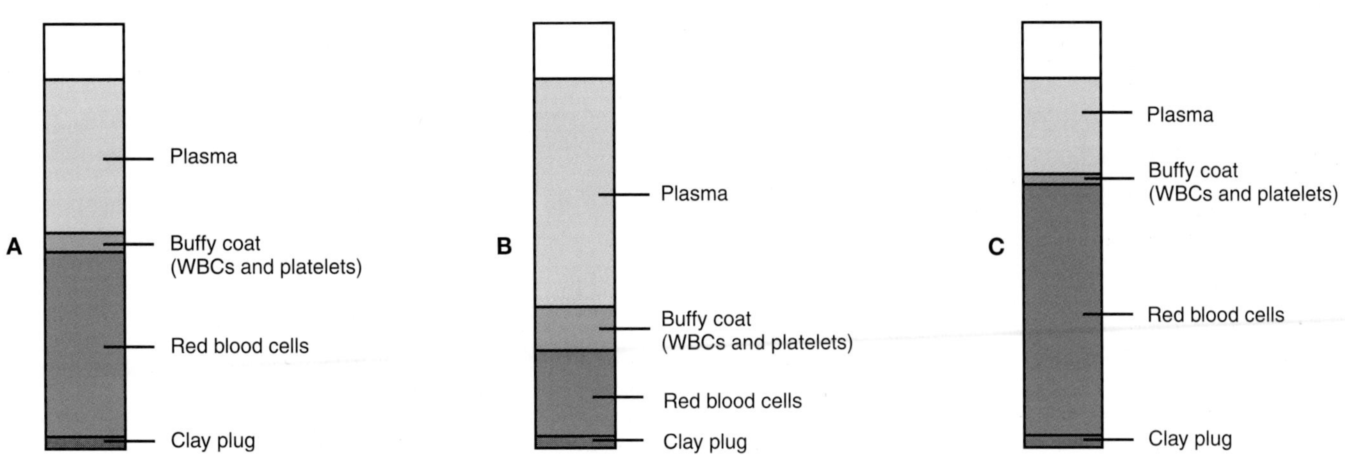

FIGURE **9-4 Hematocrit. A,** Normal blood. Normal percent of red blood cells (RBCs) and normal-thickness buffy coat. **B,** Anemia and leukocytosis. Low percent of RBCs (anemia) and thicker buffy coat (leukocytosis). **C,** Polycythemia and leukocytopenia. High percent of RBCs (polycythemia) and thinner buffy coat (leukocytopenia). *WBCs,* White blood cells.

The presence of thrombin causes the soluble fibrinogen to be converted to insoluble fibrin strands. The fibrin strands form a netlike mesh around and through the platelets. This is one of the final stages in the formation of a clot. In addition to preventing the further escape of blood, the clot also acts as a scaffolding for repair of vessel damage. At the same time the clot is being formed, other processes confine the clotting to the site of injury. Also activated are factors that will eventually dissolve the clot **(fibrinolysis)** when the endothelium has been repaired.

Life Span and Destruction

After being released from bone marrow, platelets remain in peripheral blood until they are removed by tissue macrophages because of old age or damage.

TEST YOURSELF

1. Why are platelets not considered complete cells?
2. What are the three main functions of platelets?

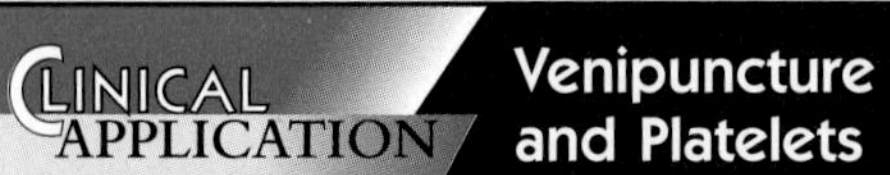

Venipuncture and Platelets

Venipuncture is performed by placing a needle into a vein to draw out a blood sample or to administer medication. This makes a hole in the vessel wall. When the needle is removed, the hole remains, and connective tissue is exposed to the inside of the vessel. This catches the attention of platelets, which congregate at the site and form a plug to prevent loss of blood through the hole. In a healthy animal, this plug will be in place within a couple of minutes. To ensure that the plug is formed as quickly as possible, once the needle has been removed from the vein, apply light pressure to the venipuncture site. Wrapping a piece of tape around the leg after a cotton ball has been placed on the venipuncture site can be helpful. Do not wipe away the blood that seeps out of the venipuncture site. Every time you rub the area, you disrupt the developing platelet plug and prolong the bleeding time.

White Blood Cells

White blood cells (WBCs) are also known as *leukocytes.* When WBCs accumulate in one place grossly, they appear white or cream colored. For example, pus is an accumulation of WBCs. Any *nucleated* cell normally found in blood is a WBC. Mature WBCs are larger than mature RBCs.

The five types of WBCs are neutrophils, eosinophils, basophils, monocytes, and lymphocytes (Table 9-2). WBCs can be classified in three different ways: type of defense function, shape of nucleus, and presence or absence of staining cytoplasmic granules (Box 9-1).

Formation

The general term for formation of WBCs is **leukopoiesis.** All WBC production starts out in the red bone marrow from the same PPSC population that produces RBCs. The stimuli that act on the PPSC determine which cell type is produced. Each type of WBC has its own stimulus for production.

All the WBCs develop in the bone marrow except for some lymphocytes (they start out in bone marrow but develop elsewhere). At the beginning of leukopoiesis, all the immature WBCs look alike. Not until the cells start developing do some of their unique characteristics show to tell them apart.

Function

The function of all WBCs is to defend the body against foreign invaders. Each type of WBC has its own unique role in this defense. If all the WBCs are functioning properly, an animal has a good chance of remaining healthy. Individual WBC functions are discussed later with each cell type.

In defending against foreign invaders, the WBCs do their job primarily out in the tissues. The WBCs use the peripheral blood to travel from their site of production (bone marrow) to their site of activity (tissue). The WBCs flow constantly out of bone marrow and into tissue in an attempt to control the millions of foreign invaders that attack a body every day. This is happening in us, too. As long as they do their job, we don't even realize what's going on, and we remain healthy.

Table 9-2 White Blood Cells

Name	Cytoplasmic Granules	Nuclear Shape	Function	Site of Action
Neutrophil	Don't stain (usually invisible)	Polymorphonuclear	Phagocytosis	Body tissues
Eosinophil	Stain red	Polymorphonuclear	Allergic reactions, anaphylaxis, phagocytosis	Body tissues
Basophil	Stain blue	Polymorphonuclear	Initiation of immune and allergic reactions	Body tissues
Monocyte (macrophage)	None	Pleomorphic	Phagocytosis and process antigens	Body tissues or blood
B lymphocyte	None	Mononuclear	Antibody production and humoral immunity	Lymphoid tissue
T lymphocyte	None	Mononuclear	Lymphokine production and cell-mediated immunity	Lymphoid tissue and other body tissues

TEST YOURSELF

1. List the five WBCs and indicate if each one is a granulocyte or an agranulocyte.
2. What is the common general function of all WBCs?
3. Which cell is the only WBC not capable of phagocytosis?

GRANULOCYTES

The granulocytes are the neutrophils, eosinophils, and basophils. They are named for the color of the granules in their cytoplasm when viewed on a stained blood smear (see earlier discussion of stains). Eosinophil granules pick up the acidic stain and appear red; basophil granules pick up the basic stain and appear blue; and neutrophils do not pick up either stain very well, and so, for the most part, the neutrophil granules are colorless on a stained blood smear.

Formation

The production of all granulocytes is called **granulopoiesis.** In the bone marrow, early granulocytes are impossible to tell apart from each other. They are all large cells with lots of cytoplasm and large, round nuclei. Initially, no cytoplasmic granules are

Box 9-1 Classification of White Blood Cells

1. Type of defense function
   Phagocytosis: neutrophils, eosinophils, basophils, and monocytes
   Antibody production and cellular immunity: lymphocytes
2. Shape of nucleus
   Polymorphonuclear (multilobed, segmented): neutrophils, eosinophils, and basophils (Figure 9-5)
   Mononuclear (single, rounded nucleus): lymphocytes
   Pleomorphic (varying shapes, nonsegmented): monocytes
3. Presence or absence of specific staining cytoplasmic granules
   Granulocytes (presence of granules): neutrophils, eosinophils, and basophils
   Agranulocytes (absence of granules): lymphocytes and monocytes

CLINICAL APPLICATION

Total White Blood Cell (WBC) Count and Differential Count

The total WBC count and differential count are used to evaluate a patient for the diagnosis or prognosis of an abnormal condition. For example, if an infection is present in the body, there will be an increased need for neutrophils to kill the microorganisms. The bone marrow responds to this need by releasing more neutrophils into the bloodstream that will travel to the tissue where the infection is located. The increased number of neutrophils in blood will increase the total WBC count. The total WBC count is equal to the sum of each of the individual WBC counts. If one cell type increases or decreases, the total WBC count will increase or decrease accordingly. Sounds simple, doesn't it? Unfortunately, it is not always that simple. If one cell type increases and another cell type decreases, the net effect could be a normal total WBC count. That's the tricky part; so the total WBC count is only one of a series of tests performed to evaluate the WBCs.

To find out which WBC(s) are affecting the total WBC count, we have to look at a stained smear of the blood. The usual method for evaluating the blood smear is to count the first 100 WBCs and to keep track of the number of each WBC type you see. This is called a *differential count* or, more commonly, "the diff." Because you're counting 100 cells, the number of each cell type you see can be expressed as a percent. For example, if you count 100 cells, and 20 of the cells are neutrophils and 80 of the cells are lymphocytes, you would report that you saw 20% neutrophils and 80% lymphocytes.

For every species of common domestic animal, there is a value range that represents a normal WBC count. There is also a normal range for individual WBC types. For example, a dog normally has between 6 billion and 17 billion WBCs per liter of blood, and 60% to 70% of the cells should be neutrophils. Cattle have between 4 billion and 12 billion WBCs/L, and only 15% to 45% of the cells should be neutrophils.

Together the total WBC count and the differential count can provide a lot of information about the animal's state of health.

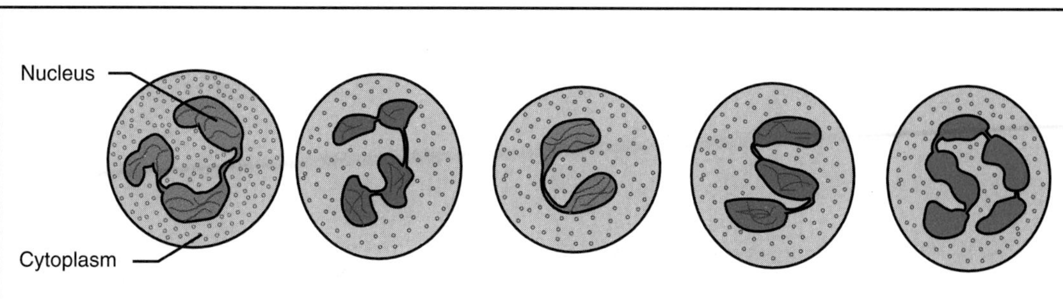

FIGURE 9-5 **Normal Neutrophil Showing Polymorphonuclear Characteristics.**

Clinical Application — Leukemia

Leukemia literally means "white blood." It is caused by an abnormal proliferation of one of the white blood cell (WBC) types. In response to some unknown stimulus, the stem cells in the bone marrow start producing abnormal cells in one cell line at an increased rate. These abnormal cells show up in peripheral blood in large numbers, many times before they are mature, and cause the total WBC numbers to increase dramatically **(leukocytosis)**. Leukemias are considered a form of malignancy or cancer and can be acute or chronic. They are classified by the type of cell involved, for example, lymphocytic leukemia, monocytic leukemia, eosinophilic leukemia.

present. As the granulocytes mature, a first set of granules is formed. These granules are the same in all three granulocytes and are called *nonspecific granules.* Gradually, the nonspecific granules are replaced by a new set of granules that is unique to each granulocyte type. These are called *specific granules.* The Golgi apparatus produces both the nonspecific and the specific granules. The substances found in its granules determine the function of a granulocyte. For example, neutrophil granules contain chemicals called *lysosomal enzymes* that aid in killing microorganisms that have been engulfed by the neutrophil. Neutrophils therefore have become a major factor in preventing the invasion of microorganisms into the body from causing disease.

An early granulocyte has blue cytoplasm, indicating that it is a metabolically active cell. As it matures the cytoplasm becomes less active and therefore does not stain as blue. Mature granulocytes in circulation contain almost colorless cytoplasm containing the specific granules. In fact, without the granules, the limits of the cell membrane would be difficult to see, making it look like the nucleus was pretty much floating around alone. This image is sometimes just how neutrophils appear because of their colorless granules.

As a granulocyte matures, its nucleus transforms from a round structure to a segmented structure that takes on many shapes (polymorphonuclear). Thin filaments connect these segments. The chromatin pattern of the nucleus starts out rather loose. As the nucleus squeezes itself down into segments, the chromatin becomes more condensed. As the cell ages and approaches death, the segments break apart and lose all evidence of any chromatin pattern. This process is called *pyknosis* and is a sign of a dead cell.

Neutrophils

Neutrophils are also known as *polymorphonuclear cells* (because their nuclei have many shapes), polymorphonuclear leukocytes (PMNs), and "segs" (because their nuclei are segmented). Even though eosinophil, basophil, and monocyte nuclei can be polymorphonuclear, the neutrophil is the only cell that is called a *PMN.* The neutrophil is the most numerous WBC in circulation in the dog, horse, and cat.

Formation. Neutrophils are produced in the bone marrow and released into blood as needed when neutrophils already in circulation leave the bloodstream and enter tissue to kill microorganisms or simply die of old age. It takes 3 to 6 days to produce a mature neutrophil under normal conditions, depending on the species. If the body has a sudden need for more neutrophils, this time can be shortened

Characteristics. Neutrophil granules do not stain with either the blue alkaline stain or the red acid stain; therefore they are said to be *neutral.* This means that they are difficult to see on a stained smear, and so identification of neutrophils is commonly based on nuclear morphology rather than granule-staining characteristics.

A mature neutrophil in peripheral blood can have from two to five nuclear segments. The segments are not separate pieces of nucleus but are joined by a thin strand of chromatin. Sometimes this strand of chromatin is difficult to see, and therefore it looks like the segments are separated. If the neutrophil is released from the bone marrow before it is mature, it will have a horseshoe nucleus without any segmentation. This is called a *band neutrophil.* When band neutrophils are seen in peripheral blood, this indicates an increased demand for neutrophils beyond what the bone marrow can supply in mature neutrophils. If the bone marrow runs out of band neutrophils and still has not met the body's demand, it will start releasing progressively more immature cells.

Function. Neutrophils are phagocytes, which means they engulf (phagocytize) microorganisms and other microscopic debris in tissues. They are the first line of defense when invading microorganisms enter the body because they can respond quickly. Neutrophil granules contain digestive enzymes that can destroy bacteria and viruses that have been engulfed. The neutrophil granules are organelles called **lysosomes.**

Neutrophils use blood as a transportation medium to take them to their site of action in tissue. Normally a neutrophil spends an average of 10 hours in the circulation before it enters the tissue. This circulation time is shorter when the demand for neutrophils in the tissue increases. Once a neutrophil enters tissue, it does not return to blood; so the circulating neutrophils need to be replaced about 2.5 times a day.

Neutrophils and other WBCs leave the blood vessel by squeezing between the cells of the endothelium in a process called **diapedesis** (Figure 9-7). Neutrophils are normally found in tissues that constantly are exposed to microorganism invasion, (e.g., the lungs and intestinal tract). Other neutrophils wander through tissue to the sites where they are needed. Neutrophils stay in tissue until they die of old age or are destroyed by the microorganisms that they are trying to destroy. Dead or abnormal neutrophils are picked up and destroyed by tissue macrophages (see later discussion of tissue macrophages in the section on monocytes). You can think of neutrophils as garbage cans and tissue macrophages as garbage trucks.

Neutrophils are attracted to a site of infection by a process called **chemotaxis.** Chemotaxis is the process by which neu-

CLINICAL APPLICATION Hypersegmented Neutrophils

If a neutrophil nucleus has more than five segments when it is seen in peripheral blood, it is called a **hypersegmented** nucleus (Figure 9-6). This indicates the neutrophil has stayed in peripheral blood longer than normal because hypersegmenting usually takes place in tissue as part of the normal aging process. The presence of hypersegmented neutrophils on a stained blood smear can mean that a pathological condition prevented neutrophils from leaving circulation or that the smear was made from old blood. Remember, blood is still living when it is removed from the animal and will continue the aging process as long as it can. Therefore hypersegmented neutrophils may be just aging normally in the tube. You can start seeing hypersegmented neutrophils within a day after the blood sample was drawn. For this reason, a smear should be made as soon as possible after the blood sample is drawn.

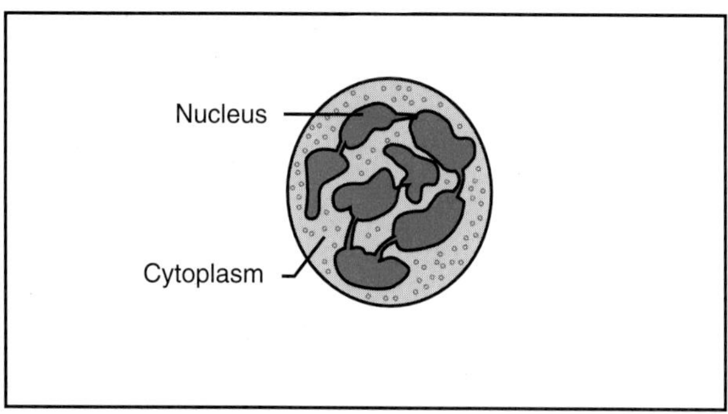

FIGURE 9-6 **Hypersegmented Nucleus.** It can indicate an older cell than is normally found in peripheral blood.

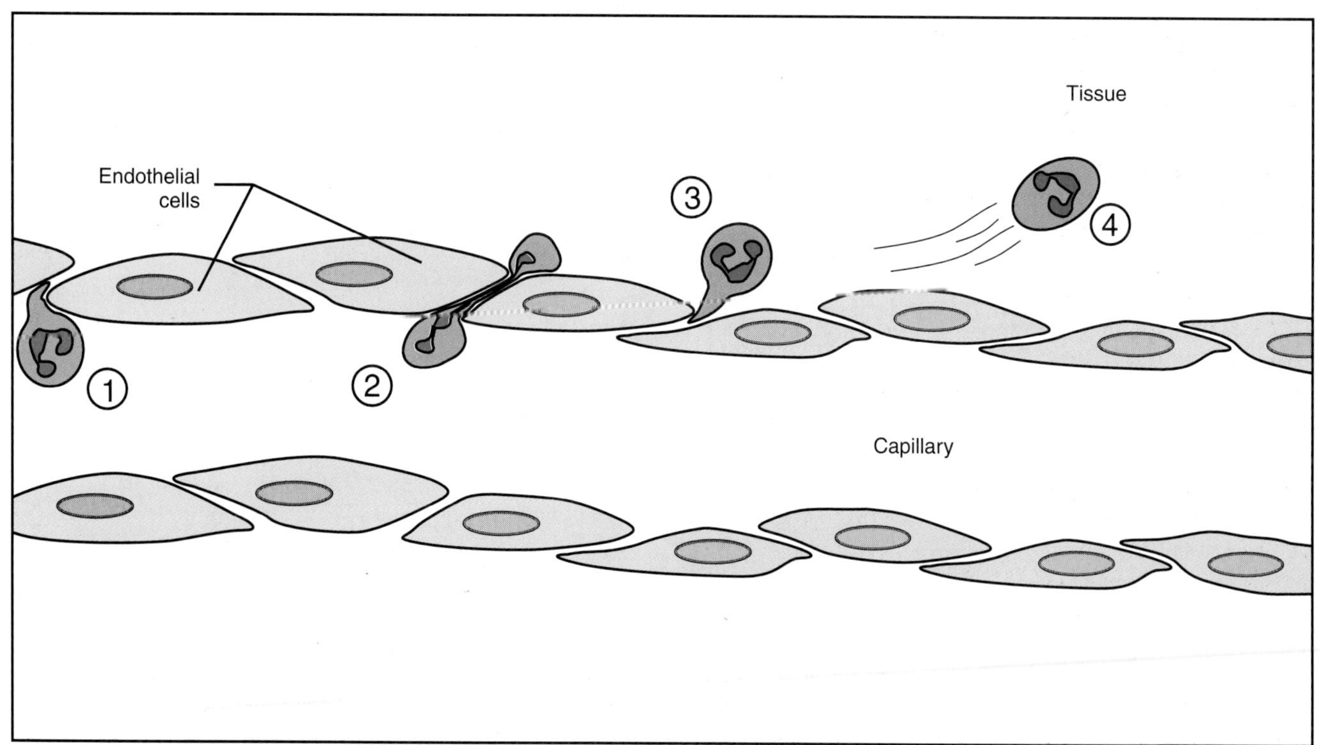

FIGURE 9-7 **Diapedesis.** *1,* Neutrophil lying against vessel wall begins to squeeze through the space between endothelial cells by flowing into pseudopod (false foot). *2,* Pseudopod continues to push its way between cells. Rest of the cell cytoplasm flows along with it. *3,* Pseudopod and rest of the cell emerge on tissue side of blood vessel. *4,* Neutrophil is off in search of foreign invaders to phagocytize.

trophils and other cells are attracted by inflammatory chemicals produced by the interaction between microorganisms and the tissues they are invading. Having arrived at the site invaded by the microorganisms, the neutrophil must recognize what to ingest. For some microorganisms, this is not problem. Others try to "hide" inside capsules that make them difficult for neutrophils to recognize. In these cases the microorganism is coated with a plasma protein, usually a specific antibody (see later discussion of antibody production in the immunity section). These plasma proteins are called **opsonins.** Coating the microorganism enables the neutrophil to recognize it as foreign and to begin phagocytosis. The coating process is called **opsonization.**

When the neutrophil recognizes foreign microorganisms, its outer membrane flows around the microorganisms and encases them within a membrane-bound phagocytic vacuole (Figure 9-8). (If you've seen the 1950s sci-fi movie *The Blob,* this is similar to how the Blob flows around anything in its way. If you haven't seen the movie, you should. It's a hoot.) The microorganisms are surrounded by the neutrophil membrane but are not really inside the neutrophil. (Think of it as a hug. When you put your arms around something, you're encasing it but not taking it inside your body.) At this point the neutrophil cytoplasmic granules move to the edge of the **vacuole** that contains the microorganisms, fuse with the membrane, and secrete their digestive contents into the vacuole.

During ingestion of microorganisms the neutrophils increase their metabolism of oxygen to produce substances that are toxic to ingested bacteria. Hydrogen peroxide is the product of oxygen metabolism that is most important for killing activity by neutrophils. Hydrogen peroxide can kill bacteria (bactericidal effect) all by itself, but its action is enhanced by the enzyme myeloperoxidase, which is released from neutrophil granules. Lysozyme from the granules also enhances the bactericidal action of hydrogen peroxide and can destroy the cell walls of microorganisms.

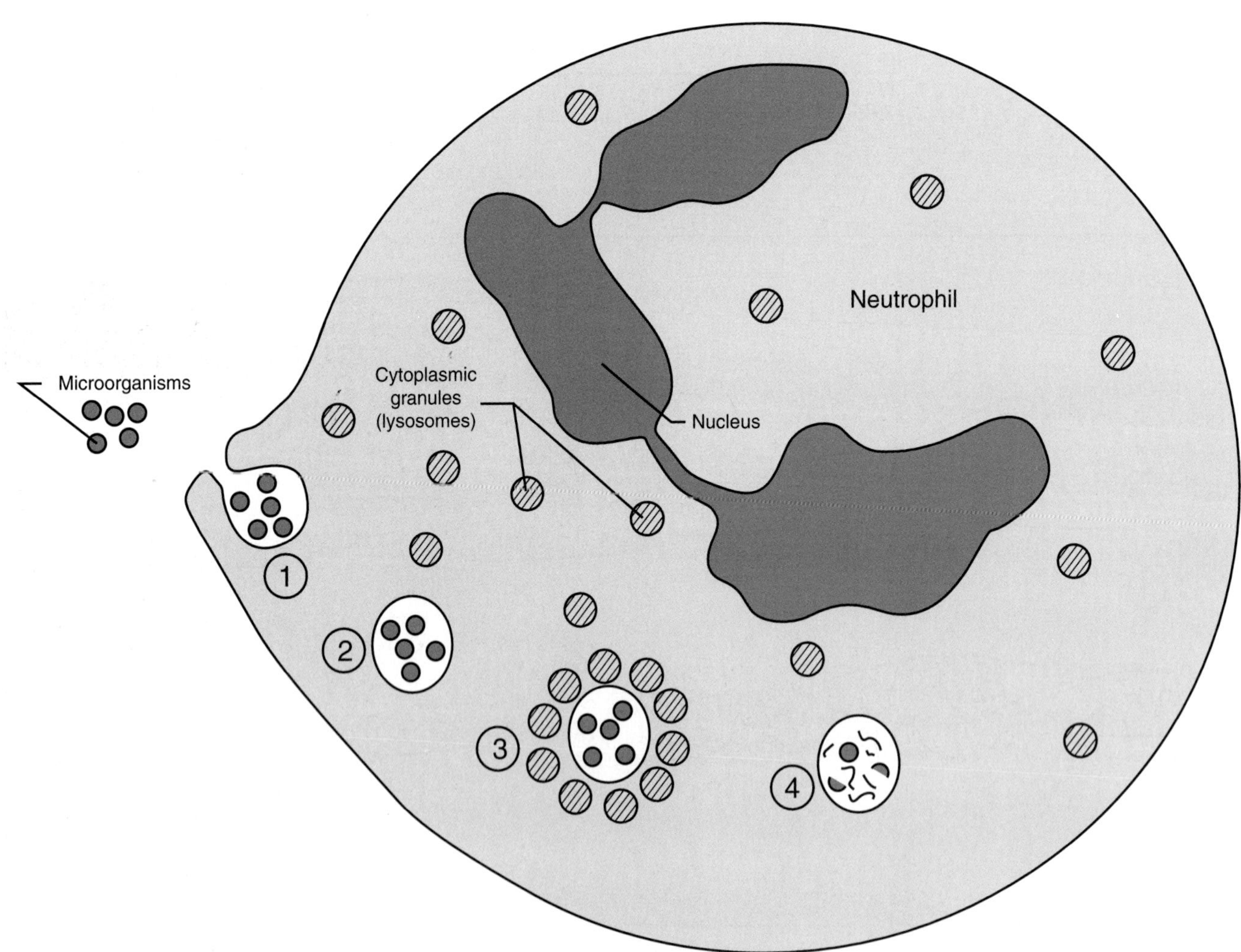

FIGURE **9-8 Phagocytosis and Destruction of Microorganisms.** *1,* Neutrophil membrane engulfs microorganisms. *2,* Phagocytic vacuole is formed. *3,* Cytoplasmic granules line up around phagocytic vacuole and empty their digestive enzymes into vacuole. *4,* Microorganisms are destroyed.

Neutrophil Count in Peripheral Blood. The neutrophil count in peripheral blood is kept within a specific range in a healthy animal. This number is controlled by the following factors:

1. Release of mature neutrophils from the storage pool in the bone marrow into the peripheral blood. The bone marrow usually has a 5-day supply (reserve or storage pool) of mature neutrophils. They are ready for immediate release if a sudden drop occurs in circulating numbers of neutrophils caused by increased movement of neutrophils into tissue.
2. Rate of escape from peripheral blood into tissue. This rate depends on the need for neutrophils in the tissue. With a massive acute infection the total neutrophil population of the peripheral blood can enter the tissue in a couple of hours (e.g., coliform mastitis in cattle).
3. The entrance of increased numbers of PPSCs into the neutrophil production line. This is a slow method of control because it takes 3 to 6 days for the neutrophils to mature and to be ready for release.

CLINICAL APPLICATION — Neutrophilia and Leukocytosis

To meet an increased demand for neutrophils in tissue, the bone marrow releases its reserve stores of mature and, if necessary, immature neutrophils into blood so that they can be transported to the site where they are needed. If a blood sample is drawn while these neutrophils are in transit, a higher than normal number of neutrophils will be included in the sample. This is called **neutrophilia** and usually is detected on a stained smear of the blood sample. The increased number of neutrophils will also increase the total number of WBCs in the blood sample. This is called *leukocytosis* and usually is detected by using an automated blood analyzer or by looking at the thickness of the buffy coat in a hematocrit tube. Leukocytosis with an accompanying neutrophilia can indicate that an infection is somewhere in the body.

CLINICAL APPLICATION — Neutropenia and Leukocytopenia

If an infection is out of control, all the reserves of neutrophils can be used up faster than the bone marrow can replace them. If this happens the number of neutrophils in circulation decreases because the neutrophils are leaving the bloodstream and entering tissue and no cells remain in the bone marrow to replace them. This condition is called **neutropenia.** The total WBC count will also decrease **(leukocytopenia).** The prognosis is poor for a critically ill animal that has neutropenia and leukocytopenia. Such a condition signifies that the body is losing the war against the invading microorganisms.

Intravascular Pools of Neutrophils. In peripheral blood, two pools of mature neutrophils are found.

1. The **circulating pool** is contained in the blood as it flows through the blood vessels. It is located in the lumen of the vessel. Blood samples that are obtained for laboratory analysis contain the neutrophils from this pool. The normal range of neutrophil numbers in peripheral blood is based on the neutrophils contained in this pool.
2. The **marginal pool** is composed of neutrophils that line the walls of small blood vessels mainly in the spleen, lungs, and abdominal organs. These neutrophils are not circulating and are not contained in blood samples obtained for laboratory analysis.

Eosinophils

Eosinophils are named for the red granules in the cytoplasm of mature cells. They make up 5% or less of the total WBC count.

Formation and Characteristics. Eosinophils are produced in the bone marrow from the same PPSC population that gives rise to all other blood cells. It takes 2 to 6 days to produce an eosinophil from a PPSC. The cytoplasmic granules take up the acidic stain eosin and appear red when seen on a blood smear. Often the segmented nucleus has only two lobes.

CLINICAL APPLICATION — Neutrophils and the Stress Response

Neutrophils can move freely between the circulating and marginal pools. At any given time in dogs, cattle, and horses, the ratio between the number of neutrophils in the circulating pool and those in the marginal pool is about 50:50. In cats the circulating pool/marginal pool ratio is about a 30:70. Cells can detach from the marginal pool and enter the circulating pool when an animal is experiencing some sort of physical or mental stress. Trauma, fear, and exercise are a few of the stresses that may lead to a temporary transfer of neutrophils from the marginal pool to the circulating pool. This predictable neutrophil response is part of a larger physiological reaction called the *stress response.* Splenic contraction also plays an important role in this movement of cells out of the marginal pool. The temporary movement of neutrophils into the circulating pool can artificially elevate the total neutrophil count (neutrophilia) and the total WBC count (leukocytosis) because the normal values are based only on the number of cells normally found in the circulating pool. These artificially elevated results can lead to a possible misdiagnosis. Remember this when you have to chase a horse around a pasture or wrestle with a cat to obtain a blood sample.

The administration of corticosteroid drugs (similar to glucocorticoid hormones [see Chapter 14]) causes the same response. Therefore a blood sample should be drawn before medications are administered.

The granules are shaped differently in various species, as described below:

- Dogs: Granules are round, their size varies from small to large within the same cell, and granules stain lightly.
- Cats: Granules are small, rod shaped, and numerous. They stain darker than canine eosinophil granules.
- Horses: Granules are very large, round, or oval and stain intensely.
- Cattle, sheep, and pigs: Granules are round and much smaller than equine granules. They stain pink to red.

The bone marrow has a good reserve of eosinophils. Circulating and marginal pools of eosinophils are also found in peripheral blood, like the neutrophil pools.

Eosinophils do not stay in peripheral blood very long but migrate into tissue in a few hours, where they spend the rest of their lives. In tissue they undergo the same aging process as neutrophils.

Function. The functions of eosinophils are not entirely understood, but like neutrophils, the functions are determined by the contents of their granules. Chemotaxis regulates their entry into tissue. They do not reenter circulation once they leave blood vessels. Large numbers of eosinophils are normally found in certain tissues in the body (e.g., skin, lung, small intestines). The functions most often associated with eosinophils are as follows:

- They are attracted to and inhibit local allergic and anaphylactic reactions. Their granules contain antiinflammatory substances that are released at the site of the allergic reaction.
- They can ingest substances associated with the humoral immune response (e.g., antigen-antibody reaction complexes).
- They have minimal phagocytotic and bactericidal functions. They are especially effective in phagocytosis of large pathogenic organisms, such as protozoa, and some parasitic worms but are not protective against most bacterial infections.

Eosinophilia and Leukocytosis. Increased numbers of eosinophils in peripheral blood **(eosinophilia)** can be seen during allergic reactions and certain parasitic infections. The increased numbers are a response to a demand created by a pathological condition in the animal. An accompanying leukocytosis may also occur, but because not very many eosinophils are normally in circulation, the increased number may not be enough to elevate the WBC count beyond the normal range.

Eosinophilia can result from the following conditions:

- Increased release of mature eosinophils from the storage pool in the bone marrow
- Migration of eosinophils from the marginal pool to the circulating pool
- Increased production in the bone marrow
- Longer time spent in peripheral blood before entering the tissue

Eosinopenia. Decreased numbers of eosinophils in peripheral blood **(eosinopenia)** are difficult to detect and evaluate because their numbers are normally low.

Basophils

Basophils are named for the blue granules in the cytoplasm of mature cells. The granules stain with the basic component of the blood stain. They are the WBC least often seen in circulation, and therefore they are also the least understood WBC.

Formation. Basophils are produced in the bone marrow from the same PPSC population as the other blood cells. Not much is known about the production and function of basophils.

Characteristics. The basophil granules are water soluble and are often washed out during the staining procedure. For this reason, they are not always readily visible on a stained smear. When they are seen, the basophil granules stain blue and fill the cytoplasm. Dogs have fewer granules than the other common domestic species. Basophils most often have a two- to three-lobed nucleus.

Basophils and Tissue Mast Cells. Basophils share some characteristics with tissue **mast cells,** but some controversy exists over the relationship between these two cells. Mast cells are normally found in tissue and do not migrate there from blood. Basophils are not commonly seen in tissue. Mast cells are larger than basophils and have more cytoplasmic granules, and the granules are not water soluble. Mast cells have a round nucleus that does not segment. The following two theories currently exist regarding this relationship:

1. Mast cells and basophils are two different cell types with similar characteristics. They are produced in two different areas of the body and do not give rise to one another.
2. Mast cells are tissue basophils. (This theory is not as popular as the first theory.)

Function. Not much is known about the function of basophils. They are the least phagocytic of the granulocytes. Basophil granules contain histamine and heparin, which are responsible for at least part of basophil function in the following ways:

- Histamine helps initiate inflammation and acute allergic reactions.
- Eosinophils are attracted to the site of an allergic reaction by eosinophilic chemotactic factor released from the granules.

- Heparin acts as a localized anticoagulant to keep blood flowing to an injured or damaged area.

Basophilia and Basopenia. Increased numbers of basophils in peripheral blood **(basophilia)** can be associated with an allergic or hypersensitivity reaction in tissue. Sometimes basophilia and eosinophilia are seen at the same time.

Decreased numbers of basophils in peripheral blood **(basopenia)** are difficult to evaluate because basophils are seen so rarely in peripheral blood. In all of the common domestic species, basophils make up less than 1% of all WBCs in peripheral blood. They are not seen at all on many blood smears.

AGRANULOCYTES

Agranulocytes are cells that do not have specific staining granules in their cytoplasm. They include monocytes and lymphocytes.

Monocytes

Monocytes make up 5% to 6% of the circulating WBCs in all common domestic species.

Formation and Characteristics. Monocytes are formed in the bone marrow from the PPSC population. They mature much faster than neutrophils (total monocyte development time is 24 to 36 hours) and stay in the blood longer (24 to 36 hours) than neutrophils. From peripheral blood they enter the tissue, where they carry out their function.

Monocytes are the largest WBCs in circulation. They have abundant cytoplasm that stains gray-blue and may contain vacuoles of varying sizes. Sometimes the cytoplasm takes on a fine granular appearance that is commonly referred to as a "ground glass" appearance. The nucleus can be round or of many different shapes (pleomorphic), but it does not split up into distinct segments like a mature granulocyte nucleus.

Function. Monocytes are major phagocytic cells. When they enter tissue, they are known as *tissue macrophages.* Monocytes in the bloodstream are less effective phagocytes than tissue macrophages. In fact, monocytes are considered immature tissue macrophages. Tissue macrophages are larger than monocytes and can be found in any tissue; however, they are most prevalent in "filter" organs, such as the liver, spleen, lung, and lymph nodes. These filter organs are responsible for removing or containing foreign invaders, damaged and old blood cells, and cellular debris. Some tissue macrophages are free and wander through tissue, whereas others become fixed in specific tissues and remain there for the rest of their life span. Collectively, the tissue macrophages and monocytes are known as the *mononuclear phagocyte system.*

Monocytes and tissue macrophages perform several specific functions:

- They clean up cellular debris that remains after the inflammation or infection clears up.
- They process certain **antigens,** making them more antigenic. Monocytes and macrophages can ingest antigens and present them on their cell membranes to the lymphocytes, which will destroy them. (This important role in the immune response is discussed later in the immunity section.)
- They ingest foreign substances. They have the same phagocytic capabilities as neutrophils and then some. They are larger than neutrophils, and therefore can engulf structures beyond the phagocytic capacity of neutrophils (e.g., fungi, protozoa, viruses, and dead neutrophils).

Monocytes enter tissue by the process of chemotaxis in response to tissue damage caused by trauma or invading microorganisms. Neutrophils respond more quickly to the tissue damage, but monocytes stay around longer once they reach the damaged site and become macrophages. Macrophages have a longer life span than neutrophils; so they are often associated with chronic infections.

Monocytes can also function in circulating blood to phagocytize damaged blood cells or microorganisms found in the blood (septicemia).

Monocytosis. An increased number of monocytes in peripheral blood is called **monocytosis.** It is often associated with a chronic inflammatory condition, possibly an infection.

Monocytopenia. A decreased number of monocytes in peripheral blood is called **monocytopenia.** It can be difficult to evaluate because of the low numbers of monocytes normally found in circulation.

Lymphocytes

Lymphocytes are normally the predominant WBC in circulation in ruminants and pigs. They are the only WBC that has no phagocytic capabilities. Most of the lymphocytes in the body actually live in what are called *lymphoid tissues* and constantly recirculate between these tissues and blood.

Formation and Function. Some controversy still exists regarding the origin and development of lymphocytes. The most popular belief is that they arise from the same stem cell in the bone marrow as other blood cells. Before they begin to mature, some of the cells leave the bone marrow to develop in other central lymphoid organs located throughout the body before settling in their permanent home in peripheral lymphoid tissue.

The following are the three different types of lymphocytes:

1. **T lymphocytes** (T cells): T lymphocytes are processed in the thymus before going to peripheral lymphoid tissue. The processing involves the formation of special proteins called **lymphokines** (some of which are called *interleukins*) on the T-cell surface. Lymphokines are responsible for a specific type of immunity called *cell-*

mediated immunity. (Cell-mediated immunity is explained later in this chapter.) The two types of T lymphocytes are killer T lymphocytes, which actually destroy cells during cell-mediated immunity, and helper T lymphocytes, which produce the lymphokines that activate killer T lymphocytes.

2. **B lymphocytes** (B cells): *B* means "bursa equivalent" and refers to bone marrow and other lymphoid tissue thought to be the equivalent of a bird organ called the *bursa of Fabricius.* These organs are where B lymphocytes are processed to produce protective proteins called *antibodies.* Each B lymphocyte is preprogrammed to produce only one specific antibody against one specific antigen (foreign protein). For example, certain B lymphocytes are preprogrammed to respond to the presence of the canine distemper virus. If a dog is exposed to the distemper virus, only the B lymphocytes that are preprogrammed to recognize the virus will respond by making antibodies against the virus. All the other B lymphocytes will be unaffected. The amazing thing is that the B lymphocytes are preprogrammed to produce antibodies against antigens to which they have never been exposed. When B lymphocytes recognize an antigen, they transform into plasma cells that release antibodies; this is called *humoral immunity.*

   Plasma cells are derived from B lymphocytes in response to an antigenic stimulus. B lymphocytes undergo a process called **blastic transformation** to become plasma cells. It is almost like reverting back to childhood because the plasma cells produce the antibodies by becoming metabolically active, much like a developing immature cell.

   Plasma cells produce, store, and release antibodies that are also known as **immunoglobulins.** Plasma cells can be found in any tissue in the body but are most numerous in tissues engaged in antibody formation (lymph nodes, spleen). Plasma cells are rarely found in peripheral blood.

3. **Natural killer (NK) cells.** These lymphocytes are neither T lymphocytes nor B lymphocytes. They do not have to be activated by a specific antigen and have the ability to kill some types of tumor cells and cells infected with various viruses. NK cells must come in direct contact with these cells before they can destroy them.

Characteristics. The lymphocytes we see in circulation are classified as large or small lymphocytes. Large lymphocytes have more cytoplasm and are thought to be younger than small lymphocytes. They gradually develop into small lymphocytes that have very little cytoplasm.

Lymphocytes contain no granules in their cytoplasm. The nucleus is round or oval and does not segment. Large lymphocytes have abundant sky-blue cytoplasm. Small lymphocytes have such a scant amount of cytoplasm that it is sometimes difficult to see. Small lymphocytes often look like nuclei without cytoplasm, or just a small amount of sky-blue cytoplasm may be visible on one side of the nucleus.

Memory Cells. Both T lymphocytes and B lymphocytes can create memory cells. These cells are clones of the original lymphocyte. They do not participate in an initial immune response to an antigen but survive in lymphoid tissue while waiting for a second exposure to the antigen. When the animal is exposed to the antigen a second time, the memory cells are all ready to respond. This response is much quicker than the initial immune response. For a more detailed description of the types of immune responses, see the later section on immunity.

Lymphocytosis and Leukocytosis. Lymphocytosis is an increased number of lymphocytes in peripheral blood. It can result from leukemia (a form of cancer of the lymphocytes), chronic infections, or epinephrine release (as part of the fight or flight response). The lymphocytosis can be significant enough to cause leukocytosis.

Lymphopenia and Leukocytopenia. Lymphopenia is a decreased number of lymphocytes in peripheral blood. It can be the result of many factors, including decreased production, the presence of corticosteroids (drugs similar to glucocorticoid hormones from the adrenal cortex), immune deficiency diseases, and acute viral diseases. In some animals, especially ruminants, in which lymphocytes are the primary WBC in circulation, lymphocytopenia can lead to leukocytopenia.

TEST YOURSELF

1. Which WBC is known as a *PMN*?
2. What is a lysosome and what is its function?
3. Which WBC is known as "the first line of defense" after a microorganism has entered the body?
4. Which WBC would you likely see increased in peripheral blood during an allergic response?
5. Which WBC is least commonly seen in peripheral blood?
6. Which WBC is the largest cell normally seen in peripheral blood?
7. What is chemotaxis?
8. What are the three types of lymphocytes?
9. What is the mononuclear phagocyte system? Why can't a neutrophil belong to this system?

THE LYMPHATIC SYSTEM

The lymphatic system is a series of vessels or ducts that carries excess tissue fluid to blood vessels near the heart, where the fluid is put back into the bloodstream. The lymphatic system also includes lymph tissue scattered throughout the body in structures such as lymph nodes, the spleen, the thymus, the tonsils, and **gut-associated lymph tissue (GALT).** The fluid carried by the lymphatic system is called **lymph.** Lymph contains very few blood cells other than lymphocytes. Some T lymphocytes circulate from blood to interstitial fluid to lymph and back to blood. B lymphocytes are found primarily in lymph tissues and rarely recirculate.

LYMPH FORMATION

Lymph starts out as excess tissue fluid that is picked up by blind-ended lymph capillaries. The excess tissue fluid exists because more fluid leaves blood capillaries than reenters them. Without the lymph vessels, the tissues of the body would all swell with the excess fluid.

Blood capillaries are very porous. Fluid can easily enter and leave them. At the arterial ends of capillaries, enough blood pressure can still force a lot of the plasma out into the tissues. The plasma carries substances such as nutrients, oxygen, and hormones out with it to bathe the cells and tissues. The blood pressure quickly dissipates in the tiny capillaries until no pressure exists at the venous end to force plasma out at all. Rather, osmotic pressure resulting from the proteins and other dissolved substances in the blood in the capillaries draws fluid back in. The problem is that this osmotic force drawing fluid in is not as strong as the blood pressure force that pushed it out. The result is an accumulation of fluid in the tissues.

Fortunately, lymph capillaries come to the rescue and carry this excess fluid away. Eventually, the fluid will be dumped back into the bloodstream. The lymph capillaries start out as blind-ended tubes that are similar to blood capillaries. They pick up the excess fluid and carry it away (Figure 9-9).

The tiny lymph capillaries join together to form larger and larger lymph vessels, many of which contain one-way valves much like those in veins. The valves allow body movements to propel lymph through the lymph vessels that eventually terminate in large vessels in the thorax called **thoracic ducts.** The thoracic ducts empty the collected lymph into major blood vessels in the thorax. By this means the lymph comes full circle from its origin in the tissues back into the bloodstream.

On its way to a thoracic duct a lymph vessel passes through at least one lymph node, where it picks up lymphocytes. If the interstitial fluid contained any microorganisms that were picked up with the lymph, they would be removed from lymph by macrophages found in the lymph nodes.

CHARACTERISTICS

By the time the lymph reaches the thoracic duct, it is a transparent or translucent liquid containing varying numbers of cells, primarily lymphocytes. The fluid is different from plasma in that it is made up of more water, sugar, and electrolytes and less of the larger proteins found in plasma (e.g., albumin, globulin, and fibrinogen).

Lymph from the digestive system is called **chyle.** After a meal the chyle contains microscopic particles of fat known as **chylomicrons** that cause the lymph to appear white or pale yellow and cloudy. These same chylomicrons also are found in blood after a meal and cause the postprandial lipemia mentioned earlier.

The following are the three compartments to the lymphoid tissue system:

1. Bone marrow where the PPSCs produce lymphocytes.
2. Central lymphoid organs. These organs process immature lymphocytes. These include the thymus, bone marrow, and GALT.
3. Peripheral lymphoid organs. These are the organs where mature lymphocytes live. They include lymph nodes, spleen, tonsils, bone marrow, GALT, and thymus.

FUNCTION

The lymphatic system has the following four primary functions:

1. *Removal of excess tissue fluid.* Plasma diffusion is how cells receive some of the nutrients carried by plasma. The fluid that enters the interstitial spaces eventually is put back into circulation. Part of the fluid is picked up directly by the capillaries in the tissues and enters the venous part of the cardiovascular system. Some of the fluid enters lymphatic capillaries. If lymph drainage to an area is inadequate, the interstitial fluid can build up, causing edema (excess fluid accumulation) of the tissues of the area. (Edema is caused by other conditions, but they relate to inadequate fluid drainage from tissue.)
2. *Waste material transport.* The interstitial fluid that enters lymphatic capillaries contains some of the cellular waste materials that will be carried to the blood in lymph and eventually be eliminated.
3. *Filtration of lymph.* Interstitial fluid that enters the lymphatic capillaries also contains microorganisms, cellular debris, and other foreign matter that has to be removed from lymph before it enters the bloodstream. This will happen as the lymph passes through lymph nodes.
4. *Protein transport.* Some large proteins, especially enzymes, are transported in lymph to blood from their cells of origin. These proteins are too large to enter the venous circulation directly. Lymph has the ability to pick up larger protein molecules than the venous capillaries and deposit them into circulation.

LYMPHATIC STRUCTURES

Lymph Nodes

Lymph nodes are sometimes called *lymph glands,* but they are not true glands. They are small, kidney-shaped structures located at various points along the lymph vessels. Lymph vessels drain fluid from specific areas of the body much like veins return blood to the heart from specific areas of the body. Therefore the lymph from a specific area always passes through the same lymph nodes.

Lymph nodes are covered with a connective tissue capsule that sends branches (trabeculae) into the body of the lymph

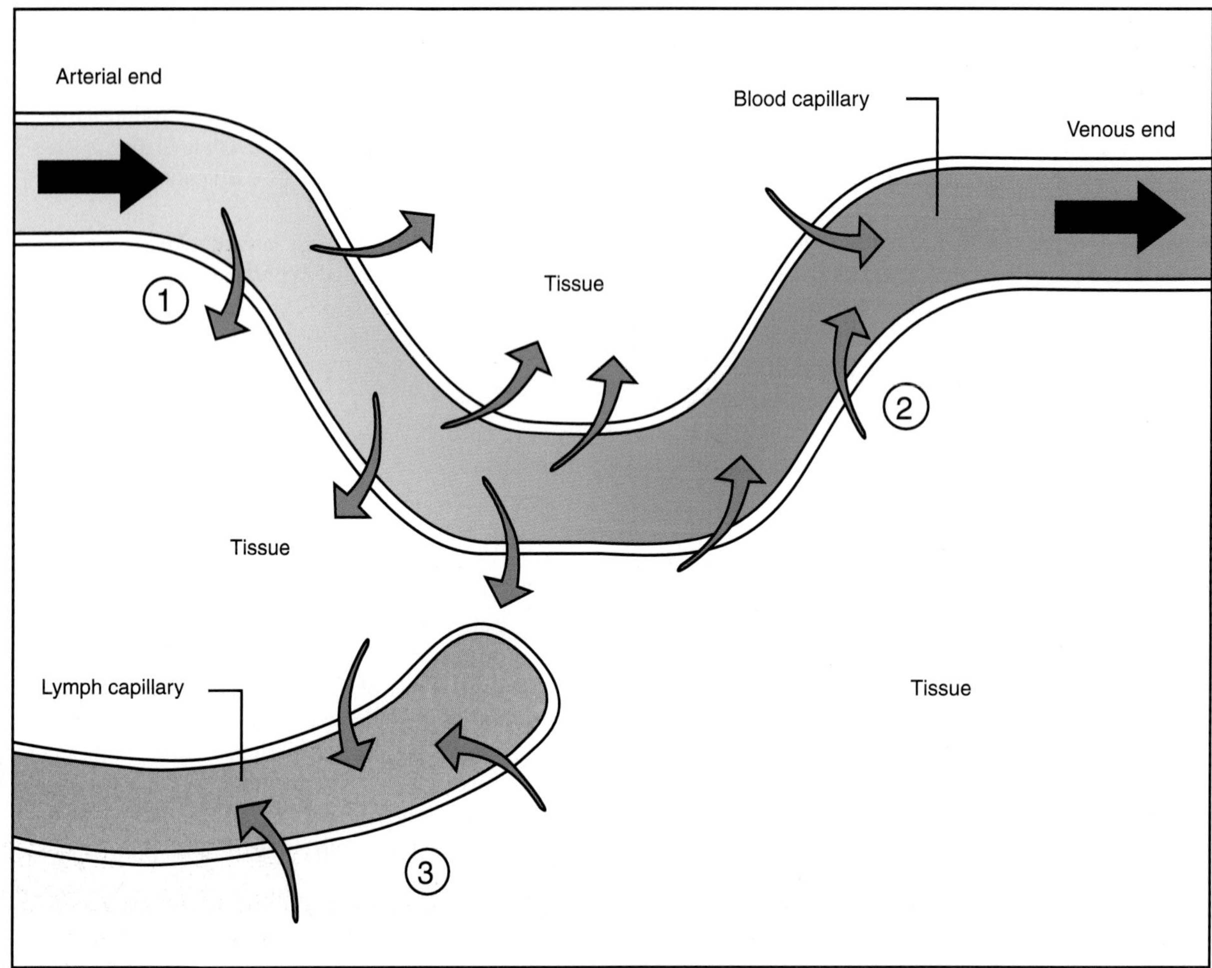

FIGURE **9-9** **Formation of Lymph.** *1,* Blood pressure forces plasma out into tissues. *2,* Osmotic pressure draws some of tissue fluid back into capillary, but not all of it. *3,* Blind-ended lymph capillary picks up excess tissue fluid and carries it off into progressively larger lymph vessels that eventually return it to bloodstream.

node. Lymph flows into the node in afferent (toward the lymph node) vessels that empty just beneath the capsule. It leaves the lymph node in efferent (away from the lymph node) vessels that exit the lymph node in the indented hilus area.

Microscopically a lymph node is divided into a cortex and a medulla. The cortex is where the lymphocytes reside. The lymphocytes are clustered in groups called *lymph nodules* that are located around the periphery of the node. The medulla forms the skeleton of the lymph node and contains many tissue macrophages embedded in a coarse, fibrous mesh. It fills the center of the node and surrounds the lymph nodules (Figure 9-10). Lymph nodes in pigs have a reversed anatomy in that the lymph nodules are at the center of the node.

On its way to the thoracic ducts, lymph will pass through at least one lymph node that will put lymphocytes or substances they produce into the lymph. As the lymph passes through the node, tissue macrophages act as filters to remove microorganisms or other foreign matter (e.g., cancerous cells that break off a tumor and are picked up by the lymphatic capillaries) in an attempt to prevent the spread of disease or cancer. If the first lymph node cannot remove all of the foreign matter, the next one along the lymph vessel will try, and so on. Therefore, when some forms of cancerous tumors are removed, a number of regional lymph nodes are also removed. By examining the lymph nodes microscopically a pathologist can determine if the cancer has moved to the regional lymph nodes and how far along the chain of lymph nodes the cancer has spread.

Spleen

The spleen is a fairly large organ that has both lymphatic and hematological (blood-related) functions. It is somewhat "tongue" shaped and is located on the left side of the abdomen. It is near the stomach in simple-stomached animals and near the rumen in ruminants. The spleen is the largest lymphoid organ in the body and is covered with a capsule made of fibrous connective tissue and smooth muscle. The capsule sends branches (trabeculae) into the soft tissue of the spleen. The trabeculae contain blood vessels, nerves, lymph vessels,

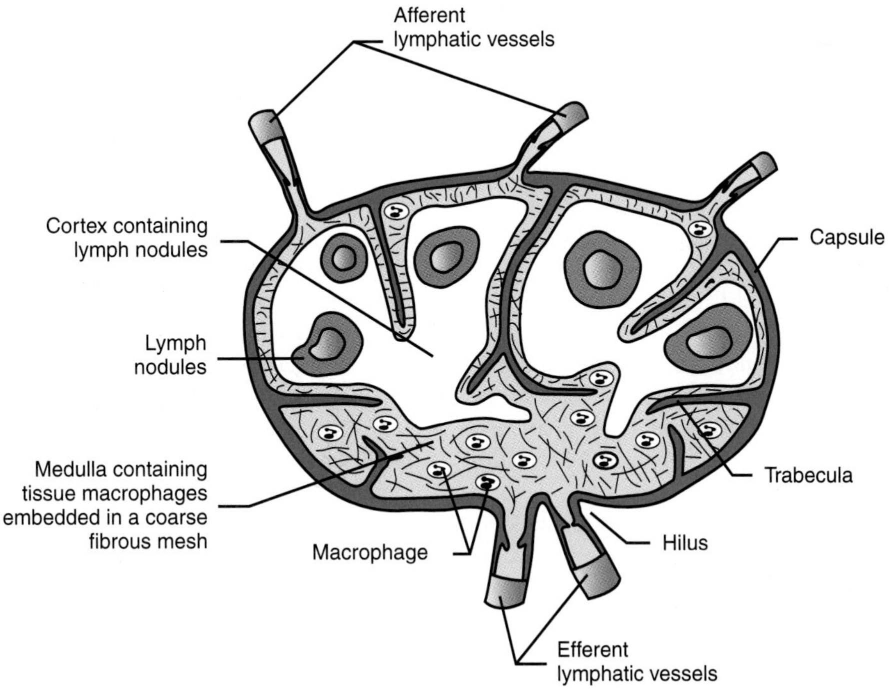

FIGURE **9-10** **Lymph Node.**

and smooth muscle cells. In carnivores the trabeculae are very muscular. In ruminants they are less muscular. When the smooth muscle cells contract, they squeeze blood out of the spleen and back into circulation. Because carnivores have more muscular branches, they can squeeze more blood out of the spleen.

The soft tissue interior of the spleen is divided into areas called **white pulp** and **red pulp** (Figure 9-11). The white pulp, which consists of localized areas of lymphoid tissue, is grossly visible. The lymphocytes that live here can clone themselves during an immune response (this topic is discussed later in more detail).

The red pulp consists of blood vessels, tissue macrophages, and blood storage spaces (sinuses). The spleen acts as a reservoir for blood when the animal is at rest and does not need large amounts of oxygen and other substances going to its muscles. When the spleen reservoir is full, the storage spaces are filled with blood and the spleen gets larger. When the body needs those "excess" blood cells (e.g., for exercising), the trabeculae contract, the blood is squeezed back into circulation, and the spleen gets smaller.

The functions of the spleen are as follows:

1. *Blood storage* in the red pulp
2. *Removal of foreign material* from circulation by the tissue macrophages in the red pulp
3. *Removal of dead, dying, and abnormal RBCs* by the tissue macrophages in the red pulp
4. *Lymphocyte cloning* in the white pulp during an immune response

CLINICAL APPLICATION — Swollen Lymph Nodes

If an infection is present in some part of the body, the causative microorganism may be picked up by a lymph vessel and carried to a lymph node. As the lymph passes through the lymph node, the macrophages attempt to remove the microorganisms. As the macrophages become more active, the lymph node becomes larger as a result of the multiplication of lymphocytes and the arrival of more macrophages. Some lymph nodes are located close to the surface of the body and can be palpated (felt) through the skin. If they are responding to an infection in their drainage area, they become larger and are more readily palpated. These enlarged lymph nodes can be used as a clue to the location of an infection if they are enlarged. You may be familiar with the mandibular lymph nodes located just behind each side of your jaw in your neck region. They are the "glands" that swell when you have a cold. The mandibular lymph nodes drain the nasal cavity, mouth, and pharynx.

The spleen is not essential for the life of an animal and can be surgically removed (splenectomy) if necessary. Trauma resulting in splenic rupture and splenic tumors is the most common reason for performing a splenectomy. After the surgery, tissue macrophages and lymphoid tissue in other areas of the body pick up the spleen's duties.

Thymus

The thymus is a lymphoid organ located in the caudal neck and cranial thoracic region lying on either side of the trachea. It is most prominent in young animals and shrinks as the animal matures. In adult animals it is usually difficult to find. The thymus is classified as a central lymphoid organ because it is here that T lymphocytes are processed before being distributed throughout the body in peripheral lymphoid tissues. Thymic function is most important in young animals because they are born without much of an immune system. The thymus helps "kick start" the normal development of the immune system.

Tonsils

Tonsils are nodules of lymphoid tissue in an epithelial surface that are not covered with a capsule. They are found all over the body, but we are most familiar with the ones in the pharyngeal (throat) region. Here they function to prevent the spread of infection into the respiratory or digestive systems.

Tonsils are classified as peripheral lymphoid tissue in which mature lymphocytes live. They are most prominent in young animals as they are developing their immune systems. Tonsils differ from lymph nodes in the following ways:

- Tonsils are found close to moist epithelial (mucosal) surfaces.
- Tonsils do not have a capsule.
- Tonsils are found at the beginning of the lymph drainage system and not along the lymph vessels like lymph nodes.

Other tonsils are found in the larynx, intestine, prepuce, and vagina.

Gut-Associated Lymph Tissue

GALT generally refers to lymphoid tissue found in the lining of the intestine. Over 25% of the intestinal mucosa and submucosa is composed of lymphoid tissue, making it the largest lymphoid organ in the body. If all the GALT were organized into a single organ contained within a capsule, it would be much larger than the spleen.

The GALT is often compared with the bursa of Fabricius in birds, in which B lymphocytes are processed before being sent to peripheral lymphoid tissue. For this reason, GALT is classified as central lymphoid tissue. It also functions as peripheral lymphoid tissue because of the many lymphocytes that it contains.

TEST YOURSELF

1. How does lymph differ from plasma?
2. Where is lymph formed?
3. What is the function of a lymph node?
4. Which lymphatic structure (organ) is composed of white pulp and red pulp?
5. Which lymphatic structure (organ) is large at birth and gradually gets smaller as the animal matures?
6. Where is the GALT located?

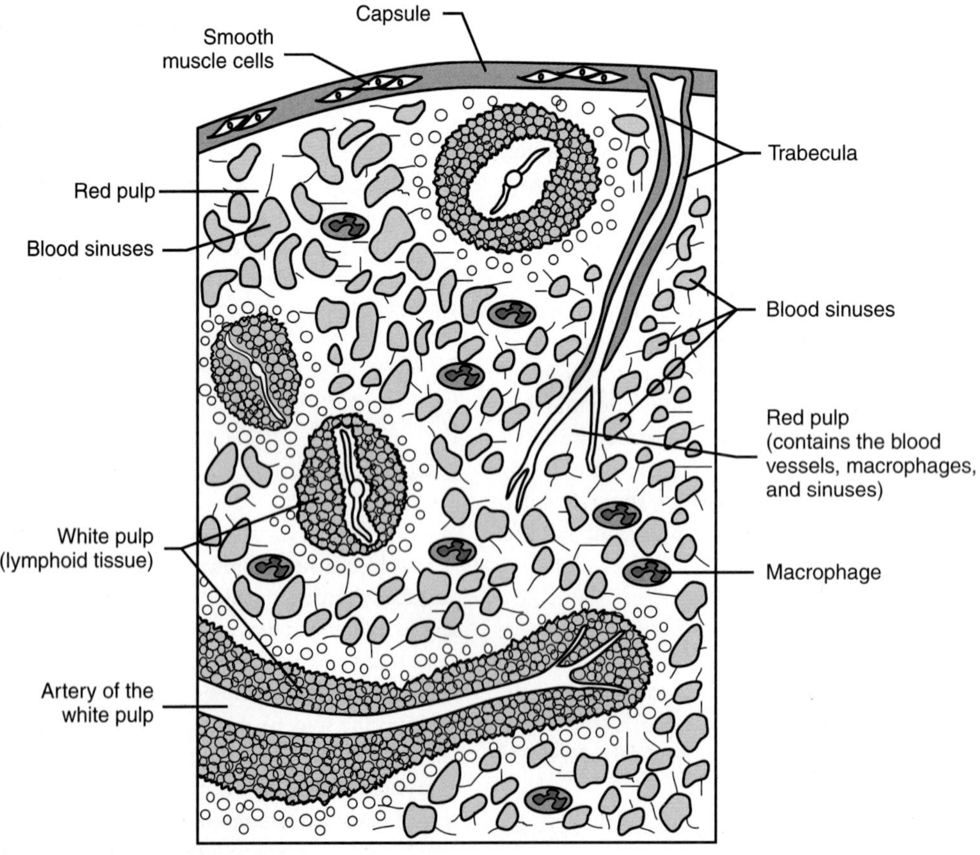

FIGURE **9-11** **Spleen.**

THE IMMUNE SYSTEM

FUNCTION

The function of the immune system is to protect the animal from anything that could cause disease or damage in the animal. It does this by recognizing and differentiating between "self" and "foreign invaders" known as *antigens* that threaten the health of an animal. The immune system can detect these antigens (e.g., microorganisms, foreign material, chemical substances) that are "not self" and employ various mechanisms to destroy them. These mechanisms include the following:

- Phagocytosis and destruction of foreign cells
- Lysis of foreign cell membranes
- Inactivation of pathogenic organisms or chemical substances
- Precipitation or clumping **(agglutination)** of cells or molecules

On occasion the immune response to antigens can go beyond being just protective and result in massive tissue damage. When this happens an immune-mediated disease results. **Anaphylaxis** (an allergic response that is often life threatening) is an example of an immune-mediated disease.

As long as the immune system is functioning in a normal protective manner, an animal is likely to remain healthy. If the immune system breaks down or is overpowered, the animal will get sick.

IMMUNE REACTIONS

Nonspecific Immunity

Nonspecific immunity involves the tissues, cells, and processes that protect an animal against anything it recognizes as foreign. Nonspecific immunity involves the following:

- Protective barrier of the skin and mucous membranes that prevent antigens from entering the body
- Inflammation (reaction of the body to tissue damage)
- Phagocytosis (neutrophils, monocytes, and tissue macrophages)

> **CLINICAL APPLICATION — Autoimmune Diseases**
>
> In some instances the immune system malfunctions and starts seeing "self" as "not self." In other words, the antigen is part of the animal's own body and not foreign to it. This results in a classification of diseases known as **autoimmune diseases.** For example, autoimmune hemolytic anemia is an autoimmune disease in which the animal starts producing antibodies against its own RBCs. The antibodies cling to the RBC membranes and cause the cells to clump together (agglutination). These clumps of cells are detected by the tissue macrophages in the spleen, removed by them, and destroyed. If enough RBCs are removed in this way, the animal will become anemic.

- NK cells (see earlier discussion on lymphocytes)
- **Interferon:** a protein produced by a cell after it has been infected by a virus that inhibits further development and spread of the virus
- **Complement:** a group of inactive enzymes in plasma that can be activated to rupture the cell membrane of a foreign cell

A nonspecific immune response is immediate (barriers provided by skin and mucous membranes) or rapid (phagocytosis, inflammation). The nonspecific immune response is a generalized response. It does not initiate a specific type of response against a specific antigen.

Specific Immunity

Specific immunity involves unique reactions aimed at destroying specific antigens. The immune system's response to a specific antigen is initiated as a reaction to proteins on the invading cell's wall that are the antigenic structures. Every type of microorganism has an antigenic structure that is unique to that type of microorganism. For example, all bovine virus diarrhea viruses have the identical antigenic structure on their surfaces. The antigenic structure is different than the antigenic structure on the surface of the canine distemper virus.

The specific immune response involves primarily lymphocytes, but in some instances this depends on the actions of other cells for activation.

Two types of specific immunity are cell-mediated immunity and humoral immunity (Table 9-3). Three properties of a specific immune response are constant regardless of which type of specific immune response is initiated:

1. The response will be initiated only after the antigen enters the body.
2. The response will be aimed specifically against the antigen present.
3. If the antigen enters the body a second time, a memory of the antigen causes the immune response to occur more quickly.

Cell-Mediated Immunity

Cell-mediated immunity is the function of T lymphocytes that attach to antigens on the surfaces of foreign cells. When T lymphocytes are processed in the thymus, they develop specific antigen receptors on their cell membranes. These receptors are unique for one antigen only, and each T lymphocyte has only one receptor on its cell membrane. After being processed in the thymus, the T lymphocytes travel via the blood to lymph nodes and the spleen.

The antigenic cells that are attacked by T lymphocytes are usually cells that have been invaded by viruses or are cancerous. They could also be cells that are part of transplanted tissues or organs. The antigen must be ingested by a macrophage and presented on the macrophage cell membrane before a T lymphocyte can attach to it.

When a T lymphocyte attaches to an antigen that fits its receptor site, it becomes an activated T lymphocyte that

Table 9-3 Humoral Immune Response vs. Cell-Mediated Immune Response

	Humoral Immune Response	Cell-Mediated Immune Response
Cell type involved	B lymphocyte that transforms into a plasma cell after antigenic stimulation	T lymphocyte that transforms into a cytotoxic T cell, helper T cell, or suppressor T cell after antigenic stimulation
Substance produced	Immunoglobulins (antibodies)	Lymphokines
Cellular mobility	B lymphocytes and plasma cells stay in lymphoid tissue; antibodies are released into plasma	T lymphocytes can enter circulation and travel to the site where an antigen entered the body
Memory cells produced?	Yes	Yes

undergoes many mitotic divisions to make numerous clones of itself. The clones travel to the site where the antigen entered the body to fight more of the same antigen. These cloned, activated T lymphocytes develop into the following three distinct populations of T lymphocytes:

1. **Cytotoxic T cells:** These cells are also known as *killer cells* or *killer T lymphocytes.* They attach to the antigenic cells and destroy them, but they are not themselves damaged.
2. **Helper T cells:** These are the most numerous of the T lymphocytes. They help the immune response by secreting substances known as *lymphokines* (sometimes called *cytokines*) into the surrounding tissue. There are many different lymphokines with many different functions. Some of these lymphokines and their functions are as follows:
    - The lymphokine that increases activation of B lymphocytes, cytotoxic T cells, and suppressor T cells
    - Interleukin 2 (IL-2): a lymphokine that stimulates the activity of other T lymphocytes
    - Macrophage migration factor: a lymphokine that attracts macrophages to the area via chemotaxis and activates them to accelerate the rate of phagocytosis. This will result in more antigens on the macrophage surfaces being presented to cytotoxic T cells.
3. **Suppressor T cells:** These cells inhibit functions of helper T cell and cytotoxic T cell by negative feedback. They also prevent B lymphocytes from transforming into plasma cells. These antagonistic actions provide a certain degree of control over the cell-mediated and humoral immune responses.

T lymphocytes leave the lymphoid tissue and recirculate through blood and lymph. B lymphocytes usually stay in lymphoid tissue and send out antibodies that are found in blood and lymph. Therefore most of the lymphocytes found in peripheral blood are T lymphocytes. However, B lymphocytes and T lymphocytes appear identical when seen on a stained blood smear; so no attempt is made to differentiate them.

Humoral Immunity

Humoral immunity is the function of B lymphocytes that transform into plasma cells and produce specific protective proteins called *antibodies* against specific antigens. When a B lymphocyte is being processed in bone marrow or GALT, it makes one specific antibody that it places in its cell membrane. This antibody has a unique shape that allows it to combine only with an antigen with the corresponding unique shape. In this way they fit together like two pieces of a jigsaw puzzle. When this specific antigen comes in contact with the antibody (in the cell membrane of the B lymphocyte) that fits its unique shape, they combine to form an antigen-antibody complex that activates the B lymphocyte. When a B lymphocyte becomes an activated B lymphocyte, it divides many times, making numerous clones of itself. These clones in turn transform into plasma cells that will produce more of the specific antibody molecules initially produced by the B lymphocyte. Plasma cells secrete the antibody molecules into plasma instead of placing them in their cell membrane. These antibodies will seek out and destroy more of the same antigen. When the antibody attaches to the antigen, several effects can result, such as the following:

- Antigens in the form of toxins that destroy cells are transformed into harmless substances.
- Antigens are agglutinated or stuck together to make large clumps that are phagocytized by macrophages.
- The antibody can change shape in a way that will activate the complement system in plasma. The group of plasma protein enzymes that make up the complement system will eventually rupture the membrane of the foreign cell.

Antibodies. An **antibody** is also known as an *immunoglobulin (Ig).* Five types of immunoglobulins that have been identified are IgG, IgM, IgA, IgE, and IgD.

- **IgG** is made during the first exposure to an antigen. It is also the first immunoglobulin made by newborns. Production of IgG is relatively slow; so the animal may become sick before the immune response can conquer the antigen.
- **IgM** is made when the animal has been exposed to an antigen for a long time or when the animal is exposed to

the antigen for the second time. The production of IgM is more rapid than the production of IgG; so the antigen may be conquered before the animal gets sick.

- **IgA** can leave blood and enter tissue fluids. It plays an important role in preventing diseases caused by antigens that may enter the body through mucosal surfaces (e.g., intestinal tract and lungs).
- **IgE** is associated with an allergic response.
- **IgD** function is unknown.

Memory Cells. When either T lymphocytes or B lymphocytes are activated to start cloning themselves, some of the cloned lymphocytes do not immediately become actively involved in the immune response. Instead, they become **memory cells.** Memory cells either circulate in blood or stay in the lymph nodes to wait for a second infection of the antigen that initially caused their formation. When that happens the memory cells mount an immune response more rapidly than with the first exposure to the antigen. Some memory cells live a few days, whereas others can live for years.

IMMUNIZATION: PROTECTION AGAINST DISEASE

Active Immunity

When an animal is exposed to an antigen for the first time, it commonly shows signs of illness before the immune system can destroy the foreign invader. The initial immune response is slow, but eventually the animal recovers. Memory T or B lymphocytes are produced as a result of this initialimmune reaction. The next time the animal is exposed to that same antigen, the immune response will occur more rapidly and probably prevent the animal from getting sick.

Animals can be protected against some diseases by activating their immune systems with vaccines. Vaccines contain modified antigens that initiate an immune response without causing the disease. This initial immune response produces memory T lymphocytes or B lymphocytes just as if the animal had been naturally infected with the **virulent** (disease-producing) antigen. When the animal is exposed to the virulent form of the same antigen that was modified in the vaccine, the memory cells initiate an immune response so quickly that the animal does not have time to get sick. Some vaccines provide protection for the life of the animal, whereas other vaccines must be periodically "boostered" to provide continuous protection.

Passive Immunity

Passive immunity involves administering preformed antibodies that were not produced by the animal's own immune system. For example, a newborn's immune system is so poorly developed that it needs the protection of antibodies from its mother for protection until it can start making its own. Antibodies produced by a mother can be passed to a fetus through the placenta (transplacentally) in some species so that the baby has some protective immunity when born. Another form of protection comes through ingestion of **colostrum.** Colostrum is the antibody-rich first milk that a mother produces at the end of her pregnancy. If a newborn is allowed to nurse immediately after birth, it will ingest and absorb these antibodies and acquire another form of passive immunity. When the newborn's immune system is fully functional, it can be vaccinated to develop an **active immunity.** Therefore we have to wait until newborns reach a certain age (the age varies with the species of animal, the pathogen involved, and type of vaccine) before we can vaccinate them. We often give a series of vaccinations in young animals because we cannot easily tell when the passive immunity from the mother has worn off sufficiently for the animal to produce its own active immunity.

Some diseases progress so rapidly that they become life threatening before the animal's immune system can respond. In these cases, antibodies that were made by another animal can be given to the sick animal in an attempt to destroy the foreign invader. For example, animals that have not been immunized against tetanus can become acutely ill if they are exposed to the toxins produced by the bacteria that cause tetanus. Administration of tetanus antitoxin that contains antibodies against the tetanus toxins can save the animal's life.

If an animal receives passive immunity, its own immune system is not activated; therefore no memory cells are produced, and the animal is not protected against future infections. For this reason, active immunity is more protective in the long run than passive immunity.

TEST YOURSELF

1. Where do plasma cells come from and what is their function?
2. How does cell-mediated immunity differ from humoral immunity?
3. How do vaccines protect an animal from developing clinical signs of a disease?
4. What is the function of memory cells?
5. Why are young animals initially given a series of vaccinations to establish immunity against a disease?

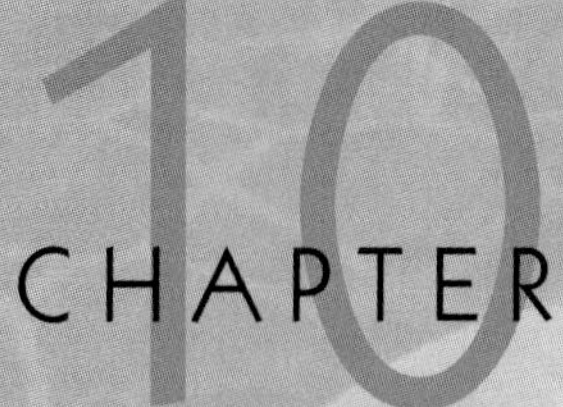

CHAPTER 10

THE RESPIRATORY SYSTEM

Thomas Colville

What do you think of when you hear the term *respiration*? Do you imagine the process of breathing—drawing air into the lungs and blowing it back out? That is certainly an important part of respiration, but it is only one component of the whole, complex process. In simplest terms, the main job of the respiratory system is to bring oxygen (O_2) into the body and carry carbon dioxide (CO_2) out of it. The body's cells need a constant supply of oxygen to burn nutrients to produce energy. Carbon dioxide is a waste product of these energy-producing reactions and has to be eliminated. In a simple, single-celled animal, these gases are exchanged between the interior of the cell and the outside environment directly through the cell membrane. In a complex animal such as a horse or dog, most of the body's cells are located too far from the outside world for that simple system to work. Regardless, oxygen somehow has to get into all of the body's cells, and carbon dioxide has to be taken away from them. These vital processes are carried out by the respiratory system working together with the cardiovascular system.

Actually, two kinds of respiration are constantly going on in the body—**external respiration** and **internal respiration.** External respiration occurs in the lungs. It is the exchange of oxygen and carbon dioxide that takes place between the *air* inhaled into the lungs and the *blood* flowing through the pulmonary (lung) capillaries. Internal respiration, on the other hand, occurs all over the body. It is the exchange of oxygen and carbon dioxide between the *blood* in the capillaries all over the body (the systemic capillaries) and all of the *cells and tissues* of the body. Internal respiration is the real "business end" of respiration. It is the means by which the body's cells receive the oxygen they need and get rid of their waste (carbon dioxide). Without external respiration, however, there would be no oxygen in the blood for the cells to absorb and no way for the cells to dump the carbon dioxide.

In this chapter, we concentrate on the organs and structures that contribute to external respiration. These are parts of what we call the respiratory system—the lungs and the complex system of tubes that connect them with the outside world. Box 10-1 lists the main components of the respiratory system in order from outside in.

In addition to its primary function of swapping oxygen for carbon dioxide, the respiratory system has some secondary functions that are also important to an animal's well-being. These include voice production, body temperature regulation, acid-base balance regulation, and the sense of smell.

- Voice production is also called **phonation.** The process usually begins in the larynx, or *voice box,* as it is commonly called. Two fibrous connective tissue bands called the **vocal cords** (also known as the **vocal folds**) stretch across the lumen of the larynx and vibrate as air passes over them. This produces the basic sound of the

Box 10-1 Main Structures of the Respiratory System

In order, from outside in, the main structures of the respiratory system are as follows:

UPPER RESPIRATORY TRACT
- Nostrils
- Nasal passages
- Pharynx
- Larynx
- Trachea

LOWER RESPIRATORY TRACT
- Bronchi
- Bronchioles
- Alveolar ducts
- Alveoli

animal's voice. Other structures, such as the thorax (chest cavity), nose, mouth, pharynx (throat), and sinuses may contribute resonance and other characteristics to the vocal sounds.

- Body temperature regulation involves many body systems, including the respiratory system. Under cold environmental conditions, the network of superficial blood vessels just under the epithelium of the nasal passages helps warm inhaled air before it reaches the lungs. (The location of these blood vessels is illustrated in Figure 10-2.) This helps prevent hypothermia (low body temperature) by avoiding chilling of the blood circulating through the lungs. Under hot environmental conditions, the respiratory system aids cooling in many animals by the mechanism of panting. The rapid respiratory movements of panting cause increased evaporation of fluid from the lining of the respiratory passages and mouth, which helps cool the blood circulating just beneath the epithelium.
- Acid-base balance is an important homeostatic mechanism in the body. For normal chemical reactions to occur in the cells, the relative acidity or alkalinity of their environment must be controlled carefully. The unit used to express relative acidity or alkalinity is **pH.** Literally, pH is a mathematical value representing the negative logarithm of the hydrogen ion concentration. More practically, pH is a number that tells us the relative acidity or alkalinity of something. The pH ranges from 0 to 14. The lower the pH number is, the more acidic the environment, and the higher the pH number, the more alkaline the environment. A pH of 7 is neutral, that is, neither acidic nor alkaline. The normal pH of the blood is 7.4, with an acceptable range of 7.35 to 7.45. A blood pH outside that narrow range spells danger for the animal's health. The respiratory system contributes to the process of acid-base control by its ability to influence the amount of CO_2 in the blood. The more CO_2 there is in the blood, the lower the blood pH and the more acidic the blood. (CO_2 dissolves in the plasma to form carbonic acid [H_2CO_3]). The respiratory system can alter the CO_2 content of the blood by adjusting how much and how fast the air is breathed in and out. We describe this process more completely in the section on the control of breathing.
- The sense of smell, also called the **olfactory sense,** is very important to many animals. The receptors for the sense of smell are contained in patches of sensory epithelium located up high in the nasal passages. More information on the olfactory sense can be found in Chapter 13.

TEST YOURSELF

1. What is the primary function of the respiratory system?
2. What are the secondary functions of the respiratory system?
3. What is the difference between internal respiration and external respiration? Which one occurs in the lungs?

STRUCTURE

Structurally, the respiratory system consists of the lungs and a system of tubes that connects them with the external environment. For this discussion, we classify all the respiratory structures outside the lungs as parts of the **upper respiratory tract** and all the structures within the lungs as parts of the **lower respiratory tract.**

UPPER RESPIRATORY TRACT

The upper portion of the respiratory tract includes the nose, the **pharynx** (throat), the **larynx** (voice box), and the **trachea** (windpipe) (Figure 10-1). All of the air that enters and leaves the lungs does so through the upper respiratory structures.

Nose

If we were air molecules being inhaled into the respiratory system of an animal, the nose would be the first respiratory structure we would encounter. It begins with the nostrils, which are also known as the **nares.** The nostrils are the external openings of the respiratory tube, and they lead into the **nasal passages.**

Nasal Passages. The nasal passages are located between the nostrils and the pharynx (throat). A midline wall called the **nasal septum** separates the left nasal passage from the right, and the hard and soft palates separate the nasal passages from the mouth.

The nasal passages are not just simple tubes. Their linings are convoluted and full of twists and turns because of the presence of the **turbinates.** Turbinates are thin, scroll-like bones covered with nasal epithelium that occupy most of the

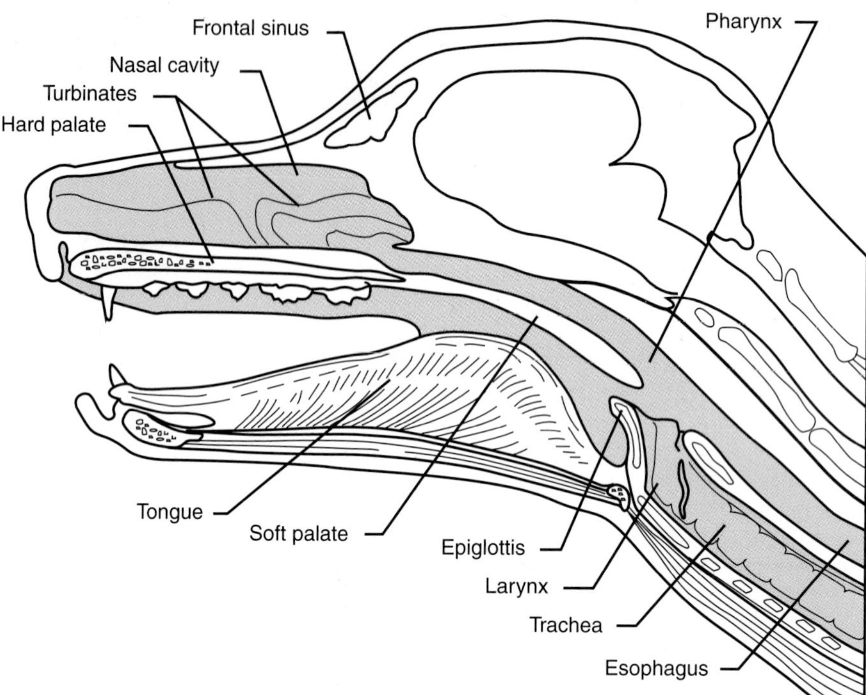

FIGURE **10-1** **Longitudinal Section of Canine Upper Respiratory Tract.**

lumen of the nasal passages. The two sets of scroll-like turbinates are found in each nasal passage: a dorsal turbinate and a ventral turbinate. They divide each nasal passage into three main passageways, each called a **nasal meatus.** (The word *meatus* means "passageway.") The ventral nasal meatus is located between the ventral turbinate and the floor of the nasal passage, the middle nasal meatus is located between the two turbinates, and the dorsal nasal meatus is located between the dorsal turbinate and the roof of the nasal passage. A small, fourth meatus, called the *common nasal meatus,* is located on either side of the nasal septum. It is continuous with the other three main nasal meatuses. See Chapter 5 for a more complete description of the turbinates.

The lining of the nasal passages is critical to their function and is illustrated in Figure 10-2. It consists of pseudostratified columnar epithelium with cilia projecting from the cell surfaces up into a layer of mucus that is secreted by many mucous glands and goblet cells. The cilia beat back toward the pharynx (throat). An extensive complex of large blood vessels lies just beneath the nasal epithelium.

Aside from housing the receptors for the sense of smell, the main function of the nasal passages is to "condition" the inhaled air that passes through them to protect the lungs. The three main conditioning roles performed by the nasal lining are warming, humidifying, and filtering the inhaled air. The scroll-like twists and turns of the turbinates tremendously increase the surface area of the nasal lining. They allow it to function as a combination radiator and humidifier. The air is warmed by the blood flowing through the complex of blood vessels just beneath the nasal epithelium and humidified by the mucus and other fluids that lie on the epithelial surface.

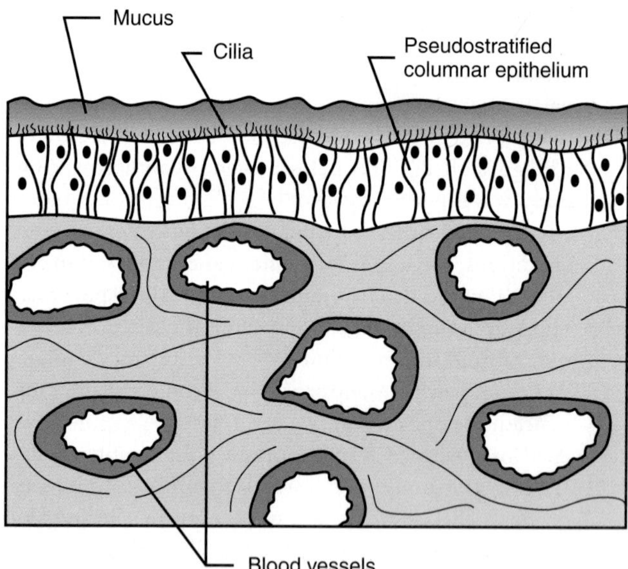

FIGURE **10-2** **Lining of Nasal Cavity.** Note cilia protruding up into overlying mucous layer and numerous large blood vessels immediately below the epithelium.

The filtering function of the nasal passages helps remove particulate matter, such as dust and pollen, from the inhaled air before it reaches the lungs. The filtering mechanism relies on the many twists and turns of the nasal passages produced by the turbinates, the mucous layer on the surface of the nasal epithelium, and the cilia that project up into it. Air easily passes along the tortuous path of the nasal lining as it is inhaled, but particles of dust and other debris do not negotiate the twists and turns as

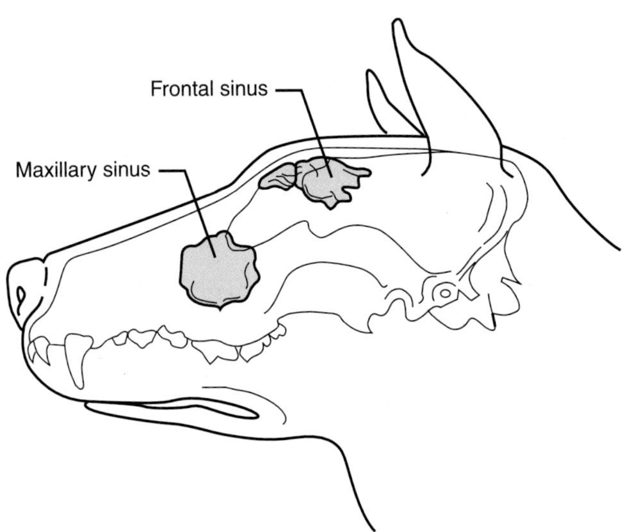

FIGURE **10-3** **Paranasal Sinuses of the Dog.**

readily and become trapped in the mucous layer. The beating of the cilia "sweeps" the mucus and the trapped foreign material back to the pharynx, where it is swallowed. One of the damaging effects of respiratory infections is that the swelling and thick inflammatory secretions "gum up" the cilia and prevent them from doing their sweeping job. Excess secretions can then build up on the epithelial surfaces, obstruct airflow, and stimulate coughing and sneezing.

Paranasal Sinuses. The **paranasal sinuses** are usually just called the **sinuses.** They are outpouchings of the nasal passages that are contained within spaces in certain skull bones. Each sinus is named after the skull bone that houses it. Most animals have two frontal sinuses and two maxillary sinuses within the frontal and maxillary bones, respectively. Figure 10-3 shows the locations of the frontal and maxillary sinuses of the dog. Some animals, including humans, have two more sinuses—the sphenoidal sinus and the ethmoidal sinus—located in the sphenoid and ethmoid bones. See Chapter 5 for more information on the skull bones that house paranasal sinuses.

The sinuses have the same kind of ciliated lining as the nasal passages. The cilia constantly sweep mucus produced in the sinuses down into the nasal passages. This sweeping action is important to prevent fluid and debris from accumulating in the sinuses and obstructing the openings into the nasal passages.

Pharynx

The nasal passages lead back to the pharynx, or what we commonly call the "throat." It is a common passageway for both the respiratory and digestive systems. At its rostral (front) end, the soft palate divides the pharynx into the dorsal nasopharynx (respiratory passageway) and the ventral oropharynx (digestive passageway). These lead back to the main part of the pharynx, which is common to both systems. At its caudal end the pharynx opens dorsally into the esophagus (digestive passageway) and ventrally into the larynx (respiratory passageway).

CLINICAL APPLICATION — Sinusitis

The sinuses can be clinically significant if they become inflamed and swollen as a result of allergies, infections, tumors, and so on. If the openings into the nasal passages swell shut or become plugged with inflammatory debris, fluids in the sinus have nowhere to go and the resulting buildup of pressure can be very painful for the animal. This condition is known as **sinusitis.** Sinusitis usually can be treated effectively with drugs, such as antibiotics to combat disease-causing microorganisms and decongestants to reduce the swelling in the lining of the sinus. However, in some severe cases, a hole must be surgically drilled into an inflamed sinus to allow fluid to drain from it.

Take a look at Figure 10-1 and note that the respiratory and digestive passageways switch places at the pharynx. The respiratory passageway (nasal passage) starts out *dorsal* to the digestive passageway (mouth) rostrally, but further caudally, the respiratory passageway (larynx) is *ventral* to the digestive passageway (esophagus). If you have ever wondered why it is so easy to choke if you try to swallow and breath or laugh at the same time, this is the reason.

Because it is a common passageway that must allow both breathing and swallowing, some delicate reflexes control the actions of the muscles around the pharynx. Breathing is easy. The pharynx just has to stay open to allow airflow. Swallowing is the tricky part. As discussed next, the larynx and the pharynx work together to prevent swallowing from interfering with breathing and vice versa. This is one of those spots in the body where timing is everything. The seemingly simple act of swallowing actually involves a complex series of actions that stop the process of breathing, cover the opening into the larynx, move the material to be swallowed to the rear of the pharynx, open the esophagus, and move the material into it. Once swallowing is complete, the opening of the larynx is uncovered and breathing resumes. It is no wonder that things occasionally don't work quite right and choking results.

Larynx

The larynx is what we commonly call the "voice box." It is a short, irregular tube that connects the pharynx with the trachea. It is made up mainly of segments of cartilage that are connected to each other and the surrounding tissues by muscles. The larynx is supported in place by the hyoid bone.

The pattern of the cartilage components of the larynx, as well as their number, varies among species. The major cartilages in the common animal species are the single **epiglottis,** the paired **arytenoid cartilages,** the single **thyroid cartilage,** and the single **cricoid cartilage.** Of these, the epiglottis and the arytenoid cartilages are most commonly of clinical importance.

The somewhat leaf-shaped epiglottis is the most rostral of the laryngeal cartilages. It projects forward from the ventral portion of the larynx, and its bluntly pointed tip is usually tucked up behind the caudal rim of the soft palate when the

CLINICAL APPLICATION: Endotracheal Intubation

Endotracheal intubation is a common clinical procedure in which a soft rubber or plastic tube, called an **endotracheal (ET) tube,** is inserted through the glottis and advanced down into the trachea. Its purpose is to provide an open airway, usually for the administration of an inhalant anesthetic, or to allow effective artificial ventilation.

Techniques for passing ET tubes vary among species. In horses and cattle, species with long heads and soft palates, endotracheal intubation is often done blindly. The unconscious animal's head and neck are extended to give a straighter path into the larynx, and the ET tube is lubricated and gently inserted into the animal's mouth. It is then slowly advanced until it passes through the glottis and into the trachea. The long, soft palate forces the tip of the tube ventrally; so it usually enters the glottis on the first try.

The soft palates of dogs and cats are generally too short for the blind technique to work. They are usually intubated with the help of an instrument called a **laryngoscope.** A laryngoscope consists of a battery-containing handle to which is attached a long, narrow blade with a small light source near the end of it. With the animal's head and neck extended, the laryngoscope blade is introduced into the mouth and advanced caudally until the epiglottis is identified. The tip of the laryngoscope blade is used to gently press the tip of the epiglottis ventrally. Once the epiglottis is out of the way, the arytenoid cartilages can be seen forming the entrance into the glottis. The tip of the lubricated ET tube is directed between the cartilages and down into the trachea. If the ET tube has an inflatable cuff (to provide a leakproof seal), the cuff is positioned just beyond the larynx to avoid passing the tube too far down into the trachea. If an ET tube is inserted too far, its tip can enter one of the two main bronchi. This can cause the other lung to collapse because it does not receive any air.

In dogs, endotracheal intubation is usually just that simple. They generally have large larynxes that are easy to pass ET tubes into. Cats, however, usually have more sensitive larynxes. As soon as an ET tube touches any part of the glottis, it typically slams shut—a condition called **laryngospasm.** The purpose of this reflex is to prevent anything but air from entering the larynx. The way to get the tube through the sensitive opening is either to time the insertion of the tube for when the opening is of maximum size during expiration or to spray a small amount of local anesthetic on the glottis. This numbs the surfaces and temporarily eliminates the protective reflex.

CLINICAL APPLICATION: Roaring in Horses

Roaring is the common name for **laryngeal hemiplegia,** a condition that is often seen in horses. *Hemi-* means "half," and *-plegia* means "paralysis"; therefore laryngeal hemiplegia literally means paralysis of half the larynx. Actually, it is a paralysis of the muscles that tighten the arytenoid cartilage and vocal cord on one side (usually the left for some reason) of the larynx. The result is that the affected vocal cord just "flaps in the wind" as the animal breathes. It usually does not cause any problems when the animal is at rest, but when the animal exercises and breathes heavily, the paralyzed vocal cord partially obstructs the glottis each time the animal inhales. This produces the characteristic "roaring" sound as the animal breathes and makes it difficult for the animal to get enough air. The lack of air causes the animal to tire quickly, thereby producing what is known as *exercise intolerance.*

The cause of roaring is a congenital (present at birth) degeneration of the left recurrent laryngeal nerve that supplies the muscles that tighten the left arytenoid cartilage. The cause of this degeneration is not known, but it may be an inheritable genetic defect. In other words, it may be a trait that can be passed on to offspring by affected parents.

The treatment of roaring usually requires surgery to stabilize the "loose" side of the larynx. The most common procedure is laryngeal ventriculectomy (removal of the lateral ventricle on the affected side). The purpose of the procedure is to produce enough scar tissue as the area heals to tighten the affected cartilage and vocal cord and hold it out of the airstream. It does not cure the condition, but it may lessen the severity of the clinical signs. More extensive (and expensive) surgical procedures are sometimes performed on affected high-value horses, such as racehorses.

animal is breathing. When the animal swallows, however, the epiglottis is pulled back to cover the opening of the larynx, much like a trapdoor being pulled shut. This keeps the swallowed material out of the larynx and helps direct it dorsally into the opening of the esophagus.

The vocal cords are attached to the two arytenoid cartilages. Muscles adjust the tension of the vocal cords by moving the cartilages. The arytenoid cartilages and the vocal cords form the boundaries of the **glottis** (the opening into the larynx).

In nonruminant animals a second set of connective tissue bands, called the **false vocal cords,** or **vestibular folds,** is present in the larynx in addition to the vocal cords. They are not involved in voice production. On each side of the larynx of these animals, blind "pouches" called the **lateral ventricles** project laterally in the space between the vocal cords and the vestibular folds. These lateral ventricles are often involved in the treatment of a condition in horses called **"roaring"** (see the Clinical Application on roaring).

Aside from its role as part of the upper airway, the larynx has three main functions: voice production, prevention of foreign material being inhaled, and control of airflow to and from the lungs.

As described earlier, the basic sound of an animal's voice originates from the vocal cords in the larynx. These two fibrous, connective tissue bands are attached to the arytenoid cartilages and stretch across the lumen of the larynx parallel to each other. As air passes over the taut vocal cords, they vibrate and produce sounds. The muscles that attach to the arytenoid cartilages control the tension of the vocal cords. They can adjust the tension from a state of complete relaxation, which opens the glottis wide and produces no sound, to a very tight condition that can completely close off the glottis and prevent airflow. Voice production requires a tension somewhere between these two extremes. In general, by lessening the tension of the vocal cords, lower-pitched sounds are made, and by tightening them, higher pitched sounds result.

The larynx also helps keep foreign material from entering the trachea and passing down into the lungs. This is accom-

CLINICAL APPLICATION Aspiration Pneumonia

Aspiration pneumonia is an inflammatory condition of the lungs produced by inhalation of foreign material. Common causes include oral liquids being administered too rapidly for an animal to swallow and inhalation of regurgitated material by an anesthetized animal. It is a much easier condition to prevent than to treat.

When large quantities of oral liquids are to be administered to an animal, care must be taken not to administer them faster than the animal can swallow. If the delivery rate is too rapid, the animal may inhale some of the fluid down into the lungs. The amount of damage caused depends on the quantity and the composition of the inhaled material. If the quantity is large or the material is irritating, the damage to the lungs can be considerable or even fatal.

An anesthetized animal must be protected from aspiration of foreign material because its swallowing reflex disappears as it becomes anesthetized. Anesthetized animals are often positioned horizontally with their heads at the same level as their stomachs; so it is easy for small amounts of stomach contents to be regurgitated up the esophagus into the pharynx. Without the protective swallowing reflex, the regurgitated material can be inhaled easily down into the lungs. The stomach contents are very acidic because of secretions from the stomach wall, so you can imagine how irritating that material can be to the delicate structures of the lungs. The biggest risk of aspiration in anesthetized animals is in those that do not have an ET tube in place. A proper size of ET tube effectively blocks foreign material from entering the larynx and trachea because it fills the lumen of the airway. Placement of ET tubes in anesthetized animals is always desirable to ensure an open airway and to prevent aspiration pneumonia. However, danger periods still arise even in animals that are intubated. During the periods just before the ET tube is inserted and just after it is removed, the animal is potentially vulnerable to aspiration of liquids from the mouth, throat, or stomach. We must monitor animals closely during these periods.

plished mainly by the trapdoor action of the epiglottis. Part of the process of swallowing consists of muscle contractions that pull the entire larynx forward and fold the epiglottis back over its opening. You can feel part of this process by putting your fingertips on your Adam's apple (the thyroid cartilage of your larynx) and swallowing. You can feel your Adam's apple move up as you swallow. This extremely effective process helps protect the delicate tissues of the trachea and lungs from trauma of inhaled foreign material.

The larynx controls airflow to and from the lungs partially through the trapdoor action of the epiglottis when swallowing occurs but also through adjustments in the size of the glottis. Small adjustments aid the movement of air as the animal draws air into its lungs and blows it out. At times, complete closure of the glottis is helpful. For example, the process of coughing starts with a closed glottis. To generate a cough, the glottis closes and the breathing muscles contract, compressing the thorax. This builds pressure behind the closed glottis. When the glottis suddenly opens, the forceful release of air that results is what we call a *cough*. The purpose of coughing is usually to clear mucus and other matter from the lower respiratory passages.

Closure of the glottis even aids nonrespiratory functions that involve "straining," such as urination, defecation, and parturition (the birth process). Straining begins with the animal holding the glottis closed while applying pressure to the thorax with the breathing muscles. This stabilizes the thorax and allows the abdominal muscles to effectively compress the abdominal organs when they contract. Without the closed glottis, contraction of the abdominal muscles merely forces air out of the lungs (exhalation).

TEST YOURSELF

1. By what mechanisms is inhaled air warmed, humidified, and filtered as it passes through the nasal passages? How do the turbinates aid these processes?
2. Describe how the respiratory and digestive passageways "switch places" in the pharynx.
3. How do the pharynx and larynx work together to keep swallowed material from entering the trachea? What role does the epiglottis play in that process?
4. How is the larynx involved in the straining process that aids functions such as defecation?

Trachea

The trachea, or windpipe, is a short, wide tube that extends from the larynx down through the neck region into the thorax, where it divides into the two main bronchi that enter the lungs. This division, called the **bifurcation of the trachea,** occurs at about the level of the base of the heart. Structurally, the trachea is a tube of fibrous tissue and smooth muscle held open by hyaline cartilage rings and lined by the same kind of ciliated epithelium that is present in the nasal passages. It is shaped like an upside-down Y. The main part of the trachea forms the base of the Y, and the bifurcation forms the arms of the Y (the left and right main bronchi that enter the lungs).

If nothing held the trachea open, it would collapse each time the animal inhaled as a result of the partial vacuum created by the inhalation process. Incomplete rings of hyaline cartilage spaced along the length of the trachea prevent this collapse. Each tracheal ring is C shaped with the open part of the C facing dorsally. The gap between the ends of each ring is bridged by smooth muscle (Figure 10-4).

The ciliated lining of the trachea is similar to that of the nasal passages. The mucous layer on its surface traps tiny particles of debris that have made it down this far into the respiratory tube. The cilia that project up into the mucous layer move the trapped material up toward the larynx. It eventually reaches the pharynx and is swallowed. If large amounts of debris are inhaled, such as might occur in a dusty environment, an increased amount of mucus is produced to help trap the foreign particles. The increased mucous accumu-

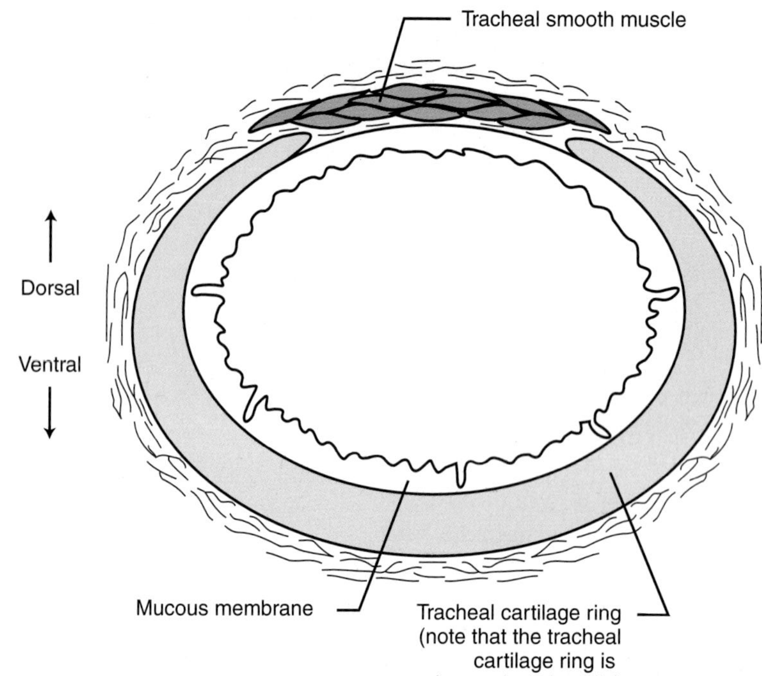

FIGURE **10-4** **Cross Section of Canine Trachea.** Note that tracheal cartilage ring is incomplete dorsally.

CLINICAL APPLICATION Tracheal Collapse

Tracheal collapse is a condition seen most commonly in toy and miniature breeds of dogs. The cause is unknown, but what happens is that the usually narrow space between the ends of several of the C-shaped tracheal rings is wider than normal. When the animal inhales, the widened area of smooth muscle gets sucked down into the lumen of the trachea and partially blocks it. This can cause a dry, honking cough and difficulty breathing (dyspnea). Because the soft tissue gets sucked down into the tracheal lumen mainly during inspiration, the breathing difficulty can be described as an *inspiratory dyspnea* (the animal has difficulty inhaling air). The clinical signs are often most severe when the animal is breathing hard from excitement or exercise. Affected animals are commonly overweight.

Therapy of tracheal collapse includes weight loss in obese animals, exercise restriction, reduction of excitement and stress, medical therapy to help control clinical signs, and surgical procedures that help hold the affected area of the trachea open.

lation irritates the lining of the trachea and stimulates coughing to help clear the passageway.

Lower Respiratory Tract

The lower respiratory tract starts with the **bronchi,** ends with the **alveoli,** and includes all the air passageways in between. Except for the two main bronchi that are formed by the bifurcation of the trachea, all the structures of the lower portion of the respiratory tract are located within the lungs.

Bronchial Tree

The air passageways that lead from the bronchi to the alveoli are often called the **bronchial tree** because they divide into smaller and smaller passageways much like the branching of a tree. Figure 10-5 gives an impression of the branching of the bronchial tree. If you imagine a bushy tree, the trunk represents the main bronchus that enters each lung. It divides into some fairly large branches, which divide into smaller and smaller branches that finally terminate in leaves. The leaves are the equivalent of the alveoli at the ends of the many branches of the bronchial tree.

After it enters the lung, each main bronchus divides into smaller bronchi, which divide into even smaller bronchi and, finally, the tiny **bronchioles.** The bronchioles continue to subdivide down to the smallest air passageways—the microscopic **alveolar ducts.** The alveolar ducts end in groups of alveoli arranged like bunches of grapes. These groups of alveoli are called **alveolar sacs** (Figures 10-5 and 10-6).

The air passageways that make up the bronchial tree are not just rigid tubes. The diameter of each one can be adjusted by smooth muscle fibers in its wall. The autonomic (unconscious) portion of the nervous system controls this smooth muscle. During times of intense physical activity, the bronchial smooth muscle relaxes, allowing the air passageways to dilate to their full, maximum diameters **(bronchodilation)** to help the respiratory effort move the greatest amount of air back and forth to the alveoli with each breath. At more relaxed times, fully dilated air passageways would actually create more physical work for the respiratory muscles to gently move air through. So, at rest, the bronchial smooth muscle partially contracts, reducing the size of the air passageways (partial **bronchocon-**

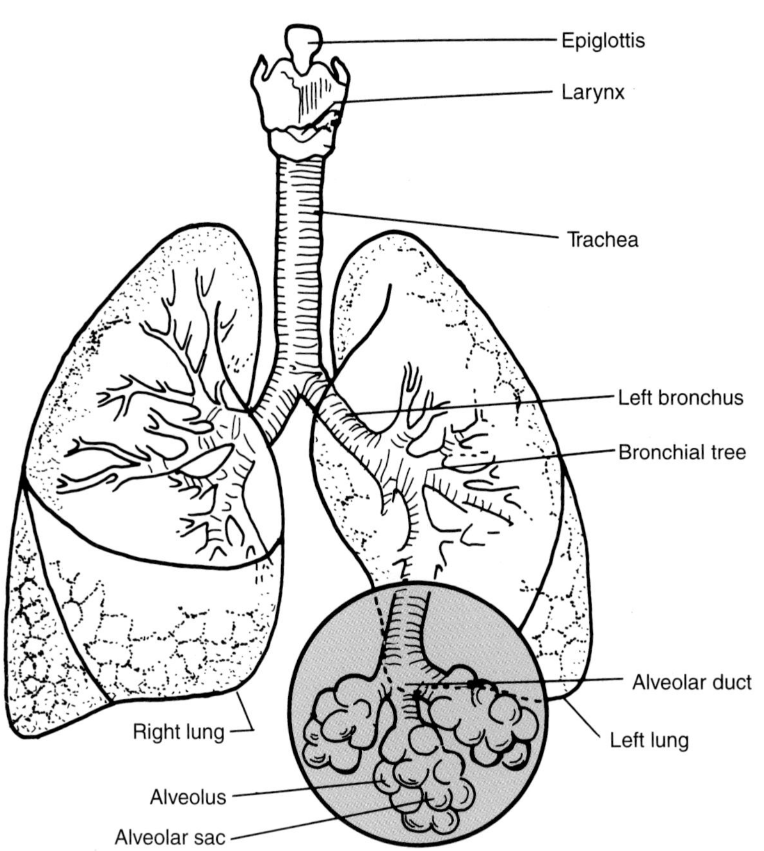

FIGURE **10-5 Lower Respiratory Tract.** (From McBride DF: *Learning veterinary terminology,* St Louis, 1996, Mosby.)

striction) to a more appropriate size. Sometimes irritants in inhaled air can stimulate severe bronchoconstriction. This can make it difficult for an animal to breathe (see the Clinical Application on asthma).

Alveoli

The alveoli are the "business end" of the respiratory system. They are where external respiration takes place, that is, where oxygen and carbon dioxide are exchanged between the blood and the air. The rest of the respiratory structures exist just to move air in and out of the alveoli.

Structurally, the alveoli are tiny, thin-walled sacs that are surrounded by networks of capillaries. Figure 10-6 shows the netlike arrangement of capillaries around alveoli. The wall of each alveolus is composed of the thinnest epithelium in the body—simple squamous epithelium. The capillaries that surround the alveoli are also composed of simple squamous epithelium. So the main physical barriers between the air in the alveoli and the blood in the capillaries are the very thin epithelium of the alveolus and the adjacent, equally thin epithelium of the capillaries. These two thin layers allow oxygen and carbon dioxide to freely diffuse back and forth between the air and the blood. We'll discuss how the movement of gases takes place shortly.

Each alveolus is lined with a thin layer of fluid that contains a substance called **surfactant.** Surfactant helps reduce the surface tension (the attraction of water molecules to each other) of the fluid. This prevents the alveoli from collapsing as air moves in and out during breathing.

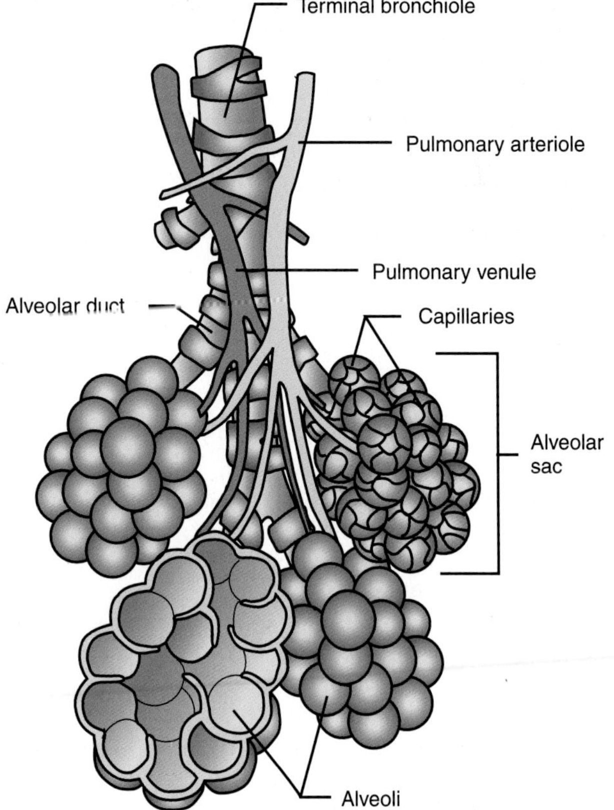

FIGURE **10-6 Alveoli and Alveolar Sacs.** Smallest terminal bronchioles divide into alveolar ducts that lead to clusters of alveoli called *alveolar sacs.*

LUNGS

The two lungs together form a shape that is somewhat like a cone. Each lung is described as having a base, an apex, and a convex lateral surface. The base of each lung is in the caudal part of the thoracic cavity and lies directly on the cranial surface of the **diaphragm** (the thin, domelike sheet of muscle that separates the thoracic cavity from the abdominal cavity). The apex of each lung is much narrower than the base and lies in the cranial portion of the thoracic cavity. Figure 10-7 shows this conelike shape. The convex lateral surface lies against the inner surface of the thoracic wall. The area between the lungs is called the *mediastinum*. It contains most of the rest of the thoracic contents, such as the heart, large blood vessels, nerves, the trachea, the esophagus, and lymphatic vessels and lymph nodes.

In most animals the lungs are divided into well-defined regions called **lobes.** These lobes are distinguished by the major branches of the bronchi rather than by externally visible grooves and clefts. The pattern of lung lobes is fairly consistent among the common domestic species. Cats, cattle, dogs, goats, pigs, and sheep all have the same basic arrangement of lung lobes. The left lung has two lobes: cranial and caudal. The right lung is divided into four lobes: cranial, middle, caudal, and a small accessory lobe. The horse is somewhat unique in that its lungs do not have lobes, except for the small accessory lobe on the right lung. Otherwise, the left and right lung each consists of just one large lobe (see Table 10-1 and Figure 10-7).

Each lung has a small, well-defined area on its medial side

Clinical Application: Asthma

Asthma is a disease that causes the bronchial tree to become overly sensitive to certain irritants. Exposure causes bronchoconstriction that can range from mild and annoying to severe and life threatening.

Asthma is seen less commonly in domestic animals than in humans. It occurs most often as an allergic condition in cats during the summer. Mild attacks can cause signs such as wheezing and coughing. More severely affected animals may show severe dyspnea (difficulty breathing), cyanosis (bluish color of the gums and lining of the eyelids), and frantic attempts to get air. Treatments include keeping affected cats indoors away from the offending allergens and administering medications to help prevent or treat the bronchoconstriction.

Clinical Application: Respiratory Tract Infections

Respiratory tract infections are common in all animals. However, a significant difference is noted between infections of the upper respiratory tract and infections of the lower respiratory tract.

An upper respiratory tract infection (URI) affects some combination of the nasal passages, pharynx, larynx, and trachea. Although they can be severe, URIs are generally less likely to be life threatening than infections of the lower respiratory tract. The main reason is the body's ability to drain excess mucus and inflammatory fluids away from infected areas in the upper respiratory tract. The body can cough up the fluids, which are either expelled through the nose or mouth or swallowed. This kind of moist cough actually accomplishes something beneficial and is referred to as a "productive" cough. We usually don't want to suppress a productive cough because it helps the animal.

A lower respiratory tract infection is usually called **bronchitis** or **pneumonia.** As its name implies, bronchitis affects the lining of the bronchial tree. Pneumonia involves the tiny bronchioles and alveoli. In either case, the animal's condition is often more severe than with a URI because inflammatory fluids tend to accumulate deep in the lungs in the small, dead-end air passageways. The fluids are more difficult to cough up, and so they often accumulate and obstruct airflow. Lower respiratory tract infections can be very serious and sometimes life threatening.

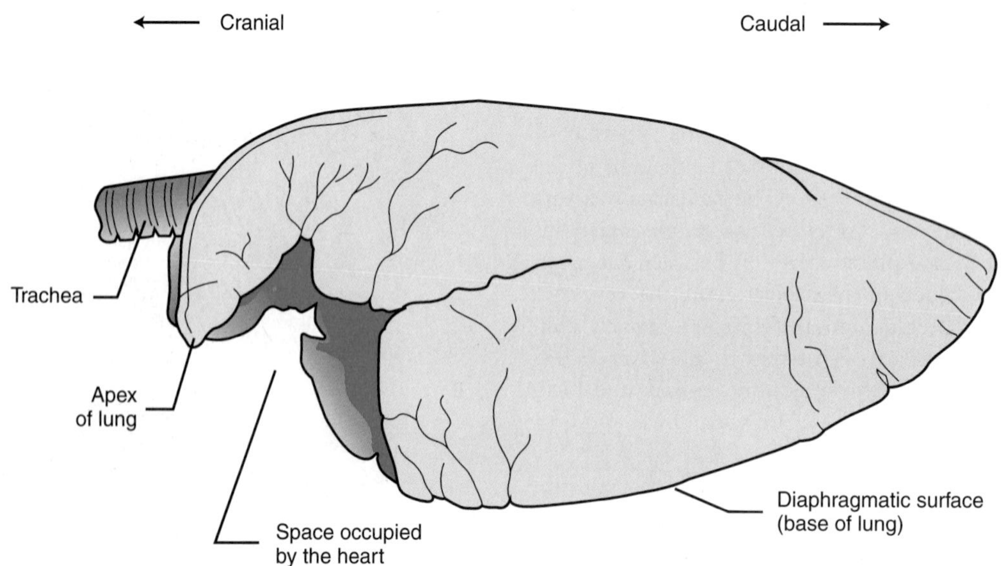

FIGURE **10-7** **Left Lateral View of Lungs of the Horse.**

called the **hilus.** This is where air, blood, lymph, and nerves enter and leave the lung, and it is the only area of the lung that is "fastened in place." The rest of the lung is free within the thorax. This physical arrangement is important to lung function and is discussed in more detail shortly.

The blood supply to and from the lungs is called the *pulmonary circulation.* (The term *pulmonary* refers to the lungs.) Blood enters the lungs through the pulmonary artery. The blood in this large blood vessel is dark red because it contains very little oxygen but a lot of carbon dioxide. It returns to the heart in the large systemic veins after delivering oxygen to the body's cells and picking up the carbon dioxide that was produced. This CO_2-rich blood enters the right side of the heart and is pumped out into the pulmonary artery by the right ventricle. The pulmonary artery splits into left and right pulmonary arteries that enter the two lungs. Within the lungs the blood vessels basically follow and subdivide along with the bronchi. Figure 10-6 shows the smallest pulmonary blood vessels as blood from pulmonary arterioles enters capillary networks around the alveoli. This is where it gets rid of its CO_2 and picks up O_2. Next it enters the pulmonary venules. The blood in the venules is bright red because of its high O_2 content and low CO_2 content. The venules join together into increasingly larger veins to eventually form the large pulmonary veins that leave each lung and enter the left side of the heart. From there this O_2-rich blood is pumped back out into the systemic circulation to supply the body's cells with oxygen and carry away their carbon dioxide.

Physically the lungs are very light with a spongy consistency. Before birth the lungs of a fetus are nonfunctional because the fetus floats in fluid as it develops. The structures of the lungs develop along with the rest of the fetus, but until birth, the alveoli do not expand into their saclike shapes. The fetal lungs have a solid consistency, much like liver. If a piece of lung from a fetus that has never breathed air is dropped into water, it will sink. Once an animal is born and takes its first breaths, the lungs expand and surfactant in the alveolar fluid prevents the expanded alveoli from collapsing again. In those first few moments after birth, the lungs of the breathing newborn change from a dense, solid consistency to the light, spongy consistency we usually associate with the lungs. If a piece of lung from an animal that has taken even one breath is dropped into water, it will float. This technique is sometimes used to determine whether a dead newborn animal was born alive and subsequently died or was born dead.

Table 10-1 Lung Lobes

Species	Left Lung	Right Lung
Cat, cow, dog, goat, pig, sheep	Cranial lobe Caudal lobe	Cranial lobe Middle lobe Caudal lobe Accessory lobe
Horse	All one lobe	All one lobe + accessory lobe

THORAX

The **thorax,** also known as the **thoracic cavity,** is the chest cavity. It is bound by the thoracic vertebrae dorsally, the ribs and intercostal muscles laterally, and the sternum ventrally. Its main contents include the lungs, the heart, large blood vessels, nerves, the trachea, the esophagus, and lymphatic vessels and lymph nodes. A thin membrane called the **pleura** covers the organs and structures in the thorax and lines the inside of the thoracic cavity. The membrane that covers the thoracic organs and structures is called the *visceral layer* of pleura, and the portion that lines the cavity is called the *parietal layer* of pleura. Between the two layers is a potential space that is filled with a small amount of lubricating fluid. The smooth surfaces of the pleural membranes lubricated with the pleural fluid ensure that the surfaces of the organs, particularly the lungs, slide along the lining of the thorax smoothly during breathing.

The **mediastinum** is the portion of the thorax between the lungs. It contains the heart and most of the other thoracic structures, including the trachea, esophagus, blood vessels, nerves and lymphatic structures. Figure 10-8 shows the posi-

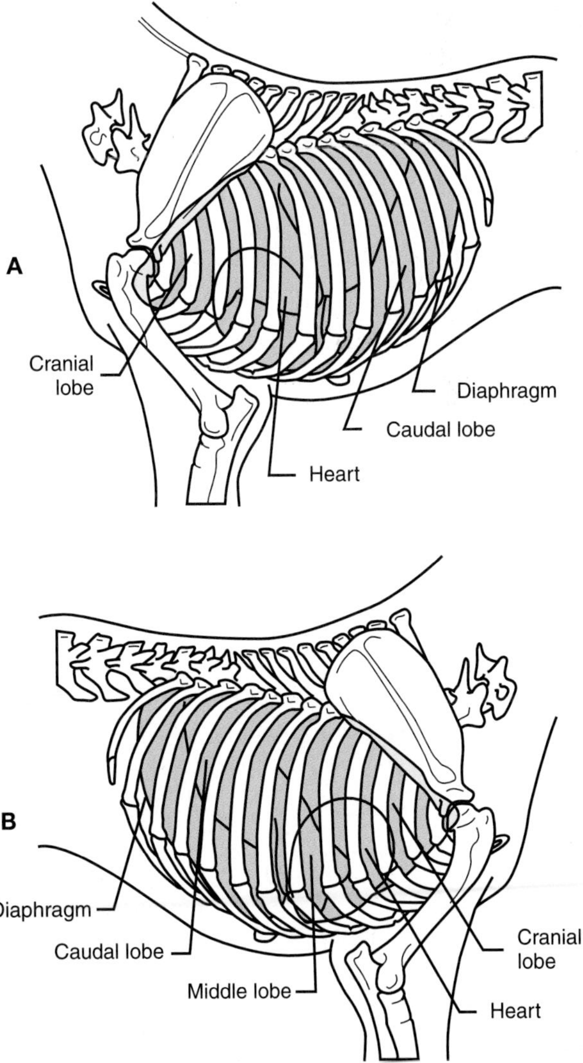

FIGURE **10-8** **Thoracic Organs of the Dog.** Note location of heart at the level of the elbow joint. **A,** Left side. **B,** Right side.

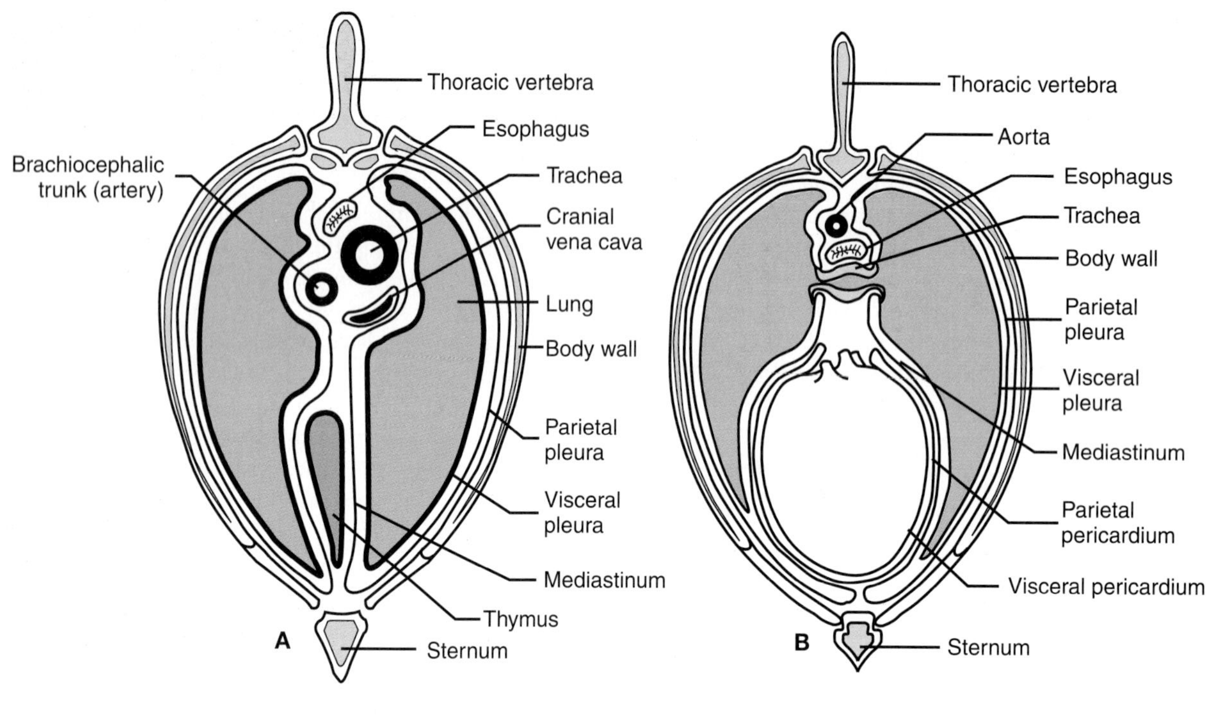

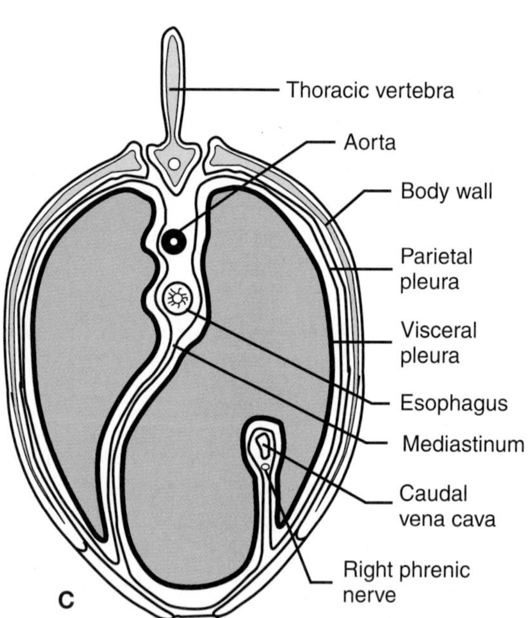

FIGURE **10-9** **Cross Sections of Thorax Showing Contents. A,** Section cranial to heart. **B,** Section through heart. **C,** Section caudal to heart.

tion of the heart in the thorax relative to the lungs. Figure 10-9 shows the contents of the thorax at three different cross-sectional levels. Note the relationship of the visceral and parietal layers of pleura and the differing contents of the mediastinum in different parts of the thorax.

The diaphragm is a thin sheet of skeletal muscle that forms the caudal boundary of the thorax and acts as an important respiratory muscle. In its relaxed state the diaphragm assumes a dome shape with its convex surface facing in a cranial direction. The bases of the lungs lie directly on the cranial surface of the diaphragmatic dome, and the liver lies just behind it. When the diaphragm contracts, its dome shape flattens out somewhat. This enlarges the volume of the thorax and helps accomplish the process of inspiration (inhalation).

TEST YOURSELF

1. Why are the hyaline cartilage rings important to the function of the trachea?
2. Describe the basic structure of the bronchial tree in the lung.
3. How do the physical characteristics of the alveoli and the capillaries that surround them facilitate the exchange of gases between the air in the alveoli and the blood in the capillaries?
4. What is the hilus of the lung and why is it important?
5. What is the *mediastinum* and what organs and structures are located there?
6. Which main pulmonary blood vessel contains bright red, high-oxygen blood: the pulmonary artery or the pulmonary vein?
7. When a piece of lung from a dead newborn animal is dropped into water, it sinks. What conclusion can be drawn about whether the newborn animal was born dead and never breathed or took some breaths before dying?
8. Why are the smooth pleural surfaces important to the process of breathing?

CLINICAL APPLICATION

Pneumothorax and Lung Collapse

Without negative intrathoracic pressure, breathing cannot take place. If air leaks into the pleural space (the space between the lungs and the thoracic wall), the partial vacuum is lost. The presence of free air in the thorax is called **pneumothorax.** It results in the lung in that area falling away from the thoracic wall because nothing is holding it in place any longer. This causes the lung to collapse, which can be a serious, life-threatening situation. The possible causes of pneumothorax and lung collapse are many, but basically the air comes either from the outside world because of a penetrating wound into the thorax or from the lung itself because of the rupture of some air-containing structure(s) as a result of lung disease or injury.

Regardless of the cause, the treatment for a collapsed lung consists of reestablishing the partial vacuum within the pleural space. This can be done in an emergency situation by sucking the air out with a needle and syringe or by placing a chest tube into the thorax that is connected to some sort of suction device. The cause of the original air leak must be identified and corrected.

FUNCTION

The process of respiration requires effective movement of air into and out of the lungs at an appropriate rate and in a sufficient volume to meet the body's needs at any particular time. Once fresh air has been drawn into the lungs, oxygen has to be moved into the bloodstream and carbon dioxide extracted from it. The "old" air must then be blown out, and the whole process repeated as long as the animal lives. The balance of this chapter is devoted to the mechanisms and controls that allow all of this to happen.

NEGATIVE INTRATHORACIC PRESSURE

The pressure within the thorax is negative with respect to atmospheric pressure. This is a fancy way of saying that a partial vacuum exists within the thorax. That partial vacuum pulls the lungs tightly out against the thoracic wall. The soft, flexible nature of the lungs allows them to conform closely to the shape of the inside of the thoracic wall. Pleural fluid between the lungs and the thoracic wall provides lubrication. As the thoracic wall goes, so go the lungs. The lungs follow passively as movements of the thoracic wall and diaphragm alternately enlarge and reduce the volume of the thorax. The whole system functions like a bellows as it pulls air into the lungs (inspiration) and blows it back out (expiration).

The negative pressure in the thorax also aids the return of blood to the heart. It helps pull blood into the large veins in the mediastinum, such as the cranial vena cava, the caudal vena cava, and the pulmonary veins. These veins return large volumes of blood to the heart but have no muscular pump to facilitate the process. The negative intrathoracic pressure helps draw blood from the midsize veins into these large veins, which then dump the blood into the atria (receiving chambers) of the heart.

INSPIRATION

Inspiration is the process of drawing air into the lungs—what we commonly call *inhalation*. The basic mechanism for inspiration is enlargement of the volume of the thoracic cavity by the inspiratory muscles. The lungs follow the enlargement passively, and air is drawn into them through the respiratory passageways.

The main inspiratory muscles are the diaphragm and the external intercostal muscles. As discussed earlier, the diaphragm is dome shaped when relaxed, with its convex surface projecting cranially into the thorax. It enlarges the thoracic cavity by flattening out its dome shape. As their name implies, the external intercostal muscles are located in the external portion of the spaces between the ribs—the intercostal spaces. Their fibers are oriented in an oblique direction so that when they contract, they increase the size of the thoracic cavity by rotating the ribs upward and forward. The lifting of the ribs is also aided by some of the muscles of the shoulder, neck, and chest that attach to the rib cage.

EXPIRATION

Expiration is the process of pushing air out of the lungs—what we commonly call *exhalation*. The basic mechanism is the opposite of inspiration in that the size of the thoracic cavity is decreased. This compresses the lungs and pushes air out through the respiratory passageways.

The main expiratory muscles are the internal intercostal muscles and the abdominal muscles. The internal intercostal muscles are located between the ribs deep to the external intercostal muscles. Their fibers run at right angles to those of the external intercostals. When the internal intercostal muscles contract, they rotate the ribs backward, which decreases the size of the thorax and helps push air out of the lungs. When abdominal muscles contract, they push the abdominal organs against the caudal surface of the diaphragm. This pushes the diaphragm back into its full dome shape and also decreases the size of the thorax. Other external muscles also contribute to the expiratory effort. Actually, expiration usually does not require as much work as inspiration because gravity pulls the ribs down, helping to decrease the thoracic cavity volume. Expiration becomes more work when breathing is fast and labored, such as when an animal is exerting itself. Then the lungs must be filled deeply and emptied quickly.

RESPIRATORY VOLUMES

The quantity of air involved in respiration can be described with some standardized terms, such as *tidal volume, minute volume,* and *residual volume.* The **tidal volume** is the volume of air inspired and expired during one breath. The tidal volume varies according to the body's needs. It is smaller when an animal is at rest and larger when it is excited or active. The **minute volume** is the volume of air inspired and expired during 1 minute. It is calculated by multiplying the tidal volume by the number of breaths per minute. For example, an animal with a tidal volume of 450 milliliters (ml) that is taking 12 breaths/min has a minute volume of 5400 ml ($450 \times 12 = 5400$), or 5.4 L. The **residual volume** is the volume of air remaining in the lungs after maximum expiration. No matter how hard the animal tries, the lungs cannot be completely emptied of air. The residual volume always remains.

EXCHANGE OF GASES IN ALVEOLI

Getting a fresh breath of air down into the alveoli of the lungs is a complex process, but the actual exchange of gases that occurs once it is down there is elegantly simple. The basic force behind the exchange is simple diffusion of gas molecules from areas of high concentration to areas of low concentration. It's as easy as rolling a ball down a hill (Figure 10-10).

Atmospheric air contains a high level of oxygen (about 21%) and very little carbon dioxide (about 0.03%). When that air is inhaled down into the alveoli of the lungs, it is only a couple of thin epithelial layers away from the blood in the surrounding capillaries. That alveolar capillary blood contains very little oxygen but a high level of carbon dioxide. Remember that it gave up its oxygen to the body's cells and picked up their carbon dioxide as it flowed through the systemic circulation. So, as this low-oxygen, high–carbon dioxide blood circulates right next to an alveolus containing high-oxygen, low–carbon dioxide air, something amazing happens. Oxygen diffuses from the alveolar air (area of high concentration) into the blood of the alveolar capillary (area of low concentration). At the same time, carbon dioxide diffuses from the blood (area of high concentration) into the alveolus (area of low concentration). The differences in the concentrations of the gases (the concentration gradient) stay fairly constant because as the blood picks up oxygen and dumps carbon dioxide, it flows away and is replaced by more low-oxygen, high–carbon dioxide blood. At the same time, the air in the alveoli is refreshed with each breath.

PARTIAL PRESSURES OF GASES

We can help you understand more clearly how and why respiratory gases diffuse as they do by explaining a physical concept called the **partial pressures** of gases. It really is not as complicated as it sounds. John Dalton, a British scientist, formulated the law of partial pressures of gases a couple hundred years ago. Dalton's law states that the total pressure of a mixture of gases is the sum of the pressures of each individual gas. The pressure of each individual gas is known as its *partial pressure.* Partial pressure is abbreviated by placing a capital letter *P* before the chemical symbol for the gas. For example, atmospheric air contains about 21% O_2. At a total atmospheric pressure of 760 mm of mercury (Hg), the partial pressure of oxygen (the Po_2) is equal to 21% × 760 mm Hg, or 159.6 mm Hg.

The concept of partial pressures holds true even for gases that dissolve in liquids, such as blood. The amount of a particular gas that dissolves in liquid exposed to a gaseous environment is determined by the partial pressure of the gas in the gaseous environment. So the partial pressure of O_2 and CO_2 in the blood of the alveolar capillaries (the liquid) is determined by the partial pressures of O_2 and CO_2 in the alveolar air (the gaseous environment). The Po_2 in the alveolar *air* is about 100 mm Hg, and the Po_2 in the *blood* of the alveolar capillaries is about 40 mm Hg. Doesn't it make sense, then, that O_2 would diffuse from the alveolar air into the blood of the alveolar capillaries? It is moving from an area of high concentration (100 mm Hg in the alveolar air) to an area of low concentration (40 mm Hg in the capillary blood). The CO_2 diffuses the other direction because its partial pressure is higher in the blood (46 mm Hg) than in the alveolar air (40 mm Hg). So the CO_2 diffuses from the alveolar capillary blood into the alveolar air.

After circulating around the alveoli and swapping gases with the alveolar air, the blood in the pulmonary veins now contains a high level of oxygen and a low level of carbon dioxide. It flows back to the heart and is ready to be pumped back out into the systemic circulation to deliver its oxygen to the cells in exchange for their carbon dioxide. And so it goes. The respiratory system takes care of the air movement, and the cardiovascular system manages the blood movement. As long as everything goes as planned, the net effect is that all of the body's cells are constantly supplied with the vital oxygen they require and relieved of the waste (carbon dioxide) they produce. However, as you can imagine, this system is rather delicate. Anything that interferes significantly with either the flow of air in the respiratory system or the flow of blood in the cardiovascular system can throw off the whole balance and endanger the health and well-being of the animal.

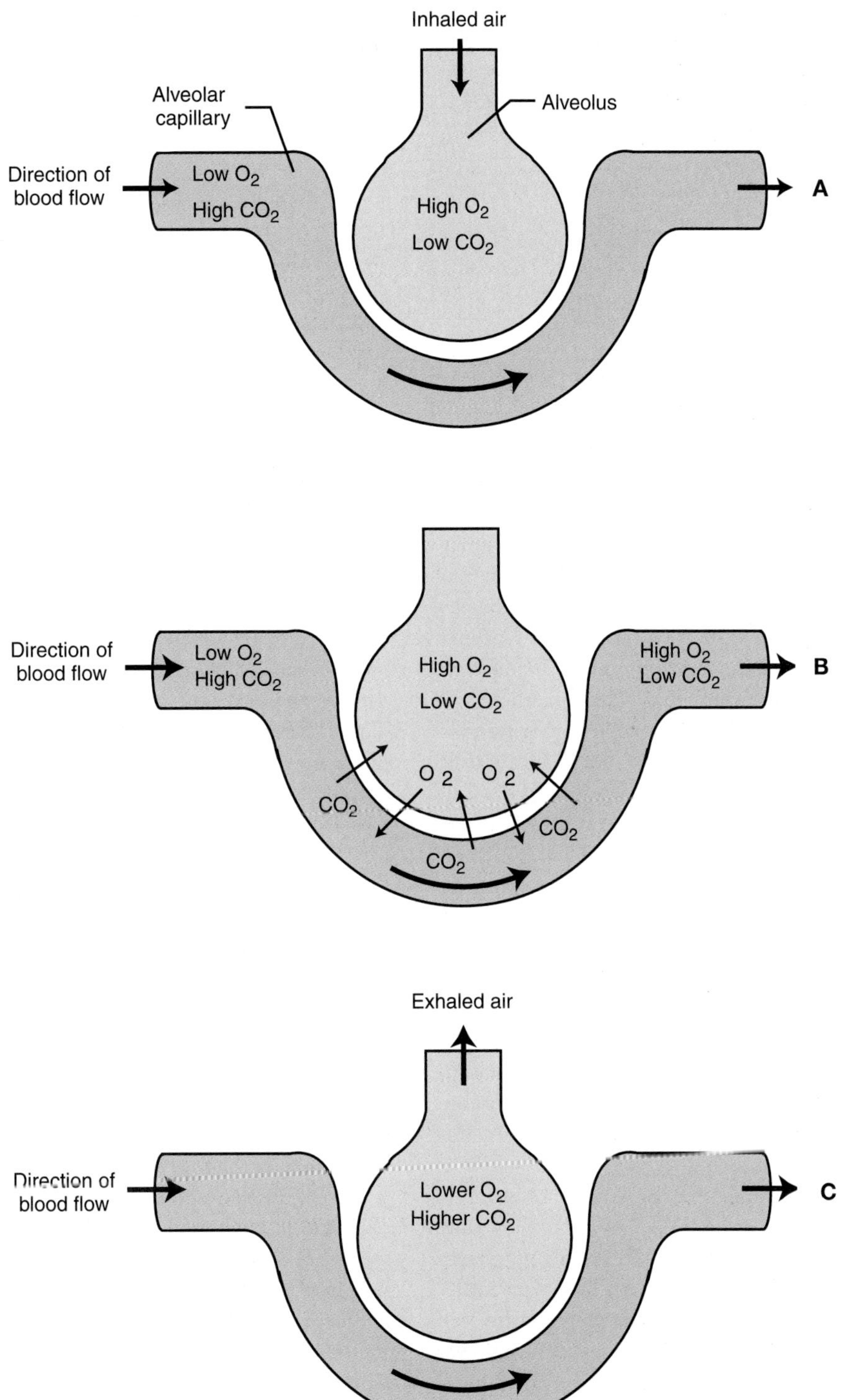

FIGURE **10-10** **Gas Exchange in Alveoli of Lung. A,** Inspiration. Inhaled air contains high level of oxygen and low level of carbon dioxide. Blood entering alveolar capillary contains low level of oxygen and high level of carbon dioxide. **B,** Gas exchange. Oxygen diffuses from air in alveolus, where its level is high, into blood in alveolar capillary, where its level is low. Carbon dioxide does the reverse, diffusing from alveolar capillary into alveolus. **C,** Expiration. Exhaled air contains less oxygen and more carbon dioxide than are present in room air. Next breath brings in fresh supply of high-oxygen air.

TEST YOURSELF

1. Why is negative intrathoracic pressure important to breathing? What happens if it is lost?
2. What are the main muscles of inspiration? How do they cause air to be drawn into the lungs?
3. What are the main muscles of expiration? How do they push air out of the lungs?
4. Describe the basic processes by which oxygen moves from the air in the alveoli into the blood in the alveolar capillaries and how carbon dioxide moves the other direction.

CONTROL OF BREATHING

Even though all of the inspiratory and expiratory muscles are skeletal muscles and therefore under voluntary control, breathing does not require conscious effort. An animal does not have to consciously think about how much and how often to inhale and exhale. It just seems to happen. Just for grins, try an experiment to put this into context. For the next few breaths, try consciously to control how often you breathe, how much air you inhale with each breath, and how much air you blow out when you exhale. After a short time, your breathing will probably become a real chore. Fortunately, by ignoring your breathing and turning your attention back to reading about it, your breathing will once again return to its normal, rhythmic pattern. So how do the voluntary respiratory muscles carry out the involuntary activity of breathing?

Breathing is controlled by an area in the medulla oblongata of the brain stem known as the **respiratory center.** Within the respiratory center are individual control centers for functions such as inspiration, expiration, and breath holding. These centers send nerve impulses out to the respiratory muscles at a subconscious level, directing them when and how much to contract. Therefore the voluntary respiratory muscles are controlled by nerve impulses from a subconscious part of the brain. Of course, this automatic system can be overridden by voluntary control from the conscious part of the brain (which is what you did if you tried the experiment of consciously controlling your breathing). Conscious control usually only lasts for a short time, however, before the automatic system kicks back in. The conscious mind just has too many other things to think about and control. (So when children threaten to hold their breath to get their way about something, never fear. They can't consciously suffocate themselves. Their automatic respiratory control system will start up after they've made a dramatic show of holding their breath for a while!)

The body has two main systems that control breathing: (1) a mechanical system that sets normal inspiration and expiration limits and (2) a chemical system that monitors the levels of certain substances in the blood and directs adjustments in breathing if they get out of balance.

Mechanical Control

The **mechanical control system** operates through stretch receptors in the lungs that set limits on normal, resting inspiration and expiration. When the lungs inflate to a certain preset point during inspiration, a nerve impulse is sent to the respiratory center, indicating that the lungs are full. The respiratory center sends out nerve impulses to stop the muscle contractions that have been producing inspiration and start the muscle contractions that will produce expiration. When the lungs deflate to another preset point during expiration, another nerve impulse is sent to the respiratory center, indicating that the lungs are sufficiently empty. The respiratory center sends out the appropriate nerve impulses to stop expiration and start the process of inspiration again. The whole process repeats itself unless some modification of the breathing process is necessary. The net effect of the mechanical control system is to maintain a normal, rhythmic, resting breathing pattern.

Chemical Control

The mechanical breathing control system is pretty much preset and automatic, whereas the **chemical control system** monitors the blood and only affects the breathing pattern if something gets out of balance. Chemical receptors in blood vessels (the carotid and aortic bodies located in the carotid artery and aorta, respectively) and in the brain stem constantly monitor various physical and chemical characteristics of the blood. Three characteristics important to the control of the breathing process are (1) the CO_2 content, (2) the pH, and (3) the O_2 content of the arterial blood. If any of these varies outside preset limits, the chemical control system signals the respiratory center to modify the breathing process to bring the errant level back into balance.

The blood level of CO_2 and the blood pH are usually linked. Earlier, in our brief discussion of acid-base balance, we explained that as the CO_2 level in the blood rises, the pH of the blood goes down, indicating that the blood is becoming more acidic. So, if the chemical control system detects a rise in the blood level of CO_2 and a decrease in the blood pH, it signals the respiratory center to increase the rate and depth of respiration so that more CO_2 can be eliminated from the lungs. If the CO_2 level falls too low, which is usually accompanied by a rise in the blood pH level, the opposite occurs, that is, respiration is decreased to allow the CO_2 level to rise back into the normal range. We sometimes see this effect clinically in anesthetized patients that have been "bagged" for a time. *Bagging* is the term used to describe manual control of an anesthetized patient's breathing by squeezing and releasing the rebreathing bag of an inhalant anesthesia machine. Bagging often hyperventilates the patient somewhat, causing more CO_2 than normal to be eliminated via the lungs. The decreased blood CO_2 level often causes the patient to hold its breath for a while when the bagging stops, until the CO_2 level rises back into the normal range. At that point, normal breathing generally resumes. Unless you know to expect this effect, it can be quite scary when it happens. (Do you see how important this normal anatomy and physiology stuff is?)

The effects of variations in the blood O_2 level are not as clear cut as the CO_2 effects. If a slight decrease in the blood O_2 level (hypoxia) occurs, the chemical control system signals the

CLINICAL APPLICATION: Coughs, Sneezes, Yawns, Sighs, and Hiccups

Coughs, sneezes, hiccups, yawns, and sighs are temporary interruptions in the normal breathing pattern. They can be responses to irritation (coughs and sneezes) or attempts to correct imbalances (yawns and sighs), or they may occur for unknown reasons (hiccups).

A **cough** is a protective reflex that is stimulated by irritation or foreign matter in the trachea or bronchi. It consists of a sudden, forceful expiration of air. Moist coughs, also known as *productive coughs,* help an animal clear mucus and other matter from the lower respiratory passages. They are generally beneficial to the animal, and we usually do not try to eliminate them with medications. Dry coughs, also known as *nonproductive coughs,* are generally not beneficial and are often treated with cough suppressant medications.

A **sneeze** is similar to a cough, but the irritation originates in the nasal passages. The burst of air is directed through the nose and mouth in an effort to eliminate the irritant(s).

A **yawn** is a slow, deep breath taken through a wide-open mouth. It may be stimulated by a slight decrease in the oxygen level of the blood, or it may just be due to boredom, drowsiness, or fatigue. Yawns can even occur in humans by the power of suggestion, such as seeing someone else yawn or even thinking about yawning. (Did you just yawn?)

A **sigh** is a slightly deeper than normal breath. It is not accompanied by a wide-open mouth like a yawn. A sigh breath may be a mild corrective action when the blood level of oxygen gets a little low or the carbon dioxide level gets a little high. It may also serve to expand the lungs more than the normal breathing pattern does. Anesthetized animals are often manually given deep sigh breaths periodically to keep their lungs well expanded. This is done to prevent the partial collapse of the lungs, which can occur in anesthetized animals as a result of respiratory system depression caused by general anesthetic drugs.

Hiccups are spasmodic contractions of the diaphragm accompanied by sudden closure of the glottis, causing the characteristic "hiccup" sound. Although hiccups can result from serious conditions, such as nerve irritation, indigestion, and central nervous system damage, most of the time they are harmless and temporary. Many "folk remedies" have been suggested for hiccups, but because they are usually self-limiting, the best approach is to just let them run their course. However, prolonged or recurrent hiccups may require medical attention.

respiratory center to increase the rate and depth of breathing so that more O_2 will be taken in. If, however, the blood O_2 level drops below a critical level, the neurons of the respiratory center can become so depressed from the hypoxia that they cannot send adequate nerve impulses to the respiratory muscles. This can cause breathing to decrease or stop completely.

The net effect of the chemical control system is to adjust the normal, rhythmic breathing pattern produced by the mechanical control system when the CO_2 content, pH, or O_2 content of the blood varies outside preset limits. In other words, the mechanical system sets a baseline respiratory rate and depth, and the chemical control system makes adjustments as needed to maintain homeostasis.

TEST YOURSELF

1. Describe how the mechanical respiratory control system maintains a normal, rhythmic, resting breathing pattern?
2. What is the basic difference between the functions of the mechanical and chemical respiratory control systems?
3. When does the chemical respiratory control system kick in and override the mechanical control system?
4. Why do animals cough, sneeze, yawn, sigh, and hiccup?

CHAPTER 11

THE DIGESTIVE SYSTEM

Robert L. Bill

The gastrointestinal (GI) tract is one of the systems that varies widely among species. More specifically, the requirements for digestion and absorption of foodstuffs vary considerably among the **herbivores** (plant-eating animals, such as cattle, sheep, and goats), the **carnivores** (meat-eating animals, such as cats), and **omnivores,** such as ourselves. In addition, species of animals are also divided between **monogastrics** (animals whose GI tract contains a single, true stomach) and **ruminants** (animals whose GI tract contains a large, fermentative compartment called the **rumen**). This chapter provides a general model of the anatomy and function of the GI tract and defines how this structure and function differ between herbivore and carnivores and between monogastrics and ruminants. For information regarding the digestive functions of birds, see Chapter 17 on avian anatomy or related references.

BASIC FUNCTION OF DIGESTIVE TRACT

The GI tract is also called the **alimentary canal,** or the *digestive tract,* which extends from the mouth through the esophagus, stomach, small intestine, and large intestine to the anus. "Gastrointestinal" is synonymous with the term *gastroenteric,* for which *gastro-* refers to the stomach (e.g., gastric ulcer) and *enteric* relates to the intestines (e.g., **enteritis** is inflammation of the intestines). The digestive tract has the following functions:

1. Prehension (grasping) of food with the lips or mouth
2. Mechanical grinding or breaking down of food (chewing)
3. Chemical digestion of food
4. Absorption of nutrients and water
5. Elimination of wastes

If any of these processes fails to function properly, the animal may fail to gain proper weight, may lose weight, and eventually may die from malnutrition. Therefore the veterinary technician needs to understand each of these processes and to comprehend how alteration of any of these functions could produce diseases or clinical signs, such as diarrhea, vomiting, weight loss, or bloat (in ruminants).

MOUTH OR ORAL CAVITY

The mouth, or oral cavity, is also called the **buccal cavity.** The mouth is where the food is initially placed and digestion actually begins. The key structures in the mouth of clinical significance include the lips, tongue, teeth, **salivary glands, hard palate, soft palate,** and **oropharynx.** The lips may play an important role as a **prehensile** organ, meaning that the animal, such as the horse, can grasp the food and pull it into the mouth. Paralysis of the lips caused by disease or trauma can result in the animal being unable to feed itself adequately. The highly sensitive nature of the lips makes them a significant sense organ in horses, cattle, and some other species. In carnivores, the lips play a more passive role in eating. **Labial** is the adjective used to describe anything pertaining to the lips.

The salivary glands produce **saliva,** which has a variety of digestive and lubrication functions. Most domestic animals have a total of three matching pairs of salivary glands: (1) the parotid salivary glands, which are located just below the ear canal and caudal to the mandible (lower jaw), (2) the mandibular salivary glands, which are located between the left and right halves of the mandible, and (3) the lingual salivary glands, which lie just under the base of the tongue. All of the glands have ducts that carry the produced saliva to the oral cavity.

TEETH

With the advancement of veterinary dentistry and dental techniques, teeth have received much more attention in small animal medicine. Because dental care and surgery are becoming more common in veterinary practice, the veterinary technician must be familiar with dental anatomy and terminology. The teeth are responsible for physically breaking down food into smaller pieces so that the surface area of the food is increased and therefore can be exposed more to digestive enzymes. The **maxilla** is the bone of the skull that contains the **upper arcade** of teeth (teeth in the upper part of the mouth), and the **mandible** contains the **lower arcade** of teeth.

Carnivore teeth are shaped differently than the teeth found in the herbivores (Figure 11-1). This difference in shape reflects the function of the teeth. The carnivore teeth are typically more pointed on their **occlusal surface** (where teeth come together) because the teeth serve important roles in holding prey (hence the teeth are slightly curved toward the back of the mouth) and tearing or shredding food. Herbivores,

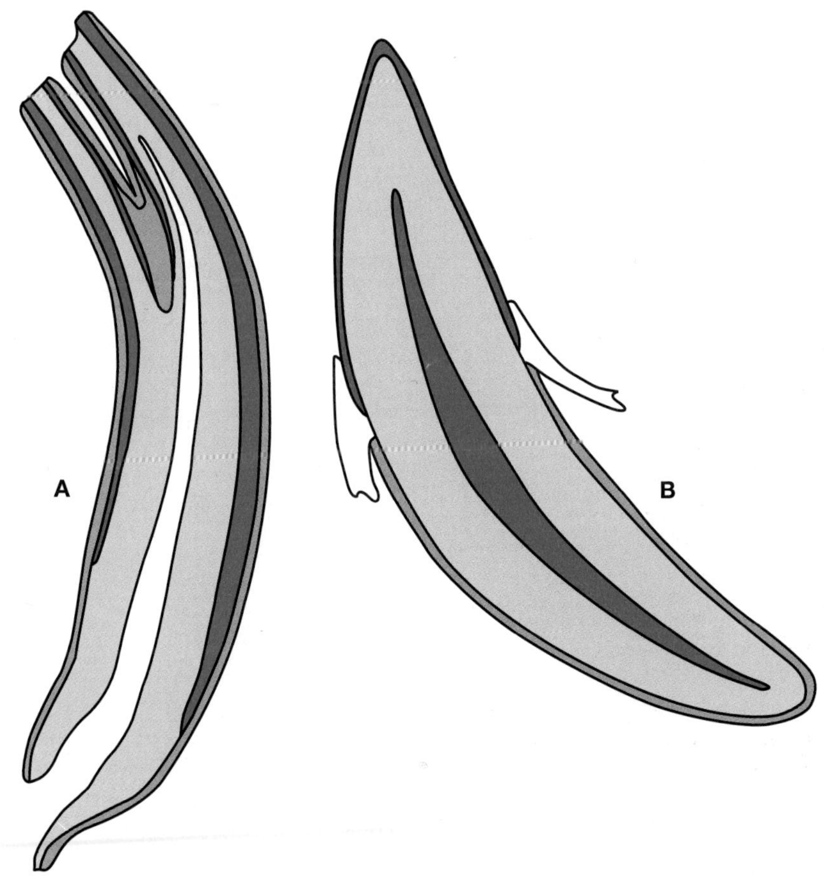

FIGURE **11-1** **Herbivore and Carnivore Teeth.** Note flat occlusive surface of herbivore (equine) tooth **(A)** compared with carnivore (dog) tooth **(B).**

in contrast, have mostly flat occlusal surfaces, which reflects the need to grind plant and grain material.

Both carnivore and herbivore teeth are classified as **incisors, canines, premolars, and molars** (Figure 11-2). The incisors are the teeth at the front **(rostral)** part of the upper and lower arcade. In both carnivores and herbivores the incisors have a narrow ridge at the tip of the tooth. The canine teeth (even in noncanine species) are typically longer than the other teeth and pointed at the tip. In some species the canines are large and form tusks. The premolars are rostral to the molars and have larger occlusal surfaces that are used for grinding by all species.

The "inner" surface of the lower arcade of teeth that faces toward the tongue is referred to as the **lingual surface** of the teeth, and the inner facing surface of the upper arcade is referred to as the **palatal surface** (meaning that it "faces" the **hard palate** at the roof of the mouth). The "outer-facing" surface of the upper and lower arcade at the front (rostral) of the mouth is called the **labial surface** (*labial* relating to the lips), and the outer-facing surface of the teeth more caudal in the mouth is called the **buccal surface** (*buccal* pertaining to the cheeks).

Typically, the number of each type of tooth found in the upper and lower arcade is represented in the **dental formula.** The dental formula uses *I* for incisor, *C* for canine, *P* for premolar, and *M* for molar, followed by two numbers separated by a slash mark (or expressed as a fraction of one number over the other). The first number represents the number of teeth in *half* (right or left half) of the upper arcade, and the second number represents the number of teeth in *half* of the lower arcade. The letters in the formula are capitalized to represent adult teeth, whereas lowercase letters *(i, c, p, m)* represent deciduous teeth (so-called baby teeth). Because the formula represents only half of the upper and lower arcade, the total number of teeth would be determined by summing all the numbers and multiplying by 2.

The dental formulas for several domestic species are shown in Table 11-1. As an example, the dental formula for the adult

Table 11-1 Dental Formulas for Several Domestic Species

Species	Dental Formula	Total Number Teeth
Canine—puppy	i3/3 c1/1 p3/3	28
Canine—adult	I3/3 C1/1 P4/4 M2/3	42
Feline—kitten	i3/3 c1/1 p3/2	26
Feline—adult	I3/3 C1/1 P3/2 M1/1	30
Equine—adult	I3/3 C1/1 P3-4/3 M3/3	40 or 42
Porcine—adult	I3/3 C1/1 P4/4 M3/3	44
Bovine—adult	I0/3 C0/1 P3/3 M3/3	32

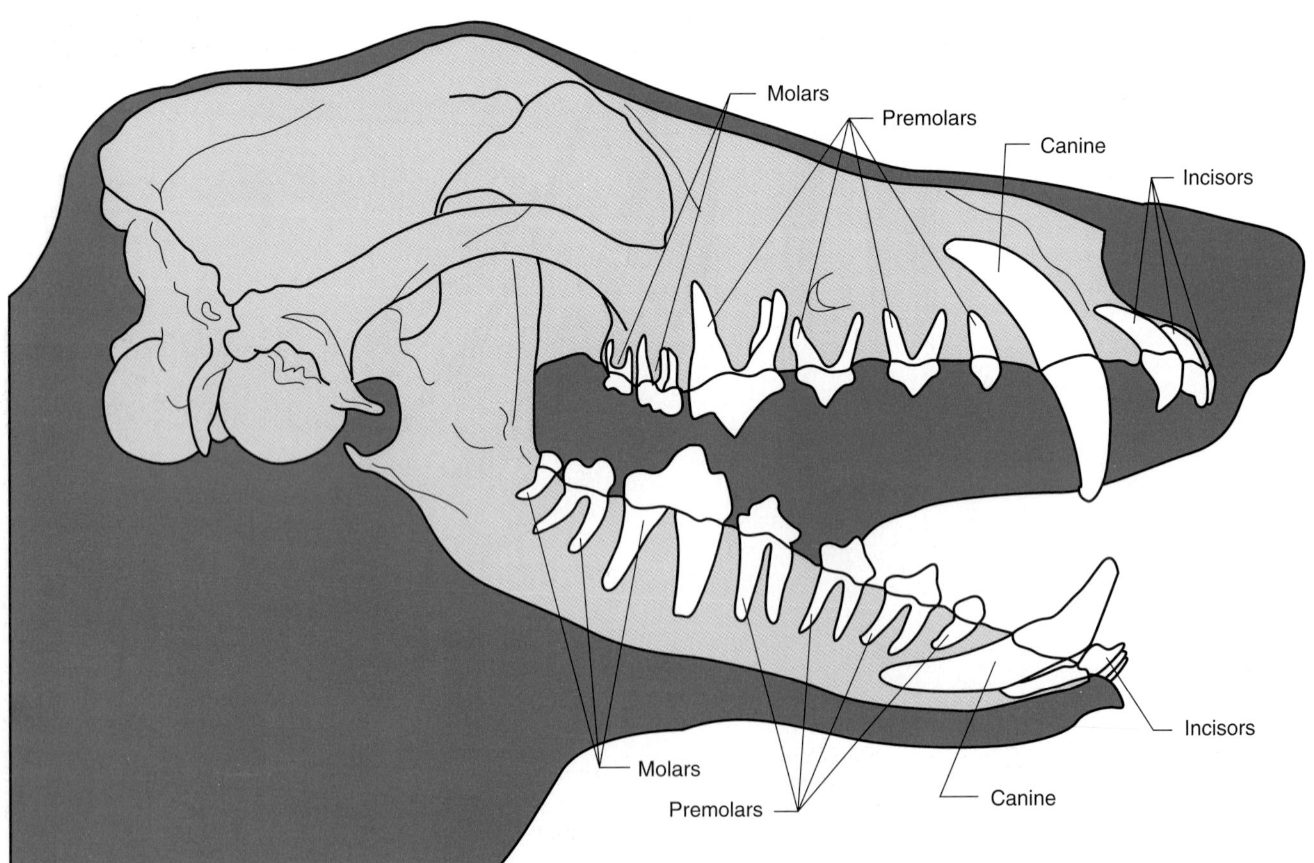

FIGURE 11-2 **Lateral View of Canine Skull Showing Types of Teeth.**

feline shows 3 incisors in each half of the upper and lower arcade (total of 12 incisors), 1 canine in each half of the upper and lower arcade (total of 4 canines), 3 premolars in the half of the upper arcade but only 2 in the half of the lower arcade (total of 10 premolars), and 1 molar in each half of the upper and lower arcade (total of 4 molars).

Note that the ruminants, as represented by cattle (bovine) in Table 11-1, do not have any upper incisors or upper canine teeth. Instead, ruminants have a **dental pad,** which is a flat, thick, connective-tissue structure on the maxilla opposite the lower incisors and canine teeth.

The first molar in the lower arcade (most rostral molar) and the fourth premolar in the upper arcade of the dog are large. These particular teeth are referred to as **carnassial teeth.** Abcesses that form at the root apex (tip) of the carnassial tooth break through the thin bone of maxilla and begin to drain through the skin just below the eye. Because carnassial teeth have such deeply entrenched roots, removing them often requires greater effort and technique than required for the other teeth.

The teeth are well supplied with nerves, blood vessels, and lymph drainage. Therefore they are susceptible to damage and severe pain in domestic animals just as they are in humans (Figure 11-3). The blood supply and nerve supply enter the **apex** of the tooth root and form a latticelike organization that comprises the **pulp** in the center of the tooth. The **dentin** surrounding the tooth pulp is more dense than bone and helps to protect the sensitive pulp. Finally, the tooth is covered with a hard **enamel** layer, which is the toughest tissue in the body.

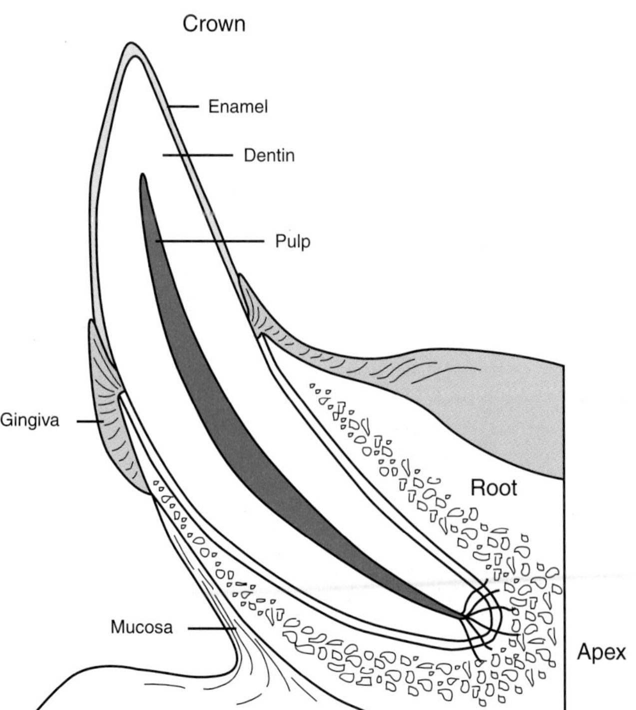

FIGURE **11-3** **Cross Section of Typical Tooth.**

The epithelial tissue that composes the "gums" is more technically called **gingiva.** The enamel covers only that part of the tooth that extends beyond the gingiva.

FUNCTION OF THE ORAL CAVITY

The purpose of the oral cavity is to **prehend** (take hold of) the food and to initiate mechanical and chemical digestion. **Mechanical digestion** is the breaking down of food into smaller particles. Breaking apart food increases the surface area available for exposure to enzymes involved in **chemical digestion** (think about how crushed ice melts faster than an equivalent weighted ice cube). Several enzymes, the proteins that serve to catalyze chemical reactions and usually recognized by the suffix *-ase,* are secreted by the body to break down different components of the food (sugars, proteins, fats, etc.).

As mentioned previously, the tearing, shredding, crushing, and grinding of food into smaller pieces in mechanical digestion is the responsibility of the various teeth. Chewing, also called **mastication,** and the addition of saliva from the salivary glands prepare the food for swallowing by softening it, moistening it, and shaping it into a form that is more readily swallowed.

Amylase is an enzyme found in the saliva of omnivore species, like rats and pigs, but is absent in carnivores, like dogs and cats. As the name implies, salivary amylase breaks down amylose, a sugar component of starch. **Lipase,** an enzyme that digests lipids (fats), also may be found in some young animals (calves) while they are nursing or on a high-milk diet.

Saliva is also involved in evaporative cooling in dogs. Panting evaporates saliva in the mouth, cooling the blood in the capillaries just below the surface of the oral mucous membranes.

Cattle rely on the high concentrations of sodium bicarbonate and phosphate buffers found in bovine saliva to neutralize

CLINICAL APPLICATION: The "Prophy" and "Floating"

In small animal medicine, many veterinary practices make teeth cleaning and scaling tartar (removal of the brown, hard plaque that builds up on the enamel) key elements of small animal wellness and prophylactic (preventive) procedures. Hence this dental procedure of cleaning and scaling is often called a **dental prophylaxis,** or the dental "prophy." Because credentialed veterinary technicians will be expected to do dental "prophies," a solid understanding of tooth anatomy is essential.

Dogs and cats get prophies, whereas horses get "floated." Horses often develop enamel points (sharp edges) on the buccal edge (edge nearest the cheek) of the occlusal surface of their upper arcade of teeth and on the lingual edge (edge closest to the tongue) of the corresponding teeth of the lower arcade. To reduce these points, as well as other occlusal-surface malformations, the surface of the teeth in horses are filed with a rasp (a coarse file). This procedure is called "floating" or "floating the teeth."

acids normally formed in the rumen and to help maintain the normal, healthy pH of their rumen. Cattle produce 25 to 50 gallons of saliva a day (think about how large a small, 10-gallon aquarium is to gain a perspective of this volume). The water and buffers in the saliva are quickly reabsorbed from the digestive tract and recycled.

The salivary glands, as well as most of the other glands in the digestive system, are controlled by the autonomic nervous system (see Chapter 7). Stimulation of the **parasympathetic nervous system** results in increased salivation. Even the anticipation of eating (the so-called cephalic phase of digestion) can cause parasympathetic stimulation of the salivary glands, resulting in copious saliva production (drooling). Sympathetic nervous system stimulation associated with fear or inhibition of the parasympathetic nervous system, as with the use of preanesthetic drugs like atropine, produces "dry mouth" because of the decrease in saliva production.

ESOPHAGUS

The esophagus extends from the oral cavity to the stomach. It is a muscular tube that actively contracts to move a **bolus** of food or liquid from the mouth into the stomach. Like most of the tubular organs in the GI tract, it contains multiple layers: (1) the innermost layer next to the **lumen** (open space inside the tubular organ) is called the **mucosa;** (2) the thicker layer underneath the mucosa that contains glands (if present) is the **submucosa;** (3) the next layer contains muscle; and (4) the outer layer is a thin, tough layer of connective tissue called the **serosa.**

The movement of food down the esophagus is accomplished by the coordinated contraction of two layers of muscles in the esophagus (and most other parts of the GI tract). The outer **longitudinal muscle** layer tends to shorten the esophagus when it contracts and results in a slight opening of the lumen. The inner **circular muscle** layer is arranged as a series of rings around the esophagus. When stimulated to contract, the circular muscle layer constricts the esophagus and reduces the size of the lumen. When a bolus of food enters the esophagus, the longitudinal muscle on the **aboral** side (the side "away from the mouth") contracts, causing a slight dilation of the esophageal lumen. Simultaneously, the circular muscles just behind the bolus (in the **oral direction**) contract, pinching the esophagus closed and forcing the bolus forward. Both the relaxation of the longitudinal muscle and the contraction of the circular muscles move the bolus toward the stomach in a wave known as **peristalsis** (similar to squeezing toothpaste out of a tube) (Figure 11-4).

When the peristaltic wave reaches the lower end of the esophagus, the shortening of the longitudinal muscle and relaxation of circular muscle contractions allow the food to pass into the stomach. The esophagus enters the stomach at an angle so that as the stomach expands with food, the fold of the stomach against the esophagus acts as a natural "valve" to close the lower end of the esophagus and reduce the risk for reflux (*reflux* is the movement of stomach contents, or ingesta, back up the esophagus). In some species, this anatomical closure can be so strong that reflux or vomiting is nearly impossible. The horse and rabbit are two species in which this occurs.

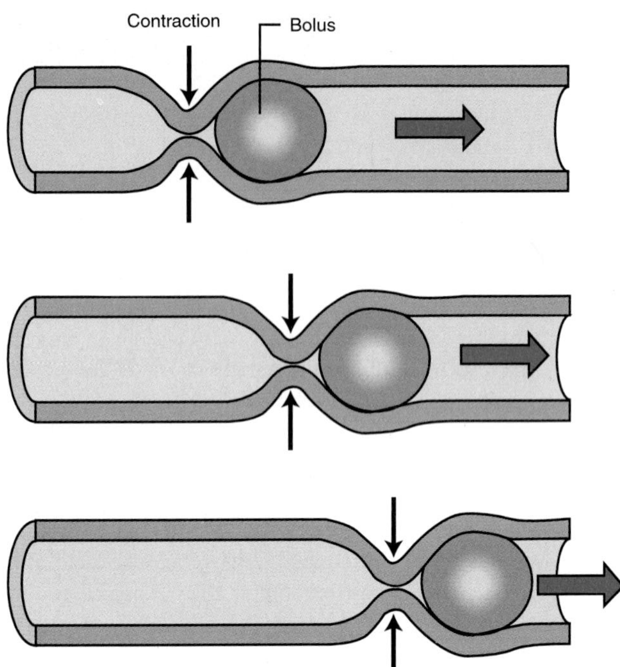

FIGURE **11-4** **Peristalsis and Segmentation.** Peristalsis is coordinated contraction and relaxation of muscle layers, resulting in movement of bolus of food or ingesta along GI tract.

TEST YOURSELF

1. How do diets differ among a herbivore, a carnivore, and an omnivore? To which group would cats, horses, cows, and humans belong to?
2. What are the "lower arcade" and "upper arcade" in reference to teeth? What bones in the skull are each of these arcades associated with?
3. What are the four types of teeth? Where are they located from rostral to caudal?
4. What is meant by the lingual surface, palatal surface, labial surface, and buccal surface of teeth?
5. What are deciduous teeth?
6. Why do ruminants have a dental formula that has zero after the *I* and *C*?
7. Where is the apex, root, pulp, dentin, and enamel of a tooth? What is the gingiva?
8. What are amylase and lipase? From where in the mouth do they come from? What do they do?
9. What effect does the parasympathetic nervous system have on the mouth? The sympathetic?
10. What are the layers of the esophagus? Which contains glands? Which provides motility?
11. What is peristalsis?

CLINICAL APPLICATION Corrosives and Megaesophagus

You may have learned in basic first-aid classes that if a child ingests a strong acid or alkali (called *corrosives* because they "corrode" the surface), they should not have vomiting induced (cause to vomit). The reason relates to the histological structure of the esophagus. As described earlier, the esophagus is mainly a muscular tube. It has little tough connective tissue or thick mucosa (the inner layer of the esophagus) to protect the muscle. If an animal swallows an acidic compound (toilet bowl cleaner, battery acid, etc.) or an alkali (drain opener, strong liquid cleansers, etc.) the inner surface of the esophagus will sustain burns the length of the esophagus. If these burns are severe enough, the esophagus can actually perforate (acquire a hole). Then, every time the animal swallows, some of the food bolus could be pushed through the perforation into the thoracic cavity (think about squeezing a tube of toothpaste that has a pinhole). If the animal that ate the corrosive chemical was forced to vomit the material, the esophagus would be exposed a second time to the chemical and further damage would occur. Thus animals that drink corrosive materials should not be induced to vomit. If you *must* have a corrosive substance inside of your body, the stomach is probably the best place to have it because it is designed to withstand the acidic environment normally found there.

Sometimes diseases result in the esophageal muscle losing its normal muscle tone. An example of this condition called *myasthenia gravis,* which is a disease in which the body produces antibodies against the nerve receptors that cause esophageal muscle contraction. Because it has little or no muscle tone, the esophagus relaxes and becomes more of a flaccid (relaxed) bag than a tight, muscular tube. Food, when swallowed, accumulates in the esophagus because not enough force is available to push the food through the anatomical closure at the end of the esophagus where it enters the stomach. This dilated esophagus is called a **megaesophagus.** With this disease the animal (usually a dog) appears to "vomit" up food. However, the food has not been digested (because it never made it to the stomach), and the animal brings the food up without the usual forceful contractions associated with true vomiting. Do animals survive with megaesophagus? Yes, they can. By feeding a diet that is of a liquid nature and making the animal eat from an elevated surface like a table or box, gravity pulls the liquid material down the esophagus and into the stomach. The risk with megaesophagus, as well as the principal reason for why many animals die from this, is that the animal often aspirates (sucks in) some of the frequently regurgitated food, resulting in a lung condition called *aspiration pneumonia.*

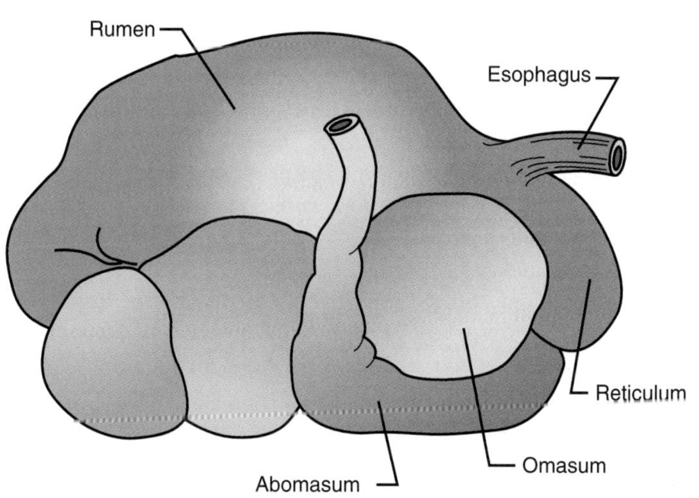

FIGURE **11-5** **Stomachs of Cow.** Location of reticulum, rumen, omasum, and abomasum as seen from right side of cow. Note that the head would be toward the right of drawing.

THE RUMINANT

Ruminants, as the name implies, ruminate their food. In other words, they swallow their food and bring it back up the esophagus to their mouth **(regurgitation)** to chew on it some more before swallowing it again. Technically this process is called **rumination.** In lay terminology, this is called "chewing the cud." Cattle, sheep, and goats are all members of the ruminant family. Unlike the monogastric (single-stomach) animals, the ruminants have a "prestomach" or "forestomach" configuration that is adapted to the herbivore (plant-eating) diet. The four compartments of the ruminant are the **reticulum,** the rumen, the **omasum,** and the true stomach—the **abomasum** (Figure 11-5).

RETICULUM

The smallest and most cranial compartment of the stomach compartments of adult ruminants is the reticulum. The reticulum is separated from the rumen by the ruminoreticular fold. The inside of the reticulum has a honeycomb appearance to it. The four- to six-sided structures of the honeycomb serve to increase the surface area of the reticulum and thus increase the absorptive surface. The muscular wall of the reticulum is continuous with the wall of the rumen, and the two compartments contract in a coordinated manner. Therefore most of the motility of the rumen and reticulum is usually discussed together as **reticulorumen** contractions.

Because of the reticulum's location, heavy objects swallowed by the cow drop into the reticulum. For example, wire,

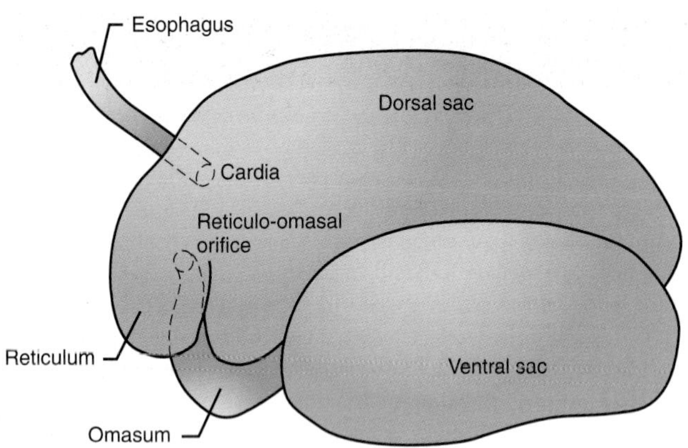

FIGURE **11-6** **Rumen Topographical Anatomy as Seen From Left Side of Cow.**

metal fragments, stones, and so on may lodge in the reticulum. When the reticulorumen contractions occur, a wire or sharp metallic object may penetrate the cranial wall of the reticulum, causing a condition known as **hardware disease.** Because the reticulum is separated from the heart by the diaphragm and a relatively short distance, an object piercing the reticulum also can penetrate the diaphragm and pericardium (outer membranous sac surrounding the heart), causing pericarditis (inflammation of the pericardium).

RUMEN

The rumen can be thought of as a large, fermentative vat inside the cow that processes plant materials into usable energy and cellular building materials for the cow (Figure 11-6). The rumen is actually a series of muscular **sacs** partially separated from one another by long, muscular folds of rumen wall called **pillars** (seen and described as grooves from the outside of the rumen). During ruminal contractions, these pillars can almost close off certain sacs of the rumen and in this way allow the effective mixing and stirring of ruminal contents. Mixing of the reticulorumen contents is essential for the fermentative function of the rumen.

In addition to providing coordinated mixing of rumen contents, the reticuloruminal contractions allow (1) partially digested plant food (the "cud") to be regurgitated up the esophagus, where it is chewed and reswallowed (rumination), or (2) built-up carbon dioxide or methane gas to be expelled from the rumen (a process called **eructation**). The rumination process facilitates the mechanical breakdown of tough plant material through multiple chewing cycles, resulting in a greater surface area on which the rumen microbes and digestive enzymes can act. The eructation is essential for dispelling excessive gas created by the fermentation process, thereby reducing the risk of too much gas being trapped in the rumen (a condition called **bloat**).

Rumen motility, like the motility in monogastric animals, is generally controlled by the **vagus nerve** of the parasympathetic nervous system. However, the rate and strength of contraction are determined by factors within the rumen (pH, presence of volatile fatty acids, consistency of the feedstuff in the rumen, stretch receptors) and feedback from the brain stem and other parts of the GI tract.

The ruminant animal derives much of its necessary sources of energy and basic cellular building blocks from the fermentation of rechewed (remasticated) plant material by bacterial and protozoal enzymes. This process is often called **fermentative digestion.** The enzymes that break down the foodstuffs in fermentative digestion come from bacteria and protozoa, in contrast to the nonfermentative processes in monogastric animals, wherein the enzymes are produced by glands in and along the intestinal tract. Thus ruminants depend on these microbes for their nutritional needs.

Enzymes produced by the digestive glands in monogastric animals cannot digest the **cellulose** and **pectin** that make up the cell wall of plant cells. However, rumen bacterial surfaces have **cellulase** enzymes that can digest cellulose effectively and transform the complex **carbohydrate** structure of cellulose into much simpler monosaccharides (simple, one-molecule sugars like **glucose**) and less complex polysaccharides (sugars made of more than one sugar molecule bound together). The glucose sugar produced by this process is *not* immediately available to the host animal. Instead, the glucose liberated from the plant materials (and other carbohydrate sources, like starch) are absorbed into the microbes and converted biochemically to **volatile fatty acids (VFAs).**

These VFAs are actually byproducts of the anaerobic ("without oxygen") fermentation process and, if allowed to accumulate, would decrease the rumen motility. However, the ruminant host rapidly absorbs these VFAs and in the liver converts selected ones (mostly **propionic acid**) to glucose. Therefore, unlike the monogastric animal that digests and absorbs glucose from its GI tract, the ruminant uses the glucose in the rumen to generate VFAs, which in turn are taken into the body and turned into glucose for use by the host's cells. The other absorbed VFAs are used to produce adipose (fat) tissue, milk fat, and other essential components required by the ruminant body.

Like carbohydrates, protein in the ruminant diet is quickly attacked by anaerobic microbial enzymes in the rumen. **Proteases** (enzymes that break down proteins) reduce the long proteins to short **peptides** (short chains of amino acids) and the **amino acid** building blocks of the peptides and proteins. Just as the breakdown of complex carbohydrates yielded simple sugars that were used by the rumen microorganisms, the amino acids and peptides from the protein breakdown are also used by the rumen's microbes. The peptides are either incorporated into the protein structure of the microbes or converted to ammonia (NH_3^+) and VFAs. The ammonia released from these microbes can be used by other microbes to create their own amino acids and proteins. The VFAs from this process are absorbed from the reticulorumen and used as previously described.

Additional nitrogen for rumen microbes comes from the ruminant's secretion of **urea** by the liver into the rumen. Urea is an end product of the liver's activity to convert possibly

CLINICAL APPLICATION A Mystery: Death at a Dairy Operation

A dairy farm manager calls to report that he has 8 dead and 12 ill Holstein heifers. The heifers were replacement heifers (12 to 24 months old) and not part of the milking herd yet. They were found dead this morning at about 6:00 AM. The last time the heifers were observed was before the evening milking of the dairy cows. The heifers were fed hay. The milking dairy herd is pastured in an adjacent lot and is fed hay and a grain mix. The milking dairy cattle seem unaffected.

A grass truck path runs along the southern edge of the property and through both pastures where the heifers are kept and where the milking herd is kept (gates are on either end to allow access to the pastures from both ends). A shallow ditch with a stream runs through the corner of both pastures and crosses the truck path. At this time of the year the ditch is usually dry. The fields adjacent to this pasture were planted in corn this year.

The veterinarian surveyed the scene and asked the dairy manager one question: "When was the corn harvested?" The manager replied, "2 days ago." The veterinarian said, "I think I know what killed your heifers." Can you figure it out? Why were the heifers affected and not the dairy cows?

THE REASON:

The ruminal flora (the mixture of microbes) changes as diets change. Some bacteria may increase in numbers while others decrease based on the availability of sugar and protein in the diet. The dead heifers in this case were not actively milking; therefore they had a relatively low-"energy" (energy = carbohydrate = sugar) diet of hay (lots of cellulose, not much readily available carbohydrates) and no grain. The milking herd, in contrast, was fed hay and grain. Grain is a readily available source of carbohydrate. The milking herd cows were accustomed to receiving more carbohydrate than the heifers, and their ruminal flora had increased to accommodate the extra microbial food.

When the veterinarian found out that the corn had been harvested 2 days ago, he walked along the truck path where it led through the two pastures. He found that the truck carrying corn from the field combine to the silo down the road always had problems going through the dry stream depression in the pastures and tended to spill several pounds of grain each trip because of the tipping.

This meant that both the heifers and the dairy herd received "extra" helpings of grain. The problem was that the heifers' ruminal flora responded to the increased available carbohydrate by churning out tremendous amounts of a different type of acid called *lactic acid* (similar to what your muscles produce when you run long distances or exercise for a long time). This large amount of lactic acid changed the flora in the rumen and killed off most of the normal microbes. The pH of the rumen rapidly became acidic and subsequently caused the blood to become acidic. The lactic acid is converted to sodium lactate (a substance that osmotically pulls water from the body into the rumen and the intestine), resulting in severe dehydration of the body. Finally, the damage to the rumen surface caused by the acidic condition allowed toxins from the rumen to enter the bloodstream and contribute to a shock syndrome and death. The dairy herd cows were unaffected because their ruminal flora was already accustomed to increased carbohydrate in the diet, and therefore they did not ingest enough carbohydrate to produce **lactic acidosis.** This syndrome is also called *grain overload* or *rumen acidosis.*

poisonous amounts of ammonia (NH_3^+) into substances that can be used by the ruminant body. Urea manufactured by the liver is secreted back into the rumen or makes it way via blood to the salivary glands, where it is secreted into the saliva. Note that urea is sometimes added to feed as a relatively cheap method of increasing the nitrogen value of poor-quality feed.

The microbes themselves are "flushed" from the reticulorumen to the omasum, abomasum, and intestines, where they are digested and provide the ruminant with its major source of protein. Thus the ruminant is quite dependent on an active, rapidly growing population of microbes in its rumen to obtain the majority of the amino acids and proteins that it needs to survive.

In addition to the VFAs and protein, the rumen also provides the host animal with B vitamins and vitamin K.

As with any fermentative process (e.g., wine fermentation, beer fermentation), the balance among the amount of substrate to be used by the microbes (glucose and peptides), the growth of the microbes, and the amount of microbial products (VFAs and ammonia) is delicate and easily prone to being upset. Changes in diet (like too much carbohydrate), illness, and even alteration in the length of hay (chopped hay vs. whole) can seriously affect the microbial production of gas, VFAs, and ammonia, resulting in the fermentation process coming to a complete halt. Therefore tremendous attention is paid to the quality and nature of the feed used in cattle and ruminant livestock operations.

OMASUM

The entrance to the omasum is off of the reticulum. When reticulorumen contractions occur, they move ingesta into the omasum. The omasum is a muscular organ, the inner surface of which contains many muscular folds. The primary mechanical function of the omasum is to break down food particles further and to convey ingesta into the abomasum. In addition, the omasum absorbs any VFAs not previously absorbed, removes bicarbonate ions from the ingesta (bicarbonate ions would alter the acid pH of the abomasum unless removed before passing on), and absorbs some water from the ingesta.

ABOMASUM

The abomasum is the "true stomach" of the ruminant. It functions in much the same way as the monogastric stomach and therefore is discussed in greater detail later in the section on the monogastric stomach.

YOUNG RUMINANT DIGESTIVE TRACT

The young ruminant's digestive tract functions primarily as a monogastric digestive system. The rumen and reticulum at birth are small (compared with the omasum and abomasum) and are essentially nonfunctional. Little or no fermentative digestion occurs while the animal is primarily receiving a milk diet (nursing). The abomasum (the true stomach) is the largest of the four stomach compartments for the first few weeks of life. Interestingly, the rate of development of the rumen and reticulum is significantly affected by the type of diet. Calves who are fed grain and roughage (hay) may begin to show signs of rumination as early as 3 *weeks* of age. However, calves kept on a liquid diet of milk or milk replacer make take over 3 *months* to fully develop their reticulorumen function.

Milk in the rumen of a young animal can disrupt normal development of the fermentative digestive process. Therefore the ability of the reticulum to convey suckled milk directly into the omasum is advantageous. The **reticular groove,** also called the **esophageal groove,** is a trough in the wall of the reticulum that extends from the esophageal opening to the opening of the omasum. When the calf nurses or suckles, the muscles associated with the groove contract and form a tubular structure that conveys swallowed liquid from the esophageal opening directly to the omasum, essentially bypassing the rumen and reticulum. The suckling act seems to be necessary for this groove to function. A calf drinking from a pail or water trough will "spill" a considerable volume of swallowed liquid from the reticular groove into the reticulum and rumen. With age and development of the rumen and reticulum, this groove formation reflex almost completely disappears.

TEST YOURSELF

1. What are the four compartments of the ruminant "stomach"?
2. What is hardware disease? With which compartment is hardware disease usually associated?
3. What is rumination vs. eructation? What purposes do they serve?
4. What is fermentative digestion? How is it different from nonfermentative digestion?
5. What is the relationship among cellulose, pectin, cellulase, glucose, and VFAs?
6. What is the relationship among proteases, peptides, and amino acids?
7. What role does urea play in the rumen function? Which organ converts ammonia to urea?
8. What is the "true stomach" of the ruminant?
9. How is the young calf's GI tract different from the adult's? What is the role of the reticular groove?

THE MONOGASTRIC STOMACH

The monogastric stomach and the ruminant abomasum are generally divided into five different areas (Figure 11-7). The **cardia** is the area immediately surrounding the opening from the esophagus into the stomach. As mentioned in the section on the esophagus, the area of the cardia has some circular muscle that maintains muscle tone to reduce reflux of stomach contents back up into the esophagus. The orientation of the esophagus as it enters the stomach also provides a natural closure for the cardia as the stomach fills and distends.

The **fundus** is the section of the stomach that forms a distensible, blind pouch that expands as more food is swallowed. The **body** of the stomach is also a distensible section in

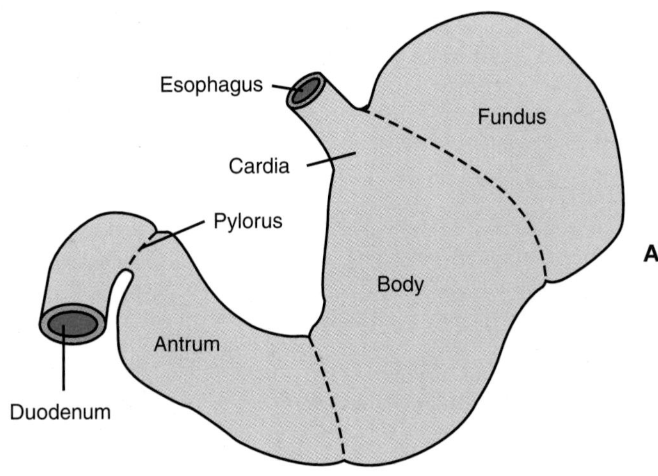

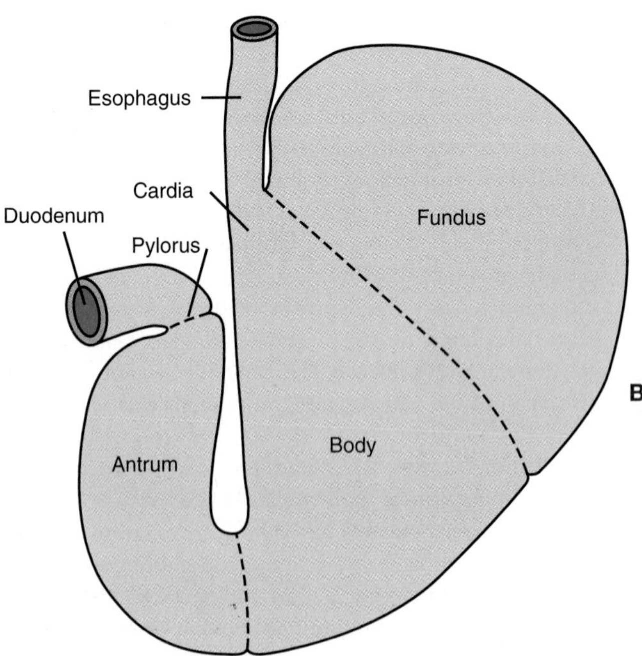

FIGURE 11-7 **Anatomy of Empty (A) and Full (B) Monogastric Stomach.**

the "middle" of the stomach. The fundus and body of the stomach are rich with glands. Typically, the gastric glands (*gastric*" refers to stomach) in this region of the stomach contain (1) **oxyntic cells,** or **parietal cells,** which produce the hydrochloric acid; (2) **chief cells,** which produce an enzyme precursor called *pepsinogen,* and (3) **mucous cells,** which produce the protective **mucus.** (Note that *mucous* is the adjective and *mucus* is the noun.)

The **antrum** is the distal part of the stomach that grinds up swallowed food and regulates the hydrochloric acid that is produced by the fundic and body parietal cells. The glands of the antrum contain endocrine cells called **G cells,** which secrete the hormone **gastrin.** Gastrin is dumped into the blood and travels, among other places, to the gastric glands in the proximal part of the stomach, where it stimulates the release of hydrochloric acid from the parietal cells. Like the gastric glands in the fundus and body, the gastric glands in the antrum also contain many mucous cells.

The **pylorus** is the muscular sphincter (ring of muscle in a tubular organ) that regulates the movement of **chyme** (digested stomach contents) from the stomach into the duodenum (first part of the small intestine) and prevents backflow of duodenal contents into the stomach.

The stomach is shaped roughly like a C on its side. The inside curve of the C is called the **lesser curvature of the stomach,** and the outside curve is called the **greater curvature of the stomach.** This terminology is often used in describing landmarks for surgical procedures involving the stomach and for anatomical location of organs immediately surrounding the stomach (e.g., spleen, pancreas).

Inside the stomach the regions just described flow seamlessly from the cardia to the pylorus. Multiple, long folds in the stomach, called **rugae,** are typically seen on endoscopic examination (a lighted, flexible tube is advanced into a body site to visually inspect structures). An empty stomach should appear pink and glistening from the copious amounts of mucus. Breaks in the surface of the mucus (the epithelium) and in underlying mucosa are called *erosions.* Deep erosions are called *gastric ulcers.* Inflammation of the stomach, called *gastritis,* often appears as a generalized reddening of the observed surface.

Gastric Motility

Each part of the stomach has different motor (muscle) functions. The proximal part of the stomach (fundus and body) tends to relax with swallowing of food, allowing the stomach to distend and fill with food (act as a reservoir). The body of the stomach also contracts to help mix food within the stomach. In contrast to the fundus, the distal part of the stomach (the antrum) increases contractions with swallowing of food. Because the antrum is responsible for most of the grinding activity of the stomach, swallowing of food stimulates vigorous mixing, grinding, and propulsive contractions that move food toward the pylorus.

Peristalsis (the wave of contractions that moves a bolus of food down the esophagus) is also present in the stomach and intestines. Like the esophagus, the stomach contains an inner mucosal layer, submucosa, muscular layer with longitudinal and circular muscle fibers, and an outer serosal layer. The longitudinal muscle fibers are continuous with the esophageal longitudinal fibers and propagate the peristaltic waves from the cardia into the body and antrum of the stomach. The circular muscle fibers encircle the antrum of the stomach and account for its strong, grinding activity.

The pylorus is a concentration of circular muscle fibers. It maintains constant tone through which liquid food (chyme) must be forced by contractions in the antrum of the stomach. The pylorus typically maintains muscle tone during stomach contractions; however, it does not completely close. By remaining partially open, liquid can move readily from the stomach into the duodenum, whereas solid or semisolid food is retained in the stomach. This preferential movement of liquid contents into the duodenum, where most substances are absorbed, helps explain why liquid poisons or medications typically have a more rapid onset of action in the body than the same substance in solid form. Eventually, the forceful contractions of the antrum move all of the stomach contents through the pylorus.

The smooth muscles that make up the muscle layer respond to several hormones, peptides, and nervous system controls. Stimulation of the stomach by the parasympathetic nervous system through the vagus nerve causes the fundus to relax (so it can fill) while increasing the contractions in the antrum and body for mixing and peristaltic movements. Although the sympathetic nevous system normally does not have much of an effect on the stomach or GI tract motility, when it is activated by stressful situations (surgery, illness, etc.), it can cause a decrease in motility that we see as **gastric atony** (decreased muscle tone in the stomach). In horses, gastric atony, or intestinal atony occurring subsequent to disease or surgery, can lead to serious problems.

Gastrin, which is produced by the G cells in the antrum of the stomach, not only increases the production of hydrochloric acid in the stomach but also inhibits the muscle activity of the fundus, resulting in relaxation and greater filling of the stomach. When food is first swallowed and begins to distend the body and antrum of the stomach, gastrin is released and signals the fundus to relax so that the food can be accommodated.

Any factors that bring about distension of the intestines or an increased acidity in the duodenum will inhibit stomach contraction, resulting in delayed gastric emptying of contents. This **enterogastric reflex** prevents the stomach from pushing contents into the duodenum before the small intestine is "ready" to handle additional chyme. **Secretin** is a hormone released from the duodenum in response to excess stomach acid being present in the small intestine. Secretin, like gastrin, can cause the fundus to relax, but it also can *inhibit* peristalsis of the body and antrum of the stomach to slow gastric emptying.

Large amount of fats or proteins present in the duodenum also slow gastric emptying by inhibiting the gastric contractions. In this case, these nutrients stimulate the release of a hormone called **cholecystokinin (CCK)** which, like secretin, decreases contraction of the antrum, body, and also (like gastrin) the fundus.

In glancing through human and veterinary physiology textbooks, you would see that many other stimulatory factors (e.g., motilin, neurotensin, bombesin) and inhibitory chemical factors (e.g., enkephalins, gastric inhibitory polypeptide [GIP], glucagon, somatostatin, vasoactive intestinal polypeptide [VIP]) play a role in controlling gastric motility. The focus of this section is to identify those that appear to have the greatest impact on gastric motility and to play a role in disease conditions or medical treatments used in veterinary medicine.

Gastric Secretions

As described previously, the submucosa of the stomach contains many gastric glands. The secretions of these glands include hydrochloric acid, enzymes, mucus, and an additional protein called **intrinsic factor.** In several species, intrinsic factor must combine with vitamin B_{12} in order for this vitamin to be absorbed from the small intestine. An anemia resulting from a lack of vitamin B_{12} caused by surgical removal of the stomach (e.g., from cancer) is reported in humans but has not been reported in domestic animals.

Pepsinogen is secreted by chief cells and is a precursor for the enzyme **pepsin.** Pepsinogen is cleaved by hydrochloric acid into the proteolytic (protein-digesting) pepsin, which, in turn, can further activate more secreted pepsinogen to produce additional pepsin. The proteins degraded by pepsin form chains of amino acids (polypeptides and peptides) but are not broken down into the elemental amino acids themselves. This is done later on in the intestine. The presence of peptides in the antrum of the stomach stimulate the G cells to release more gastrin, which in turn stimulates more hydrochloric acid and pepsinogen release. Once the pepsin moves from the acidic pH of the stomach to the more alkaline pH of the duodenum, it is inactivated by the change in pH and stops functioning.

The mucus produced by the gastric glands is actually a complex of many substances that provides a gelatinous, protective coating for the stomach. **Mucins** are complex molecules produced by the goblet cells in the gastric glands and are the main constituent of the mucous coating. In addition to the mucin, **bicarbonate ion** is also secreted onto the surface, making the mucous coat more alkaline. By alkalinizing the mucus, the hydrochloric acid contacting it is neutralized to some degree. The mucous coating is essential to protect the stomach cells from the harsh, acidic environment of the stomach (pH of 2 to 3). A pH of 2 normally would remove paint from many surfaces and cause etching of metal.

The mucus itself is not digested by the pepsin but is fragmented by the hydrochloric acid in the stomach. For the stomach to be continually protected, all the components of the mucus must be secreted continuously. Failure to do so sets the stomach up for gastritis and gastric ulcers.

The oxyntic or parietal cells secrete hydrogen (H^+) and chloride (Cl^-) ions separately into the stomach. Once these ions are secreted into the stomach, they combine to produce the hydrochloric acid that accounts for the acidic pH of the stomach. The secretion of hydrogen and chloride ions is an active process involving energy expenditure by the cell and an active transport mechanism. For this reason, the body can tightly control the acid-producing process.

The parietal cell has three receptors on the "blood" side of the cell (as opposed to the stomach lumen side of the cell) that regulate acid production. These receptors are for gastrin, **acetylcholine** (the neurotransmitter of the parasympathetic nervous system), and **histamine.** Stimulation of all three of these receptors results in the optimum amount of hydrogen and chloride secretion (hence hydrochloric acid production). When the body and antrum of the stomach are stretched by food entering the stomach or when more acetylcholine from the parasympathetic nervous system is released at the G cells, gastrin is released from the G cells of the antrum, causing relaxation of the fundus and simultaneous production of increased amounts of hydrochloric acid. How does the body know when "enough" acid has been added to the stomach? When the pH of the stomach contents in the antrum drops below 3, gastrin release is inhibited. With the inhibition of gastrin release, one of the three key stimulants for hydrogen and chloride production is terminated, and hydrochloric acid production declines.

Selectively blocking any one of these receptors markedly decreases the production of stomach acid. This is the mechanism by which systemic antacid drugs, like cimetidine (Tagamet) or ranitidine (Zantac), work. These drugs are called *H_2 blockers* in reference to the histamine receptor, which is designated as an H_2 receptor (to differentiate it from the H_1 receptors in the respiratory tract that produce the red, itchy eyes and nose associated with allergies and respiratory inflammation). By blocking the H_2 receptor, the amount of acid produced by the parietal cells is decreased significantly, and therefore the acidity of the stomach is lessened. Atropine, a drug commonly used as a preanesthetic medication, occupies and blocks the acetylcholine receptor on the parietal cells and, as a side effect, decreases the acid production by the stomach. Atropine is not used as an antacid drug because of its wide range of activity through most of the body's other systems.

Role of Prostaglandins in Gastric Health

Prostaglandins (PGs) are small molecular structures released by the body that have a wide variety of effects. Typically, we associate the action of PGs with inflammation. They are the end product of a cascade of steps in inflammation that ultimately results in the redness, swelling, and heat associated with injury from trauma or disease. Nonsteroidal antiinflammatory drugs (NSAIDs), such as aspirin, ibuprofen, and others, produce their antiinflammatory effect by blocking the production of these inflammatory PGs.

Not all PGs are associated with inflammation. Many have beneficial activities, including regulating the blood supply to the kidney, regulating the normal estrous cycle, and maintaining the normal health and stability of the GI tract. PGs type E

Clinical Application

Because the prostaglandins (PGs) in the stomach play such a critical role in the stomach's normal maintenance of the mucous barrier and ability to repair itself, anything that decreases these beneficial PGs poses the potential to cause great harm. Nonsteroidal antiinflammatory drugs (NSAIDs) commonly used in veterinary medicine (e.g., aspirin, phenylbutazone ["bute"], ketoprofen [Ketofen], meclofenamic acid, flunixin [Banamine]) and in human medicine (ibuprofen [Motrin, Advil], naproxen [Aleve], but *not* acetaminophen [Tylenol]) often list "stomach upset" as a common side effect. Dogs and cats are especially sensitive to the antiprostaglandin effect of these drugs on the GI tract. The net result of the decreased mucous layer and increased acidity caused by these drugs can be gastritis (stomach inflammation), gastric erosions (epithelial layer of stomach is eroded away by the acid), or gastric or duodenal ulcers. Because NSAIDs and glucocorticoids (antiinflammatory "steroids," including cortisone, prednisone, etc.), affect the mucous protective layer *and* the ability of the stomach to heal itself, the ulcers caused by these drugs can perforate ("make a hole through") the stomach, resulting in a fatal condition called *septic peritonitis.* Newer antiinflammatory drugs like carprofen (Rimadyl) and etodolac (EtoGesic) are designed to have more impact on the PGs involved in inflammation and less impact on the PGs responsible for GI health and function. This selective inhibition of PG production theoretically should reduce the gastric side effects associated with the more nonselective NSAIDs. However, the new drugs are not totally selective for the "bad" PGs; therefore gastric side effects still can and do occur with these drugs. Veterinary technicians must keep current on the most recent information regarding these drugs because this area of veterinary medicine will continue to expand.

and I (PGE and PGI) reduce the stomach's hydrochloric acid production by inhibiting gastrin release from the G cells. They are also thought to directly inhibit the parietal cells. PGs also stimulate the cells in the gastric glands to produce the bicarbonate ion, which helps make the mucous layer capable of neutralizing the stomach acid to some degree. Not only do PGE and PGI help maintain the barrier that protects the stomach wall from the gastric acid, but they also enhance blood flow to the stomach, stabilize potentially destructive lysosomes within the gastric cells, and regulate the activity of macrophages and mast cells. All of these functions help the stomach to rapidly repair any damage to the stomach epithelial lining caused by a break in the mucous barrier.

TEST YOURSELF

1. What are the cardia, fundus, antrum, and pylorus? What are each of their functions?
2. Describe what each of these cells produces: parietal cells, chief cells, mucous cells, and G cells. What do their products do?
3. How does motility differ in the fundus vs. the body or antrum?
4. Explain the effect that each of the following has on gastric motility: gastrin, increased acidity in the duodenum, secretin, and cholecystokinin (CCK).
5. What is the relationship between pepsinogen and pepsin? What does pepsin do?
6. What is the relationship between mucus, mucous, and mucin? What role does bicarbonate play in the mucous layer?
7. What are the three receptors on the parietal cells that stimulate hydrochloric acid production?
8. How does the stomach "know" when to stop producing acid?
9. What effect do prostaglandins have on mucus production, gastric blood flow, and the ability of the stomach to heal itself?
10. Explain how NSAIDs produce side effects in the GI tract.

SMALL INTESTINE

The small intestine is divided into three general segments: **duodenum, jejunum,** and **ileum.** The jejunum makes up the majority of the small intestine. (Note that the ileum [with an *e*] in the intestinal tract is not to be confused with the ilium [with an *i*] that is part of the bony pelvis.) A clear demarcation is not evident between segments of the small intestine, and all three can perform peristalsis and absorb fluids and nutrients. The ileum enters the **colon** (large intestine) and is separated from the colon by the **ileocecal sphincter** (*-cecal* relates to the term **cecum,** which is the blind pouch of the large intestine). This sphincter is an anatomical and functional muscle that regulates movement of materials from the small intestine into the colon or cecum.

Like other components of the intestinal tract, the parasympathetic nervous system (vagus nerve mostly, with some nerves from the sacral-vertebral area) provides the stimulatory role for small intestinal motility, secretions, and blood flow, whereas the sympathetic nervous system tends to decrease circulation to the intestine but has little effect on motility or secretions. Decreased motility and secretions result more from a decrease in parasympathetic activity rather than an increase of sympathetic activity.

The structure of the small intestine is similar to other segments of the GI tract; thus it includes an inner mucosal layer, a submucosal layer, a muscular layer, and an outer serosal layer. The relative thickness of these layers changes depending on the segment of intestine; however, the general pattern remains consistent. The mucosa in the small intestine is adapted to provide tremendous surface area for absorbing nutrients, thanks to the folds in the intestinal wall and the millions of cylindrical, fingerlike projections called **villi** (*singular,* villus) (Figure 11-8). In addition to the folds and the villi, each villus contains thousands of very small villi of its own called **microvilli.** The microvilli are so plentiful that they

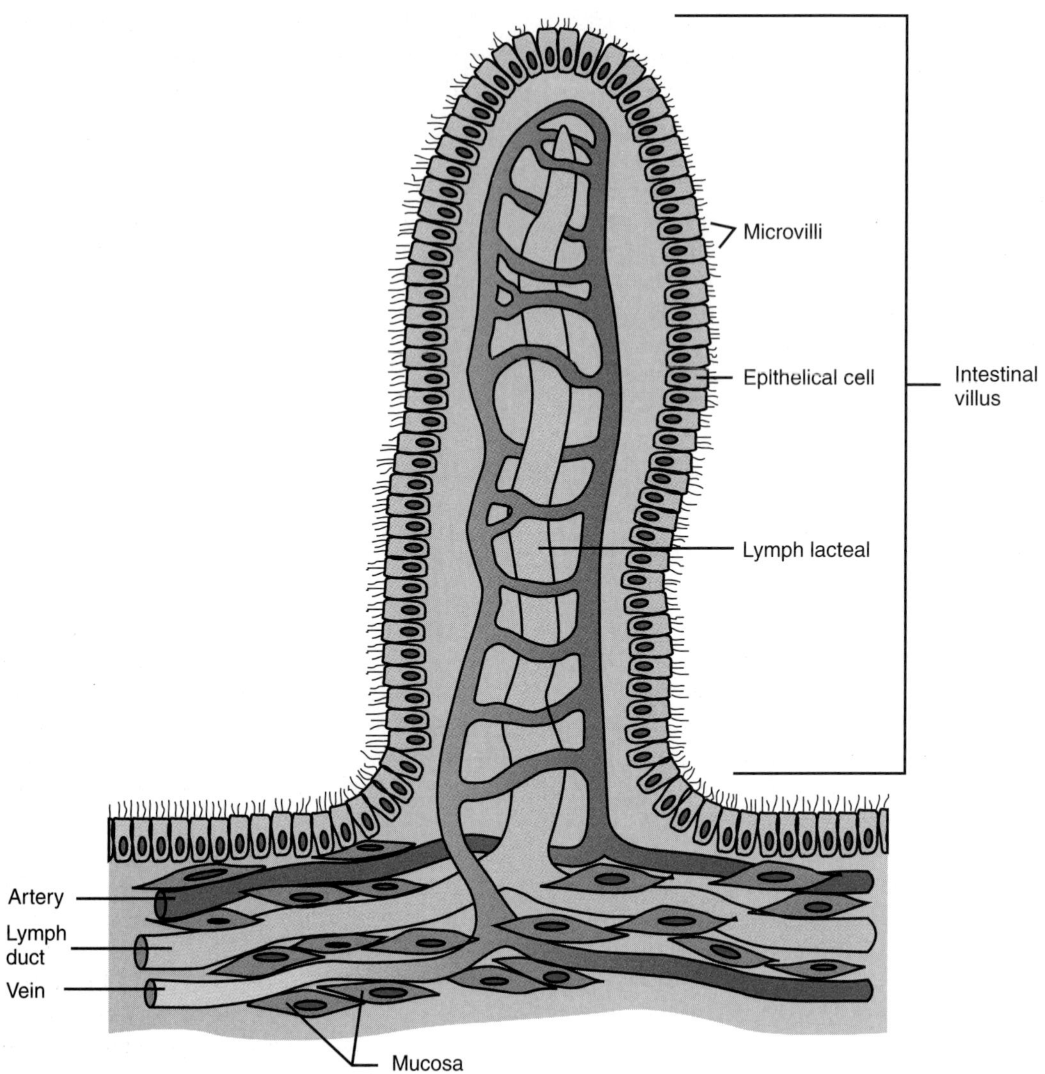

FIGURE **11-8** **Microanatomy of Intestinal Villus.**

microscopically resemble short bristles on a brush; hence the layer of microvilli is often called the **brush border.** The cells of this brush border have many digestive enzymes and carrier molecules embedded in their cell membranes for digestion and absorption of nutrients, minerals (sodium, etc.), and vitamins.

The cells of each villus are constantly replenished. Surrounding each villus are invaginations in the intestinal mucosa called **crypts.** The crypts constantly produce the cells that are pushed up from the bottom of the crypt to the villus to replace those cells sloughed off at the tip of the villus. Diseases such as transmissible gastroenteritis (TGE) in pigs or parvovirus in dogs attack the villus or the crypt cells, resulting in severe damage to the villi and greatly reducing the ability of the animal to digest and absorb nutrients from the intestinal tract.

Goblet cells, like those found in the stomach, are present in the intestine. They produce mucus that helps protect the intestinal mucosa from the ingesta.

SMALL INTESTINE MOTILITY

Similar to the rest of the digestive tract, the small intestine has peristaltic waves, which are associated with the coordinated contractions of the longitudinal and circular muscle layers, and **segmental contractions,** which mix the intestinal contents and slow movement of liquid ingesta through the length of the intestines. The segmental contractions churn the ingesta, ensuring that digestive enzymes secreted into the lumen of the intestine are mixed well with the contents. The churning motion of the segmental contractions also brings digested materials into contact with the surface of the intestinal tract for absorption.

Segmental contractions also slow the movement of ingesta through the intestinal tract. Slowing the movement allows enough time for the ingesta to contact the intestinal wall and be absorbed. Because peristaltic movements push ingesta forward, absorption of contents and consistency of the stool depend partly on the balance between peristalsis and segmental contractions. Many cases of diarrhea in dogs and cats are not due to an overactive peristalsis but instead are due to a lack of segmental contractions. Thus the intestinal tract resembles a garden hose through which contents can rapidly "slide." The result is a high-volume, small bowel diarrhea. Antidiarrheal drugs, like the opioid compounds (diphenoxylate [Lomotil] or loperamide [Imodium AD]), slow diarrhea by decreasing intestinal secretions and increasing the segmental contractions.

The peristaltic movements of the intestine are stimulated by reflexes in response to dilation of a segment of the bowel. This local stretch reflex is mostly independent of any overall control of the GI tract by the parasympathetic nervous system; however, increased stimulation by the parasympathetic nervous system can increase the degree of reflex response.

A decrease in peristaltic waves can result in the ingesta moving too slowly through the intestinal tract. Disease and stress (sympathetic nervous system) inhibit peristalsis and can result in a condition of decreased movement of ingesta called **ileus.** Ileus is often encountered in horses after surgery or in susceptible animals receiving strong antiparasympathetic drugs (e.g., atropine).

Unlike its role in the stomach where it serves to decrease gastric emptying, cholecystokinin (CCK) is thought to stimulate intestinal motility. The CCK is secreted by cells in the intestinal mucosa when fats and proteins are present in the lumen of the intestine. PGs are thought to increase GI motility and secretions, which helps explain some of the colic side effects observed in mares given PG drugs for reproductive problems. Like gastric motility, a wide variety of other compounds and hormones increase or inhibit intestinal motility. (For further information on the roles of tachykinins, VIP, GIP, or other motility-modifying compounds, refer to a veterinary internal medicine or veterinary gastroenterology textbook.)

Small Intestine Digestion

Electrolytes (sodium, chloride, potassium, etc.), water, and vitamins can be absorbed intact across the small intestine wall, whereas carbohydrates, proteins, and fats must be chemically digested to be absorbed. After mechanical breakdown by mixing contractions, food in the intestine is chemically digested in two general steps: (1) by enzymes in the lumen of the intestine and (2) by enzymes associated with the microvilli brush border. The end result is a basic "unit" of the foodstuff that can be transported by carrier molecules or passive diffusion across the intestinal tract membrane.

Carbohydrate Digestion

Starch, glycogen, and various sugars constitute the complex carbohydrates, or **polysaccharides** (meaning "many sugars"), normally present in domestic animal foods. The ruminant processing of carbohydrates in the fermentative process has been described already. Amylase (an enzyme that is produced in the saliva in some but not all species and secreted by the **pancreas** into the lumen of the duodenum) converts starch into smaller sugar segments called **disaccharides** (meaning "two sugars"). These disaccharides, which include *sucrose, maltose, isomaltose* (also called *dextrin*), and *lactose,* are further digested into **monosaccharides** (meaning "one sugar") by the enzymes *sucrase, maltase, isomaltase,* and *lactase,* which are found in the cell membranes of the microvilli. The resulting monosaccharides (*glucose, galactose,* and *fructose*) are transported across the brush border cell membrane and absorbed into the body.

Note that the number of enzymes on the brush border varies with the diet. Nursing animals typically have a large number of lactase enzymes to digest the lactose sugar found almost exclusively in milk. However, once carnivores stop nursing, the lactase enzyme all but disappears from the brush border. If adult dogs or cats are suddenly given milk after not having had any for some time, enough lactase will not be present to digest the lactose sugar. This would result in the lactose sugar remaining in the intestinal lumen, osmotically holding water in the intestinal lumen, and producing a small bowel diarrhea.

Sucrose is normally not found in large amounts in domestic animal diets. However, dogs or cats on "soft moist" diets ingest significant amounts of sucrose used to give the soft texture and composition of these types of foods. Suddenly switching from a dry meal diet to a soft, moist-type food could produce a similar diarrhea described for the lactose-intolerant animal earlier. Within a few days, however, the brush border would increase the number of enzymes to match the increased molecules of sugar, resulting in resolution of the diarrhea.

Protein Digestion

Proteins are large molecules and must be reduced by proteases to their elemental form of amino acids or dipeptides (two amino acids linked together) before they can be absorbed. As previously mentioned, gastric pepsin breaks apart some of the protein chains into smaller chains called *polypeptides* (also called **oligopeptides**). However, because proteins have so many different types of amino acids and because different amino acids have different types of chemical bonds with other amino acids, many different proteases are required to complete the chemical digestion of proteins.

The pancreas produces five basic proteases: **trypsin, chymotrypsin, elastase, aminopeptidase,** and **carboxypeptidase.** Each of these pancreatic enzymes is released as an inactive precursor much in the same way that gastric pepsin is released as pepsinogen. The key precursor and activator is **trypsinogen,** which is activated by an intestinal enzyme to trypsin. Trypsin then activates other trypsinogen molecules, as well as the other pancreatic enzyme precursors. Aminopeptidase and carboxypeptidase proteases start breaking apart protein molecules at either their amino end (—NH_2) or their opposite carboxyl end (—COOH). Trypsin, chymotrypsin, and elastase all break apart the protein at bonds in the middle of the protein.

The chemical digestion of protein is completed at the brush border, where the partially digested peptide strings of amino acids are digested by **peptidases** embedded in the cell membranes of brush border cells. Cleaved amino acids, dipeptides, and even some tripeptides (three amino acids) are then absorbed across the cell membrane.

CLINICAL APPLICATION — Exocrine Pancreatic Insufficiency and Trypsinlike Immunoreactivity

Exocrine pancreatic insufficiency (EPI) is a disease in which the ability of the pancreas to secrete enzymes is markedly reduced. The result is poor digestion of carbohydrates, proteins, and, especially, fats. Animals affected by EPI lose weight and have chronic, pale, foul-smelling, and greasy diarrhea. The presence of undigested fats in the stool is called **steatorrhea** (from the Latin *steato,* meaning "of fat or oil").

Animals with this disease are often given powdered forms of the enzymes with their meals. However, because the lipase requires a certain body temperature and pH and is so easily inactivated, most animals with EPI receiving enzyme supplementation continue to have greasy stools.

Diarrhea resulting from EPI has been diagnosed more often using the **trypsinlike immunoreactivity (TLI) test.** This test looks for the presence of both trypsin and trypsinogen in the *blood,* a place where they are not normally secreted; but they leak into the blood from the pancreas at a fairly predictable rate. Because animals with EPI produce little trypsinogen, their degree of reactivity of their blood to trypsin and trypsinogen is also low. Therefore a low TLI test result suggests EPI and can be used to differentiate diarrhea caused by EPI from other chronic forms of diarrhea.

Fat Digestion

As anyone who has ever tried to mix oil with water knows, fats and water do not mix. In an aqueous environment, fats clump together to form globules. In the intestinal tract, these globules have a relatively small surface area on which enzymes can act. Hence for fats to be adequately digested, these fat globules must be broken down into smaller pieces. This process is called **emulsification** and **micelle formation.** In the stomach the agitation of the antrum breaks the fat globules into small droplets (like shaking a bottle of water and oil). As this emulsified liquid of fat droplets passes into the small intestine, **bile acids** (secreted into the duodenum from the liver's bile duct) combine with the droplets to keep them from forming back into globules. Bile acids have a hydrophilic (water-loving) end and a hydrophobic ("water-fearing" or fat-loving) end. The bile acid sticks the hydrophobic end into the fat droplet, leaving the hydrophilic end exposed to the environment of the intestinal tract. In doing so, it makes the resulting fat droplet "water soluble." Pancreatic lipases (fat-digesting enzymes) penetrate the bile acid coating and digest the fat molecule **(triglycerides)** to produce *glycerol, fatty acids,* and **monoglycerides.** This results in the droplet fragmenting into smaller pieces called **micelles.** These bile acid–lipid component micelles allow the lipid components to diffuse readily through the water contents of the intestine and to come in contact with the brush border of the intestinal wall, where they are absorbed. Fat-soluble vitamins A, D, E, and K are often incorporated into the micelles and absorbed with them.

DIETARY CHANGES

As mentioned in the section on carbohydrate digestion, the ability of the animal to digest the components of any particular diet changes with the diet itself. Thus changing back and forth between two diets of different composition can result in transient periods of diarrhea. This is caused by "up regulation" (increasing numbers of enzymes) or "down regulation" (decreasing numbers of enzymes) of digestive enzymes to match the "demand." Switching from canned food to soft, moist food or dry food or switching from one brand that uses a high corn protein to another form of protein or carbohydrate often results in a greater amount of food being incompletely digested. Thepresence of these undigested molecules osmotically retains water within (and may even draw water into) the lumen of the intestine, producing diarrhea. The best bet when switching diets is to introduce the food over a 5- to 7-day period to allow adjustment to the different dietary components.

TEST YOURSELF

1. What are the three segments of the small intestine? Which is usually the longest?
2. What does the ileocecal sphincter do?
3. What are villi, microvilli, brush border, and crypts? How do they aid digestion and absorption of food?
4. What is the role of segmental contractions in the small intestine? Why do animals get diarrhea if segmental contractions are decreased?
5. What is ileus? What causes it? Why would antiparasympathetic drugs like atropine cause it?
6. What do CCK and prostaglandins do to the small intestine?
7. What are polysaccharides, disaccharides, and monosaccharides? Give examples of each. What enzymes break down each of these?
8. What are the five proteases produced by the pancreas? What protease is produced by the stomach? What effect do these have on polypeptides?
9. Explain how each of the following plays a role in digestion of fats: emulsification, bile acids, liver, pancreatic lipase, triglycerides, glycerol, fatty acids, monoglycerides, and micelles.
10. Why do some animals get diarrhea when their diet is changed suddenly?

LARGE INTESTINE

Although the general functions of the large intestine (cecum and colon) are to recover fluid and electrolytes and to store feces until they can be eliminated, the large intestine is another organ of the GI tract that can vary greatly among species. In the carnivores the colon is a rather simple, tubular organ that uses segmental contractions and peristaltic contractions to

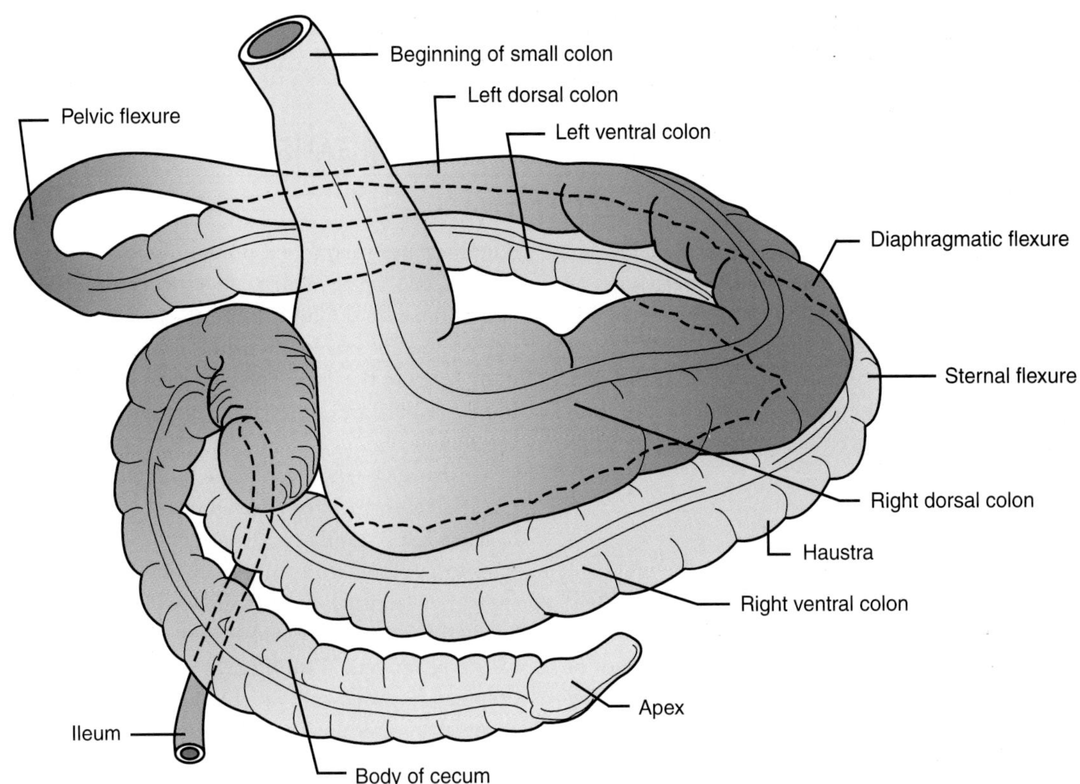

FIGURE **11-9** **Topographical Anatomy of Colon and Cecum of Horse.** The head would be to the right of figure.

control movement of feces through it. The cecum, or blind sac located at the ileocecal junction, is poorly developed in the carnivore but is slightly more developed and larger in the ruminant. Some microbial action on digested foodstuffs occurs in the colon in almost all species. Parasympathetic nervous system stimulation generally causes increased motility in the colon and increased mucous secretion in most species.

The exception to the preceding description of the colon is found in the nonruminant, herbivore species and best represented by the horse. The "hindgut " (colon and cecum) in the equine species is tremendously developed compared with the small intestine and has a greater capacity for fermentation of foodstuffs than in the other species.

The equine hindgut consists of four sections: the cecum, ventral colon (right and left halves), the dorsal colon (right and left halves), and the small colon (Figure 11-9). Ingesta from the small intestine passes through the ileocecal sphincter and enters the cecum, which in the horse is a large, blind sac consisting of the base, the main body, and the apex (point of the blind end). The cecum is located on the ventral floor of the peritoneal cavity. Like the dorsal and ventral colon, the cecum has longitudinal bands that separate the structure into a series of lined-up sacs called **haustra.** The cecum is separated from the colon by a distinct opening called the **cecocolic orifice.**

Contractions of the cecum from the apex and body to the base force ingesta from the cecum into the right ventral colon. Ingesta flows cranially from the right to the left ventral colon through the **sternal flexure.** Ingesta is moved caudally in the left ventral colon, and at the caudal end of the peritoneal cavity, the left ventral colon narrows into the **pelvic flexure,** which reflects on itself and opens into the left dorsal colon. Once again the ingesta flows cranially to the **diaphragmatic flexure,** where it enters the right dorsal colon and begins flowing caudally to the small colon. The relatively narrow flexures and small colon are areas of potential obstruction. However, impaction can occur in just about any segment of the equine colon. Colonic impaction is considered to be one of the most common forms of colic in horses.

Like the ruminant forestomachs, the nonruminant herbivore hindgut requires carbohydrates and protein for sustaining the microbes. Because the horse's small intestine is relatively inefficient in digesting and absorbing carbohydrates, a significant percentage of ingested carbohydrates makes it through the small intestine to the cecum and colon. Proteins are digested more efficiently in the horse's small intestine; thus less protein nitrogen is available to the colonic microbes than would be available to rumen microbes. However, like the ruminant, the nitrogen needs of the colonic microbes are supplemented by the liver's secretion of urea into the GI tract.

VFAs produced by the microbes are absorbed from the cecum and colon for energy needs just like they are from the rumen in ruminants. One of the differences between the rumen and the equine colon, however, is that acids must be buffered by secretion of bicarbonate directly into the colon and cecum (the bicarbonate ions secreted in ruminant saliva buffers the rumen).

The role of the small colon is to absorb electrolytes, water, and VFAs not previously absorbed by the colon. Little to no VFA production occurs in this segment of the GI tract of the horse.

Besides the horse, several other species, including guinea pigs, rats, rabbits, and swine, rely on hindgut fermentation to provide their energy needs. These nonruminant herbivores all have modifications of the cecum and colon that are quite different from the carnivore GI tract and reflect the difference in diet required to sustain the animal. Note that ruminants, even with their incredible fermentation process in the forestomachs, also rely on some degree of fermentation of VFAs in their hindgut.

RECTUM AND ANUS

The process of expelling feces is called **defecation.** Many animals voluntarily decide when to defecate for purposes of living with humans, for marking territory, or for preventing detection by scent. The rectum is the terminal portion of the colon, and the anus is composed of an internal and external muscular sphincter that allows controlled passage of fecal material.

Because the rectum is largely an extension of the colon, most control mechanisms over rectal motility and secretions are similar to that of the colon. Like the colon, the rectum has numerous mucus-secreting glands. The rectum has many sensory receptors that detect stretching or distension, and this expansion typically stimulates the defecation response.

The anus has an internal sphincter that is under autonomic control and an external sphincter that is under voluntary control. The parasympathetic nervous system normally causes relaxation of the internal sphincter, which would correspond with the parasympathetic stimulation of colonic motility. The sympathetic nervous system causes constriction of the internal smooth muscle sphincter.

As the rectum fills and distends, the stretch receptors in the rectum cause partial relaxation of the internal sphincter. This allows fecal contents to move briefly into the internal sphincter canal, where they make contact with the anal mucosa and stimulate mucosal receptors. This increases the sense or need for defecation. As the rectum distends further, the internal sphincter opens for longer periods, allowing more time for anal mucosa contact with fecal material and further increasing the conscious need for defecation. When defecation finally occurs, the voluntary motor impulses to the external sphincter are inhibited, allowing the external sphincter to relax.

The muscle and nerve supply of the anal region is easily disrupted by surgery in the perianal ("around the anus") area or by trauma to the spinal nerves in the area, such as occurs with avulsion of the tail. Diseases like perianal adenomas or adenocarcinomas (cancers of the perianal area) can infiltrate or disrupt the integrity of the anal sphincter, rendering the animal fecally incontinent (unable to control defecation).

OTHER ORGANS RELATED TO DIGESTION

Liver

The liver was mentioned previously in regard to the production of bile acids, which aid fat digestion. The liver is the largest organ in the body (with the exception of skin, which is considered an "organ" by some physiologists). The term **hepatic** refers to the liver. The liver is divided into several **hepatic lobes,** which are divided further into microscopic **hepatic lobules.**

In mammals the liver plays an important role in filtering materials absorbed from the GI tract before they have a chance to reach the systemic circulation. The blood vessel system that transports blood from capillaries in the intestines to hepatic capillaries (actually, hepatic sinusoids, or blood-filled cavities) is called the **hepatic portal system.** Lining the hepatic sinusoids are phagocytic ("eating cells") that remove bacteria, toxins or poisons, worn-out red blood cells, and other infectious agents that enter the body through the wall of the GI tract. In addition, nutrients like glucose, amino acids, and some vitamins and minerals absorbed from the GI tract are stored or metabolized by the body in the liver.

Bile is produced by hepatic cells. It contains bile acids (or bile salts), cholesterol, and bilirubin (a pigment broken down from the heme pigment in hemoglobin that is released when red blood cells are destroyed). The bile produced is secreted into small canaliculi ("small canals") that merge to form bile ducts. The bile ducts form the **hepatic duct,** which (in those species that have one) combines with the cystic duct that leads to the **gallbladder.** The horse does not have a gallbladder. The gallbladder is a storage compartment for bile acids. Stimulation of the gallbladder by CCK during digestion causes the gallbladder to contract, thereby forcing bile down the **common bile duct** into the duodenum. In some species the common bile duct fuses with the pancreatic duct before entering the duodenum.

The liver is the major source for important blood proteins, such as **albumin.** Albumin plays an important role in maintaining the proper fluid balance within the blood. A decrease of albumin as a result of liver failure allows water to leak out of the capillaries, resulting in fluid moving into the tissues, pleural cavity (thorax), abdomen (peritoneal cavity), or other body cavities. The pictures of starving children with potbellied appearances show how a lack of protein in the diet can reduce albumin, causing fluid to leak from the capillaries and accumulate in the abdomen. The accumulation of fluid in the abdomen is called **ascites.**

The glucose absorbed from the GI tract may be stored in the liver as glycogen through a process called **glycogenesis.** There the glycogen acts as a storage pool for glucose molecules. If the body needs glucose, the glycogen is broken down by the liver (a process called **glycogenolysis**) and the glucose moved into the blood. Glucose also can be made in the liver from amino acids through a process called **gluconeogenesis.** Thus the liver plays an important role in providing glucose in those species that are heavily dependent on glucose for energy sources.

PANCREAS

The pancreas is an exocrine gland (secretes substances to the "outside" of the body through a duct) and an endocrine gland (dumping hormones directly into the blood without going through a duct). The exocrine function was detailed in the small intestine, where pancreatic amylase, proteases (trypsin, etc.), and lipase played a critical role in the normal enzymatic digestive process.

In addition to the enzymes, the pancreas also secretes significant amounts of bicarbonate into the duodenum, which helps to neutralize the acid contents coming from the stomach, and maintains a pH in the duodenum at which the pancreatic enzymes can function.

The pancreatic endocrine function also is covered elsewhere in this text. However, suffice it to say that **insulin** and **glucagon** are two hormones that help regulate blood glucose levels from food that has been digested and absorbed. The **beta cells** in the **islets of Langerhans** (or pancreatic islets) produce insulin. Insulin is released in response to elevated blood glucose levels; its action is to move the glucose from the blood into the tissues of the body, thereby effectively supplying the cells with the nutrition they need to function and lowering the concentration of glucose in the blood. A lack of insulin, or a lack of cellular response to insulin, results in an elevated glucose level in the blood and a condition called *diabetes mellitus.*

Glucagon, produced by the **alpha cells** in the pancreas, antagonizes insulin in that it mobilizes glucose from the liver via gluconeogenesis and glycogenolysis. The combined effect of insulin and glucagon results in blood glucose being tightly regulated in a specific concentration range despite varying demands for glucose by the body and changes in carbohydrate in the diet.

TEST YOURSELF

1. How does ingesta flow from the small intestine to the anus in nonruminant herbivores like the horse? Include the different flexures.
2. What are haustra?
3. How do microbes in the colon and cecum use carbohydrate and protein differently than microbes in the rumen?
4. What role do stretch receptors, the internal and external sphincters, and receptors in the anal mucosa play in defecation?
5. What does it mean to be fecally incontinent?
6. What are hepatic lobes, lobules, and the hepatic portal system?
7. What produces bile? Where is it stored? How does it reach the intestine? What stimulates it to be secreted into the small intestine?
8. What is glycogenesis, glycogenolysis, and gluconeogenesis? Where do these occur? What is produced by each process?
9. In addition to digestive enzymes, what else does the pancreas secrete into the duodenum? What is the role of this secretion?
10. What impact do insulin and glucagon have on blood glucose concentrations?

CHAPTER 12

THE MUSCULAR SYSTEM

Thomas Colville

When we think about an animal's body moving, it all seems so simple and automatic. The animal wants to move forward; so it moves its legs appropriately to walk, trot, or run in that direction. At the same time, things are moving inside its body too. Blood is being pumped through the blood vessels, food is being moved along the digestive tract, and little adjustments are being made all over to help keep the body operating smoothly. All this just seems to happen, but all these activities and many more are produced by the work of the muscular system.

Muscle is one of the four basic tissues of the body. (Epithelial tissue, connective tissue, and nervous tissue are the other three.) It is made up of cells that can shorten or contract. When we hear the word *muscle* we usually think of large muscles, like the biceps or gluteal muscles. Actually, three different types of muscle make up the muscular system: **skeletal muscle** (the most familiar kind), **cardiac muscle,** and **smooth muscle** (Figure 12-1 and Table 12-1). Skeletal muscle is controlled by the conscious mind and moves the bones of the skeleton so that the animal can move around. This type is what we usually think of as muscle. The other two types are a little less obvious.

Cardiac muscle is found only one place in the body—the heart. It starts the heart beating long before an animal is born and keeps it up until the animal dies. It has some interesting features, which we'll discuss in this chapter.

Smooth muscle is found all over the body in places such as the eyes, the air passageways in the lungs, the stomach and intestines, the urinary bladder, the blood vessels, and the reproductive tract. It carries out most of the unconscious, internal movements that the body needs to maintain itself in good working order.

In general the nervous system gives the orders, and the muscular system carries them out. This is certainly true of the skeletal muscles, although things are different for cardiac muscle and smooth muscle. They do not require stimulation from nerves to carry out their basic functions; instead, this kind of activity is "built in" to the cardiac and smooth muscle cells. The nervous system influences cardiac and smooth muscle cells but only to adjust and modify their basic activities, not to start them. We'll talk more about that fun stuff shortly.

Like most parts of the body the muscular system is associated with some strange and unique terminology. The term *myo-* refers to muscle generally, and *sarco-* more specifically refers to muscle cells. For example, *myo*logy is the study of muscles, and *myo*sitis is inflammation of muscle tissue. Down at the cellular level, the cytoplasm of a muscle cell is called the *sarco*plasm. We use these terms fairly often in this chapter.

Table 12-1 Comparison of Muscle Features

Feature	Skeletal Muscle	Cardiac Muscle	Smooth Muscle
Location	Skeletal muscles	Heart	Internal organs, blood vessels, eye
Action	Move the bones, generate heat	Pump blood	Produce movements in internal organs and structures
Nuclei	Multiple	Single	Single
Striations	Present	Present	Absent
Cell shape	Long, thin fiber	Branched	Spindle
Nerve supply	Necessary for function	Modifies activity, not necessary for function	Visceral—modifies activity, not necessary for function Multiunit—necessary for function
Control	Voluntary	Involuntary	Involuntary

TEST YOURSELF

1. What is muscle?
2. What are the three types of muscle and what are some of the general characteristics of each type?

SKELETAL MUSCLE

Skeletal muscle is the type that usually comes to mind when we hear the word *muscle.* It is called *skeletal muscle* because it moves the bones of the skeleton, which in turn move the animal around. You might also hear it referred to by an old name—**voluntary striated muscle** (called *voluntary* because it is under the control of the conscious mind). However, not every movement an animal makes is a conscious one. That would be very cumbersome because so many of them are going on all the time. Actually, many skeletal muscle movements, such as maintaining balance and an upright posture, are governed by built-in "cruise control" settings that involve sensory structures, the central nervous system, nerve fibers, and muscle fibers. This kind of system allows animals to breathe, swallow, and stand upright without having to consciously think about each part of the process. To illustrate this yourself, try to consciously control your breathing—how often you breathe, how much air you take in with each breath, how long you hold it in, and how much air you exhale. Pretty soon the process of breathing becomes a chore. The antidote is to think about other things and let your cruise control kick back in. By the time you read the next few paragraphs, your breathing cruise control will probably take over again.

The **striated** part of skeletal muscle's alias (voluntary striated muscle) comes from its microscopic appearance. Even under low-power magnification, skeletal muscle cells are obviously striped (striated) (Figure 12-2). Alternating, crosswise dark and light bands run the length of each cell. Under higher magnification, the pattern of bands appears more complex than just dark and light bands. We'll look into what gives skeletal muscle that kind of appearance when we discuss its microscopic anatomy.

GROSS ANATOMY OF SKELETAL MUSCLE

By *gross anatomy* we mean those features that can be seen with the unaided eye, that is, without microscopes or magnifying glasses. (Some people think all anatomy is gross, but that's another story.)

Muscles

When we talk about "muscles," we are referring to well-defined organs composed of groups of skeletal muscle cells surrounded by a layer of fibrous connective tissue. Some muscles are tiny and delicate, and others are large and powerful. They come in a variety of shapes and sizes, but they usually have a thick, central portion called the **"belly"** of the muscle and two or more attachment sites, which join them to whatever they move when they contract.

Muscle Attachments

Most muscles are attached to bones at both ends by tough, fibrous connective tissue bands called **tendons.** However, as usual, a few oddballs exist. Instead of bandlike tendons, some muscles are attached by broad sheets of fibrous connective tissue, called **aponeuroses,** to bones or to other muscles. The most prominent aponeurosis is the **linea alba** (white line) that runs lengthwise between the muscles on an animal's ventral midline. It connects the abdominal muscles from each side together and is a common site for surgical entry into the abdomen (see the Clinical Application on abdominal incisions).

One of a muscle's attachment sites is generally more stable (moves less) than the other. This more stable site is called the ***origin*** of the muscle. It does not move much when the muscle contracts. The site that undergoes most of the movement when a muscle contracts is called the ***insertion*** of the muscle. For example, the origin of the triceps brachii muscle (the muscle on the back of the upper arm) is on the scapula and proximal humerus, and its insertion is on the olecranon process of the ulna (the point of the elbow). When the triceps muscle contracts, its pull on the olecranon process straightens (extends) the elbow joint.

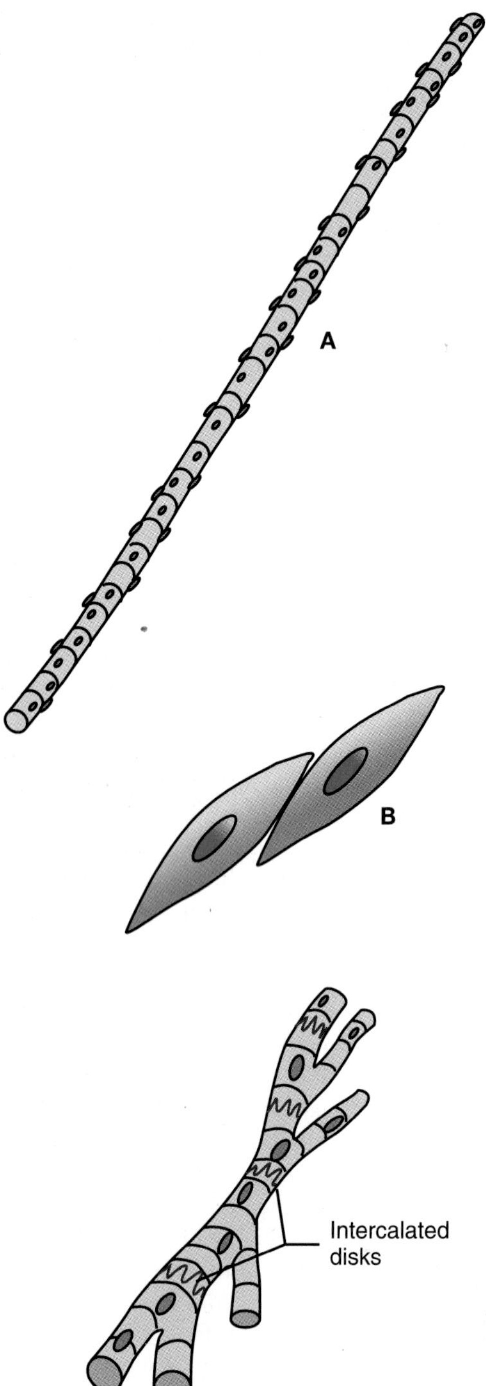

FIGURE 12-1 **Muscle Cell Shapes (Not to Scale). A,** Skeletal muscle cell. Note multiple nuclei. **B,** Smooth muscle cell. **C,** Cardiac muscle cell. Note branching network of cells and intercalated disks connecting cells. Note long, fiberlike shape of skeletal muscle cell; tapered, spindlelike shape of smooth muscle cell; and branching network of cardiac muscle cell.

> **TEST YOURSELF**
>
> 1. What is the difference between a tendon and an aponeurosis?
> 2. What is the origin of a muscle? The insertion?
> 3. Why might it be of clinical importance to know the origin and insertion of a muscle?

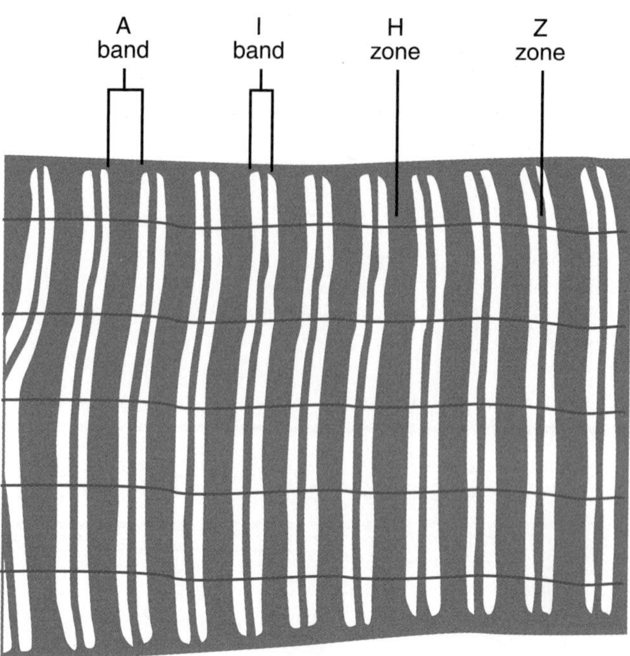

FIGURE 12-2 **Section of Highly Magnified Skeletal Muscle Fiber Showing Characteristic Light and Dark Bands.**

Muscle Actions

A muscle only does one thing, but it does it really well. When stimulated by a nerve impulse, a muscle contracts (shortens). By pulling on its attachment sites (its origin and insertion), the contraction of a muscle produces movement of bones and other structures. Muscles rarely contract singly, however. They usually work in groups, with certain muscles producing most of the desired movement and others stabilizing nearby joints and providing smooth control over body movements. The term **prime mover** (or agonist) is used to describe a muscle or muscle group that directly produces a desired movement. An **antagonist** is a muscle or muscle group that directly opposes the action of a prime mover. Through partial contractions, antagonists can help smooth out the movements of prime movers, or they can contract forcefully at the same time as the prime mover, resulting in rigidity and lack of motion. For example, the biceps brachii muscle that flexes (bends) the elbow and the triceps brachii muscle that extends (straightens) the elbow can each act as a prime mover or antagonist, depending on the movement desired. A **synergist** is a muscle that contracts at the same time as a prime mover and assists it in carrying out its action. For example, the digits of the front limb are flexed (bent) by the deep digital flexor muscle while the superficial digital flexor muscle acts as a synergist to aid the motion. **Fixator** muscles stabilize joints to allow other movements to take place. For example, some of the muscles that flex the digits also can flex the carpus. If a muscle that extends the carpus contracts at the same time as a digital flexor muscle, it fixes the carpus in place (prevents it from moving) while the digits are pulled into a flexed position. You can demonstrate this by starting with the fingers of one of your hands extended and then flexing them into a fist while feeling your forearm muscles with your other hand. You will be able to feel the muscles on the underside of your forearm contracting to flex your fingers, but you will also feel muscles on the top of your forearm contracting to stabilize your wrist (carpus).

Movements of the body are complex; so each muscle may fulfill all four of these roles at one time or another. For one type of movement a muscle may act as the prime mover, but for others, it may act as an antagonist, a synergist, or a fixator.

Muscle-Naming Conventions

Among the biggest causes of misery for students of anatomy are the odd and seemingly random names given to muscles. Surely anatomists must be sadistic ogres who delight in thinking up the most obscure and complicated names possible for body structures, especially muscles. (*Author's note:* I can't speak for all anatomists, but I have known a few who showed signs of being normal human beings.) Actually, some logic can be found behind the names given to most muscles. They are often named for physical characteristics, such as the following:

- *Action*: A portion of a muscle's name is often related to its function. Muscles that flex a joint are often called *flexor muscles.* For example, the action of the superficial digital flexor muscle is fairly apparent by its name. It flexes (bends) the digits when it contracts. Extensor muscles do the opposite in that they extend (straighten) joints.
- *Shape*: A muscle's name can reflect its distinctive shape, such as with the deltoid muscle. The term *deltoid* means triangular shaped, and so the deltoid muscle is a triangular-shaped muscle of the shoulder region.
- *Location*: A muscle's name can indicate its physical location in the body. For example, the biceps brachii muscle is located in the brachial (upper arm) region.
- *Direction of fibers*: The term *rectus* means straight. The rectus abdominis muscles are two straplike muscles on either side of the linea alba on the ventral abdomen. (When someone who lifts weights is referred to as having "washboard abs." the rectus abdominis muscles are being noticed.) The fibers of the rectus muscles run straight lengthwise with the long axis of the body and parallel to each other.
- *Number of heads or divisions*: The number of "heads" refers to the number of attachment sites that a muscle has to its origin. From the term *cephal,* meaning "head," comes the combining form *-cep.* So the *biceps* brachii muscle has two heads, the *triceps* brachii muscle has three heads, and the *quadriceps* femoris muscle has four heads.
- *Attachment sites*: Origin and insertion sites are used to name some muscles. For example, the origin of the sternocephalic muscle is the sternum and its insertion is the back of the head. (Remember that *–cep* or *cephal* refers to head.)

Selected Muscles

Animals have several hundred muscles in their bodies. Complete descriptions of each of them can be found in larger anatomy textbooks. Rather than attempting to catalog all the muscles in the common domestic animal species, we discuss some muscles that are of clinical importance or that can be used as reference points or landmarks on an animal's body. See Figure 12-3 for the locations of many of the superficial muscles in the horse. The general arrangement of muscles in other species is similar.

Cutaneous Muscles. Have you ever watched an animal twitch its skin to get rid of an annoying insect? If so, you have seen that animal contracting one of its **cutaneous** (skin) **muscles.** Actually, the muscles are not in the skin itself but are in the connective tissue (fascia) just beneath it. Unlike most muscles, the cutaneous muscles have little or no attachment to bones. They are thin, broad, and superficial and just serve to twitch the skin. (It's a pity we humans don't have cutaneous muscles. They could save us a lot of swatting during mosquito season.)

Head and Neck Muscles. The muscles of the head have a lot of roles. They control facial expressions; enable chewing (mastication); and move sensory structures, such as the eyes and ears. The muscles of the neck help support the head and allow the head and neck to flex, extend, and move laterally. The large *masseter muscle* in the cheek area of the skull is the most powerful of the chewing muscles. Its main action is to close the jaw. Two of the main muscles that extend (raise) the head and neck are the *splenius* and *trapezius muscles*, which are located on the dorsal (upper) part of the neck. Another muscle that extends the head and neck and also pulls the front leg forward is the *brachiocephalic muscle.* It is a fairly large, straplike muscle that runs from the proximal area of the humerus up to the base of the skull. Neck flexor muscles are located on the ventral (lower) portion of the neck. The *sternocephalic muscle* is a smaller, straplike muscle that extends from the sternum to the base of the skull and acts to flex (lower) the head and neck. Flexors of the head and neck do not have to be particularly large or strong because gravity helps them lower the head and neck.

Abdominal Muscles. The most obvious function of the abdominal muscles is to support the abdominal organs. However, that's not all they do. They also help flex (arch) the back and participate in various functions that involve straining. These include the expulsion of feces from the rectum (defecation), the expulsion of urine from the urinary bladder (urination), the expulsion of the newborn from the uterus (parturition), and the processes of vomiting and regurgitation. Abdominal muscles also play a role in respiration. We discuss their respiratory role more in the section on respiratory muscles.

The abdominal muscles are arranged in layers. From outside in they are the *external abdominal oblique muscle*, the *internal abdominal oblique muscle*, the *rectus abdominis muscle,* and the *transversus abdominis muscle.* The left and right parts of each muscle come together on the ventral midline at the linea alba (an aponeurosis that extends from the xiphoid process [caudal end] of the sternum to the cranial brim of the pubis). The oblique muscles are given that name because their fibers run in

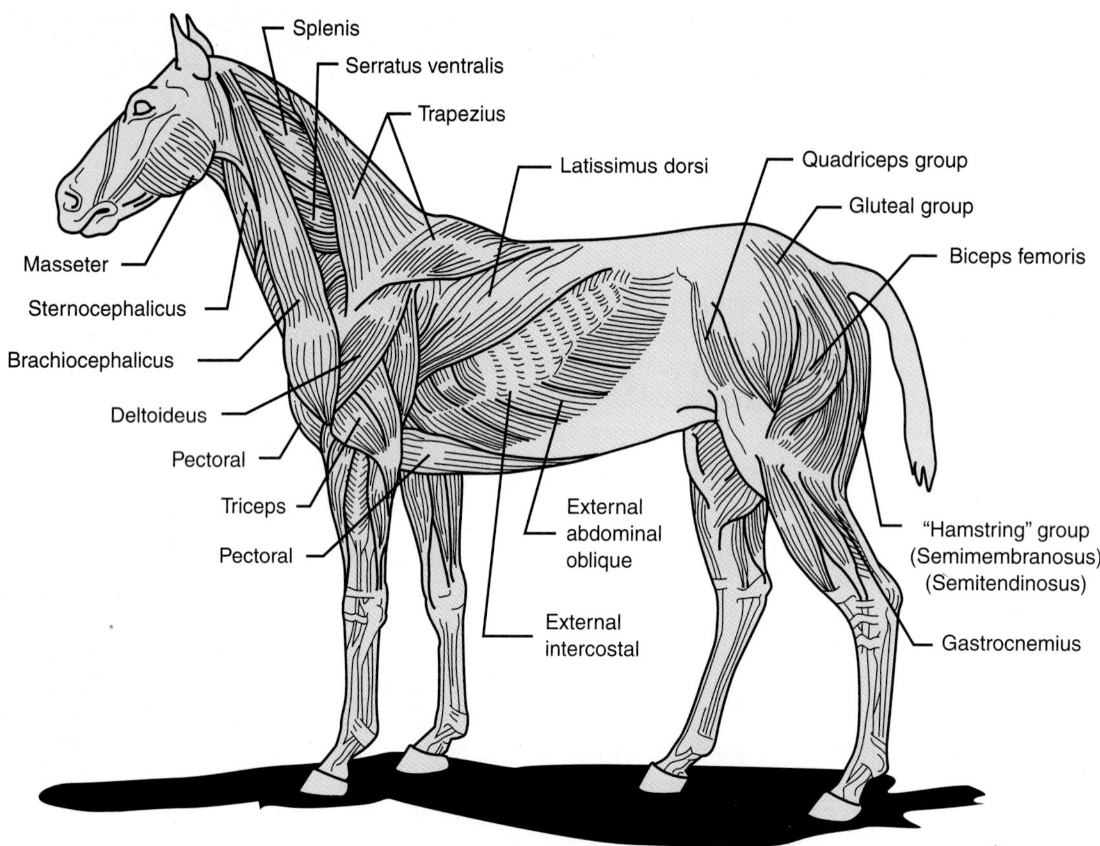

FIGURE **12-3** **Major Superficial Muscles of Horse.**

oblique directions to the long axis of the body and opposite to each other. The fibers of the *external abdominal oblique muscle* run in a caudoventral (backward and downward) oblique direction. The *internal abdominal oblique muscle's* fibers run in the opposite oblique direction, that is, cranioventral (forward and downward). The *rectus abdominis muscle* forms the floor (ventral portion) of the muscular abdominal wall. It consists of two straplike muscles on either side of the linea alba that run from the ribs and sternum back to the brim of the pubis. The *transversus abdominis muscle* is the deepest of the abdominal muscles. Its fibers run directly downward in a ventral direction to insert on the linea alba.

Thoracic Limb Muscles. The muscles of the thoracic (front) limb function mainly in locomotion, thereby allowing the animal to walk and run and generally move around its environment. The primary muscles that we'll discuss are the large muscles of the shoulder and brachial (upper arm) regions, although we do touch on the smaller but very important muscles of the lower leg.

The superficial muscles of the shoulder region are the *latissimus dorsi muscle*, the *pectoral muscles,* and the *deltoid muscle.* The *latissimus dorsi muscle* is a broad, triangular muscle that extends from the spinal column down to its insertion on the humerus. It flexes the shoulder, which helps propel the body forward. Usually two *pectoral muscles,* one superficial and one deep, are located on each side. They both extend from the sternum to the humerus and act as adductors (inward movers) of the front leg, helping to keep the front legs under the animal and preventing them from splaying out to the sides. The *deltoid muscle* is also triangular shaped and extends from the lateral portion of the scapula down to the humerus. It abducts (moves outward) and flexes the shoulder joint.

The names of the *biceps brachii muscle* and *triceps brachii muscle* reveal their general location and their basic physical appearance. Both are muscles of the **brachium,** or upper arm region, and they have opposite actions on the elbow joint. The *biceps brachii muscle* has two proximal attachments (two "heads") and extends from the distal end of the scapula to the proximal end of the radius. When it contracts, it flexes (bends) the elbow joint. The *triceps brachii muscle* has three heads and extends from the distal scapula and proximal humerus down to the olecranon process of the ulna (the point of the elbow). When it contracts, it extends (straightens) the elbow joint.

The muscles distal to the elbow joint are an important collection of carpal and digital flexors and extensors that play important roles in locomotion. Their names often reveal their actions and something about their location. They have names like *extensor carpi radialis muscle* (extends the carpus and is

CLINICAL APPLICATION Abdominal Incisions

Abdominal surgery is commonly performed on veterinary patients. From rumenotomies in cattle to ovariohysterectomies (spays) in dogs, abdominal surgical procedures have one thing in common—the surgeon must make an incision somewhere in the abdominal muscles to expose the contents of the abdomen. The location of the incision is usually carefully selected to offer maximum exposure of the organ(s) or structure(s) to be worked on and to allow a secure closure when the operation is over and the incision is sutured shut.

The positions and arrangements of the abdominal muscles and the direction their fibers run are important considerations when choosing the site for an abdominal incision. The most common abdominal incision site is the ventral midline, where the linea alba is located. It offers several advantages over other sites, such as excellent exposure of abdominal organs, easy closure, and few sensory nerves. Nearly all abdominal organs and tissues can be reached through a ventral midline incision. Also, because all of the abdominal muscles come together at the linea alba, an incision through it opens the abdomen in one cut. When it is time to close the abdomen, one layer of sutures (stitches) in the linea alba can effectively and securely close the abdominal cavity. The linea alba contains less sensory nerves than the adjacent muscles; therefore less postoperative pain is involved with a ventral midline incision than with other abdominal incision sites. The only real disadvantage of a ventral midline incision is that the weight of all the abdominal contents presses on it during the healing process; so it must be closed with very secure sutures.

At times, however, a ventral midline incision is not practical, such as when a cesarean section must be performed on a cow. The complicated digestive system of a ruminant animal like a cow can make it dangerous to position the animal on its back for a surgical procedure. Therefore abdominal surgery in cattle is often done with the animal standing and wide awake by use of local anesthetic blocks to numb the flank (side) area. The incision is usually made in an up-and-down (dorsal-ventral) direction in the flank area. This means that three layers of muscle (the *external abdominal oblique, internal abdominal oblique,* and *transversus abdominis muscles*) must be cut to gain access to the abdominal cavity. To minimize trauma and allow normal function after surgery, many surgeons separate each muscle layer individually according to the direction that its fibers run. Optimal closure of this type of incision requires a separate layer of sutures for each muscle incision, which entails a lot more work than suturing a ventral midline incision closed.

Several other common abdominal incisions can be used, such as the paramedian incision (parallel to but beside the ventral midline), the paracostal incision (parallel to and just behind the last rib), and the transverse incision (crosswise, perpendicular to the linea alba). The abdominal muscles present at each incision site determine how the abdominal cavity should be entered and how it can be sutured closed most securely. (See, this anatomy stuff is important even after you're done with your anatomy class!)

located over the radius) and *deep digital flexor muscle* (flexes the digit and is located down beneath some of the other digital flexor muscles). Despite the general similarities in these muscles among species, their precise locations, names, and actions vary greatly. (We suggest that you consult more in-depth anatomical references if more information about these muscles is needed.)

Pelvic Limb Muscles. Like the thoracic limb muscles, the pelvic limb muscles are mainly involved in locomotion. The large *gluteal muscles* and the "hamstring" muscle group are extensor muscles of the hip joint. These powerful muscles help propel the body forward by extending the hip joint (pulling the leg backward). The gluteal muscles extend from the bones of the pelvis down to the trochanters of the femur. The hamstring muscles are three muscles located on the back of the "thigh" region: the *biceps femoris muscle,* the *semimembranosus muscle,* and the *semitendinosus muscle.* They not only help extend the hip joint but also are the main flexors of the stifle joint. They are powerful muscles that are very important in propelling the animal forward when it walks or runs.

The *quadriceps femoris muscle* is the main extensor muscle of the stifle joint. It is located on the front of the "thigh" region. When an animal has taken a stride with its hind leg, the *quadriceps femoris muscle* helps bring the leg forward to prepare for the next stride. As its name implies, it is composed of four heads or parts.

The flexors and extensors of the tarsus and digit are similar to the flexors and extensors of the carpus and digit of the front leg. One important landmark muscle in some species is the *gastrocnemius muscle,* which is the equivalent of our main calf muscle. It extends from the caudal portion of the distal end of the femur and inserts on the calcaneal tuberosity of the fibular tarsal bone (the point of the hock). The distal gastrocnemius tendon in humans attaches to our heel and is called our *Achilles tendon.* The *gastrocnemius muscle* is a powerful extensor muscle of the hock. It also helps propel the body forward as an animal takes a stride.

Muscles of Respiration. The muscles of respiration increase and decrease the size of the thoracic cavity to draw air into and push air out of the lungs. Because drawing air into the lungs is called *inspiration,* the muscles that increase the size of the thoracic cavity when they contract are called **inspiratory muscles.** Pushing air out of the lungs is called *expiration;* so the muscles that decrease the thoracic cavity size are called **expiratory muscles.**

The main inspiratory muscles are the *diaphragm* and the *external intercostal muscles.* The diaphragm is a thin, dome-shaped sheet of muscle that separates the thoracic cavity from the abdominal cavity. The convex surface of its dome shape protrudes into the thoracic cavity. The caudal-most lobes of the lungs are in contact with the diaphragm, and the liver is just behind (caudal to) it. When the diaphragm contracts, it flattens

Clinical Application: Intramuscular Injection Sites

Because skeletal muscles have large blood supplies, drugs injected into them are absorbed into the bloodstream and carried off to the rest of the body fairly quickly. This method of drug administration is called an **intramuscular injection,** and it is commonly used particularly when a fairly rapid drug effect is desired.

In theory we should be able to use any skeletal muscle for an intramuscular injection. In practice, however, only a few muscles are suitable in each species. Many muscles are either too small or too thin or have other prominent structures (such as nerves) nearby that could be damaged by the injection. To be useful for an intramuscular injection, a muscle must be fairly large, must be easily accessible, and must have a sufficiently thick "belly" into which we can deposit the drug.

The following are some common intramuscular injection sites used in domestic animals:

Cats and Dogs

Pelvic limb	Gluteal muscles
	Quadriceps femoris muscle
	Gastrocnemius muscle
	Hamstring group (biceps femoris, semimembranosus, and semitendinosus muscles)
Thoracic limb	Triceps brachii muscle

Cattle and Goats

Pelvic limb	Gluteal muscles
	Hamstring group (biceps femoris, semimembranosus, and semitendinosus muscles)
Thoracic limb	Triceps brachii muscle
Neck	Trapezius muscle

Horses

Pelvic limb	Gluteal muscles
	Hamstring group (biceps femoris, semimembranosus, and semitendinosus muscles)
Thoracic limb	Triceps brachii muscle
Neck	Trapezius muscle
Chest	Pectoral muscles

Swine

Pelvic limb	Semitendinosus muscle
Neck	Brachiocephalicus muscle
	Trapezius muscle

out somewhat. This pushes the abdominal organs caudally. It also increases the size of the thoracic cavity, causing air to be drawn into the lungs.

The *external intercostal muscles* have the same general inspiratory effect, but they accomplish it by a different mechanism. The word *intercostal* means between ribs. Animals have two sets of intercostal muscles located between each set of adjacent ribs. The *external intercostal muscles* are inspiratory muscles, and the deeper *internal intercostal muscles* are expiratory muscles. The difference is due to the orientation of their fibers. The fibers of the *external intercostal muscles* are directed in an oblique direction so that when they contract, they rotate the ribs upward and forward. This increases the size of the thoracic cavity and causes air to be drawn into the lungs.

Expiration (pushing air out of the lungs) does not require as much effort as inspiration because mechanical forces, such as gravity, and the elastic nature of the lungs help collapse the rib cage and push air out. Nonetheless, two sets of expiratory muscles that aid the process are the *internal intercostal muscles* and the abdominal muscles. The fibers of the *internal intercostal muscles* run at right angles to those of the *external intercostal muscles*. When the *internal intercostal muscles* contract, they rotate the ribs backward, which decreases the size of the thorax and pushes air out of the lungs. When abdominal muscles contract, they push the abdominal organs against the caudal side of the *diaphragm*. This pushes the *diaphragm* back into its full dome shape and decreases the size of the thorax. The contributions of the abdominal muscles to breathing become important mainly when animals are breathing hard and fast, such as when they are exerting themselves physically.

Microscopic Anatomy of Skeletal Muscle

Skeletal Muscle Cells

Skeletal muscle cells are huge. They are not very wide, but they sure are long. Most body cells are a few micrometers (μm) in length or diameter (1 μm = 0.001 millimeter [mm]). Skeletal muscle cells can be several *inches* long. An inch is equal to about 25 mm, or 25,000 μm, which is really large on a cellular scale. Despite being really long, skeletal muscle cells are very thin (up to 80 μm in diameter). This gives them an overall threadlike or fiberlike shape. In fact, skeletal muscle cells are usually called **skeletal muscle** ***fibers*** rather than skeletal muscle *cells*.

Aside from their large size, skeletal muscle fibers have some other strange characteristics. Instead of having just one nucleus like most cells, skeletal muscle fibers have many. Large ones can have 100 or more nuclei per cell, all located out at the edge of the cell just beneath the **sarcolemma** (muscle cell membrane). This reflects their development from numerous primitive muscle cells that fused. The interior of a muscle fiber is even more interesting. Most of the volume of a skeletal muscle fiber is made up of hundreds or thousands of smaller **myofibrils** packed together lengthwise that are themselves composed of thousands of even tinier protein filaments. Prominent organelles between the myofibrils in a muscle fiber include many energy-producing mitochondria, an extensive network of **sarcoplasmic reticulum** (similar to the endoplasmic reticulum of other cells), and a system of tubules called **transverse** or **T tubules** that extend in from the sarcolemma (cell membrane). We'll look at the important roles that these organelles play in muscle cells when we discuss how they contract.

To set the stage for our discussion of how and why muscle fibers contract, we need to get down to the nitty-gritty small stuff in a muscle fiber. The myofibrils that make up the muscle fiber (cell) are composed of thousands of tiny, contractile protein filaments. The two primary proteins that make up the filaments in the myofibrils are thin **actin filaments** and thick

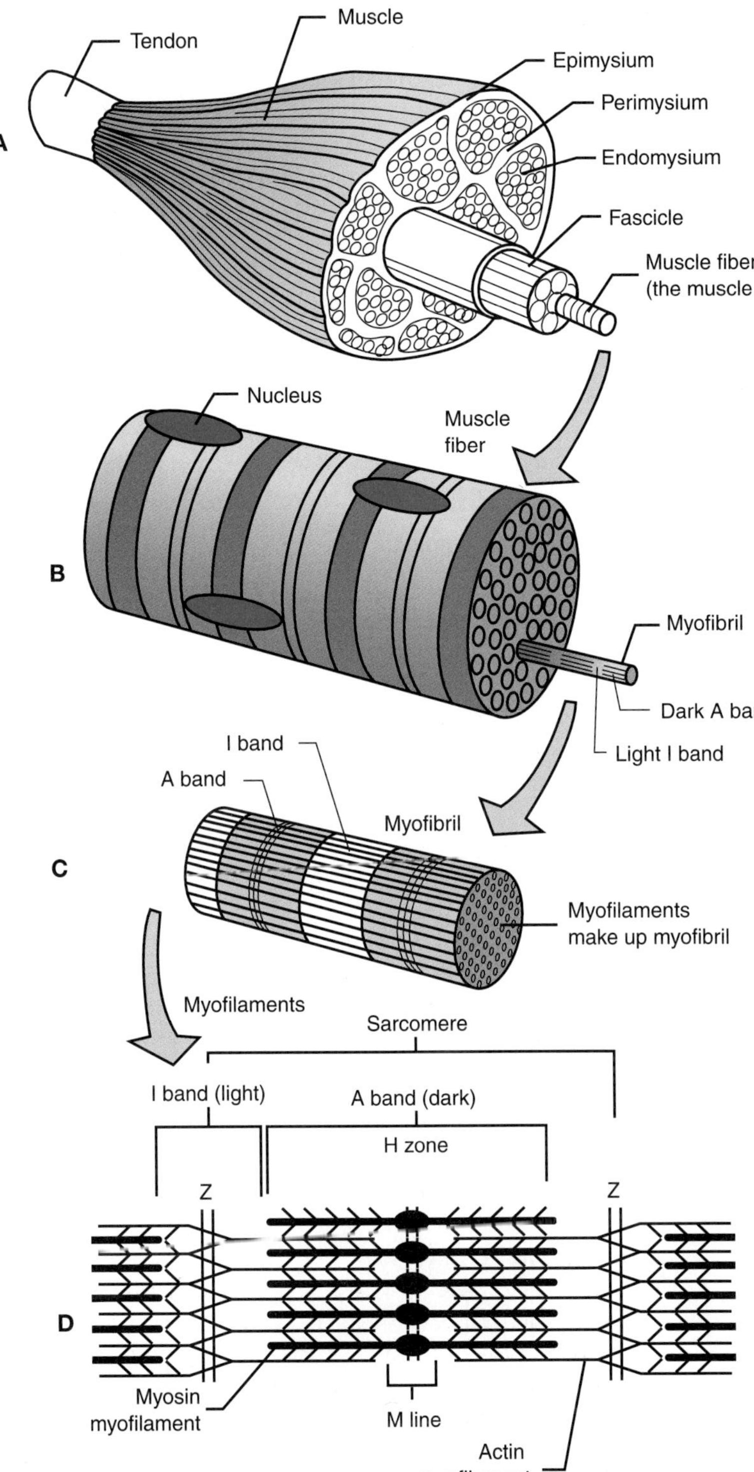

FIGURE **12-4** **Structure of Skeletal Muscle.** **A,** Skeletal muscle composed of bundles of muscle fibers. **B,** Magnified view of single muscle fiber made up of smaller myofibrils. **C,** Highly magnified view of myofibril made up of even smaller protein myofilaments. **D,** Ultrahigh-magnification view of the myofilaments that make up the myofibril. Note how thin actin myofilaments, thick myosin myofilaments, and the structures to which they are attached make light and dark bands visible in Figure 12-2.

myosin filaments. Figure 12-4 illustrates the structure of skeletal muscle from a large muscle down to the individual protein filaments.

If we put a thin section of skeletal muscle under a microscope and look at it under low-power magnification, we will see the alternating dark and light bands that give it part of its other name—voluntary striated muscle (see Figure 12-2.) At higher magnification, we can see a thin dark line in the center of the large light band and a lighter band in the center of the dark band. What we are actually viewing is the attachments and overlapping of the tiny actin and myosin filaments that make up the myofibril. Figure 12-3 shows that the large dark band (the **A band**) is made up of thick myosin filaments. The large light band (the **I band**) is made up of thin actin filaments.

The dark line in the center of the I band is called the **Z line.** It is actually a disk that looks like a line when viewed on end (like a coin viewed edgewise). It is the attachment site for the actin filaments. The area from one Z line to the next Z line is called a **sarcomere** and is the basic contracting unit of skeletal muscle. Each myofibril is made up of many sarcomeres lined up end to end. Each sarcomere only shortens slightly when the fiber is stimulated to contract, but when all the sarcomere contractions are added together, the muscle fiber shortens considerably.

TEST YOURSELF

1. Describe a skeletal muscle cell in terms of cell size, shape, number of nuclei, and appearance under the microscope.
2. What are the differences among a skeletal muscle fiber, a skeletal muscle myofibril, and a skeletal muscle protein filament?
3. Which contractile protein filaments make up the dark bands of skeletal muscle cells? Which make up the light bands?
4. What is a sarcomere and what are its components?

Neuromuscular Junction

Skeletal muscle is under conscious, voluntary control. Unless it receives nerve impulses, it does not do anything. If a skeletal muscle's nerve supply is interrupted for a lengthy period as a result of injury, the muscle will shrink down through a process called *atrophy.* The sites where the ends of motor nerve fibers "connect" to muscle fibers are called **neuromuscular junctions.** However, the word *connect* is not literally accurate because actually a very small space, called the *synaptic space,* exists between the end of the nerve fiber and the sarcolemma (cell membrane) of the muscle fiber. Figure 12-5 shows a neuromuscular junction.

Within the end of a nerve fiber in a neuromuscular junction are tiny sacs called *synaptic vesicles* that contain the chemical neurotransmitter acetylcholine. When a nerve impulse comes down the fiber, it causes the release of acetylcholine, which diffuses across the synaptic space and binds (attaches) to receptors on the sarcolemma. This starts the process that leads to the contraction of the muscle fiber. (We explore this process more fully in the section on skeletal muscle physiology.) The effect of

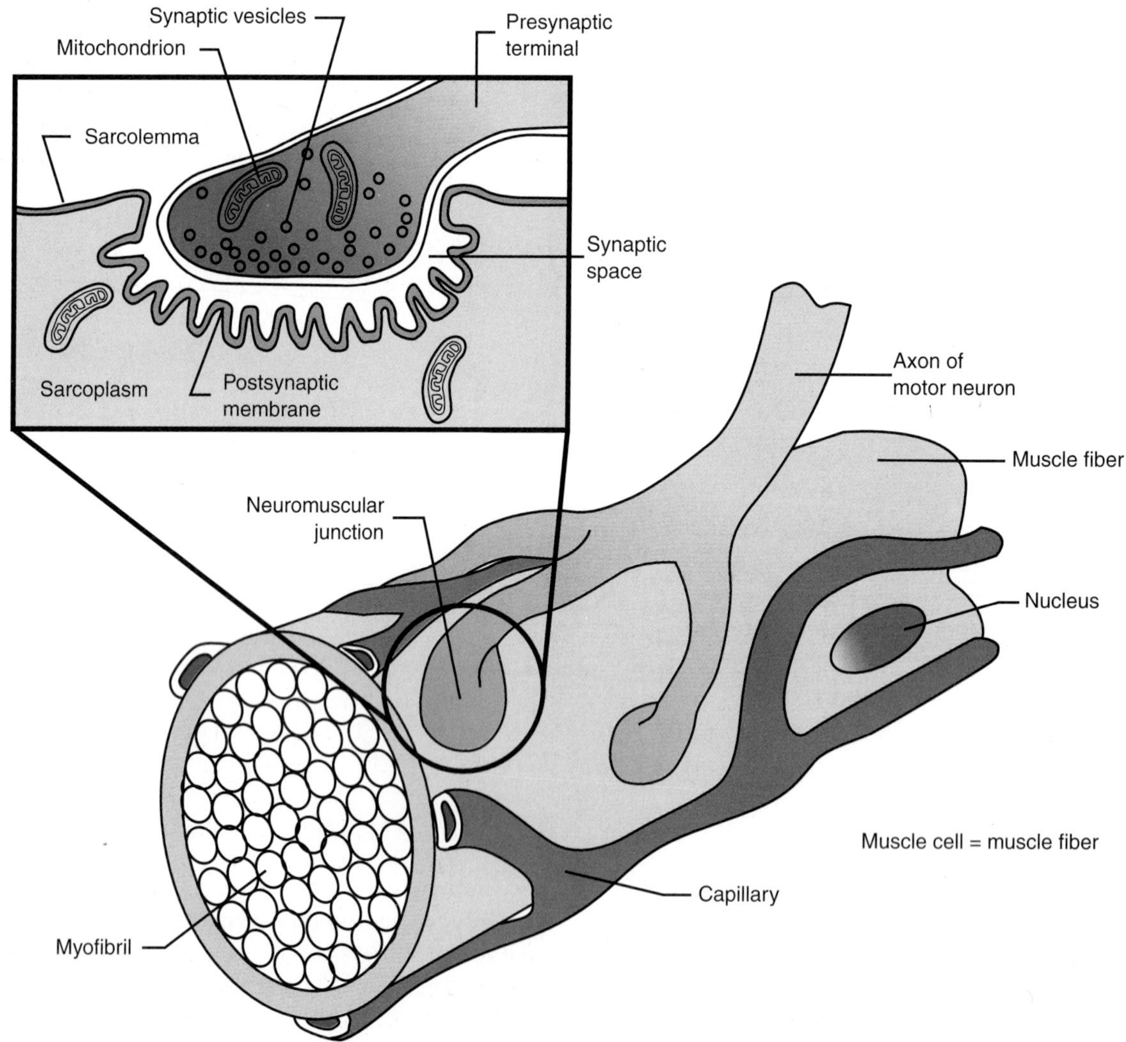

FIGURE **12-5** **Neuromuscular Junction.**

the acetylcholine on its receptor is very short, however. An enzyme in the synaptic space, acetylcholinesterase, quickly removes the acetylcholine molecule from its receptor and splits it apart. This ends the effect of that nerve impulse. If the body needs to contract that muscle fiber again, it must send down another nerve impulse.

Each nerve fiber innervates (sends impulses to) more than one muscle fiber. The number of muscle fibers per nerve fiber determines how small a movement will result from a nerve stimulus. The term **motor unit** is used to describe one nerve fiber and all the muscle fibers it innervates. Muscles that must make very small, delicate movements, such as the muscles that position the eyes, may only have a few muscle fibers per nerve fiber in each motor unit. On the other hand, large, powerful muscles, such as leg muscles, may have a hundred or more muscle fibers per motor unit. This allows the nervous system to control the activities of the skeletal muscles in an economical manner. If each nerve fiber attached to only one skeletal muscle fiber, immense numbers of nerve impulses would be constantly necessary to control the muscles' activities. That would require so much work that the nervous system could not do anything else.

Connective Tissue Layers

Because they exert a lot of force when they contract, skeletal muscle fibers must be securely fastened together and securely fastened to the structures (usually bones) they move. Each individual skeletal muscle fiber is surrounded by a delicate connective tissue layer composed of fine, reticular fibers called the **endomysium.** Groups of skeletal muscle fibers, called **fascicles,** are bound together by a tougher connective tissue layer, called the **perimysium,** which is composed of reticular fibers and thick collagen fibers. Groups of muscle fascicles are surrounded by **epimysium,** a fibrous connective tissue layer composed largely of tough collagen fibers. The epimysium is the outer covering of entire muscles. These three connective tissue layers are continuous with the tendons or aponeuroses that connect the muscle to bones or other muscles. So they not only hold the components of the muscle together but also help fasten the muscle firmly to its attachment mechanisms.

Aside from holding the muscle firmly together and attaching it to the appropriate structures, the connective tissue layers of a muscle also contain the blood vessels and nerve fibers that supply the muscle fibers. They commonly contain varying amounts of adipose tissue, or fat. The fat deposits are often visible grossly in meat and are called the **"marbling"** of the meat.

Physiology of Skeletal Muscle

Initiation of Muscle Contraction and Relaxation

When a nerve impulse comes down a motor nerve fiber and reaches the end bulb at the neuromuscular junction, acetylcholine is released into the synaptic space. The acetylcholine molecules bind to receptors on the surface of the sarcolemma (cell membrane) of the muscle fiber, which starts an impulse that travels along the sarcolemma and through the T tubules to the interior of the cell. When the impulse reaches the sarcoplasmic reticulum, it causes the release of stored calcium ions (Ca^{++}) into the **sarcoplasm** (cytoplasm). As the Ca^{++} diffuses into the myofibrils, it turns on the contraction process, which is powered by high-energy molecules of **adenosine triphosphate (ATP).** (ATP's function of providing cells with energy was discussed with cell metabolism in Chapter 3. We'll discuss its role in muscle contraction later in the section on the chemistry of muscle contraction.)

Almost as soon as the sarcoplasmic reticulum releases its Ca^{++} into the sarcoplasm, it begins pumping it back in again. This pulls the Ca^{++} out of the myofibrils, and the contraction process shuts down. The elasticity of the muscle fiber then returns it back to its original length, relaxing the fiber. Pumping the Ca^{++} back into the sarcoplasmic reticulum requires energy, which is also supplied by ATP molecules. So not only does muscle *contraction* require energy, but muscle *relaxation* does too.

The amount of calcium in the muscle fiber is determined largely by the level of calcium in the bloodstream. If the blood calcium level is too high or too low, abnormalities in skeletal muscle function can result. (See Chapter 14 for a discussion of the two hormones, calcitonin and parathyroid hormone, that control the blood calcium level, as well as the Clinical Application on hypocalcemia [too low a blood calcium level].)

Mechanics of Muscle Contraction

When a muscle fiber is in a relaxed state, the actin and myosin filaments overlap only a little. When the fiber is stimulated to contract, small levers on the myosin filaments, called **cross bridges,** ratchet back and forth and pull the actin filaments on both sides toward the center of the myosin filaments. This sliding of the filaments over each other shortens the sarcomere. The combined shortening of all the end-to-end sarcomeres in a muscle fiber results in what we call a *muscle contraction.*

Characteristics of Muscle Contraction

An individual muscle fiber either contracts completely when it receives a nerve impulse or it does not contract at all. This is known as the **all-or-nothing principle.** We know this is not true of whole muscles; so how does the body produce movements that vary in range and strength when individual muscle fibers are doing all or nothing? It does so by carefully controlling the number of muscle fibers it stimulates for a particular movement. Small, fine movements require only a few muscle fibers to contract. Larger, more powerful movements, on the other hand, require contraction of many muscle fibers. The nervous system is calling the shots; therefore it must predict how large and powerful a movement needs to be and must send the appropriate nerve impulses down to the appropriate muscle fibers in the appropriate muscle(s).

Getting down to the basics of muscle contraction, a single muscle fiber contraction (called a **twitch contraction**) can be divided into three phases: (1) the latent phase, (2) the contracting phase, and (3) the relaxation phase. The latent phase is the brief hesitation between the nerve stimulus and the beginning of the actual contraction. It lasts about 0.01 second (10 milliseconds [ms]). The contracting phase lasts about 0.04 second (40 ms), and the relaxation phase lasts about 0.05 second (50 ms). The entire contraction cycle takes about 0.1 second (100 ms). So maximum contraction efficiency occurs if nerve impulses arrive about 0.1 second apart. This results in a series of complete muscle fiber twitches. Whole muscles rarely contract by twitching; so how do they contract smoothly? They do so mainly by careful timing of the nerve impulses to the various motor units of the muscle. Twitches of individual muscle fibers are stimulated out of phase with each other; that is, they each occur at slightly different times. Some muscle fibers are contracting while others are relaxing. When all the muscle fiber activity is averaged out, smooth sustained muscle contractions result. Pretty tricky, eh?

Chemistry of Muscle Contraction

The considerable mechanical work of muscle contraction must be powered by a plentiful supply of energy. The immediate energy source that powers the sliding of the actin and myosin filaments is the compound ATP, which is produced by the many mitochondria in muscle fibers. ATP molecules are like tiny batteries that can release energy and then be recharged so that they can do it again. As their name implies, ATP molecules have three phosphate groups attached to a central adenosine core. When one of the phosphate groups is split off (forming **adenosine diphosphate, [ADP]**) a considerable amount of energy is released that powers the sliding of the actin and myosin filaments. This also "discharges" the ATP molecule. Another energy source has to reattach the phosphate group to "recharge" the ATP and get it ready to supply energy again.

The "battery charger" that converts ADP back to ATP is another compound in the muscle fiber and is called **creatine phosphate (CP).** When the CP molecule splits, the energy that is released adds a phosphate group to the ADP, converting it back to ATP. The newly recharged ATP molecule is ready to provide energy for further muscle contraction or relaxation (by helping pump Ca^{++} back into the sarcoplasmic reticulum).

The ultimate source of energy used to produce ATP and CP and keep the whole system operating comes from the catabolism (breakdown) of nutrient molecules. The two main compounds involved are glucose and oxygen. Glucose is a sugar molecule that is the primary energy source for most body cells, including the muscle cells. The muscles have a very large blood supply that constantly brings new supplies of glucose and oxygen to the muscle fibers.

Muscle fibers can also store glucose and oxygen for a rainy day when the supplies are plentiful and the cells are fairly inactive. Glucose is stored in the fibers in the form of glycogen, and oxygen is stored attached to large protein molecules called **myoglobin.** Like hemoglobin, myoglobin is red and can store and release large quantities of oxygen. When strenuous muscle contractions begin to deplete the oxygen supply to a muscle fiber, myoglobin can release its stash of oxygen molecules to resupply the fiber. As long as the oxygen supply is adequate to keep up with the energy needs of the fiber, the process is known as **aerobic** (oxygen-consuming) **metabolism,** and the maximum amount of energy is extracted from each glucose molecule.

Sometimes, particularly during periods of strenuous activity, the need for oxygen exceeds the available supply and muscle fibers must shift to what is called **anaerobic** (non–oxygen dependent) **metabolism** to produce the energy required for continued activity. Anaerobic metabolism is not as efficient as aerobic metabolism and results in **lactic acid** formation as a byproduct of incomplete glucose breakdown. The lactic acid can accumulate in the muscle tissue and cause discomfort. (Have your muscles ever felt sore after physical activities that were more strenuous than you were used to? That was the lactic acid making its presence known.) After the burst of activity is over, some of the lactic acid diffuses into the bloodstream and goes to the liver, where it is converted back to glucose by a process that requires oxygen. So, after a strenuous burst of exercise, an animal may continue to breathe heavily for awhile as its body repays its so-called oxygen debt.

TEST YOURSELF ✓

1. What ion, released from the sarcoplasmic reticulum by a nerve impulse, starts the contraction process in a muscle fiber?
2. What molecules in muscle act as the "batteries" to power the sliding of the actin and myosin filaments? What molecules function as the "battery chargers?"
3. If individual muscle fiber contractions obey the "all-or-nothing law," how does an animal control the size and strength of its muscular movements?
4. What is myoglobin and why is it important?
5. Why does an animal breathe heavily for awhile after heavy exercise?

CLINICAL APPLICATION — Rigor Mortis

Rigor mortis is Latin for "stiffness of death." We use this term to describe the stiffness of skeletal muscles that occurs shortly after an animal dies. It would seem more sensible for the muscles to go limp after death because all nerve stimulation ceases, but chemical reactions at the cellular level send things in another direction. When the animal dies, lack of oxygen to the cells causes normal activities and barriers within the cells to break down. One of the things that happens in skeletal muscle cells is that most of the Ca^{++} spills out of the sarcoplasmic reticulum. This causes contraction of many of the muscle fibers that is fueled by the last of the ATP molecules in the sarcoplasm. All the ATP is used up in the contraction, and no more is being made (because the animal is dead); therefore no energy source is available to relax the muscles. So the muscles get "stuck" in the contracted position, resulting in what we call *rigor mortis.*

Heat Production

Like all machines, muscles are less than 100% efficient at converting energy to useful work, or motion in this case. A considerable amount of the energy produced in muscles is in the form of heat. In fact, muscular activity is one of the major heat-generating mechanisms that the body uses to maintain a constant internal temperature. If heat production exceeds body needs, the excess must be eliminated by mechanisms such as panting or sweating. Under cold conditions, the body may need to increase the production of heat to avoid hypothermia (too low a body temperature). It often does this by producing the small, spasmodic muscle contractions we know as *shivering*.

CARDIAC MUSCLE

Cardiac muscle is also known as **involuntary striated muscle.** It is called *involuntary* because its contractions are not under conscious control. The *striated* part is so named because under the microscope its cells have the same kind of striped appearance as skeletal muscle cells.

Gross Anatomy of Cardiac Muscle

Cardiac muscle is found in only one place in the body—the heart. It forms most of the volume of the heart and makes up the majority of the walls of the cardiac chambers (the atria and the ventricles). Instead of being organized into distinct muscular structures like skeletal muscle, cardiac muscle cells form elaborate networks around the cardiac chambers. The arrangement and physical characteristics of cardiac muscle allow it to start contracting early in the embryonic period before birth and to continue contracting without a rest until the animal dies. To get a feel for how amazing that is, make a fist and, for the next minute or two, clench it tightly and then relax it about once per second. Before too long the forearm muscles that tighten your fist will become fatigued. The heart does this same kind of work, but it does not get any rest periods. Isn't that amazing?

Microscopic Anatomy of Cardiac Muscle

Cardiac muscle cells are striated (striped) like skeletal muscle cells and contain many of the same organelles and intracellular structures, such as myofibrils. However, cardiac muscle cells and skeletal muscle cells are otherwise very different. Cardiac muscle cells are *much* smaller than skeletal muscle cells and have only one nucleus per cell. They are not shaped like the long, thin fibers of skeletal muscle. They are longer than they are wide and often have multiple branches. They are securely attached to each other end to end to form intricate, branching networks of cells. The firm end-to-end attachments between cardiac muscle cells are visible under the microscope as dark, transverse lines between the cells (see Figure 12-1). These attachment sites are called **intercalated disks.** The intercalated disks securely fasten the cells together and also transmit impulses from cell to cell to allow large groups of cardiac muscle cells to contract in a coordinated manner. In fact, the networks of cardiac muscle cells around the cardiac chambers function as if they were each a large, single unit instead of a whole bunch of individual cells.

Physiology of Cardiac Muscle

Muscle Contractions

If we looked through a microscope at individual cardiac muscle cells being grown in a tissue culture flask, we would see something amazing. Each cell would be contracting rhythmically with no external stimulation at all. Furthermore, each cell would be contracting at a constant rate set by its own internal metronome—some rapidly and others more slowly. However, if two cells touch, the slower contracting cell adopts the faster cell's contraction rate. This demonstrates two unique and important things about cardiac muscle: (1) it contracts without any external stimulation, and (2) groups of cardiac muscle cells adopt the contraction rate of the most rapid cell in the group.

These self-starting and self-controlling aspects of cardiac muscle enable the heart to function as a very efficient pump. Rather than large numbers of muscle cells contracting at the same time, as in skeletal muscle, cardiac muscle cells contract in a rapid, wavelike fashion. The impulse that coordinates the contractions spreads from cell to cell across the intercalated disks like a wave. That rapid, wavelike contraction effectively squeezes blood out of the cardiac chambers much like milk being squeezed out of a dairy cow's teat at milking time.

For these wavelike contractions of cardiac muscle to effectively move blood through the chambers and valves of the heart and out into the rest of the body, they must be carefully initiated and controlled. This is the role of the heart's internal impulse conduction system, which functions like a "mini nervous system." This impulse conduction system consists entirely of cardiac muscle cells. The impulse that starts each heartbeat begins in the heart's "pacemaker," or the **sinoatrial (SA) node** located in the wall of the right atrium. Why does the SA node have so much control over things? The reason goes back to that business about cardiac muscle cells adopting the contraction rate of the most rapidly contracting cells in the group. The contraction rate of the cardiac muscle cells in the SA node is faster than those in the walls of the atria or ventricles therefore its rate takes precedence. The impulse that starts in the SA node follows a carefully controlled path through the conduction system of the heart. Structures in the system transmit, delay, and redirect each impulse so that the cardiac muscle cells in the walls of the heart chambers contract in the coordinated, effective manner necessary to pump blood around the body. (Details of the cardiac impulse conduction system can be found in Chapter 8.)

Nerve Supply

Although it is not needed to *initiate* the contractions of cardiac muscle, the heart has a nerve supply that can *modify* its activity. We know from successful heart transplants that the heart's nerve supply is not essential to its function. (The nerves to the heart are severed when it is removed from the donor.) So what role does the heart's nerve supply play in controlling the beating of the heart?

The nerves to the heart are from both divisions of the autonomic portion of the nervous system, that is, the sympathetic and parasympathetic systems. Sympathetic fibers stimulate the heart to beat harder and faster as part of the "fight or flight response" that kicks in when an animal feels threatened. Parasympathetic fibers do the opposite in that they inhibit cardiac function, thereby causing the heart to beat more slowly and with less force when the body is relaxed and resting. The two opposing systems strike a balance that keeps the heart's activity appropriate for what is going on inside and outside the animal at any particular time. (More information about the autonomic portion of the nervous system and its effect on cardiac function can be found in Chapter 7 and Chapter 8.)

TEST YOURSELF

1. Describe a cardiac muscle cell in terms of cell size, shape, number of nuclei, and appearance under the microscope.
2. What are intercalated disks and why are they important to the functioning of cardiac muscle?
3. Describe the effect of its nerve supply on the functioning of cardiac muscle.
4. What is the general effect of sympathetic nervous system stimulation on cardiac muscle? Parasympathetic nervous system stimulation?

SMOOTH MUSCLE

Smooth muscle is also called **nonstriated involuntary muscle,** or sometimes just **involuntary muscle.** Like cardiac muscle, it is called *involuntary* because its contractions are not under conscious control. The *smooth* part is so named because its cells do not have the striped appearance under the microscope that skeletal muscle and cardiac muscle cells have. It is really very different from the other two types of muscle.

GROSS ANATOMY OF SMOOTH MUSCLE

Smooth muscle is found all over the body but not in distinct structures like the skeletal muscles and the heart. Rather, it is found in two main forms: (1) large sheets of cells in the walls of some hollow organs **(visceral smooth muscle)** and (2) small, discrete groups of cells **(multiunit smooth muscle).**

MICROSCOPIC ANATOMY OF SMOOTH MUSCLE

Smooth muscle cells are small and spindle shaped (tapered on the ends) with a single nucleus in the center. They have a smooth, homogeneous appearance under the microscope because their filaments of actin and myosin are not arranged in parallel myofibrils as in skeletal and cardiac muscle. Rather, small contractile units of actin and myosin filaments crisscross the cell at various angles and are attached at both ends to **"dense bodies"** that correspond to the Z lines of skeletal muscle (Figure 12-6). When these contractile units shorten, they cause the cell to "ball up" as it contracts. Because their contractile units are not organized into regular, parallel sarcomeres, individual smooth muscle cells can shorten to a greater extent than skeletal or cardiac muscle cells.

PHYSIOLOGY OF SMOOTH MUSCLE

Visceral Smooth Muscle

Visceral smooth muscle is found in the walls of many soft, internal organs, which are also known by the general name **viscera.** Its cells are linked to form large sheets in the walls of organs such as the stomach, intestine, uterus, and urinary bladder. Fine movements are not possible with visceral smooth muscle; rather, it shows large, rhythmic waves of contraction. These contractions can be quite strong, as in the peristaltic contractions that move food along the gastrointestinal tract and the uterine contractions that push the newborn animal out into the cold, cruel world at parturition (birth).

Like cardiac muscle, visceral smooth muscle contracts without the need for external stimulation. It does react to stretching, however, by contracting more strongly. This is useful in the gastrointestinal tract, where the presence of food in the lumen stretches the tube and the smooth muscle in its wall responds with increased contractions that help move the food along. Something similar happens in the urinary bladder; however, the slow, gradual stretching of the bladder wall caused by urine accumulation does not trigger contraction of the smooth muscle in its wall until the bladder is fairly full. In the pregnant uterus it is very important that the smooth muscle in its wall *does not* contract as the fetus grows and stretches the uterine wall. The result would be premature loss of the fetus and termination of the pregnancy. The uterus must be kept quiet as the fetus enlarges and develops. This is done through hormones, such as progesterone, that inhibit the smooth muscle in the uterine wall from contracting during pregnancy. When the time comes to give birth, the level of the progesterone in the bloodstream plummets dramatically. This removes the inhibition of the uterine smooth muscle, and a combination of factors, including rising levels of other hormones (such as estrogens and oxytocin) stimulate the smooth muscle to contract. This starts the process of labor.

Like cardiac muscle, visceral smooth muscle has a nerve supply that is not necessary to initiate contractions but serves to modify them. Also like cardiac muscle, the nerve supply to smooth muscle consists of the sympathetic and parasympathetic divisions of the autonomic nervous system. The effects of the two are reversed from their effects in cardiac muscle, however. Sympathetic stimulation decreases visceral smooth muscle activity, and parasympathetic stimulation increases it. This makes sense if we think about sympathetic and parasympathetic functions. Sympathetic stimulation prepares an animal for intense physical activity. Blood is diverted away from the viscera and redirected to the heart, skeletal muscles, and brain to help deal with whatever threat initiated the fight or flight response. Decreasing gastrointestinal motility as a part of this

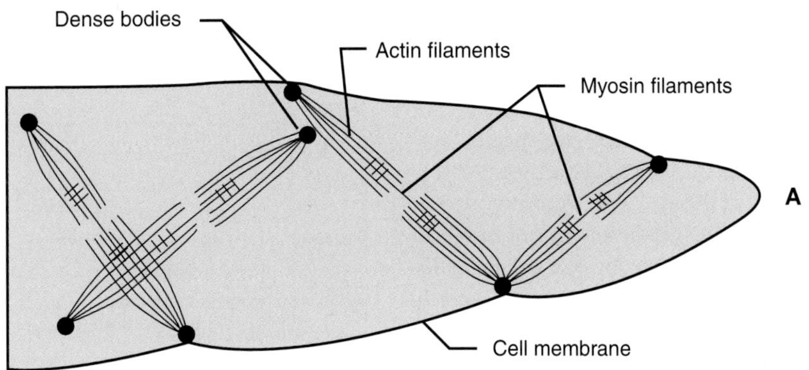

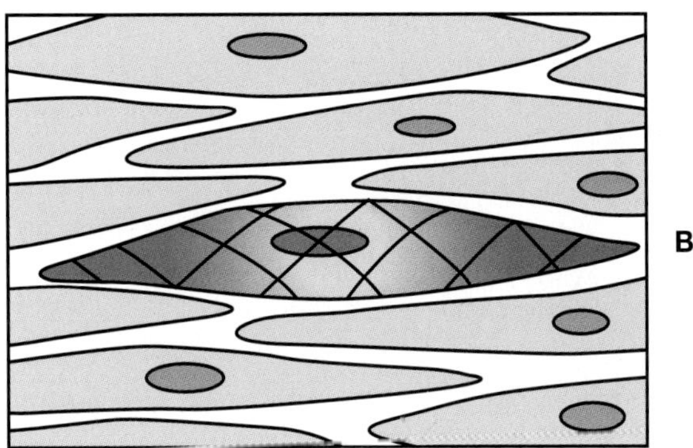

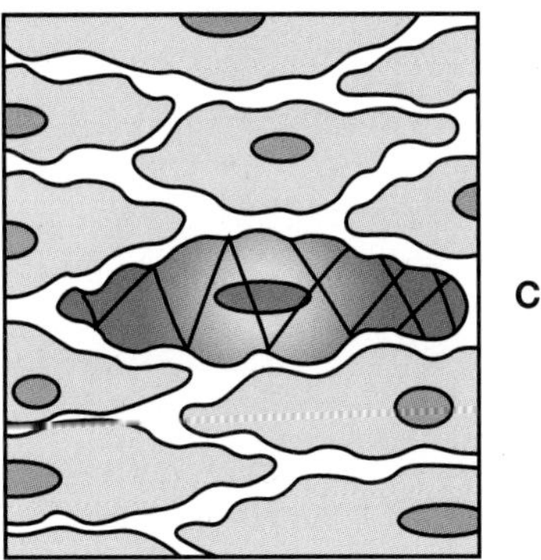

FIGURE **12-6** **Smooth Muscle. A,** Arrangement of actin and myosin filaments in crisscrossing contractile units. **B,** Relaxed smooth muscle cells. **C,** Contracted smooth muscle cells.

response makes sense. Digestion is not a priority at that point. On the other hand, when the animal is relaxed and resting, the parasympathetic system predominates and enhances functions such as gastrointestinal activity to help supply nutrients to the body cells during this "down time." As with the heart, the two opposing autonomic divisions strike a balance to keep smooth muscle activity at an appropriate level for the body's ever-changing needs.

Multiunit Smooth Muscle

Where visceral smooth muscle is large and relatively powerful, **multiunit smooth muscle** is small and delicate. Instead of being formed into large sheets that function as a single, large unit, multiunit smooth muscle is made up of individual smooth muscle cells or small groups of cells. It is found where small, delicate contractions are needed, such as the iris and ciliary body of the eye, the walls of small blood vessels, and around small air passageways in the lungs. Also unlike visceral smooth muscle, contractions of multiunit smooth muscle are not automatic. They require specific impulses from autonomic nerves to contract.

The actions of multiunit smooth muscle are specific and carefully controlled. This allows fine control of actions, such as adjusting the size of the pupil of the eye or the accommodation (focusing) of the lens. It also allows delicate control of blood flow throughout the body and airflow through the lungs by adjusting the size of blood vessels and air passageways according to the body's needs.

TEST YOURSELF

1. Describe a smooth muscle cell in terms of cell size, shape, number of nuclei, and appearance under the microscope.
2. What are the main differences between visceral smooth muscle and multiunit smooth muscle?
3. Describe the effect of nerve stimulation on the functioning of visceral smooth muscle and multiunit smooth muscle.
4. What is the general effect of sympathetic nervous system stimulation on visceral smooth muscle? Parasympathetic nervous system stimulation?
5. What are the main differences in the structures and functions of skeletal muscle, cardiac muscle, and smooth muscle?

CHAPTER 13

SENSE ORGANS

Thomas Colville

How many senses do animals have? Tradition says five: hearing, seeing, feeling, smelling, and tasting. Anatomy and physiology say they have a whole bunch of senses. How's that for scientific precision? Actually, coming up with a precise number is difficult because so many different kinds of sensations can be identified and the total number depends on how we separate or group them. However, the total is definitely more than five.

Before we try to sort through the sensory numbers game, let's look at what sense organs are. In simplest terms, they are extensions of the central nervous system (CNS) that allow it to monitor what is going on inside and outside the animal. At the heart of all sense organs are various kinds of specially modified nerve endings called **sensory receptors.** When triggered by an appropriate stimulus, a sensory receptor generates a nerve impulse that travels to the CNS and is interpreted as a particular sensation.

The sensory receptors of common domestic animals are sensitive to the following four general types of stimuli:

1. Mechanical stimuli (e.g., touch, hearing, balance)
2. Thermal stimuli (e.g., hot and cold)
3. Electromagnetic stimuli (e.g., vision)
4. Chemical stimuli (e.g., taste and smell)

All of the sensations that an animal can perceive start with one or more of these four types of stimuli. Therefore the CNS has to do a lot of work to correctly interpret the resulting sensory nerve impulses. For instance, one type of mechanical stimulus is a pesky cat rubbing against a dog's leg. Another type of mechanical stimulus is the sound of a can opener being used to open a can of dog food. The distinction is important to a hungry dog. Fortunately, its CNS is preprogrammed to correctly identify the many sensory nerve impulses it receives.

So how many senses are there? Would you believe 10? That's right; we are going discuss 10 senses or categories of sensation in this chapter—five general senses and five special senses. The general and special senses are listed in Table 13-1.

GENERAL SENSES

The **general senses** are visceral sensations, touch, temperature, pain, and proprioception. Some of them are not exactly household names. As their name implies, general senses are distributed generally throughout the body. Their receptors tend to be fairly simple structures, and they transmit sensory information to the CNS through peripheral and autonomic nerve fibers. Because their receptors tend to be widespread on the inside and outside of the body, the general senses keep the CNS informed about the overall prevailing conditions inside and outside the body.

Although they are important to the well-being of an animal, the general senses are rarely involved in clinical disease or treatment. So we will give them a quick once-over, but we won't discuss them in detail. Additional information about the general senses can be found in more in-depth anatomy and physiology references.

VISCERAL SENSATIONS

Visceral sensations make up a somewhat miscellaneous category of "interior" body sensations. Most are vague and poorly localized. They include the sensations of hunger and thirst, which indicate deficiencies of nutrients and water. The result

Table 13-1 General and Special Senses

Sense	What Is Sensed	Type of Stimulus
General Senses		
Visceral sensations	Hunger, thirst, hollow-organ fullness	Chemical, mechanical
Touch	Touch and pressure	Mechanical
Temperature	Heat and cold	Thermal
Pain	Intense stimuli of any type	Mechanical, chemical, or thermal
Proprioception	Body position and movement	Mechanical
Special Senses		
Taste	Tastes	Chemical
Smell	Odors	Chemical
Hearing	Sounds	Mechanical
Equilibrium	Balance and head position	Mechanical
Vision	Light	Electromagnetic

is the initiation of behaviors designed to secure the needed substances and restore nutrient and fluid balance (homeostasis) in the body.

Other visceral sensations originate in internal organs, particularly hollow organs such as the gastrointestinal tract and portions of the urinary system. Interestingly, these organs have only certain, specific kinds of receptors, particularly stretch receptors. Anything that stretches the wall of the organ, such as a bubble of gas in the intestine or a stone (calculus) in the ureter, can be intensely painful. On the other hand, these same organs can be handled, cut, or crushed without any apparent pain. This can be a problem on those rare occasions when an abdominal surgical incision breaks down (called *surgical wound dehiscence*) and internal organs come out through the defect. The animal actually can traumatize its own organs without feeling any apparent discomfort.

The urinary bladder is an exception to the rule that "stretching causes severe pain," which holds true for most other hollow internal organs. The job of the urinary bladder is to store urine as it is produced by the kidneys and release it periodically to the outside. The sensation of a filling bladder reaches the conscious mind, but it is not an acutely painful event. Rather, it triggers reflex centers in the spinal cord that cause the smooth muscle in the wall of the bladder to contract. Urination then may take place, or it can be delayed if the animal contracts the voluntary sphincter muscle that surrounds the neck of the bladder.

The pleura and peritoneum (membranes that line and cover the contents of the thorax and abdomen, respectively) are well supplied with sensory receptors. As long as conditions are normal and the pleural and peritoneal surfaces are sliding over each other smoothly, no sensation is felt. However, if the surfaces become roughened by inflammation and infection, the resulting pleuritis or peritonitis is very painful. Pleuritis and peritonitis most often result from penetrating wounds from the outside or from ruptures or perforations of internal organs. When opening thoracic or abdominal organs surgically, we must be very careful to suture them closed securely to prevent leakage, which could lead to pleuritis or peritonitis.

Touch

We include **touch** and **pressure** together, even though they are sometimes classified as separate senses by nitpickers (aka "real" anatomists and physiologists). Touch, also known as the **tactile sense,** is the sensation of something being in contact with the surface of the body. It can be difficult to differentiate touch from pressure, which is the sense of something pressing on the body surface. Different kinds of specific touch and pressure receptors produce sensations of light contact, deep pressure, vibration, or hair movement. The overall effect is to give the CNS a picture of what, where, and to what extent objects from the outside environment are physically in contact with the surface of the body. The touch and pressure sensations operate almost at an unconscious level unless the contact is abrupt or the pressure severe. Once physical contact or pressure is initially sensed, it quickly fades into the sensory background unless it changes or is extreme.

If you are sitting down while reading this, take a moment to think about where the chair is contacting your body—probably in the areas of your lower back, buttocks, and the backs of your thighs. Until you thought about those areas, you probably were not consciously aware of the pressure on them, unless you are sitting in a very uncomfortable chair. The CNS has too much information to process to keep track of everything that is or is not in contact with every square millimeter of the skin's surface. Usually, only when things change do the sensations of touch and pressure rise to the level of the conscious mind.

Temperature

The **temperature sense** is the monitoring half of the body's temperature control (temperature homeostasis) system. Temperature receptors detect increases or decreases in body temperature and transmit the information to the CNS. The CNS can activate mechanisms to correct conditions of **hypothermia** (a too low body temperature) or hyperthermia (a too high body temperature).

Temperature receptors fall into two categories: superficial and central. Superficial temperature receptors are located in the skin and detect upward or downward changes in skin temperature. Heat receptors increase their generation of nerve impulses when the temperature increases, and cold receptors increase theirs when the temperature falls. These increased impulses get the attention of the conscious mind and let it know that things are out of balance. At constant temperatures the receptors generate steady, low-level streams of nerve impulses that are sensed at the subconscious level and do not intrude on the conscious mind.

Central temperature receptors keep track of the core (interior) temperature of the body by monitoring the temperature of the blood. Central temperature receptors are located in the hypothalamus, a small but very important area of the brain. (See Chapters 7 and 14 on the nervous and endocrine systems for information on other important functions of the hypothalamus.) An animal's rectal temperature indicates its core temperature.

By monitoring the temperature of the body both superficially and centrally, the nervous system can initiate corrective actions if things become too hot or cold. By controlling functions such as blood flow in and beneath the skin, sweating, piloerection (hairs "standing on end" to increase insulation by trapping air), shivering, and even thyroid hormone production, the nervous system can set in motion mechanisms that can help bring body temperature back into balance. It can also initiate behaviors to help heat or cool the animal as needed. If the animal is too hot, it may seek out shade or cool water. If it is too cold, it might seek out warmth or increase its muscular activity to generate more heat.

PAIN

Pain receptors, also called **nociceptors,** are the most common and widely distributed sensory receptors inside and on the surface of the body. They are found almost everywhere. They consist of simple, free nerve endings that respond to intense stimuli of all types. Their purpose is to protect the body from damage by alerting the CNS to potentially harmful stimuli. Interestingly, the only place in the body where pain receptors are *not* found is the brain. It is not uncommon for certain types of human brain surgery to be performed on wide-awake patients who have had local anesthesia so that the brain could be exposed.

Pain can be classified in a number of ways. One useful system classifies pain as superficial (skin and subcutaneous areas), deep (muscles and joints), and visceral (internal organs). Another system classifies pain as acute (sharp and intense) or chronic (dull and aching).

We cannot get inside the head of a dog or a horse to find out precisely how they perceive pain, but behavioral and physiological responses suggest that they experience pain much the same way we do. The difference is often in how they *react* to the pain. Humans often tend to dwell on pain they are experiencing, which often seems to make the overall experience even more stressful, whereas nonhuman animals seem to accept the current situation as how things are supposed to be. This is not to say that they do not suffer pain; rather, they just do not seem to have the same kind of emotional reaction to it that humans do. They often seem to hide it well, which can be a problem for us clinically when we are trying to assess the degree of pain a patient is experiencing. Actually, hiding signs of pain is a survival instinct for most animals. An animal that shows signs of pain is showing signs of weakness that might encourage other animals, including predators, to attack it.

Visible reactions to pain vary greatly among species, breeds, and animals. Some animals are very sensitive to pain and become stressed by even mildly painful stimuli. Others hardly seem to react at all until pain becomes severe. Prevention and relief of pain are becoming increasingly important in veterinary medicine as we learn more about its harmful effects and how to prevent them. Research studies are providing the knowledge necessary to detect the subtle signs of pain that many animals show. This information is allowing us to become more proactive in our efforts to prevent and treat pain in ill and injured patients.

CLINICAL APPLICATION: Heatstroke and Hypothermia

Normal cellular functions in warm-blooded animals depend on the core body temperature remaining fairly constant. This is because chemical reactions, including all the metabolic reactions that occur in the body, are temperature dependent. Higher temperatures speed up chemical reactions, and lower temperatures slow them down. Significant variations in the core temperature of the body, such as might occur in **heatstroke** (significantly elevated body temperature) or hypothermia (significantly decreased body temperature), can have serious consequences and endanger the life of the animal.

Heatstroke can result from prolonged exposure to high environmental temperatures. The core temperature of the affected animal climbs to dangerously high levels. Early on the animal typically appears weak and confused; as things progress, it may lapse into unconsciousness that can lead to convulsions and even death. The very rapid heart and respiratory rates that occur in affected animals are signs of the abnormally accelerated metabolic reactions in the body. If the animal is not cooled in time, the distorted metabolic reactions, particularly in the brain, can reach a point at which brain damage and possibly death can result. The maximum body temperature compatible with life is about 10° F (5° C) above the animal's normal body temperature level.

Hypothermia results from an abnormally low body temperature that slows all the metabolic processes. Heart and respiratory rates of affected animals slow as their core temperatures drop. If not warmed, affected animals can lose consciousness and die. Hypothermia can result from prolonged exposure to cold environmental temperatures, but it also can occur in the veterinary hospital in animals under general anesthesia. Most general anesthetic drugs anesthetize the temperature control centers in the brain along with the conscious mind. This often results in a slow fall in body temperature during anesthetic procedures that can be accelerated by contact with cold environmental surfaces, such as metal surgery tables. The falling core temperature slows metabolic reactions in the animal's body, including those that metabolize or eliminate the anesthetic agent at the end of the procedure and allow the animal to wake up. This can prolong the time it takes for the animal to recover from the anesthetic. For this reason, we generally try to keep anesthetized and recovering animals warm through means such as table and cage warmers, towels, blankets, and hot water bottles.

PROPRIOCEPTION

Without looking at them, can you tell what positions your arms and legs are in? Of course you can, although precisely

Clinical Application — Anesthesia and Analgesia

Esthesia is the ability to perceive sensations, that is, to feel things. (The study of the sensory system can be called *esthesiology*.) ***An*****esthesia** is the loss of esthesia, or the complete loss of sensation. In clinical veterinary medicine, we use two basic types of anesthesia to carry out procedures that would be painful for patients: general anesthesia and local anesthesia.

General anesthesia involves a complete loss of sensory perception accompanied by loss of consciousness. The animal is placed into a controlled sleep that prevents it from feeling painful procedures. We produce it by administering general anesthetic drugs either by injecting them or by having animals breathe them from an inhalant anesthesia machine. Animals under general anesthesia must be monitored closely because the drugs depress cardiovascular and respiratory functions along with the CNS.

Local anesthesia produces loss of sensation from a specific, localized area of the body without affecting consciousness. It is produced by injecting a local anesthetic drug into an area through which sensory nerve fibers pass. The drug blocks the transmission of nerve impulses through the site, which prevents sensory information from reaching the brain. Otherwise painful procedures can be performed without having to put the animal completely out.

Analgesia is a related state in which the perception of pain is decreased but not completely absent. The pain is dulled but not completely gone. A drug that produces analgesia is called an *analgesic* drug. Aspirin, ibuprofen, and morphine are all examples. Analgesic drugs are often used to make animals with severe pain more comfortable.

how you do it may not be clear. You just seem to know where all your body parts are. Actually, you are making use of your **proprioception** sense, which is the sense of body position and movement. This sense operates largely at the subconscious level and is very important in allowing an animal to stand upright and make accurate, purposeful movements as it interacts with its environment. During the examination of an animal with suspected nervous system damage, a veterinarian often evaluates proprioception by bending the animal's foot so that it is upside down and seeing how long it takes the animal to right it. Animals with normal proprioception almost immediately bring the foot up into a normal standing position,

The heart of the proprioception sense is the variety of stretch receptors located in skeletal muscles, tendons, ligaments, and joint capsules. These receptors keep the CNS informed about the movements of limbs, the positions of joints, the state of contraction of muscles, and the amount of tension being exerted on tendons and ligaments. This information is important to the CNS so that it can send out the right combination of motor nerve impulses, which are appropriate in range and strength, to produce smooth body movements.

TEST YOURSELF

1. Why are visceral sensations important to the survival of an animal?
2. Why do touch and pressure sensations fade so rapidly from the conscious mind unless they change or are severe?
3. If a dog walks out of an air-conditioned house and lies in the sun on a hot summer day, which of its temperature receptors will signal the brain first that the dog is getting hot—superficial receptors or central receptors?
4. Which category of temperature receptors is most critical to the long-term survival of an animal in very hot or very cold environmental conditions—the superficial receptors or the central receptors? (Hint, which is more critical to an animal's survival—keeping its skin and extremities from getting too hot or cold or keeping the core of its body from getting too hot or cold?)
5. Why do you suppose mild to moderate pain often does not seem to significantly affect the mood or behavior of domestic animals?
6. Why is the proprioception sense so important to the maintenance of balance and an upright posture?

SPECIAL SENSES

The **special senses** are taste, smell, hearing, equilibrium, and vision, that is, most of the "traditional" senses. In contrast with the general senses, the special senses are organized into specific, often complex sensory organs and structures that are all located in the head. Because of their locations, structures, and functions, the special sense organs often are involved in clinical illnesses and injuries.

Taste

The sense of **taste,** also called the **gustatory sense,** is a chemical sense. Its receptors are located in the mouth in structures called *taste buds.* When they detect chemical substances dissolved in the saliva, the taste receptors generate nerve impulses that travel to the brain and are interpreted as tastes.

The majority of the taste buds are located on the sides of certain small, elevated structures on the tongue called *papillae,* although a few can be found in the lining of the mouth and throat (pharynx). As seen in Figure 13-1, taste buds are tiny, rounded structures made up of gustatory (sensory) cells and supporting cells. Tiny openings on the surface of each taste bud, the taste pores, allow dissolved substances to enter the taste buds and contact the sensory receptors. The sensory receptors are tiny, hairlike processes from the gustatory cells that project up into the taste pores. When appropriate chemical substances dissolved in the saliva come in contact with the sensory processes, nerve impulses are generated that travel to the brain and are interpreted as particular tastes.

In humans the four primary taste sensations are sweet, sour, salty, and bitter. Each has a particular area of the tongue that

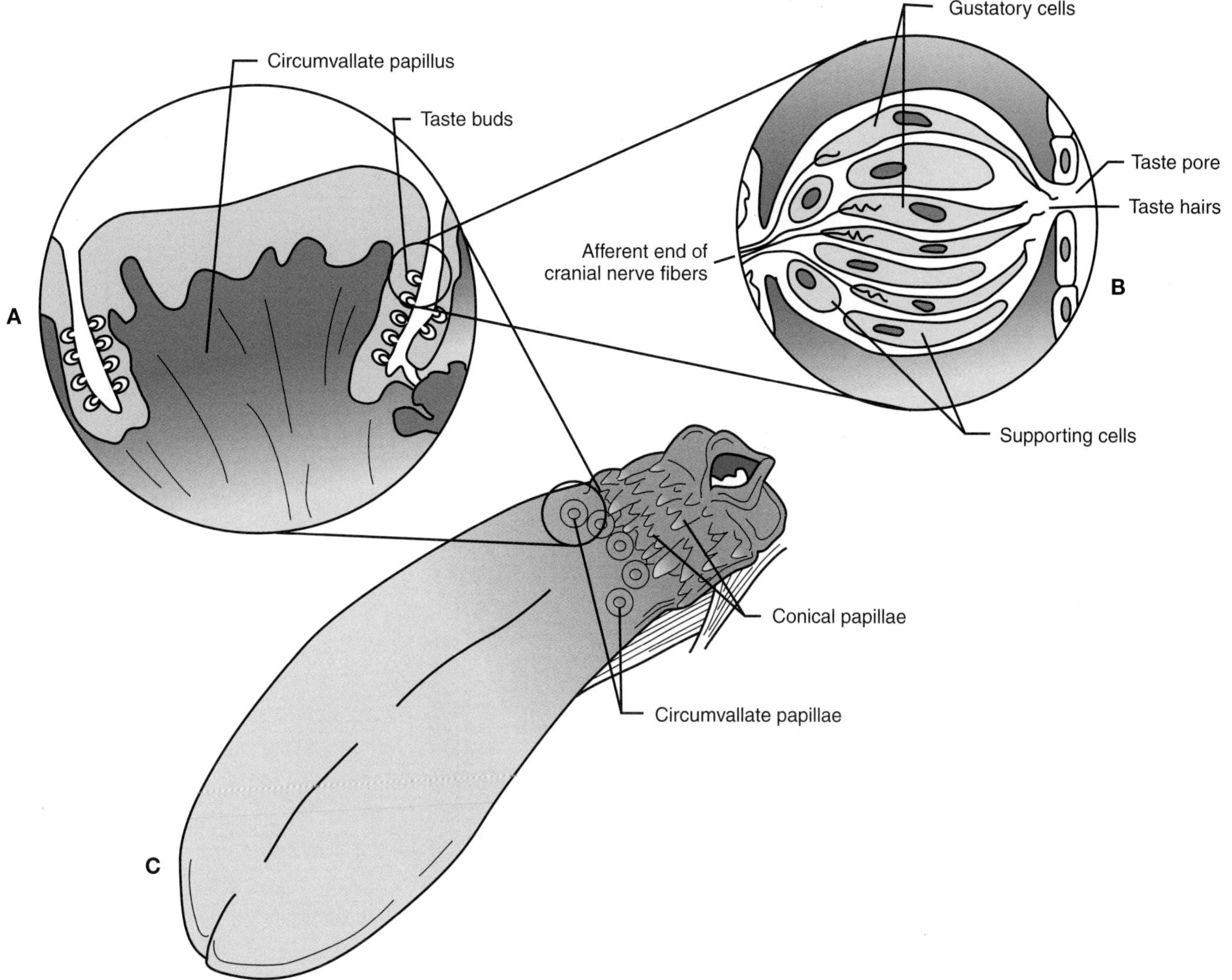

FIGURE **13-1** **Taste Buds on Tongue.** **A,** One magnified papilla showing locations of taste buds. **B,** Taste bud structure. **C,** Tongue showing a few of the many papillae that contain taste buds.

responds most strongly to that taste. The ability to detect many different kinds of tastes is due to combinations of the four basic taste sensations and interactions with the sense of smell. We cannot know if nonhuman animals experience tastes in the same way, but taste sensations most likely vary among animal species.

SMELL

The sense of **smell** is also called the **olfactory sense.** It is a chemical sense very similar to taste. The sense of smell is more important in most nonhuman animals than it is in humans. We live in a sight-oriented world. Although we have a decent sense of smell, our keen vision is more important to us as we interact with our environment. In contrast, many nonhuman animals have less sensitive eyesight but a highly sensitive sense of smell. They live in more of a smell-oriented world. This can be difficult for us to relate to, but dogs obtain a huge amount of information from sniffing the air or an object, such as a fire hydrant. For reasons that we will discuss shortly, they probably do not see colors like we do, but they can smell "colors" that we cannot even imagine. So the next time you are walking a dog and it decides to stop and do a thorough "sniff-examination" of something, do not immediately yank on its leash to get it moving. It is busy "reading" messages left for it by every other dog that has visited there. Take a moment to appreciate the amazing communication process you are witnessing. The dog will appreciate it.

The sense of smell is organized in two patches of olfactory epithelium located up high in both nasal passages. Figure 13-2 shows the location and some of the structure of the olfactory epithelium. Sensory (olfactory) cells are mixed with supporting cells in these epithelial

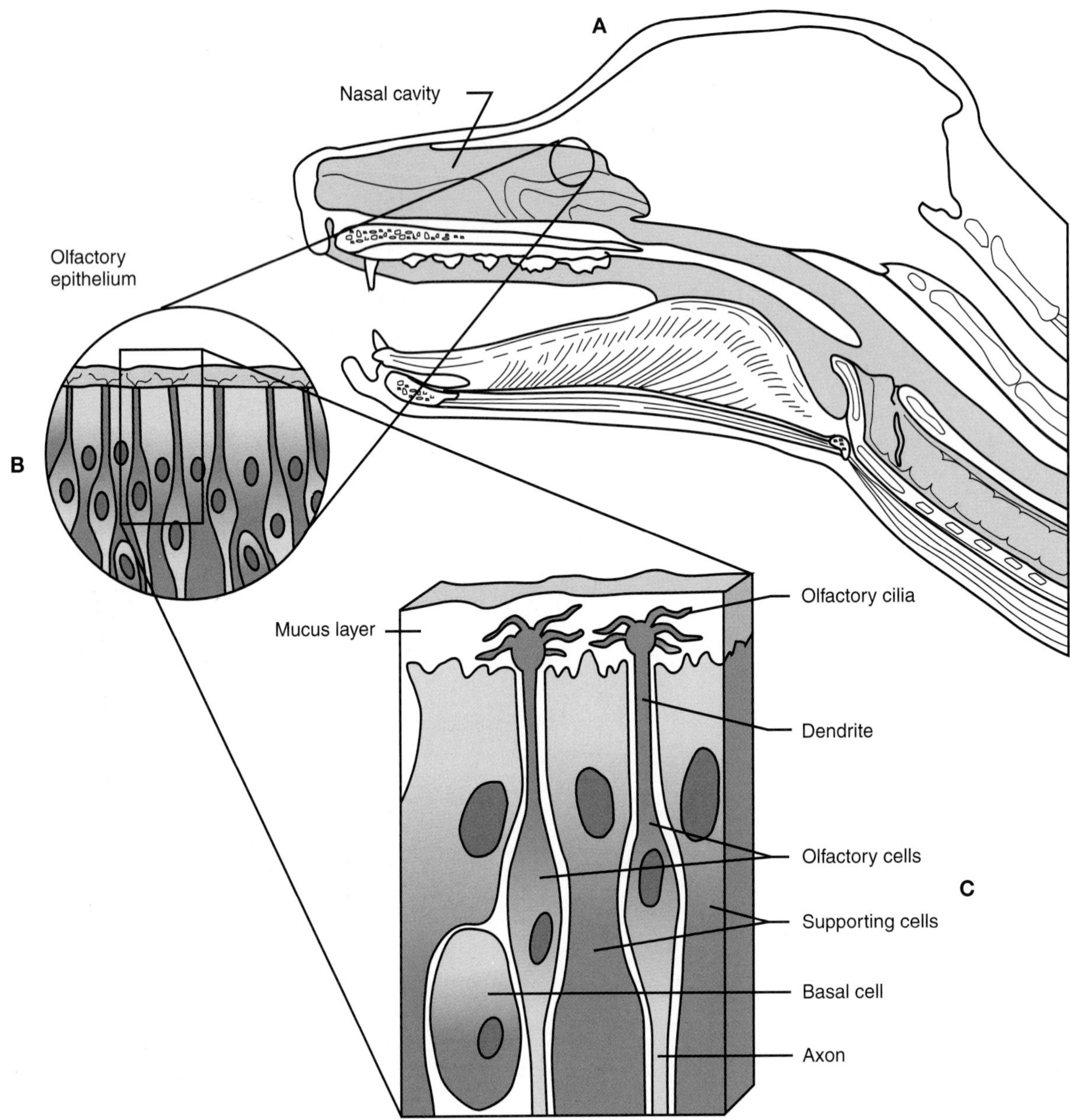

FIGURE **13-2** **Olfactory Region of Dog. A,** Location of olfactory region high in nasal passage. **B,** Olfactory epithelium. **C,** Detail of olfactory epithelium showing olfactory cilia projecting up into overlying mucous layer.

patches. Hairlike processes from the surfaces of the olfactory cells project up into the mucous layer that covers the nasal epithelium. When odor molecules dissolve in the mucus and contact the sensory processes, nerve impulses are generated that travel to the brain and are interpreted as particular smells.

TEST YOURSELF

1. How are the senses of taste and smell similar? How are they different?
2. Why do nonhuman animals often greet others by sniffing them?

Hearing

Hearing, also called the *auditory sense,* is a mechanical sense that converts vibrations of air molecules into nerve impulses that are interpreted by the brain as sound. The ear, the organ of hearing, can be divided into three physical and functional areas: the **external ear,** the **middle ear,** and the **inner ear.** The external ear acts as a funnel to collect sound wave vibrations and direct them to the eardrum. The middle ear amplifies and transmits the vibrations from the eardrum to the inner ear. The inner ear contains the actual sensory receptors that convert the mechanical vibrations to nerve impulses, along with receptors for the equilibrium sense.

Most of the ear structures are housed within the temporal bones of the skull. The external ear canal, the middle ear

CLINICAL APPLICATION Upper Respiratory Tract Infections

Upper respiratory tract infections are caused by disease-causing organisms such as viruses and bacteria. They affect primarily the nasal passages and pharynx (throat) and result in coughing, sneezing, sore throat, and discharges from the eyes and nose. The common cold is a human upper respiratory tract infection. What sometimes makes upper respiratory tract infections dangerous for domestic animals is their affect on the animals' senses of smell—they effectively eliminate it. Think back to your last cold. You probably did not have much of a sense of smell, which rendered most foods bland and tasteless. The effect on animals that live in a smell-oriented world is even more drastic. They often stop eating and drinking completely because they cannot smell anything. If this continues for very long, they can be in real danger from dehydration. Therefore we often have to administer fluids either orally or by injection to animals with upper respiratory tract infections. By keeping them properly hydrated while we provide other necessary medical and nursing care, we often can help them fight off the infection.

cavity, and the inner ear structures all occupy hollowed-out areas in the temporal bones that are lined with soft tissue membranes. The processes of collecting, transmitting, and converting sound wave vibrations all take place within these membrane-lined bony cavities. Figure 13-3 shows the main structures of the external, middle, and inner portions of the ear.

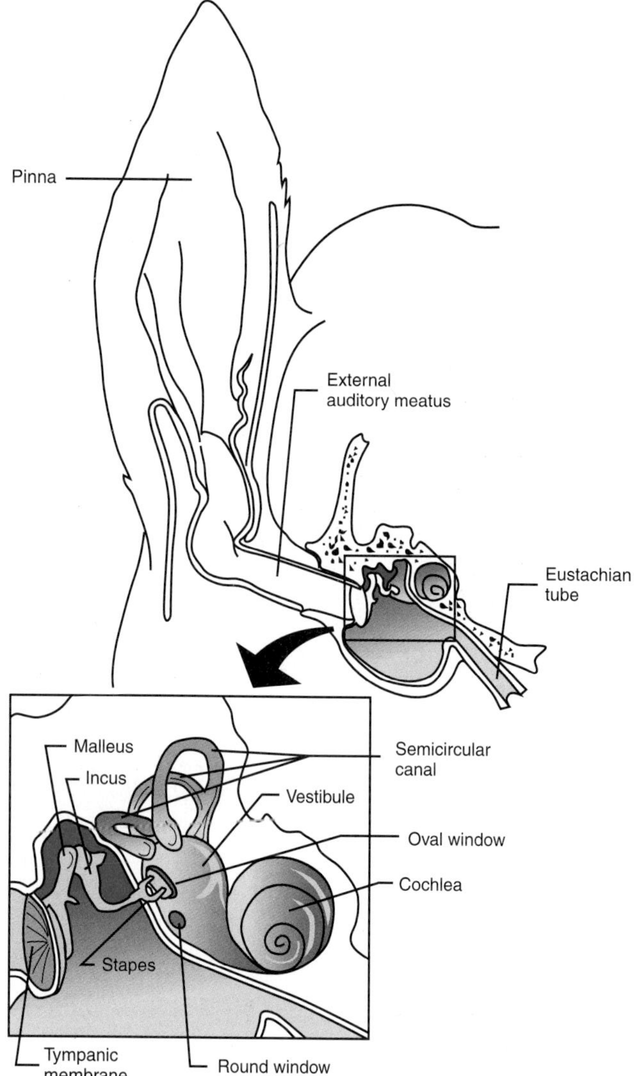

FIGURE **13-3** **Cross Section of Dog's Ear Structures With Middle and Inner Ear Regions Enlarged.**

External Ear

The external ear consists of structures that collect sound waves and transmit them to the middle ear. Its main parts are the **pinna,** the **external auditory canal,** and the **tympanic membrane (eardrum).**

The pinna is the part of the ear that we can see from the outside. It is a funnel-like structure composed mainly of elastic cartilage and skin that collects sound wave vibrations and directs them into the external auditory canal. In many animals the pinna is very mobile and can be aimed in the directions of sounds. For instance, watch the ears of a horse in a strange environment. Its ears will probably be scanning the area like a couple of little radar dishes. This ability is particularly useful in animals with erect ears.

The external auditory canal is a soft, membrane-lined tube that begins at the base of the pinna and carries sound waves to the tympanic membrane (eardrum). In most domestic animal species, it is somewhat L shaped, with an outer vertical portion and an inner horizontal portion. It ends blindly at the tympanic membrane.

The tympanic membrane is commonly called the *eardrum.* It is a paper-thin, connective tissue membrane that is tightly stretched across the opening between the external auditory canal and the middle ear cavity. When sound wave vibrations strike it, the tympanic membrane vibrates at the same frequency through a process called *sympathetic vibration.* (*Author's note:* Another example of sympathetic vibration is the annoying audible vibration of a snare drum that occurs when certain notes are played by a band or orchestra. If you have ever been in a band or orchestra, you know what I am talking about.)

Middle Ear

The middle ear cavity is a hollowed-out area of the temporal bone that is lined by soft tissue membranes. It is filled with air and contains three small bones called **ossicles** and the opening of the **eustachian tube,** which connects it with the pharynx (throat). Laterally it is separated from the external ear by the tympanic membrane, and medially it is separated from the inner ear by the membranes that cover the oval and round windows of the cochlea.

The three small ossicles link the tympanic membrane with the **cochlea** of the inner ear, where the receptors for hearing are located. The individual ossicles are named for some past

CLINICAL APPLICATION — Ear Hematomas

The pinna is basically just elastic cartilage and some small blood vessels covered by skin. Sometimes irritation in the ear canal (such as otitis externa [see the following Clinical Application]) will cause an animal to vigorously shake its head. In some animals, particularly floppy-eared dogs, this movement can rupture small blood vessels under the skin of the pinna, usually on the inside surface. The resulting bleeding between the cartilage and skin can cause an accumulation of blood, called an *ear hematoma.* (A hematoma is an abnormal accumulation of free blood in an area.) An ear hematoma usually is not painful or dangerous to an animal, but it is heavy and swollen and often seems to bother the animal. If left untreated, the blood will be reabsorbed slowly, but the ear probably will be permanently deformed by scar tissue, resulting in what is called a "cauliflower ear." Treatment of ear hematomas usually involves surgically draining the material from the hematoma and placing sutures through the pinna to hold the skin tight against the cartilage and prevent the fluid from reaccumulating. The underlying cause of the head shaking should be determined and treated also to prevent recurrence.

CLINICAL APPLICATION — Otitis Externa

Otitis externa is an inflammation of the skin of the external ear canal that occurs most commonly in dogs, cats, and rabbits. It is often caused by parasites, such as ear mites, foreign bodies, or microorganisms such as bacteria and yeasts. The irritation in the ear canal causes redness, pain, itching, and fluid accumulation. The owner usually notices that the animal shakes its head a lot and spends time pawing at its ears. When the affected ear is examined, the ear canal is often red, moist, swollen, and painful and often has a characteristic pungent odor.

The basic anatomy of the external ear canal adds a challenge to the treatment of otitis externa. Inflammatory fluids tend to drain down and accumulate in the horizontal portion of the canal next to the tympanic membrane. Because topical medications are commonly used to treat otitis externa, the ear canals must be cleaned thoroughly and carefully to remove the discharges before the medications are instilled. Because the ear canals are often swollen and painful, this process can be difficult for at least the first few days. Therapy for otitis externa often must be continued for many weeks to bring the condition under control.

anatomist's fanciful impression of their shapes. The outermost bone, the **malleus** (hammer), is attached to the tympanic membrane. The malleus forms a complete synovial joint with the middle bone, the **incus** (anvil), which in turn forms a joint with the medialmost bone, the **stapes** (stirrup). The other end of the stapes is attached to the membrane that covers the **oval window** of the cochlea. How this attachment to the cochlea contributes to hearing is described further in the section on the inner ear.

The ossicles act as a system of levers that transmit the sound wave vibrations from the tympanic membrane to the cochlea. In doing so, they decrease the amplitude (size) of the vibrations but amplify their force. This helps transmit the vibrations accurately to the very sensitive receptor structures in the cochlea, hopefully without causing damage. Another mechanism that helps prevent damage to the hearing receptors is a tiny muscle, the *tensor tympani,* that attaches to the malleus. It adjusts the tension of the tympanic membrane and helps deaden the transmission of extremely loud sound vibrations to the cochlea. Another tiny muscle, the *stapedius,* assists the damage-control process by restricting the movement of the stapes by loud sounds.

The eustachian tube (also called the *auditory tube*) connects the middle ear cavity with the pharynx. Its purpose is to equalize the air pressure on the two sides of the tympanic membrane. Without this structure, every time the atmospheric (barometric) pressure changed (as it often does; watch the next weather forecast), the tympanic membrane would bulge in or out, depending on which way the barometric pressure changed. This would be painful (the tympanic membrane is liberally supplied with pain receptors) and would decrease sound wave transmission. Fortunately, the eustachian tube comes to the rescue. The slitlike opening of the tube in the pharynx is stretched open whenever the animal swallows or yawns. This allows air to enter or leave as necessary to equalize the pressure in the middle ear cavity with that of the outside air. (This system is put to the test when we engage in activities that rapidly change the pressure on the outside of the tympanic membrane, such as flying or scuba diving. Consciously swallowing or yawning often helps correct the resulting pressure imbalance.)

Inner Ear

The inner ear is made up of structures that contribute to both hearing and equilibrium. The hearing portion of the inner ear is contained in a snail shell–shaped spiral cavity in the temporal bone called the cochlea (Figure 13-4). Within the hollowed-out bony cavity of the cochlea is a soft, multilayered, fluid-filled portion that contains the receptor organ of hearing—the **organ of Corti**. The organ of Corti runs the length of the cochlea in a long tube called the **cochlear duct** that is filled with a fluid called **endolymph.** A U-shaped tube containing another fluid, **perilymph,** lies on either side of the cochlear duct. Membrane-covered openings at the ends of the U, called the **oval window** and the **round window,** are located at the base of the cochlea. The "bottom" of the U is located at the tip of the cochlea. Nothing lies against the round window, but the stapes (one of the ossicles) is attached to the oval window.

The organ of Corti runs along the cochlear duct, on a shelf called the *basilar membrane,* like a long ribbon. Its main parts are hair cells, supporting cells, and the **tectorial membrane.** The hair cells are the receptor cells of hearing. They have tiny, hairlike projections on their surfaces. The gelatin-like tectorial membrane lies gently on top of the "hairs" like a long, soft

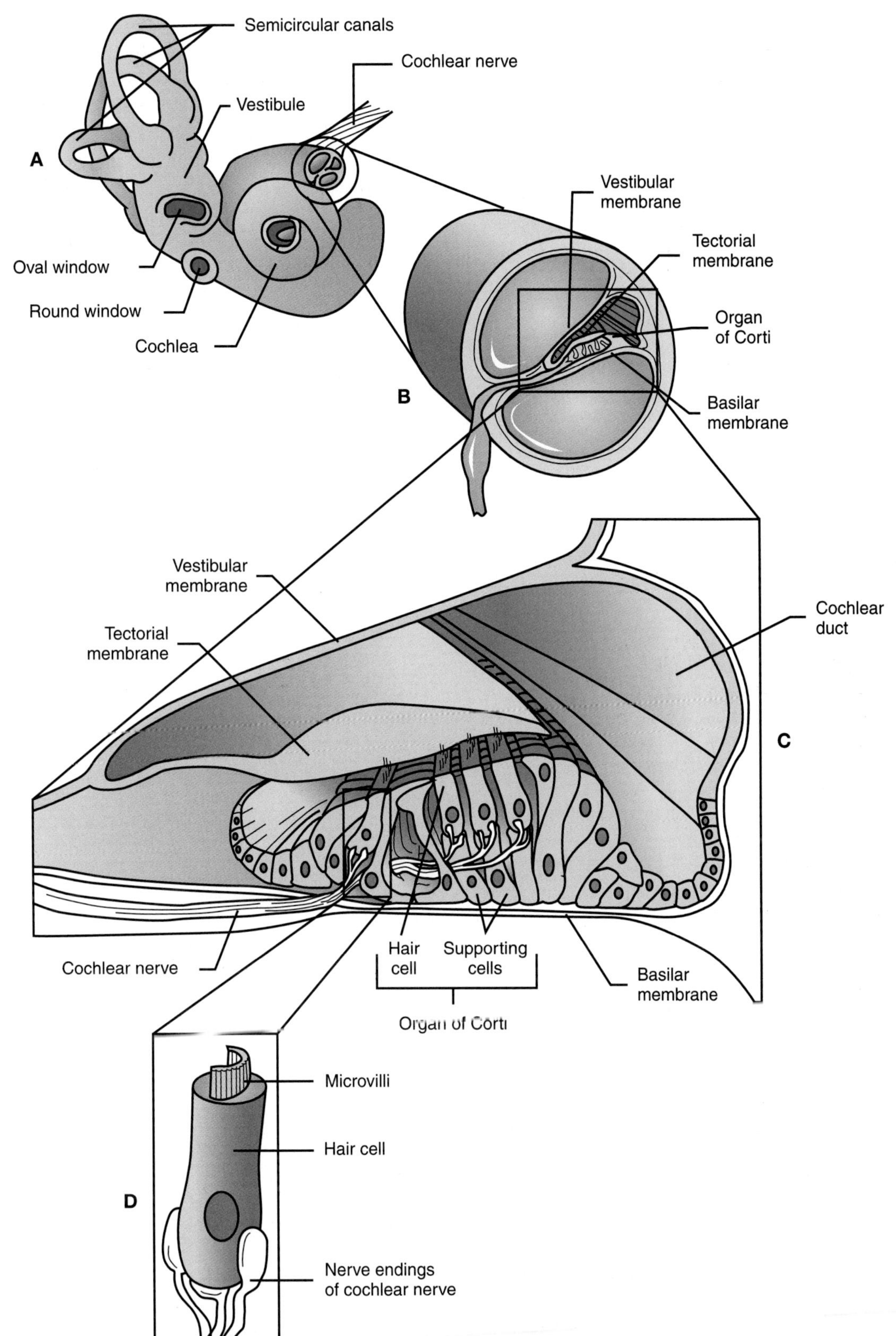

FIGURE **13-4** **Inner Ear Structures With Detail of Cochlear Anatomy. A,** Inner ear structures. **B,** Enlarged cross section of cochlea. **C,** Detail of organ of Corti. **D,** Greatly enlarged single sensory hair cell.

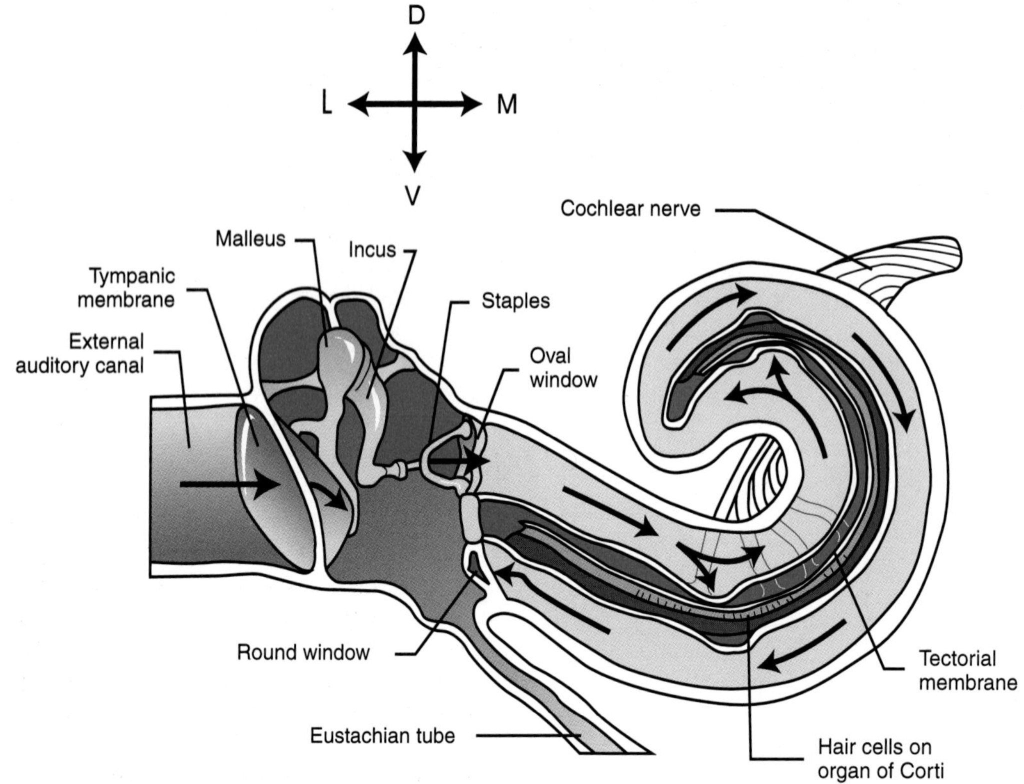

FIGURE **13-5** **Effect of Sound Waves on Cochlear Structures.** Sound waves cause tympanic membrane and ossicles to vibrate. As the stapes vibrates back and forth, it pushes and pulls on membrane covering the oval window of the cochlea. This sets fluid in the cochlea in motion, which causes hair cells and tectorial membrane to rub against each other. This bends sensory hairs, generating nerve impulses that are transmitted to the brain and interpreted as sound.

strip lying on top of a broad series of brush bristles. As their name implies, the supporting cells provide physical support to the hair cells.

Sound wave vibrations cause the tympanic membrane and the ossicles in the middle ear to vibrate. As the stapes vibrates back and forth, it alternately pushes and pulls on the membrane covering the oval window of the cochlea. This causes the perilymph around the cochlear duct to vibrate back and forth. (The membrane covering the round window acts as a pressure relief mechanism by alternately bulging in and out as the fluid moves back and forth.) This process is summarized in Figure 13-5. The movement of the perilymph causes the cochlear duct to move, which causes the tectorial membrane and the hair cells of the organ of Corti to rub against each other. This bends the sensory hairs, which generates nerve impulses that travel to the brain and are interpreted as sound. Different frequencies of sound wave vibrations stimulate different areas along the length of the organ of Corti. Areas near the oval window respond best to high-frequency (high pitched) sounds, and areas at the tip of the cochlea respond best to low-frequency (low-pitched) sounds. This physical process generates nerve impulses in different parts of the organ and helps the brain differentiate high- and low-pitched sounds.

TEST YOURSELF

1. Which skull bone houses the middle and inner ear structures?
2. Why would keen hearing be important to the survival of a potential prey animal? How about a predator animal?
3. How would rupture or perforation of an eardrum affect hearing?
4. How would arthritis in the tiny joints of the ossicles affect hearing? Could this possibly affect the hearing of older animals?
5. How would an animal with a middle ear infection that caused the opening of the eustachian tube to swell closed probably feel?
6. How might a lot of exposure to loud sounds lead to progressive hearing loss?

Equilibrium

As the head goes, so goes the rest of the body. At least that is the principle behind the sense of **equilibrium.** This mechanical sense helps the animal maintain its balance by keeping track of the position and movements of the head. Its receptors are located in portions of the inner ear called the **vestibule** and the **semicircular canals.**

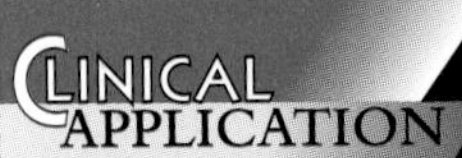

Recovery From General Anesthesia

The importance of head position to overall body posture and balance can be seen in an animal that is recovering from general anesthesia. One of the first things that a recovering animal tries to do as it regains consciousness is to raise its head into an upright position and steady it there. It has to accomplish that position before it can start trying to raise its body. Primitive instincts for survival prompt many animals to try and stand before they are steady and coordinated enough to support themselves. This can lead to stumbling and falling, as well as injury. By taking advantage of our knowledge of the sense of equilibrium, we can prevent an animal from trying to get up prematurely by gently holding its head down in a horizontal position until it has enough strength and coordination to rise. This can be particularly important in larger animals, such as horses. By holding a recovering horse's head down with a gentle hand or knee on its neck just behind the skull, we can keep the animal from trying to get up too soon. Once we feel it has regained enough strength, we can allow it to raise its head and prepare to help steady it as it rises to its feet.

Actually, maintaining balance is a complicated process that involves information from the equilibrium receptors, as well as from the eyes and the proprioceptors around the body. (See the Clinical Application on motion sickness for an explanation of what happens when the information from these various sources does not agree about what is happening.)

Vestibule

The vestibule is the portion of the inner ear that is located between the cochlea and the semicircular canals. It is made up of two saclike spaces, called the **utricle** and the **saccule,** that are continuous with the cochlear duct of the cochlea and are filled with the same endolymph fluid. Like the cochlear duct, the utricle and saccule are surrounded by perilymph.

In each utricle and saccule is a patch of sensory epithelium called the **macula** (Figure 13-6). It consists of hair cells and supporting cells covered by a gelatinous matrix that contains tiny crystals of calcium carbonate called **otoliths.** (The word *otolith* literally means "ear stone.") The hair cells are similar to the hair cells of the organ of Corti in the cochlea. They have hairlike processes on their surfaces that the gelatinous matrix sits on. Gravity causes the otoliths and the gelatinous matrix to put constant pressure on the hairs as long as the head stays still. Movement of the head bends the sensory hairs, which generate nerve impulses that give the brain information about the position of the head.

Semicircular Canals

The semicircular canals are located on the other side of the vestibule from the cochlea. Each canal is semicircular and oriented in a different plane at right angles to the other two. If you are indoors in a room with square walls, look up in a corner where two walls and the ceiling come together. Each of the walls and the ceiling is in a different plane at right angles to the other two. This is the basic arrangement of the semicircular canals.

Within each bony semicircular canal is an endolymph-filled membranous tube that is surrounded by perilymph. (Each of the endolymph-filled structures in the inner ear is continuous with the others, as are the perilymph-filled structures.) Near the utricle end of each semicircular canal is an enlargement, called the **ampulla,** that contains the receptor structure—the **crista** (full name, **crista ampullaris**).

The crista is similar to the macula of the vestibule. It consists of a cone-shaped area of supporting cells and hair cells with their processes sticking up into a gelatinous structure called the **cupula** (Figure 13-7). However, there are no otoliths to weigh down the cupula. It functions as a float that moves with the endolymph in the membranous canal.

When the head moves in the plane of one of the semicircular canals, inertia causes the endolymph to lag behind the movement of the canal itself. The same principle is at work if you quickly rotate a glass containing liquid and ice cubes. The glass turns, but the liquid and ice cubes lag behind. The relative movement of the endolymph pulls on the cupula, which bends the hairs. This generates nerve impulses that give the brain information about motion of the head, particularly rotary motion.

So the vestibular system senses rotary motion of the head with the semicircular canals and linear motion and position of the head with the vestibule. By integrating this information, the brain forms a picture of what is happening to the animal's head, and by extension, to its body as a whole.

TEST YOURSELF

1. How is the functioning of the vestibule and the semicircular canals similar? How is it different?
2. What are otoliths and why are they important to the equilibrium sense?
3. How is the physical concept of inertia important to the functioning of the semicircular canals?
4. What is the basic cause of motion sickness?

VISION

The eyes have a lot in common with electronic cameras. They have lens covers (the eyelids), a front "window" to let light in (the cornea), an adjustable diaphragm to control the amount of light that enters (the iris), a lens that can be focused, light detectors on which the image is formed (rods and cones in the retina), and a cable to carry the images to a recorder (the optic nerve).

As complicated as the eye seems, most of its components exist to help *form* an accurate visual image, not *detect* it. The actual **photoreceptors** that detect the image, and generate visual nerve impulses are in a single layer of cells in the retina (the structure that lines the back of the eyeball). In our discussion of vision, we'll deal mostly with the image-formation structures of the eye.

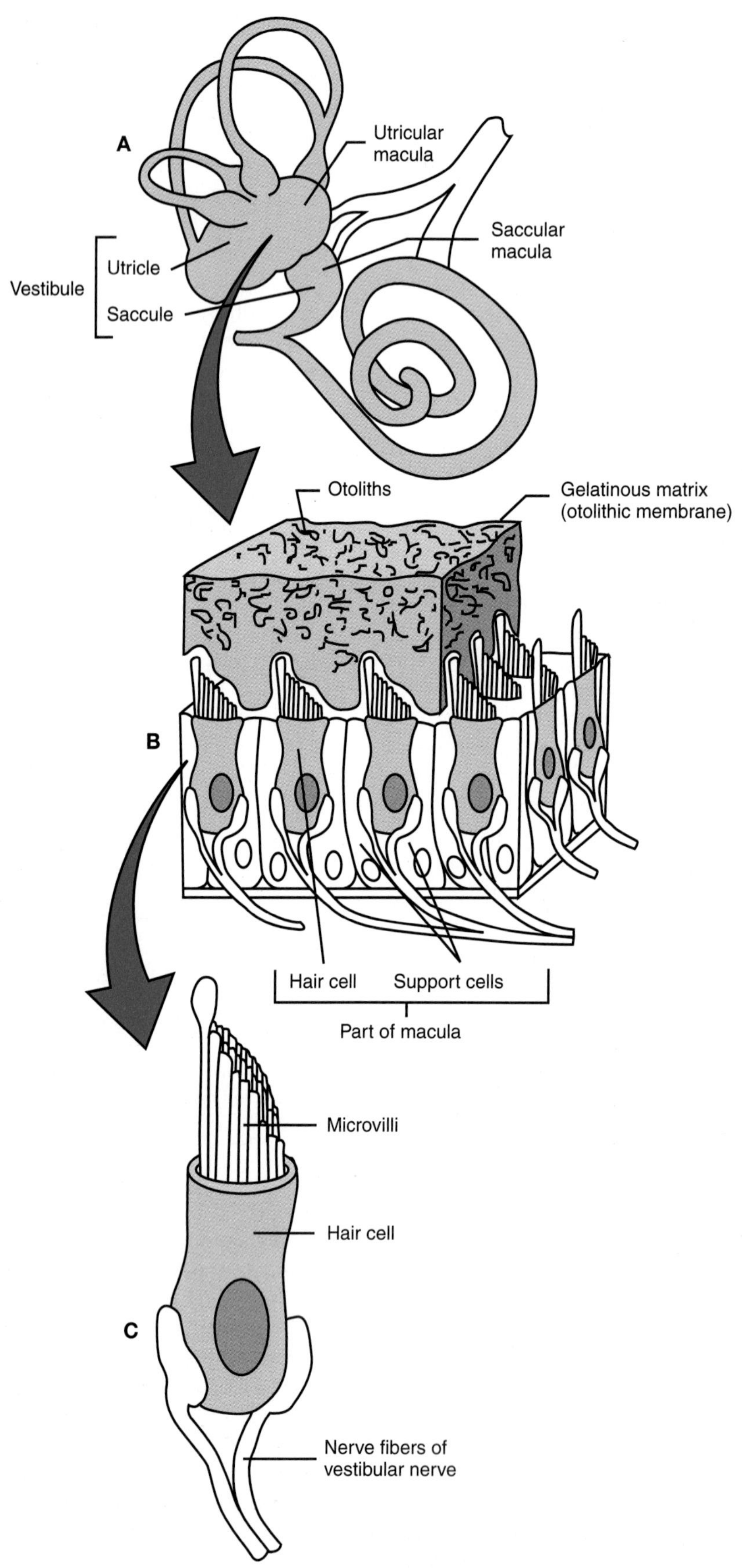

FIGURE **13-6 Inner Ear Structures With Detail of Vestibular Anatomy. A,** Inner ear structures. Note utricle and saccule, which make up the vestibule, and locations of macula (sensory epithelium) in each. **B,** Enlarged view of macula showing sensory hair cells, gelatinous matrix, and otoliths. **C,** Greatly enlarged sensory hair cell.

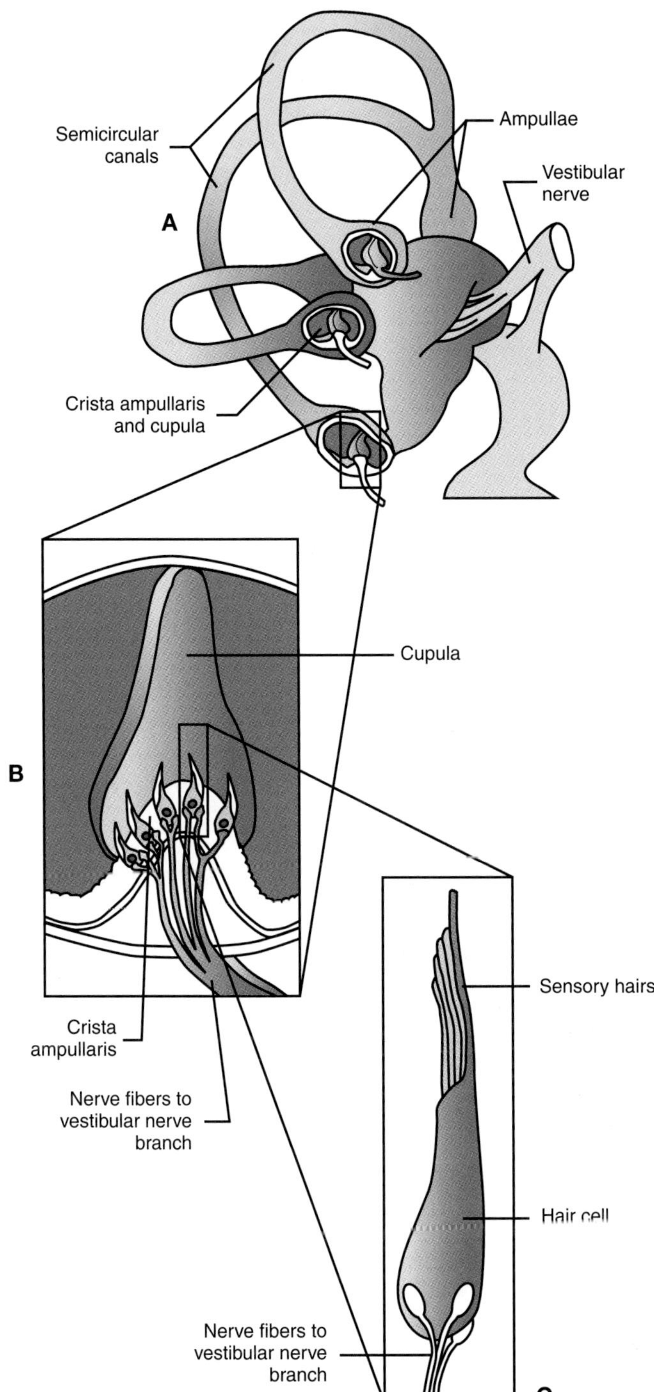

FIGURE **13-7** **Semicircular Canals With Detail of Ampulla and Crista Ampullaris. A,** Semicircular canals showing locations of ampullae. **B,** Enlarged view of crista ampullaris in an ampulla showing sensory hair cells and cupula. **C,** Greatly enlarged sensory hair cell.

Terminology

Two general terms are used to refer to the eye: the word *ocular* and the combining form *ophthalm-*. For example, ocular anatomy refers to the anatomy of the eye, ophthalmic medications are used to treat the eye, and ophthalmology is the study of the eyes.

CLINICAL APPLICATION Motion Sickness

The brain relies on the vestibular system, the eyes, and the proprioceptors around the body for information about how and where the body is moving so that it can keep the animal upright and maintain balance. Usually the information the brain receives from these sources agrees—the animal is either moving or it is not. This is fine as long as it is standing or moving around on the ground (assuming the ground is not moving). When we put an animal into a moving car, boat, airplane, or a vehicle in space, however, things become more complicated. The eyes look around the interior of the vehicle and see that nothing is apparently moving, but the equilibrium receptors and proprioceptors detect motion (or, in the case of space travel, the absence of gravity). This disagreement between the sensory receptors can result in the unpleasant sensations of motion sickness, such as headache, nausea, and vomiting. This often occurs in dogs and cats (and humans) that travel by car, boat, or plane. Medications often can be used to prevent motion sickness, but they usually must be administered before traveling. Motion sickness is easier to prevent than it is to treat in midjourney. Veterinary clinics often dispense anti–motion sickness medications to clients who must travel with animals prone to motion sickness.

A form of motion sickness is common in astronauts as well. "Space adaptation syndrome" occurs in a high percentage of astronauts, particularly during the first few days of a space flight. It causes symptoms similar to normal motion sickness, such as headache, nausea, and cold sweating. The symptoms often disappear after a day or two, indicating that the brain adjusts to the conflicting signals. Ongoing research is trying to find ways to prevent this annoying and sometimes debilitating disorder. It seems more complicated to deal with than traditional earth-bound motion sickness.

Major Layers of the Eyeball

The eyeball consists of three major layers: the outer fibrous layer, the middle vascular layer, and the inner nervous layer. Figure 13-8 illustrates the main structures of each layer.

Outer Fibrous Layer. The outer fibrous layer of the eye admits light to its interior and gives strength and shape to the eyeball. Its two components are the **cornea** and the **sclera.** The cornea is the transparent "window" that admits light to the interior of the eye. It consists of an orderly arrangement of collagen fibers and contains no blood vessels. Its transparency is maintained by careful control of the amount of water it contains. Too much water (corneal edema) or too little water (corneal dehydration) causes the cornea to become cloudy and opaque. The cornea is richly supplied with pain receptors, making it one of the most sensitive tissues of the body. The sclera is the "white" of the eye. It consists of dense, fibrous connective tissue and makes up the majority of the outer fibrous layer of the eye. The junction of the cornea and the sclera is called the **limbus.** It can be used as a landmark to describe the position of lesions (abnormalities) on the cornea or sclera.

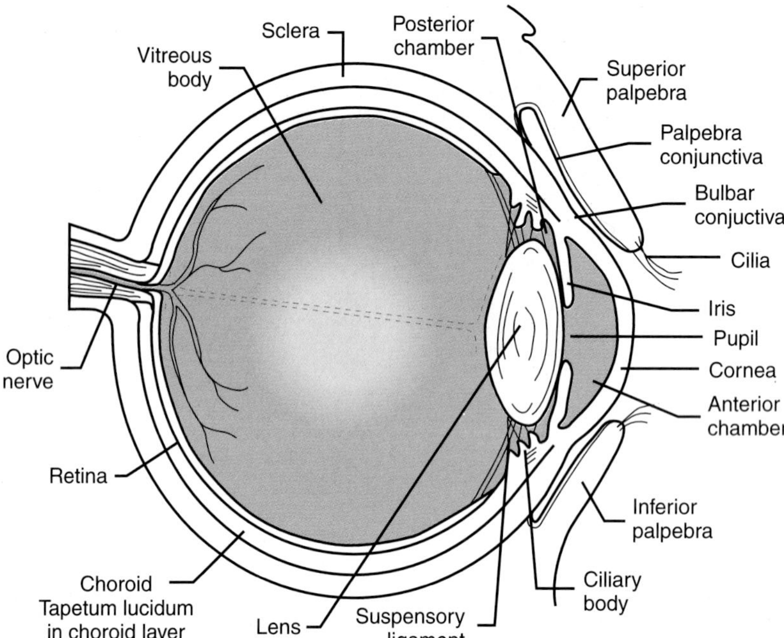

FIGURE **13-8** **Cross Section of Eye.**

Middle Vascular Layer. The middle vascular layer is also called the **uvea.** It has several parts, including the **choroid,** the **iris,** and the **ciliary body**.

The choroid is sandwiched between the sclera and the retina. It consists mainly of pigment and blood vessels that provide blood to the retina. Most of the pigment is dark melanin, but in most domestic animals, except swine, the choroid forms a highly reflective area in the rear of the eye called the **tapetum.** (Sometimes it is called the **tapetum lucidum.**) The tapetum is like a brightly colored mirror and is responsible for the bright light that seems to shine from an animal's eyes in the dark when a light is directed into them. Its purpose seems to be to act as a light amplifier to aid dim light vision. After light has passed through the photoreceptors (the rods and cones) in the retina, it reflects off the tapetum and passes back through the photoreceptors again, stimulating them a second time. Therefore most animals can see better in dim light than we can. Humans and pigs do not have a tapetum.

At the front of the eye, the middle vascular layer is modified into the iris and the ciliary body. The iris is the "colored part" of the eye. If we speak of an animal as having blue eyes, it is the color of its irises that we are talking about. The iris is a pigmented muscular diaphragm that controls the amount of light that enters the posterior part of the eyeball. The opening at its center is called the **pupil.** The pupil enlarges in low light conditions and gets smaller in bright light. Two types of multiunit smooth muscle fibers make up the iris: (1) radially arranged fibers (oriented like the spokes of a wheel) that enlarge the pupil when they contract and (2) circularly arranged fibers that constrict the pupil when they contract. The nerve supply for the smooth muscle cells of the iris comes from the autonomic nervous system.

The ciliary body is a ring-shaped structure located immediately behind the iris. It contains the tiny muscles that adjust the shape of the lens to allow near and far vision. The muscles of the ciliary body (the **ciliary muscles**) are also multiunit smooth muscles. They are contained within small processes (called, amazingly enough, the *ciliary processes*) that are attached to the periphery of the lens by tiny **suspensory ligaments.** The ciliary muscle fibers are oriented so that when they are relaxed, the suspensory ligaments pull on the periphery of the lens, stretching it into a flattened shape. When they contract, they move the ciliary body forward and inward. This action takes tension off the suspensory ligaments, allowing the lens to assume its natural, more rounded shape. (We discuss this focusing process more in the section on the lens.)

Inner Nervous Layer. The inner nervous layer is the **retina,** which lines the back of the eye. It is like the film in the camera of the eye. It contains the actual sensory receptors for vision—the rods and cones. (We discuss the retina in more detail shortly.)

TEST YOURSELF

1. An animal has an area of inflammation located at the dorsal limbus of its right eye. Where is the lesion located?
2. Why is the cornea transparent whereas the sclera is opaque?
3. Which layer of the eyeball are the iris and ciliary body part of?
4. How does the tapetum aid dim light vision in animals that have it?
5. What is the function of the iris of the eye?
6. Which layer of the eyeball contains the photoreceptors?

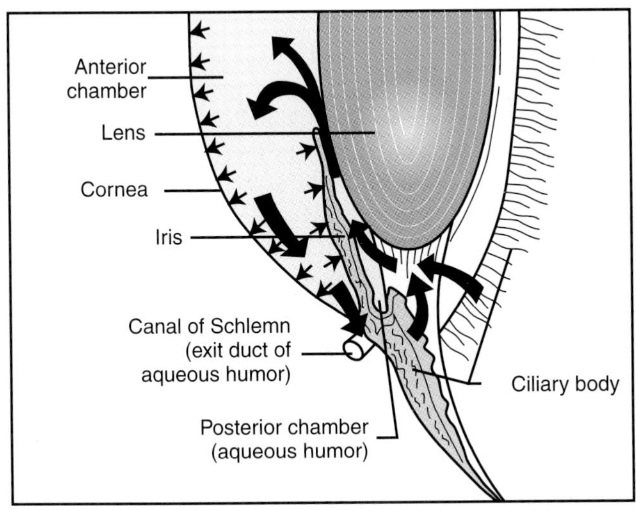

FIGURE **13-9** **Formation of Aqueous Humor.** Aqueous humor *(large arrows)* is formed in posterior chamber by cells of ciliary body. It slowly circulates through the pupil into the anterior chamber from which it is drained by canal of Schlemm, located at the junction between cornea and iris. Pressure of aqueous humor is indicated by small arrows.

Major Compartments of the Eyeball

The interior of the eyeball is made up of two fluid-filled compartments: one in front of the lens and ciliary body and the other behind it. The **aqueous compartment** is in front of the lens and ciliary body and contains a clear, watery fluid called **aqueous humor.** The **vitreous compartment** is behind the lens and ciliary body and contains a clear fluid with the consistency of soft gelatin called **vitreous humor.** The term *humor* is an old anatomical term meaning "fluid." The eye is the only part of the body for which this archaic term is still commonly used.

When we look into an animal's eye, we are looking into its aqueous compartment. Actually, to be more precise, we are looking into the anterior chamber of its aqueous compartment. The aqueous compartment is subdivided into two parts by the iris. The space in front of the iris is the **anterior chamber,** and the space behind the iris (between it and the lens) is the **posterior chamber.** The anterior chamber is the only portion of the eye's interior that we can see clearly without special instruments.

Within the aqueous compartment, aqueous humor is constantly being produced and drained. It is produced in the posterior chamber by cells of the ciliary body. It then passes very slowly through the pupil into the anterior chamber, where it is drained by the **canal of Schlemm** and the fluid returned to the bloodstream. The canal of Schlemm is a ringlike structure located way out at the edge of the anterior chamber where the iris and the cornea meet (Figure 13-9).

The vitreous compartment of the eye is considerably larger than the aqueous compartment. It fills the whole back of the eyeball behind the lens and ciliary body. It contains vitreous humor (sometimes called the *vitreous body*), which is a clear fluid that has a soft, gelatinous consistency.

CLINICAL APPLICATION — Glaucoma

Glaucoma is not one simple disease. Rather, it is a group of diseases characterized by increased intraocular pressure (pressure within the eye) that causes pain and can lead to blindness. In domestic animals, glaucoma is most often diagnosed in dogs, partly because it is seen fairly commonly in that species but partly because other species are not commonly tested for it. An instrument called a *tonometer* is used to test for glaucoma by measuring the intraocular pressure.

Glaucoma can have many origins, but the basic mechanism is that aqueous humor is being produced at a faster rate than it is being drained from the eye. This causes the intraocular pressure to rise. Most often the problem is due to insufficient drainage of aqueous humor rather than overproduction. Therapy of glaucoma usually involves medical or surgical treatments designed to increase the rate at which aqueous humor drains from the anterior chamber.

The treatment of glaucoma usually is not as successful in domestic animals as it is in humans. The reason is that the glaucoma is often in a very advanced stage when veterinary patients are presented for treatment. Unfortunately, glaucoma comes on very slowly and gradually with few, if any, clinical signs noticed early in the process, when treatment would be most beneficial. By the late stages, when the eyeball becomes noticeably enlarged and painful, it is often too late to save vision. In many cases the affected eye must be surgically removed.

Lens

The lens of the eye is a soft, transparent structure made up of layers of microscopic fibers that are arranged like the layers of an onion. It is elastic and biconvex (it bulges out on both sides). Its normal shape is fairly rounded, but it can be pulled into a flatter shape if tension is applied equally around its equator. The front surface of the lens is in contact with aqueous humor, and its back surface is in contact with vitreous humor. Its main role is to help focus a clear image on the retina regardless of whether the object being viewed is close up or far away. It does this with the help of the muscles of the ciliary body through a process called **accommodation.**

Accommodation is the process by which the shape of the lens is changed to allow close-up and distant vision. When the muscle fibers of the ciliary body are relaxed, the suspensory ligaments that attach it to the periphery of the lens exert tension on the lens, pulling it into a flattened shape that allows clear distant vision (greater than about 20 feet). For close-up vision, the ciliary muscles must contract to take tension off the suspensory ligaments. This allows the lens to assume its naturally more rounded shape. So close-up vision requires muscle contractions in the ciliary body, but distant vision does not. This explains why we often suffer eyestrain when we do close-up work (like reading this book, for example) for long periods. Fortunately, we can take advantage of our knowledge of how accommodation works to relieve the eyestrain; that is, we just need to look off into the distance periodically to rest our ciliary muscles.

CLINICAL APPLICATION: Cataracts

A cataract is an abnormal condition of the eye whereby the lens becomes opaque. Instead of having a normal transparent appearance, a cataract lens appears milky. This impairs vision, particularly in dim light. Cataracts can be a normal part of the aging process. As a result, they are often seen in older animals in which they can lead to total or near-total blindness. In younger animals, they can be genetically inherited or develop secondary to conditions such as infection, trauma, diabetes mellitus, or excessive exposure of the eyes to ionizing radiation (such as x-rays). Usually the only effective treatment for a cataract is surgical removal of the affected lens.

Retina

The retina is the business end of the eye—the film in the camera, so to speak. It is where the visual image is formed, sensed, and converted to nerve impulses that are decoded in the brain to re-form the image in the conscious mind. The whole reason the rest of the eye structures exist is to produce as accurate and clear an image as possible on the retina.

The retina is a complex, multilayered structure that lines most of the vitreous compartment of the eye. Its main components are three layers of neurons, the outermost of which is the actual layer of sensory cells. Figure 13-10 is a diagram of the major layers of the retina. From outside in, the layers of the retina are a thin pigment layer, the photoreceptor layer, the bipolar cell layer, the ganglion cell layer, and a layer of nerve

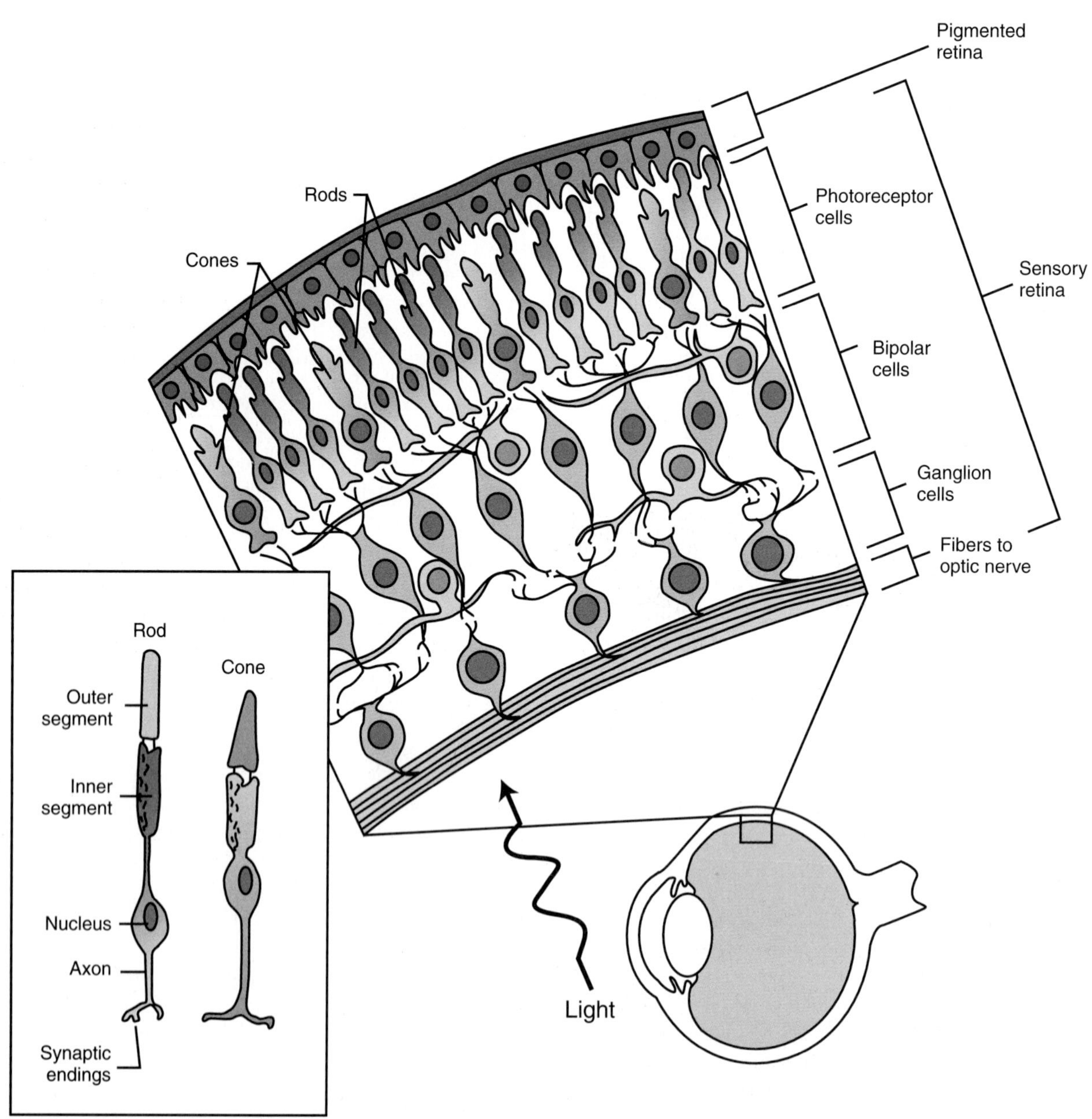

FIGURE 13-10 **Cell Layers of Retina With Detail of Rod and Cone (Photoreceptor) Cells.**

fibers on their way to the optic nerve. The bipolar cells and ganglion cells are neurons that integrate and relay nerve impulses from the photoreceptor cells to the optic nerve. Because the photoreceptor cells are the outermost layer of neurons, light rays must pass through the other layers before reaching them. Fortunately, these layers are basically transparent to light.

The nerve fibers on the inside surface of the retina all converge at the **optic disc.** This is where they leave the eye to form the optic nerve that carries visual information to the brain. The optic disc contains only nerve fibers and a few blood vessels but no photoreceptor cells (so no visual images are formed there). It is the blind spot of the eye.

Photoreceptor cells are neurons also, but their dendrites have been modified into the actual sensory receptors for light. Two receptors of different shapes are found among the photoreceptor cells: (1) thin, rodlike receptors and (2) thicker, cone-shaped receptors. They are usually referred to as **rods** and **cones** and actually have different sensory roles (Table 13-2). Rods are more sensitive to light than are the cones, but they produce a somewhat coarse image in shades of gray. The cones are more sensitive to color and detail than are the rods, but they do not function well in dim light. So rods are the main receptors for dim light vision, and cones perceive color and detail. (The next time you are in dimly lit conditions, notice that you see little or no color and that things do not appear very sharp. Your rods are doing most of the work.)

Domestic animals are often described as being color blind. This is not really an accurate way to describe their vision because color blindness implies a defect in color reception that sometimes occurs in humans. Most domestic animals *can* see colors to some extent, but because most have a lot of rods and very few cones, colors probably appear washed out to them. Their color vision probably looks like an old color photograph that has been exposed to too much direct sunlight; the colors are there, but are they are pale and faded.

Domestic animals also do not seem to perceive detail as sharply as we do for another physical reason. Humans and other primates have a dense accumulation of cones in a small depression called the *fovea centralis* in the center of the retina. This is the area of clearest vision and the one you are using to read these words. Domestic animals do not have a fovea; so their vision is apparently less sharp. Focus your eyes on the center of this page. The way the top, bottom, and sides of the page appear to you is probably as sharp as the world appears to most animals. That might seem like a severe handicap to us sight-oriented humans, but that's not a good way to think of it. Remember that animals are equipped with sense organs that are appropriate for them. They would probably consider our limited sense of smell as much of a handicap as their visual limitations seem to us.

CLINICAL APPLICATION: The Blind Spot of the Eye

To detect the blind spot of your eye, mark an "X" on a piece of paper and about 2 inches to the right of it, mark an "O." Now close or cover your left eye, focus your right eye on the "X," and hold the paper about 12 inches from your face. Slowly move the page toward your eye. At some point the image of the "O" will disappear. When that happens, it has fallen on your optic disc, where there are no photoreceptors. So its image disappears! Interestingly, the brain normally fills in the blind spot area; so the conscious mind is not generally aware of that "hole" in the visual field.

Table 13-2 Photoreceptor Characteristics

Receptor	Sensitivity to Light	Sensitivity to Detail	Sensitivity to Color
Rods	High	Low	Absent
Cones	Low	High	High

Formation of a Visual Image

For the eye to transmit a clear visual image to the brain, a clear image must be formed on the retina. This is done by structures in the eye that refract (bend) light rays so that they come into focus on the retina. Refraction is the bending of light rays and occurs as they pass obliquely from one medium to another that has a different optical density (speed of light transmission). The more oblique the angle, the greater the degree of refraction. Because eye structures are curved, most light rays (except those directly in the center) strike the ocular surfaces at an angle.

Four refractive media in the eye help form a clear image on the retina: the cornea, the aqueous humor, the lens, and the vitreous humor. All contribute to the creation of a clear visual image, but the cornea does the majority of the refractive work. Its curved shape and the extreme difference between its optical density and that of the air in front of it result in significant refraction of light rays as they pass through it. The other refractive media, even the adjustable lens, just fine-tune the image that the cornea has formed. Interestingly, the image formed on the retina by these refractive structures is upside down. The brain somehow inverts the image so that the conscious mind sees everything right side up.

TEST YOURSELF

1. Where is aqueous humor produced? Where is it drained from the aqueous compartment of the eye?
2. Which type of vision requires more muscular effort: close-up vision or far-away vision? Why?
3. Why is the optic disc the blind spot of the eye?
4. What kind of vision do the rods in the retina perceive? What do cones perceive?
5. What is the main refractive structure of the eye? Why?

Extraocular Structures

Extraocular structures are not part of the eye itself, but they play important roles in its protection and functioning. They

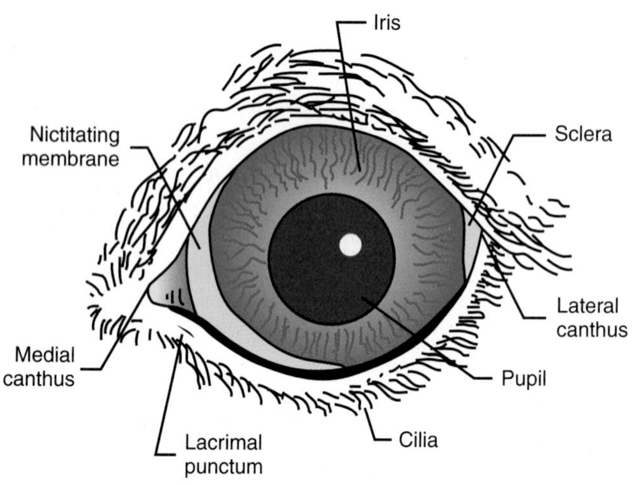

FIGURE **13-11** **External View of Dog's Left Eye.**

> **CLINICAL APPLICATION — Conjunctivitis**
>
> Conjunctivitis is inflammation of the conjunctiva of the eye. It is one of the most common eye diseases and occurs in all common domestic animal species. Signs include redness (hyperemia) and swelling (chemosis) of the conjunctiva, ocular discharge, and discomfort. The ocular discharge seen with conjunctivitis can range from watery (serous) to bloody (sanguineous) or pussy (purulent). Causes include bacterial and viral infections, as well as physical and chemical irritants. Conjunctivitis is often seen in dogs that have been swimming in pools containing chlorinated water or hanging their heads out car windows. Often the precise cause (etiologic factor) is not known. In mild cases of conjunctivitis, medical treatment may not be necessary. In more severe cases, antibiotic ointments or drops, which often contain corticosteroids to lessen the inflammation, are administered topically. Most cases of conjunctivitis respond quickly to treatment.

include the conjunctivae, the eyelids, the tear production and drainage system, and the muscles that delicately move and position the eyeballs. Figure 13-11 shows many of the externally visible extraocular structures.

Conjunctiva. The **conjunctiva** is a thin, transparent membrane that covers the front portion of the eyeball and lines the interior surfaces of the eyelids. The portion covering the front of the eyeball is called the **bulbar conjunctiva** (*bulbar* refers to the eyeball), and the portion lining the eyelids is called the **palpebral conjunctiva** (*palpebral* refers to the eyelids). The transparency of the conjunctiva allows the underlying tissues to show through; so it can be used as a window to see the blood vessels that are hidden elsewhere in the body by opaque structures, such as the skin. By looking through the conjunctiva at the lining of the eyelid, we can often detect abnormalities such as anemia (pale color caused by decreased blood flow) and jaundice (yellowish color).

The space between the bulbar and palpebral portions of the conjunctiva (between the eyelid and the eyeball) is called the **conjunctival sac.** It is normally only a potential space moistened by tears, but the conjunctival sac can be a useful place to deposit ophthalmic medications.

Eyelids. The **eyelids** consist of an upper and lower fold of skin that is lined by the thin, moist conjunctivae. The lateral and medial corners where the eyelids come together are called the lateral and medial **canthus.** Along the margin of each eyelid are the tiny openings of the **tarsal glands** (also known as **meibomian glands**). They can be seen as a line of little "dots" along the eyelid margin. They produce a waxy substance that helps prevent tears from overflowing onto the face. Eyelashes (cilia) are most prominent on the upper lid of most animals. Lower eyelashes are usually more sparse and thin if they are present at all.

Domestic animals also have a **third eyelid** (also called the **nictitating membrane**) located medially between the eyelids and the eyeball. It consists mainly of a T-shaped plate of cartilage covered by conjunctiva. On its ocular surface (the surface in contact with the eyeball) are lymph nodules and an accessory lacrimal (tear-producing) gland. No muscles attach to the third eyelid. Its movements are entirely passive.

Lacrimal Apparatus. The **lacrimal apparatus** includes the structures that produce and secrete tears and the structures that drain them away from the surface of the eye. Tears are an important part of the overall liquid film that moistens and protects the surface of the eye. They are produced by the lacrimal glands and the accessory lacrimal glands of the third eyelids. The **lacrimal glands** are the primary source of tears. They are located dorsal and lateral to each eye inside the bony orbits that protect the eyeballs. Several small ducts from each gland deposit tears in the dorsal conjunctival sacs, from where they wash down over the surface of the eyes aided by blinking movements of the eyelids. Figure 13-12 illustrates the position of the lacrimal glands.

The overall liquid film that moistens and protects the surface of the eye actually is made up of three main layers, only one of which comes from the lacrimal glands. The layers are an inner mucous layer, a middle tear layer, and an outer oily layer. The inner mucous layer comes from cells in the conjunctiva. It contains antibacterial substances that help protect the eye from infection. The middle tear layer comes from the lacrimal glands and the accessory lacrimal glands of the third eyelids. It serves to keep the cornea moist. The outer oily layer comes from the tarsal (meibomian) glands. It helps reduce evaporation of the underlying tear layer and prevents tears from flowing over the lid margin.

Tears are constantly being produced; so they must constantly be drained from the surface of the eye to prevent them from spilling down the animal's face. The tear drainage system is illustrated in Figure 13-12. Two small openings, one each in the upper and lower eyelid margins, drain the tears away from the surface of each eye. The openings are called the **lacrimal puncta** (*singular,* punctum), and they are located near the medial canthus of each eye. From the lacrimal puncta on each

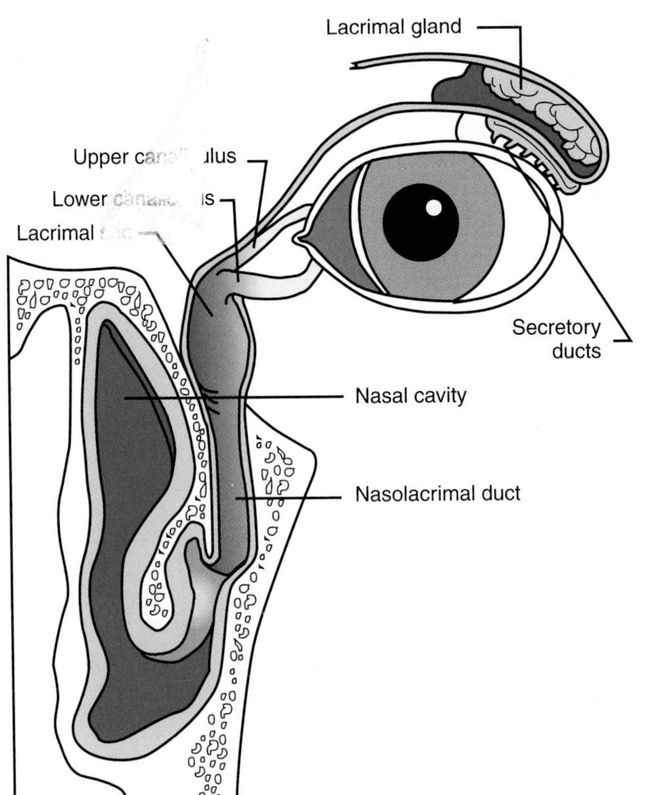

FIGURE **13-12** **Lacrimal Apparatus.** Tears produced by lacrimal gland flow down over surface of eye and drain into lacrimal puncta. From there they pass into lacrimal sac and down nasolacrimal duct to nasal passage.

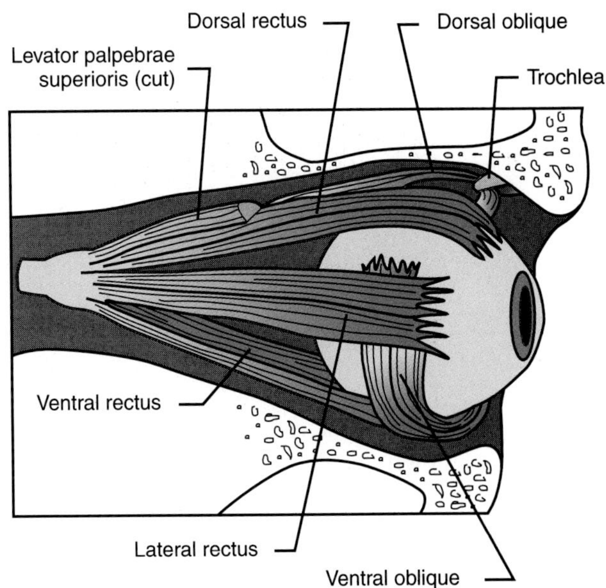

FIGURE **13-13** **Extraocular Muscles of Right Eye.**

side the tears flow down two small ducts to the **lacrimal sac** and then down a single duct, the **nasolacrimal duct,** to the nasal cavity. This is why, when your eyes water for any reason, you get the sniffles. Those excess tears have to go somewhere, and they drain down into your nasal cavity.

Eye Muscles. The **extraocular eye muscles** attach to the sclera of the eye (Figure 13-13). They are the small skeletal muscles that hold the eyeballs in place and delicately and accurately move them. They are capable of a wide range of movements that allow the eyes to track and examine objects with great precision. As you are reading this, note that your eyes track along the lines of words. If you concentrate, you can cause your eyes to move from letter to letter instead of word to word. That's pretty delicate muscle control!

Humans share six extraocular muscles with domestic animals: four straight muscles and two oblique muscles. The four straight muscles are called the *rectus muscles.* (The word *rectus* means "straight.") They are the dorsal, ventral, medial, and lateral rectus muscles. Their names indicate where they attach to the eyeball. The two oblique muscles are the dorsal and ventral oblique muscles. Many animals also have a seventh extraocular muscle—the retractor bulbi muscle. It retracts the eyeball slightly deeper into the orbit when it contracts. This may assist the activity of the other muscles by enhancing their mechanical advantage. Most movements of the eye involve a combination of several of these muscles contracting together.

TEST YOURSELF

1. How might examination of the bulbar and palpebral portions of the conjunctiva be useful as part of the overall physical examination of an animal?
2. An animal can intentionally blink its eyes. Can it intentionally cover its eye with its third eyelid? Why or why not?
3. How would an animal with a plugged nasolacrimal system appear? Why?
4. If the medial rectus muscle of an animal's eye were damaged and lost its ability to contract, what would the effect be on the positioning of the affected eye? Why?

CHAPTER 14

The Endocrine System

Thomas Colville

The animal body is a large, complex, living machine. Its various parts and functions must be controlled and coordinated carefully to keep everything working smoothly. Two body systems share the responsibility for this control and coordination: the endocrine system and the nervous system.

Put most simply, the endocrine and nervous systems help maintain **homeostasis** (balance) in the body. They constantly send instructions to the rest of the body, telling it how to respond to changing internal and external conditions.

Similarities and differences between the endocrine and nervous systems are summarized in Table 14-1, but let's discuss some of the main ones. Both systems use chemicals to transmit their messages, but they do it by different means. The endocrine system messengers, **hormones,** are produced by endocrine gland cells, or modified neurons. They travel through the bloodstream to distant cells and tissues where they produce their effects. The nervous system messengers, neurotransmitters, are produced only by neurons. They travel very short distances across synaptic spaces to produce their effects. The targets of hormones are all of the cells and tissues in the body. The targets of neurotransmitters are generally only muscle cells and glands. The endocrine system reacts slowly to changes but can sustain its responses for long periods. The nervous system reacts more quickly to changes but cannot sustain prolonged responses.

The basic units of the endocrine system are **endocrine glands.** Located throughout the body, endocrine glands secrete tiny amounts of hormones directly into the bloodstream. This method of secretion gives them their nickname of "ductless glands." This feature differentiates them from **exocrine glands,** which secrete their products onto epithelial surfaces (*exo-* meaning "out" or "external") through tiny tubes called *ducts.* The hormones produced by the endocrine glands circulate throughout the body and produce effects whenever they find friendly receptors they can attach to in or on cells.

Endocrine glands are found throughout the body, and the list of them grows as we learn more about **endocrinology.** In this chapter we focus mostly on the major endocrine glands. Table 14-2 summarizes the major endocrine glands and their hormones, and Figure 14-1 shows their relative locations in the body. Like many other parts of the body, hormones and endocrine structures are known by more than one name or abbreviation. We use common clinical veterinary usage as our guide, with alternative terms included where appropriate for clarity.

Table 14-1 Comparison of Endocrine and Nervous System Characteristics

Characteristic	Endocrine System	Nervous System
General function	Regulation of body functions to maintain homeostasis	Regulation of body functions to maintain homeostasis
Reaction to stimuli	Slow	Fast
Duration of effects	Long	Short
Target tissues	Virtually all body cells and tissues	Muscle and glandular tissues
Chemical messenger	Hormone	Neurotransmitter
Messenger producing cells	Endocrine gland cells or modified neurons	Neurons
Distance from chemical message production to target	Long (via bloodstream)	Short (across synaptic space)

Table 14-2 Major Endocrine Glands

Gland	Hormone	Target	Action
Anterior pituitary	Growth hormone	All body cells	Growth, metabolic regulation
	Prolactin	Female—mammary gland	Lactation
		Male—no known effect	None
	Thyroid-stimulating hormone	Thyroid gland	Thyroid hormone production
	Adrenocorticotropic hormone	Adrenal cortex	Adrenal cortical hormone production
	Follicle-stimulating hormone	Female—ovary (follicles)	Oogenesis
		Male—testis (seminiferous tubules)	Spermatogenesis
	Luteinizing hormone	Female—ovary (follicle/corpus luteum)	Ovulation and corpus luteum production
		Male—testis (interstitial cells)	Testosterone production
	Melanocyte-stimulating hormone	Unknown	Unknown
Posterior pituitary	Antidiuretic hormone	Kidney	Water conservation
	Oxytocin	Female—uterus	Contraction at parturition
		Mammary gland	Milk letdown
		Male—no known effect	No known effect
Thyroid	Thyroid hormone	All body cells	Growth, metabolic regulation
	Calcitonin	Bones	Prevents hypercalcemia
Parathyroid	Parathyroid hormone	Kidneys, intestines, bones	Prevents hypocalcemia
Adrenal cortex	Glucocorticoid hormones	Whole body	Increased blood glucose, blood pressure maintenance
	Mineralocorticoid hormones	Kidneys	Sodium and water retention, potassium elimination
	Sex hormones	Whole body	Minimal effects
Adrenal medulla	Epinephrine and norepinephrine	Whole body	Part of "fight or flight" response
Pancreas (islets)	Insulin	All body cells	Movement of glucose into cells and its use for energy
	Glucagon	Whole body	Increased blood glucose
Testis	Androgens	Whole body	Anabolic effect, development of male secondary sex characteristics
Ovary	Estrogens	Whole body	Preparation for breeding and pregnancy
	Progestins	Uterus	Preparation for and maintenance of pregnancy

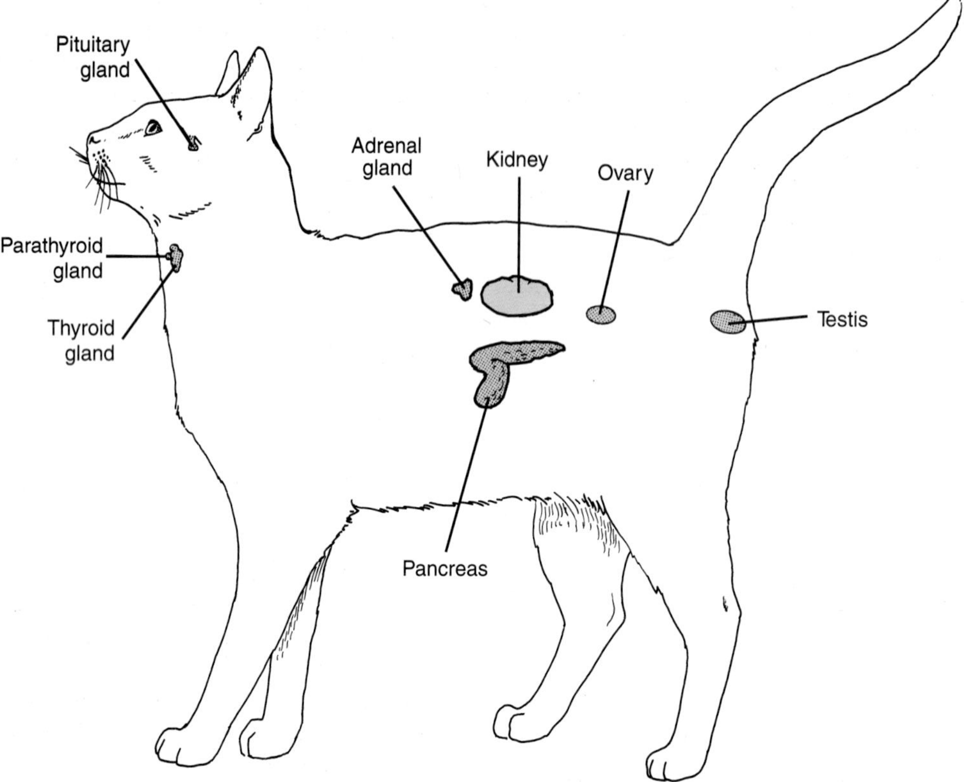

FIGURE **14-1** **Relative Locations of Major Endocrine Glands in Cat.** (From McBride DF: *Learning veterinary terminology,* ed 2, St Louis, 2002, Mosby.)

TEST YOURSELF

1. How do endocrine glands differ from exocrine glands?
2. In what ways are the functions and characteristics of the endocrine system similar to those of the nervous system? In what ways are they different?

HORMONES

Characteristics

Hormones are chemical messengers produced by endocrine glands and secreted directly into blood vessels. They travel in the bloodstream to all parts of the body and produce effects when they find their receptors in or on cells. Each body cell has specific receptors to a variety of hormones. These receptors are like locks into which only specific keys (hormones) can fit. When a hormone (key) binds to its receptor (lock) in or on a cell, it changes some activity of that cell. If a cell does not have receptors to a particular hormone, that hormone just flows by without producing any effect on that cell. A cell that has receptors for a particular hormone is referred to as a **target** of that hormone.

Control of Hormone Secretion

Hormone secretion is usually controlled by what are called *negative feedback systems* that function like thermostatically controlled heaters. When the thermostat is set to a temperature higher than the current temperature, the heater is turned on, heating the air. When the room's temperature reaches the thermostat setting, the heating device is turned down or off. Without a source of heat, the air in the room cools. When its temperature falls below the thermostat setting, the heater is turned back on again, and so forth. The rising temperature of the room air "feeds back" to the thermostat and has a negative effect on the heater in that it is turned down or off. This is how it gets the name of the "negative feedback system." Hormone secretion is often controlled in a similar fashion. For example, the thyroid gland produces its hormone as a result of stimulation by another hormone—the thyroid-stimulating hormone (TSH) from the anterior pituitary gland. When the level of thyroid hormone drops below needed levels (below the "thermostat setting"), the anterior pituitary produces more TSH, which stimulates the thyroid gland to produce more of its hormone. This is like turning on the heater (thyroid gland) to produce more heat (thyroid hormone.) The rising level of thyroid hormone in the bloodstream eventually reaches the level required in the body. Once that level is reached, the production of TSH by the anterior pituitary is turned down. This reduces the stimulation of the thyroid gland, causing it to produce less thyroid hormone (the heater has been turned down). When the level of thyroid hormone drops below what the body needs again, the anterior pituitary turns its production of TSH back up, which turns the production of thyroid hormone back up, and the process continues.

Some endocrine glands use another control mechanism for hormone secretion—direct stimulation from the nervous system. For example, the secretion of hormones from the medulla of the adrenal gland is stimulated by sympathetic nerve impulses when an animal feels threatened. The adrenal medullary hormones that are released into the bloodstream as a result of this stimulation contribute to the whole-body "fight or flight" response that prepares the animal's body for intense physical activity. (The adrenal gland is discussed more fully later in this chapter.)

TEST YOURSELF

1. What is a hormone target?
2. How does a negative feedback system control the secretion of many hormones?

THE MAJOR ENDOCRINE GLANDS

THE HYPOTHALAMUS

Characteristics

The **hypothalamus** is actually a part of the brain. It is located in the ventral part of the brain stem just caudal to the optic chiasma (where the optic nerves cross). It has many important nervous system functions, including appetite control, body temperature regulation, and control of wake-sleep cycles. It also links the conscious mind with the rest of the body by connecting the cerebral cortex with lower brain centers and the endocrine system. This link with the endocrine system is accomplished through the control the hypothalamus has over the activities of the pituitary gland. This makes it a very important bridge between the nervous system and the endocrine system.

Relationship With Pituitary Gland

The **pituitary gland** is an endocrine gland that is attached to the hypothalamus ventrally by a slender stalk. Blood vessels and nerve fibers in the stalk enable the hypothalamus to control the activity of the pituitary gland and therefore most of the rest of the body.

A system of tiny blood vessels called a **portal system** links the hypothalamus with what is called the *anterior portion* of the pituitary gland. Figure 14-2 shows this pituitary portal system. Modified neurons in the hypothalamus secrete hormones into these portal blood vessels. The hormones travel the short distance down to the anterior pituitary and regulate much of its function. These hypothalamic hormones, called *releasing* and *inhibiting factors,* are each specific for a particular anterior pituitary hormone. As their names imply, a releasing factor causes the anterior pituitary to produce and release a particular hormone, and an inhibiting factor has the opposite effect of inhibiting the production and release of a hormone. Because some anterior pituitary hormones influence all of the body's cells, the hypothalamus indirectly affects the whole body by regulating anterior pituitary gland functions. In part, this is how the state of an animal's mind can influence its susceptibility and reaction to illnesses.

The effect of the hypothalamus on the posterior part of the pituitary gland is more direct. Modified neurons in the hypothalamus produce two hormones, antidiuretic hormone and oxytocin, that are transported down nerve fibers to the posterior pituitary gland, where they are stored. They are then released into the bloodstream by nerve impulses from the hypothalamus. Figure 14-3 illustrates this process.

THE PITUITARY GLAND (HYPOPHYSIS)

Characteristics

The pituitary gland (hypophysis) is often called the "master endocrine gland" because many of its hormones direct the activity of other endocrine glands. Physically the pituitary gland is about the size of a small pea or bean. It is connected to the hypothalamus above it by a slender stalk, and it is securely housed in a small pocket, the pituitary fossa, of the sphenoid bone of the skull.

Although it looks like one structure, the pituitary gland is actually two separate glands with completely different structures, functions, and embryological origins. The rostral (front) portion is called the **anterior pituitary,** or adenohypophysis. It develops from glandular tissue and looks like normal glandular tissue under the microscope. The caudal (rear) portion is called the **posterior pituitary,** or neurohypophysis. It develops from the nervous system and looks like nervous tissue under the microscope.

The functions of the two parts of the pituitary gland are as different as their appearances. The anterior pituitary produces seven known hormones when stimulated by the hypothalamus and direct feedback from target organs and tissues. The posterior pituitary does not produce any hormones. Rather, it stores and releases two hormones that are produced up in the hypothalamus and transported down to the posterior pituitary along nerve fibers.

The Anterior Pituitary (Adenohypophysis)

The following are the seven known anterior pituitary hormones:

1. Growth hormone
2. Prolactin
3. Thyroid-stimulating hormone
4. Adrenocorticotropic hormone
5. Follicle-stimulating hormone
6. Luteinizing hormone
7. Melanocyte-stimulating hormone

Growth Hormone. Growth hormone (GH) is also known as *somatotropin* and *somatotropic hormone.* Its name comes from its

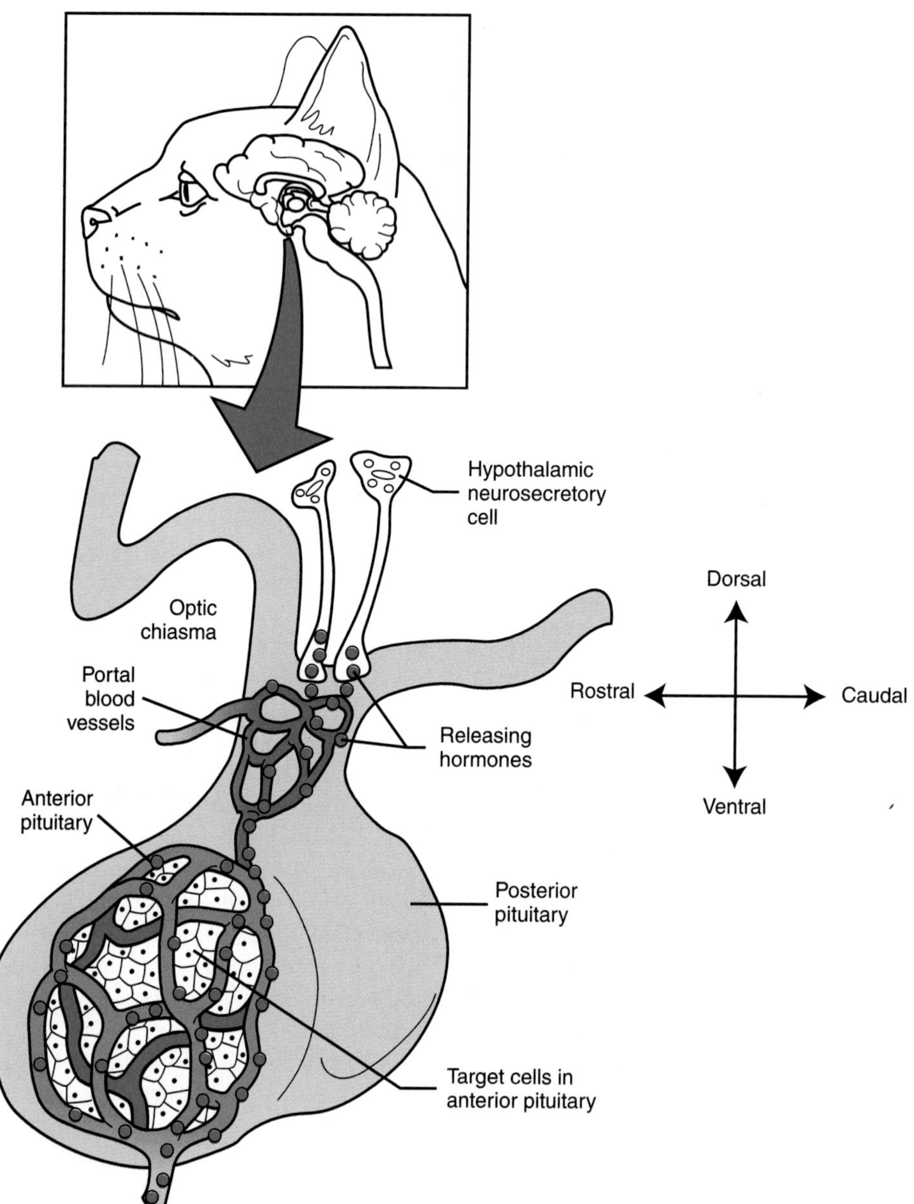

FIGURE **14-2** **Relationship of Hypothalamus and Anterior Pituitary.** Releasing and inhibiting hormones from the hypothalamus are secreted into portal blood vessels that carry them to the anterior pituitary. There they cause or inhibit release of anterior pituitary hormones.

most obvious effect—the promotion of body growth in young animals, particularly the growth of bone and muscle. It has other important roles in animals of all ages, however. It helps regulate the **metabolism** of proteins, carbohydrates, and lipids in all of the body's cells.

The effect of GH on protein metabolism is to encourage the **anabolism,** or synthesis, of proteins by body cells. This supplies the materials for growth, as well as for the ongoing regeneration and repair of body tissues that have undergone injury or normal wear and tear.

The effects of GH on carbohydrate and lipid metabolism are linked. GH causes the mobilization (release) of lipids from storage in adipose tissue and their **catabolism** (breakdown) in body cells for energy production. At the same time, it discourages the cells from using carbohydrates, principally the sugar glucose, as energy sources. Because less glucose is removed from the blood by the cells, the level of glucose in the blood tends to rise. This is called a *hyperglycemic effect.* This effect is opposite to that of the pancreatic hormone insulin, which tends to lower blood glucose levels. Because glucose is such an important energy source for the body's cells, a balance between GH and insulin is important to maintain homeostasis of glucose levels in the blood.

Prolactin. Prolactin is named for its effect in the female. It helps trigger and maintain **lactation**—the secretion of

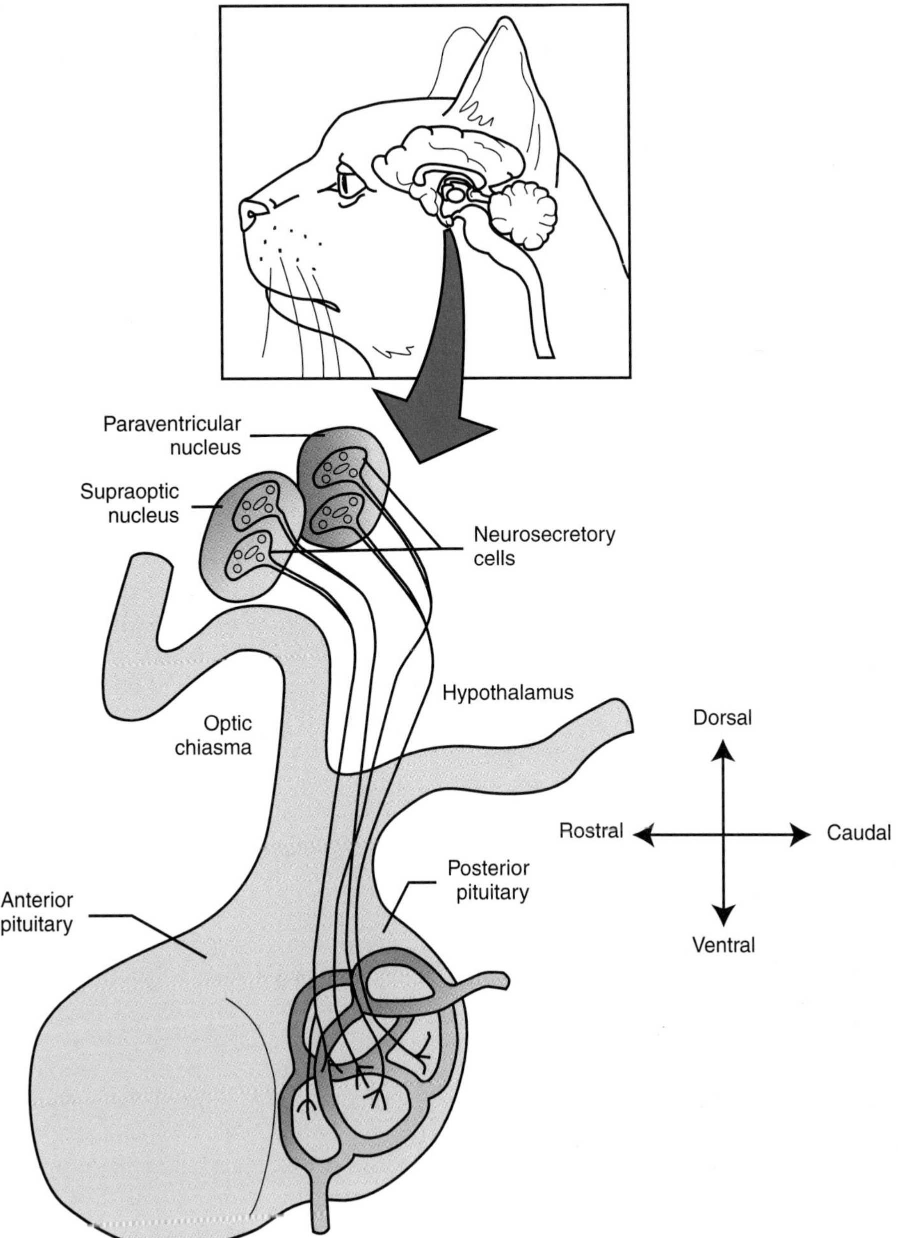

FIGURE **14-3** **Relationship of Hypothalamus and Posterior Pituitary.** Neurosecretory cells (modified neurons) in hypothalamus produce hormones that are transported down nerve fibers to posterior pituitary, where they are stored. Their release is controlled by nerve impulses from the hypothalamus.

CLINICAL APPLICATION Growth Hormone (GH)

Because of its "whole-body" effects, deficiencies or excesses of GH can produce some very obvious effects. The most pronounced effect of a GH deficiency is dwarfism, a condition in which a young animal does not grow normally. Other, less dramatic effects of GH deficiency relate to its metabolic effects and interrelationships with other hormones and endocrine glands. These can include alopecia (hair loss); thin skin; and development of secondary abnormalities of thyroid, adrenal, and reproductive hormones. Animals with GH deficiencies often respond to the therapeutic administration of GH.

An excess of GH can result in a form of giantism referred to as **acromegaly.** This condition is often caused by a pituitary gland tumor.

A synthetic GH-like drug is also used to increase milk production in dairy cows. The drug bovine somatotropin (BST) is used for its generalized anabolic effect, which enhances the production of milk by the mammary glands. As is often the case with hormone-related drugs, some potentially serious side effects are associated with the use of BST. The drug is known to elevate animals' body temperatures, reduce conception rates, increase the risk of mastitis (mammary gland infection) development, and increase the risk of digestive disorders.

milk by the mammary glands. Once lactation has begun, prolactin production and release by the anterior pituitary gland continue as long as the teat or nipple continues to be stimulated by nursing or milking. If nursing or milking ceases, the production of prolactin will cease as well. Without stimulation from prolactin, the mammary gland "dries up." Milk production stops, and the mammary gland shrinks back to its nonlactating size. In the male, prolactin has no known effect.

Thyroid-Stimulating Hormone. TSH is also known as *thyrotropic hormone.* As its name implies, it stimulates the growth and development of the **thyroid gland** and causes it to produce its hormones. Increased TSH secretion increases thyroid hormone production and vice versa. TSH secretion is regulated by feedback from its target organ—the thyroid gland. This occurs both through direct effects on the anterior pituitary gland and through changes in TSH-releasing factor produced by the hypothalamus. If thyroid hormone levels rise higher than the body needs, TSH production diminishes. With less stimulation, the thyroid gland decreases its hormone production, causing the thyroid hormone level in the bloodstream to drop. If the level drops too low, TSH production increases, stimulating the thyroid gland to increase its hormone production again. Homeostasis of thyroid hormone production is maintained through this interaction among the hypothalamus, anterior pituitary gland, and thyroid gland.

Adrenocorticotropic Hormone. **Adrenocorticotropic hormone (ACTH)** stimulates the growth and development of the **cortex** (outer portion) of the **adrenal gland** and the release of some of its hormones. Its production is generally regulated by feedback from the hormones of the adrenal cortex in much the same manner as TSH production is regulated by feedback from thyroid hormones. In times of sudden stress to an animal, however, ACTH can be released quickly as a result of stimulation of the hypothalamus by other parts of the brain. When stimulated in this way, the hypothalamus sends a burst of ACTH-releasing factor down to the anterior pituitary through the portal system of blood vessels that links them and causes ACTH to be released quickly.

Follicle-Stimulating Hormone. **Follicle-stimulating hormone (FSH)** is another hormone that is named for its effect in the female. It stimulates the growth and development of **follicles** in the ovaries. Each follicle is an "incubator" for a single, large female reproductive cell (the oocyte), which develops and matures as the follicle enlarges. This process is termed **oogenesis.** FSH also stimulates the lining cells of the follicles to produce and secrete estrogens, which are the female sex hormones. Estrogens are responsible for the physical and behavioral changes that prepare the female for breeding and pregnancy.

In the male, FSH has an effect similar to one of its effects in the female. It stimulates **spermatogenesis**—the development of male reproductive cells (the spermatozoa) in the seminiferous tubules of the testes.

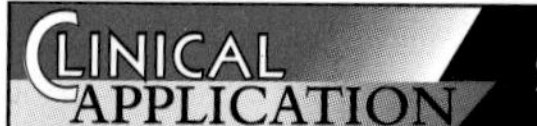

Superovulation

FSH-like drugs are often used to "superovulate" animals in preparation for embryo transfer. They cause the ovaries to produce more follicles and ova than normal. This is called **superovulation.** Once the animal is bred, the resulting embryos are retrieved from the uterus (usually by flushing) before they implant in its wall. They can then be transferred to several other recipient animals, whose estrous cycles have been synchronized with the donor animal, for the remainder of the gestation (pregnancy) period. This allows females of particularly good genetic stock to produce more offspring in their lifetimes than normal reproductive mechanisms would allow.

Luteinizing Hormone. **Luteinizing hormone (LH)** is yet another hormone whose name is derived from its effect in the female. (Are you sensing a pattern here?) LH completes the process of follicle development in the ovary that was started by FSH. As a follicle grows, it produces increasing amounts of estrogens that feed back to the anterior pituitary. They cause the production of FSH to decrease and the production of LH to increase. By the time a follicle is fully mature, LH levels reach a peak. In most animal species this causes ovulation, or rupture of the mature follicle and release of the reproductive cell. Once ovulation has occurred, the high LH level stimulates the cells left behind in the empty follicle to multiply and develop into another endocrine structure—the **corpus luteum.** The corpus luteum produces progestin hormones, principally progesterone, which will be necessary for the maintenance of pregnancy should it occur. In the male, LH stimulates cells in the testes called *interstitial cells* to develop and produce the male sex hormone testosterone. Therefore LH is sometimes called **interstitial cell–stimulating hormone (ICSH)** in the male.

FSH and LH are sometimes grouped together under the term **gonadotropins** because they stimulate the growth and development of the gonads—the ovaries and testes.

Melanocyte-Stimulating Hormone. Everything in the animal body exists for a reason, although the reason may just be that something is left over from some long-ago time in the species' history. That seems to be the case with our little toe and a horse's splint bones. **Melanocyte-stimulating hormone (MSH)** may be another remnant of an earlier time, but we have no conclusive evidence one way or the other.

MSH is associated with control of color changes in the pigment cells (melanocytes) of reptiles, fish, and amphibians—animals that can rapidly change colors and color patterns. Administration of artificially large amounts of MSH to higher mammals can cause darkening of the skin from melanocyte stimulation, but its effect at normal physiological levels is not known. Does it have some important role(s) that we are not aware of? We're just not sure yet.

The Posterior Pituitary (Neurohypophysis)

Unlike the very busy anterior pituitary, the posterior pituitary does not produce *any* hormones. Instead, it serves as a place for two hormones produced in the hypothalamus to be stored for periodic release into the bloodstream. The antidiuretic hormone and oxytocin are transported down to the posterior pituitary along nerve fibers and stored in nerve endings. Nerve impulses from the hypothalamus tell the nerve endings when to release them into the bloodstream.

Antidiuretic Hormone. The name of **antidiuretic hormone (ADH)** tells us what it does. It helps prevent **diuresis,** which is the loss of large quantities of water in the urine. Put more plainly, it helps the body conserve water in times of short supply by acting on the kidneys. ADH causes them to reabsorb more water from the urine they are producing back into the bloodstream. The resulting urine is more concentrated than it would have been otherwise. It has a deeper color and a stronger odor.

ADH is released when the hypothalamus detects a water shortage in the body. When an animal becomes a little dehydrated, the osmotic pressure of the blood increases (it becomes more concentrated), producing a condition called *hemoconcentration*. Receptors in the hypothalamus detect this change, resulting in nerve impulses that travel down to the posterior pituitary and cause the release of ADH. The ADH travels to its target organ, the kidney, and causes it to conserve water by producing more concentrated urine.

An interesting side note is that ADH release is inhibited by alcohol and caffeine. So, if we attempt to relieve thirst by drinking alcoholic beverages or caffeine-containing drinks such as colas or coffee, we will actually produce the opposite effect. By putting the brakes on ADH release, these substances allow more water to flow out of the body in the urine. This worsens the hemoconcentration, making the thirst worse instead of better in the long run. So your mother's advice is accurate: The best thing to drink when you are thirsty is water! Moms are pretty smart.

A deficiency of ADH in the body causes the disease **diabetes insipidus.** Affected animals produce large quantities of very dilute urine **(polyuria)** and drink large quantities of water **(polydipsia).** Other disease conditions also produce polyuria and polydipsia; therefore a complete diagnostic workup is necessary to confirm the diagnosis of diabetes insipidus. The condition is treated by administering a drug with ADH activity for the rest of the animal's life.

Oxytocin. The two targets for the hormone **oxytocin** are the uterus and the mammary glands. In the uterus, oxytocin causes contraction of the **myometrium** (the muscle of the uterus) at the time of breeding and at parturition. At the time of breeding, oxytocin induces uterine contractions that aid the transport of spermatozoa up to the oviducts. When **parturition** (the birth process) begins, oxytocin stimulates strong uterine contractions that aid in the delivery of the fetus and the placenta. During a prolonged or difficult labor, oxytocin, in the form of an injectable drug, is sometimes given to dams to help strengthen weak uterine contractions. However, the myometrium may be "burned out" by overstimulating it with oxytocin; so good clinical judgment should govern its use.

The effect of oxytocin on active (milk-producing) mammary glands is to cause what is called **milk letdown,** or the movement of milk down to the lower parts of the gland. As milk is produced, it accumulates in the alveoli (milk-producing structures) and small ducts in the upper part of the mammary gland. Stimulation of the teat or nipple by nursing or milking causes oxytocin to be released into the bloodstream. The oxytocin circulates down to the mammary gland and causes the musclelike **myoepithelial cells** around the alveoli and small ducts to contract. This squeezes milk down into the lower parts of the gland, where it is accessible for nursing or milking. Usually a lag time lasts from a few seconds to a minute or two from when teat stimulation starts to when milk flow caused by milk letdown begins. This is how long it takes for the sensory stimulation to reach the brain and signal the hypothalamus to release oxytocin from the posterior pituitary and for the oxytocin to reach the mammary gland via the blood circulation.

TEST YOURSELF

1. Through what mechanisms does the hypothalamus control the production or release of hormones from the pituitary gland? How do its effects on the anterior and posterior portions of the pituitary differ?
2. Why is the pituitary gland referred to as the "master endocrine gland?"
3. Other than promoting growth in young animals, what are some of other effects of GH?
4. What stimulates the continued release of prolactin during lactation?
5. Do FSH and LH play important roles in male animals? If so, what are they?
6. Does ADH help promote or prevent the loss of large amounts of water in the urine? What effect would the inhibition of ADH release have on the body?
7. When milking a cow by hand, why does it take a minute or two of teat stimulation before milk starts to flow freely?

The Thyroid Gland

Characteristics

The thyroid gland consists of two parts called *lobes* that are located on either side of the larynx. The lobes may be connected by a narrow band called an *isthmus,* depending on the animal species. Figure 14-4 shows how the thyroid glands appear in several species. Microscopically the thyroid gland has an odd appearance. It is composed of tens of thousands of tiny *follicles,* where thyroid hormone is produced. Each follicle consists of a little sphere of simple cuboidal glandular cells surrounding a globule of thyroid hormone **precursor** (the raw material for thyroid hormone) they have produced. The thy-

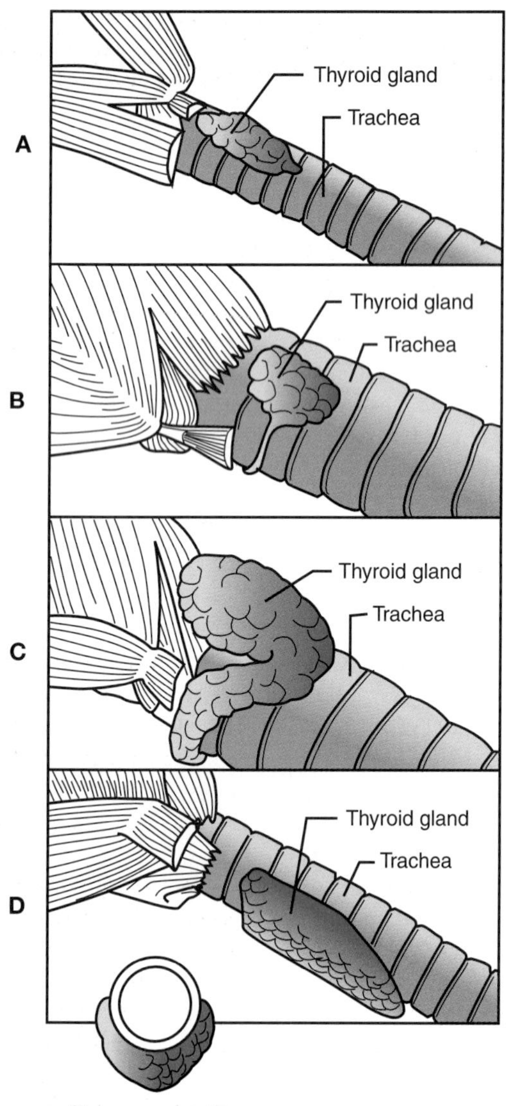

FIGURE **14-4 The Thyroid Glands of Several Species.** The inset cross section shows the ventral connection of the thyroid glands in the pig. **A,** Dog. **B,** Horse. **C,** Ox. **D,** Pig.

roid hormone precursor in the globule is called *colloid.* The thyroid gland is the only endocrine gland that stores large amounts of hormone precursor for later use.

The thyroid gland produces two hormones: (1) **thyroid hormone,** which mainly helps regulate the body's metabolic rate, and (2) **calcitonin,** which helps regulate blood calcium levels.

Thyroid Hormone

Thyroid hormone is produced when TSH from the anterior pituitary gland reaches the thyroid gland. It is actually two hormones: T_3 **(triiodothyronine)** and T_4 **(tetraiodothyronine, or thyroxine).** They are named according to how many iodine atoms each molecule of hormone contains. T_3 contains three iodine atoms per molecule, and T_4 contains four. The thyroid gland produces more T_4 than T_3, but T_3 is considered the main thyroid hormone. T_4 is mostly converted to T_3 before producing effects on target cells.

Calorigenic Effect. Thyroid hormone's **calorigenic** effect helps heat the body. It regulates the metabolic rate of all the body's cells, that is, the rate at which they "burn" nutrients to produce energy. Thyroid hormone's influence over the metabolic rate of the body's cells allows an animal to generate heat and maintain a constant internal body temperature when the temperature of the outside world changes. The production of thyroid hormone increases with exposure to cold temperatures. This response increases the body's metabolic rate, which generates more heat. It also causes nutrients to be burned at a faster rate; so animals housed outdoors in very cold temperatures need to be fed a lot more food than when kept in warmer temperatures to prevent significant loss of body weight. The level of thyroid hormone can be thought of as the body's "temperature setting."

Thyroid hormone production can be inhibited by emotional or physical stresses on an animal. Under cold conditions, this effect can cause animals to have difficulty maintaining their body temperatures. This in turn can compound the stress and open the door to disease. In otherwise healthy animals, cold temperatures alone usually do not cause disease outbreaks. However, if stress is added, animals become more susceptible and disease outbreaks often occur.

Effect on Protein, Carbohydrate, and Lipid Metabolism. Thyroid hormone also affects the metabolism of proteins, carbohydrates, and lipids much like GH does. It encourages the anabolism, or synthesis, of proteins if the animal's diet contains adequate energy sources. If the diet is deficient in energy foods or if the amount of thyroid hormone is excessive, the opposite can occur—protein catabolism or breakdown. The effect on carbohydrate metabolism is a hyperglycemic effect. Through several mechanisms, thyroid hormone helps maintain homeostasis of the blood glucose level by helping to prevent it from dropping too low. The effect on lipids is to encourage their catabolism, or breakdown.

Effect on Young, Growing Animals. Thyroid hormone is necessary for normal growth and development in young animals. In particular, it influences the development and maturation of the central nervous system and the growth and development of muscles and bones.

Calcitonin

Calcitonin, the other hormone produced by the thyroid gland, has an entirely different role. It is produced by C cells located between the thyroid follicles. Calcitonin is involved in maintaining homeostasis of blood calcium levels. Calcium is a vital substance in the body. It is involved in many important body functions, such as muscle contraction, blood clotting, milk secretion, and formation and maintenance of the skeleton. The level of calcium in the bloodstream must be kept within a

CLINICAL APPLICATION Thyroid Dysfunctions

Because of its many important roles, **dysfunctions** (abnormal functioning) of the thyroid gland can have serious effects on the health and well-being of an animal. Three conditions most commonly seen are goiter, hypothyroidism, and hyperthyroidism.

Goiter manifests itself as a nonneoplastic (noncancerous), noninflammatory enlargement of the thyroid gland. It usually results from an iodine-deficient diet. Because iodine is an important component of thyroid hormone, a deficiency of iodine results in a deficiency of thyroid hormone. The anterior pituitary attempts to compensate for this by producing more thyroid-stimulating hormone (TSH). The elevated TSH levels overstimulate the thyroid and cause **hyperplasia** (overdevelopment) of the gland. This causes it to enlarge, resulting in what we call *goiter.* Although goiter can be treated with iodine supplementation, it is more easily prevented than treated. In areas known to be iodine deficient, iodized salt should be added to animals' diets.

Hypothyroidism results from a deficiency of thyroid hormone. It is most commonly seen in dogs, although it can be seen in any species. Because thyroid hormone influences the functioning of all cells, organs, and systems, hypothyroidism affects the whole body. This results in clinical signs that are vague and nonspecific. They relate primarily to a slowing of the body's metabolism. Common clinical signs include **alopecia** (hair loss, usually bilaterally symmetrical), dry skin, lethargy, reluctance to exercise, and weight gain without any increase in appetite. Affected animals often seek out sources of heat because deficient thyroid hormone levels cause the animal to have difficulty maintaining its body temperature. Most cases of hypothyroidism occur in middle-age animals, but if it occurs in a young animal, dwarfism (impaired growth) and impaired mental development occur along with the other common signs. Hypothyroidism often can be treated effectively by administering thyroid hormone supplements to affected animals. These usually have to be continued for the rest of the animals' lives.

Hyperthyroidism is the opposite problem. It results from too much thyroid hormone production. It is most commonly seen in cats although it is seen occasionally in dogs. Excessive amounts of thyroid hormone speed up cellular metabolism all over the body. This results in signs such as nervousness, excitability, weight loss, increased appetite, **tachycardia** (abnormally fast heart rate), vomiting, diarrhea, polyuria (excessive urine production), and polydipsia (excessive thirst). Hyperthyroidism is usually treated by surgical removal of the thyroid gland (thyroidectomy) or by long-term administration of a thyroid-inhibiting drug.

narrow range to allow these functions to take place without any difficulty.

The action of calcitonin is to help prevent **hypercalcemia** (an excessively high blood calcium level) by decreasing the blood calcium level if it gets too high. It does this mainly by encouraging the excess calcium to be deposited in the bones. It's kind of like putting money in the bank knowing that you can go back and take it out later if you need it. The bones are the body's "calcium bank."

CLINICAL APPLICATION Hypocalcemia

The hypocalcemia-preventing action of parathyroid hormone can sometimes be overwhelmed by the loss of calcium in the milk of lactating animals. The hypocalcemia that results can be a serious, potentially life-threatening condition. The most obvious clinical signs relate to disturbances in skeletal muscle function caused by the lack of calcium. In cattle the condition is called **milk fever** and results in generalized muscle weakness. In mild cases tremors and weakness are seen. As the condition becomes more severe, the animal may lie down and be unable to rise. Such an affected animal is often referred to as a "downer cow." In dogs and cats the condition is called **eclampsia** and causes muscle tremors and spasms that can progress to full-blown seizures if left untreated. Treatment in both cases is aimed at rapidly increasing the level of calcium in the blood by infusing a calcium solution intravenously.

THE PARATHYROID GLANDS

Characteristics

The **parathyroid glands** got their names because of their physical relationship with the thyroid gland. They are several small, pale nodules in, on, or near the thyroid glands. The precise location and appearance of the parathyroid glands vary quite a bit.

Parathyroid Hormone

Parathyroid hormone (PTH) is also conveniently called *parathormone.* It helps maintain blood calcium homeostasis by exerting an opposite effect to calcitonin. PTH helps prevent **hypocalcemia** (a blood calcium level that is too low) by increasing the blood calcium level if it gets too low. It does this through its effects on the kidneys, the intestine, and the bones. It causes the kidneys to retain calcium, the intestine to absorb calcium from food, and it withdraws calcium from the calcium bank (the bones).

TEST YOURSELF

1. What hormone plays an important role in helping an animal maintain its body temperature under cold environmental conditions? How does it work?
2. How do the clinical signs of hypothyroidism and hyperthyroidism relate to the normal functions of thyroid hormone?
3. What two hormones play important roles in maintaining homeostasis of blood calcium levels in the body? Which one prevents hypercalcemia? Which prevents hypocalcemia?

THE ADRENAL GLANDS

Characteristics

The adrenal glands are named for their proximity to the kidneys (*renal* refers to kidneys). The two adrenal glands are located near the cranial ends of the kidneys (note their locations in Figure 14-5). Like the pituitary gland, they appear to

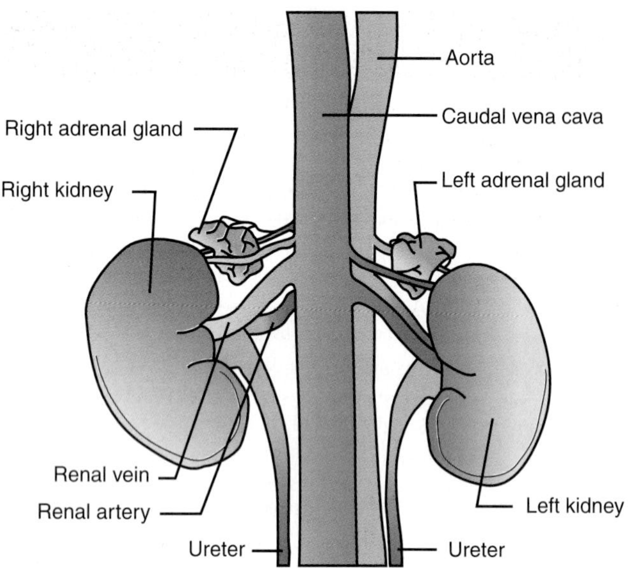

FIGURE **14-5** **Adrenal Glands of Dog: Ventral View.**

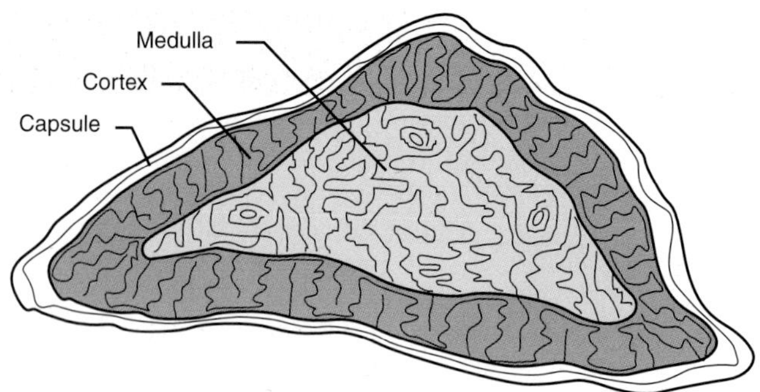

FIGURE **14-6** **Adrenal Gland: Cross Section Showing Cortex and Medulla.**

be single structures, but each is actually two glands, with one wrapped around the other like chocolate wrapped around a peanut (Figure 14-6). The two glands, the outer adrenal cortex and the inner adrenal **medulla,** come from different embryological origins and have very different structures and functions.

Adrenal Cortex

The **adrenal cortex,** the outer gland, develops from glandular tissue and looks like normal endocrine tissue microscopically. Under the direction of ACTH from the anterior pituitary gland and other mechanisms, the adrenal cortex produces a whole bunch of hormones that are classified into three main groups: glucocorticoids, mineralocorticoids, and sex hormones. All are referred to as *ster*oids because their basic chemical structure is similar to chole*ster*ol.

Glucocorticoid Hormones. The name of the **glucocorticoid** group of hormones comes from its effect on the blood glucose levels. These hormones, such as cortisone, cortisol, and corticosterone, have a general hyperglycemic effect; that is, they cause the blood glucose level to rise. Several mechanisms are involved, including the breakdown (catabolism) of proteins and lipids. Most of the breakdown products are ultimately converted to glucose in the liver through a process called **gluconeogenesis.** Other effects of glucocorticoids include helping to maintain blood pressure and helping the body resist the effects of stress.

Mineralocorticoid Hormones. **Mineralocorticoid hormones** regulate the levels of some important electrolytes (mineral salts) in the body. The principal mineralocorticoid hormone, **aldosterone,** affects the levels of sodium, potassium, and hydrogen ions in the body. Its target is the kidney, where it causes sodium ions to be reabsorbed from the urine back into the bloodstream in exchange for potassium and hydrogen ions, which pass out of the body in the urine. The level of sodium in the body must be maintained at a fairly high level normally, but much less potassium is needed. Potassium actually can be toxic if it accumulates to a level that is too high. Some drug preparations used to euthanize animals contain very high levels of potassium, which stops the beating of the heart. Hydrogen ions affect the body's acid-base balance, which must be controlled carefully. Aldosterone also affects water levels in the body in that water accompanies sodium back into the bloodstream when sodium ions are reabsorbed.

Sex Hormones. The adrenal cortex in both females and males produces small amounts of **sex hormones.** Both androgens (male sex hormones) and estrogens (female sex hormones) are produced. The amounts are very small, and their effects are minimal.

Adrenal Medulla

The **adrenal medulla,** the inner gland, develops from nervous tissue and resembles nervous tissue microscopically. Its hormone-secreting cells are modified neurons that secrete directly into the bloodstream. Two very similar hormones are produced: **epinephrine** and **norepinephrine.**

Hormone secretion by the adrenal medulla is under the control of the sympathetic portion of the autonomic nervous system—the "threat control" system. When an animal feels threatened, its sympathetic system kicks in, producing what is termed the **"fight or flight" response.** This reaction prepares the body for intense physical activity. Sympathetic nervous system effects include increased heart rate and output, increased blood pressure, dilated air passageways in the lungs, and decreased gastrointestinal function. These effects are produced partly by direct sympathetic nerve stimulation of target tissues and partly by the epinephrine and norepinephrine released into the bloodstream by the adrenal medulla. The adrenal medullary hormones circulate around the body, helping to produce the whole-body fight or flight effect. After the threat has passed, it takes the body awhile to "come down" from its excited state. This delay is due to the epinephrine and norepinephrine circulating in the bloodstream. It takes some time for them to be metabolized and removed from circulation.

CLINICAL APPLICATION: Glucocorticoid-Related Drugs

Drugs modeled after glucocorticoid hormones are commonly used therapeutically in animals, usually for their antiinflammatory effect. This general class of drugs is commonly known as *corticosteroids* or *glucocorticosteroids* and includes drugs such as hydrocortisone, prednisone, dexamethasone, and triamcinolone. Because they mimic many of the effects of natural glucocorticoid hormones and are given in amounts much greater than the natural hormones, these powerful drugs have many potential side effects. These include the following:

- *Suppression of the immune response,* which can lower an animal's defenses and make it more susceptible to infection.
- *White blood cell count alteration.* As a result of corticosteroid drug administration, neutrophil numbers go up, and lymphocyte, eosinophil, and monocyte numbers go down. This mimics the body's natural "stress" response. If we're going to administer corticosteroid drugs to an animal around the time that blood is to be drawn for a complete blood count (CBC), the blood should be drawn before the drug is given. This approach avoids confusion in interpreting the results.
- *Slowing of wound healing* because of inhibition of scar tissue–producing fibroblast cells.
- *Catabolic effect.* After long-term corticosteroid drug use, the catabolism (breakdown) of protein can result in thinning of the skin, loss of hair, and a general loss of muscle mass.
- *Premature parturition.* Administration of corticosteroid drugs to pregnant animals can cause abortion of fetuses.
- *Hyperglycemia.* This condition can be significant in an animal with diabetes mellitus because it can change the animal's insulin requirement.
- *Suppression of adrenal cortex stimulation.* The body's normal feedback mechanisms interpret the high levels of corticosteroid drug in the bloodstream as high levels of glucocorticoid hormones. This causes a cascade effect from the hypothalamus to the anterior pituitary gland to the adrenal cortex. The hypothalamus decreases its production of ACTH-releasing factor, which causes the anterior pituitary gland to decrease its production of ACTH. This results in diminished stimulation of the adrenal cortex. Long-term, high-level corticosteroid drug use actually can cause **atrophy** (physical shrinkage) of the adrenal cortex. If corticosteroid drug administration were then suddenly withdrawn, the animal would be left with a severe deficiency of glucocorticoid hormones. This would result in signs of hypoadrenocorticism (see the following Clinical Application). Therefore long-term use of corticosteroid drugs should not be terminated suddenly but tapered off gradually to give the adrenal cortex a chance to recover.
- ***Iatrogenic*** (caused by the treatment) hyperadrenocorticism can result when excessive levels of corticosteroid drugs are administered. Signs mimic naturally occurring hyperadrenocorticism (see the following Clinical Application).

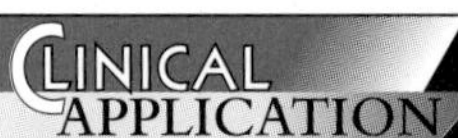

Glucocorticoid-Related Diseases

Hyperadrenocorticism (sometimes called *Cushing's syndrome*) is a condition that results from too much glucocorticoid hormone being produced by the adrenal cortex. Initial clinical signs include polyuria (excess urine production), polydipsia (excess water consumption), and polyphagia (increased appetite). Long-term signs include hair loss, muscle wasting, and slow wound healing. The signs of naturally occurring hyperadrenocorticism can be mimicked by excessive administration of corticosteroid drugs.

Hypoadrenocorticism (sometimes called *Addison's disease*) is a condition caused by a deficiency of adrenal cortical hormones. Clinical signs are somewhat nonspecific, including weakness, lethargy, vomiting, and diarrhea. It is usually a progressive condition that can lead to circulatory and kidney failure. The effects of the disease can be mimicked if long-term corticosteroid drug administration is suddenly stopped.

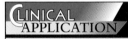

TEST YOURSELF

1. What three groups of hormones are produced in the adrenal cortex?
2. How are the hormones of the adrenal medulla involved in producing the "fight or flight" response?

THE PANCREAS

The pancreas is a long, flat, abdominal organ located near the duodenum that has both exocrine and endocrine functions. Most of its mass is made up of exocrine glandular tissue that produces important digestive enzymes. Its endocrine component makes up only a small percentage of the total volume of the organ, but one of its hormones, insulin, is vital to the life of an animal.

The Pancreatic Islets

The endocrine portion of the pancreas is organized into thousands of tiny clumps of cells scattered throughout the organ. These clumps of cells are called **pancreatic islets,** or *islets of Langerhans.* The main endocrine cells of the pancreatic islets are alpha cells, which produce the hormone glucagon; beta cells, which produce insulin; and delta cells, which produce somatostatin.

Pancreatic Hormones

The pancreatic islets produce three main hormones. Two of them, insulin and glucagon, play important roles in controlling the metabolism and use of glucose and have opposite effects. The third hormone, somatostatin, inhibits the secretion of insulin and glucagon, as well as GH, and diminishes the activity of the gastrointestinal tract.

Clinical Application: Diabetes Mellitus

Diabetes mellitus is a disease caused by a deficiency of the hormone insulin. Without sufficient insulin in the body, glucose does not move into body cells. It builds up in the blood, resulting in excessively high blood glucose levels (hyperglycemia), which spill over into the urine, thereby producing **glycosuria** (glucose in the urine). At the same time, the body's cells are starved for energy because they cannot absorb and use the glucose that surrounds them.

The clinical signs of diabetes mellitus usually develop gradually. They include polyuria (excess urine production), polydipsia (excessive thirst), **polyphagia** (increased appetite), weight loss, and weakness. Laboratory tests reveal hyperglycemia (too high a level of glucose in the blood) and glycosuria. The condition can be fatal if left untreated.

Diabetes mellitus is not presently curable, but it often can be controlled effectively through appropriate treatment. This approach usually involves careful management of the animal's diet and amount of exercise, administration of insulin injections once or twice a day, and frequent monitoring of the animal's urine and blood glucose levels. The dose of insulin must be carefully controlled because an overdose can result in **hypoglycemia** (too low a level of glucose in the blood), which can lead to weakness and collapse of the animal.

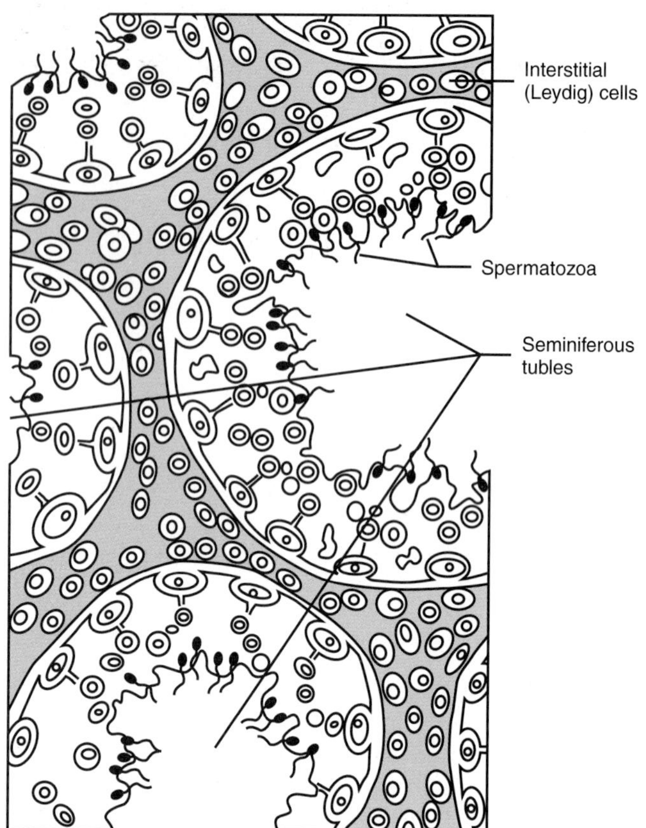

FIGURE **14-7** **Interstitial Cells of Testes.** Interstitial cells of testes produce androgens, principally testosterone, under stimulation by luteinizing hormone from the anterior pituitary.

Insulin. The hormone **insulin** is essential for life. It causes glucose, amino acids, and fatty acids in the bloodstream to be absorbed through cell membranes into body cells and used for energy. Because its overall effect on glucose is to move it out of the bloodstream and into cells, insulin acts to lower the level of glucose in the blood.

Glucagon. **Glucagon** has an effect opposite to insulin. Insulin lowers the blood glucose level, whereas glucagon raises it. This hyperglycemic effect is accomplished by two main mechanisms. Glucagon stimulates liver cells to convert glycogen (a storage form of glucose) to glucose. It also stimulates gluconeogenesis (the conversion of fat and protein breakdown products to glucose). The net effect of both is to raise the level of glucose in the blood. Because other hormones, such as GH (from the anterior pituitary gland) and glucocorticoid hormones (from the adrenal cortex), have similar hyperglycemic effects, a deficiency of glucagon is not as devastating to the body as a deficiency of insulin.

The Gonads

The **gonads** are the reproductive organs—the testes in the male and the ovaries in the female. They produce the male and female reproductive cells and important hormones.

The Testes

The two **testes** are housed in the scrotum, a sac of skin in the inguinal region. The majority of each testis is made up of coiled seminiferous tubules, where spermatozoa are produced. Scattered between the seminiferous tubules are clumps of endocrine cells, called the **interstitial cells** (Figure 14-7), which produce **androgens,** the male sex hormones. The production of androgens by the interstitial cells is stimulated by the anterior pituitary hormone LH, or ICSH in the male. The principal androgen that the interstitial cells produce is **testosterone.** It is responsible for the development of male secondary sex characteristics such as the muscular male body shape and the male libido, or the sex drive. Testosterone also stimulates the development of the male accessory sex glands, activates spermatogenesis (spermatozoa production), and stimulates the growth of the penis. Testosterone is a steroid hormone with an overall anabolic effect in that it stimulates the buildup of proteins in muscle and bone.

The Ovaries

The two **ovaries** are located in the abdomen up near the kidneys. Unlike the testes, which produce spermatozoa and hormones continuously, the ovaries produce ova (the female reproductive cells) and hormones in cycles. The ovarian cycles are controlled by two anterior pituitary hormones: FSH and LH. The main hormone groups produced in the ovaries are estrogens and progestins.

Estrogens. **Estrogens,** such as estradiol and estrone, are the female sex hormones. They are produced when FSH from the

CLINICAL APPLICATION Anabolic Steroid Drugs

Anabolic steroid drugs, which are related to testosterone, are used to help debilitated animals regain strength and weight after surgery or long illnesses. Unfortunately, they are sometimes abused by people seeking a shortcut to muscular development and performance enhancement. Because of their similarity to the hormone testosterone, they have many undesirable side effects that alter reproductive functions, behavior, and other body systems.

anterior pituitary gland stimulates follicles to develop in the ovaries. Follicles are fluid-filled structures in which the female reproductive cells develop. The cells that make up the follicles produce and release the estrogens into the bloodstream. Estrogens are responsible for the physical and behavioral changes that prepare the female for breeding and pregnancy and signal the male that the time for breeding is approaching.

As an ovarian follicle grows, the amount of estrogens it produces grows as well. The increasing estrogen levels accelerate the physical and behavioral changes that are occurring and feed back to the anterior pituitary gland. The feedback causes the anterior pituitary gland to reduce the production of FSH and increase the production of LH. As the follicle continues to grow, the amount of FSH in the bloodstream gradually decreases and the LH level increases. When the follicle is fully mature, the LH level peaks and, in most animal species, ovulation occurs. Ovulation is the rupture of the blisterlike follicle with release of the ovum into the oviduct. (See Chapter 16 for a more complete description of the whole process of follicle development and rupture.)

Progestins. After ovulation has taken place, the high LH level stimulates the cells of the now-empty follicle to multiply and develop into a solid, hormone-producing structure—the corpus luteum. The term *corpus luteum* literally means "yellow body" because of its pale yellow color. The corpus luteum produces several hormones that are collectively called **progestins.** The principal progestin is **progesterone,** whose name means "pregnancy-promoting steroid hormone." Progesterone helps prepare the uterus to receive the fertilized ovum and is necessary for pregnancy to be maintained once the fertilized ovum implants in the uterus.

If the female animal is bred and becomes pregnant, the corpus luteum receives a hormone signal from the uterus and is maintained in the ovary. If pregnancy does not occur, no hormone signal is sent from the uterus, and the corpus luteum shrinks up and disappears.

Progestin-related drugs are often used therapeutically, especially in horses. They are most commonly used to delay the onset of estrus (the heat period), to synchronize the estrous periods in a group of mares so that they can be bred together, and to help maintain pregnancy in mares that have deficient natural progesterone levels.

CLINICAL APPLICATION Hormones as Drugs

Because of their powerful and often widespread effects, hormones and hormonelike substances are used as drugs to treat illnesses or produce particular desired effects in animals. When natural hormone levels are too low, hormones can be given therapeutically to help correct the imbalance. This is often the case with hypothyroidism (deficiency of thyroid hormone), diabetes insipidus (deficiency of antidiuretic hormone), and diabetes mellitus (deficiency of insulin). In other cases, drugs derived from natural hormones are used to produce particular effects, such as an antiinflammatory effect (glucocorticoid-like drugs) or stimulation of uterine contractions (oxytocin), cardiovascular stimulation (epinephrine), or to synchronize estrous cycles (prostaglandin $F_{2\alpha}$).

Because the production and effects of natural hormones are so interrelated, the therapeutic use of hormones and hormonelike drugs can produce some potent and widespread problems, along with beneficial effects. The amounts of hormones used therapeutically are usually very large compared with the normal physiological hormone levels in the body; therefore the potential for undesired side effects increases accordingly. For example, use of a hormonelike drug can inhibit production of the natural hormone it mimics. Later when the drug is to be discontinued, the animal should be gradually weaned off it so that the natural hormone production mechanisms can gradually take over again. Suddenly stopping the drug after long-term administration can produce disastrous results. In general, hormone therapy must be carefully planned and closely monitored so that the benefits outweigh the consequences.

TEST YOURSELF

1. Which four hormones have a direct hyperglycemic effect in the body? What is the only hormone that acts to lower the blood glucose level?
2. Which hormone are anabolic steroid drugs related to?
3. How do the basic actions of estrogens and progestins differ?

OTHER ENDOCRINE ORGANS

Hormone production is not restricted to the major endocrine glands that we have just discussed. Other organs and tissues produce hormones that also play important roles in maintaining homeostasis in the body. We discuss the most important and well-understood ones next.

THE KIDNEYS

In addition to their blood-filtering duties, the kidneys produce the hormone **erythropoietin,** which stimulates red bone marrow to increase production of oxygen-carrying red blood cells. The production of erythropoietin is stimulated by a decrease in the oxygen content of the blood, a condition called **hypoxia.** As the production of red blood cells increases in response to the erythropoietin, the increased oxygen level in the blood feeds back to the kidneys and slows the production of erythropoietin. This helps maintain the long-term homeostasis of the blood's oxygen-carrying ability.

One of the conditions that often accompanies serious kidney disease or kidney failure is anemia, which is a deficiency of red blood cells. It results from the damaged kidneys' inability to produce enough erythropoietin. The deficiency of erythropoietin causes the patient to become increasingly hypoxic because old, worn-out red blood cells continue to be removed from the bloodstream but not enough new red blood cells are being produced to replace them. Blood transfusions are often necessary to support patients with kidney failure while other forms of therapy are administered. Synthetic forms of erythropoietin are available and are often used therapeutically in human patients with kidney failure. Their high cost limits their use in veterinary medicine.

THE STOMACH

Cells in the wall of the stomach produce the hormone **gastrin.** It is a somewhat oddball hormone because it is produced in the stomach wall and acts on the stomach wall too. Its secretion is stimulated by the presence of food in the stomach. When released, gastrin stimulates gastric (stomach) glands to secrete hydrochloric acid and digestive enzymes, and it encourages muscular contractions of the stomach wall.

THE SMALL INTESTINE

Cells in the lining of the small intestine produce two hormones when partially digested material from the stomach (chyme) enters the first portion of the small intestine (the **duodenum**). One of the hormones, **secretin,** stimulates the pancreas to secrete fluid rich in sodium bicarbonate into the duodenum to neutralize the acidic **chyme** from the stomach. The other hormone, **cholecystokinin,** stimulates the release of digestive enzymes from the pancreas into the duodenum. Both secretin and cholecystokinin also act on the stomach to inhibit gastric gland secretions and stomach motility. This slows the movement of chyme into the small intestine. They also stimulate the gallbladder of the liver to contract, sending bile down into the small intestine to aid the digestion and absorption of fats and fat-soluble vitamins.

THE PLACENTA

The **placenta** is the life support system that surrounds a developing fetus during pregnancy and acts as an interface with the maternal circulation. It is also an important endocrine organ. Its secretions vary among species, but the hormones it produces have the general effect of helping to support and maintain pregnancy. Small amounts of estrogen and progesterone are often produced, as well as significant amounts of **chorionic gonadotropin** in some species, most notably the human and the horse. Detection of chorionic gonadotropin is the basis of over-the-counter pregnancy tests for humans and blood tests for the detection of pregnancy in horses. Other species, such as dogs, cats, and cattle, produce too little chorionic gonadotropin to make it useful as a method of pregnancy diagnosis.

THE THYMUS

The **thymus** is an organ that helps "kick start" the immune system early in an animal's life. It shrinks up and nearly disappears when the animal reaches adulthood. In a young animal the thymus is fairly large. It extends cranially from the level of the heart in the thorax up into the neck region along both sides of the trachea, often to the level of the larynx. After puberty, however, the thymus begins to atrophy (shrink). By the time the animal reaches adulthood, it is hard or impossible to find any remnant of the thymus.

The thymus is an important part of the animal's developing immune system—the system that helps fight off foreign invaders, such as disease-causing bacteria and viruses. Part of its functioning seems to involve hormones or hormonelike chemical substances, such as **thymosin** and **thymopoietin.** These substances seem to cause primitive cells in the thymus and other lymphoid organs to be transformed into T (for "thymus-derived") lymphocytes. T lymphocytes are often just called *T cells.* They are an important part of the animal's **cell-mediated immunity**—the portion of the immune system that produces "killer cells" that directly attack foreign invaders (see Chapter 9).

THE PINEAL BODY

The **pineal body** is a part of the brain located at the caudal end of the deep cleft that separates the two cerebral hemispheres and just rostral to the cerebellum. Its functions are not well understood yet, but it is known to influence cyclic activities in the body, or the body's biological clock. It produces a hormonelike substance called **melatonin** that seems to affect moods and wake-sleep cycles. It may also play a role in the timing of seasonal estrous cycles in some species. We still have a lot to learn about the roles of the pineal body and its secretions.

PROSTAGLANDINS

Prostaglandins are hormonelike substances that are derived from **unsaturated fatty acids.** They are produced and exert their effects within a variety of body tissues. Because they only travel a short distance from where they are produced, prostaglandins are sometimes called "tissue hormones." Typical hormones regulate the activities of tissues and organs at some distance from where they are produced. Prostaglandins do not go very far from home. They regulate the activities of neighboring cells.

The name *prostaglandin* actually came about by mistake. The first prostaglandin was isolated from semen, and its origin was incorrectly identified as the **prostate gland,** hence the name *prostaglandin.* We now know that the **seminal vesicles,** not the prostate, produce that particular compound.

Prostaglandins are now known to be produced in a variety of body tissues, including the skin, intestine, brain, kidney, lungs, reproductive organs, and eyes. Based on their molecular structure, they are organized into nine main groups—prostaglandins A through I. Subscript numbers and Greek letters are added to designate subgroups.

Prostaglandins exert some powerful effects in the body, including influences on blood pressure, gastrointestinal tract function, respiratory function, kidney function, blood clotting, inflammation, and reproductive functions. The E group of prostaglandins (PGEs) is known to play a role in the initiation of inflammation in the body. **Nonsteroidal antiinflammatory drugs,** such as aspirin, produce some of their effects by inhibiting PGE synthesis. Another clinically important prostaglandin is prostaglandin F_2-alpha ($PGF_{2\alpha}$). If administered to a female animal that has a functional corpus luteum in the ovary, $PGF_{2\alpha}$ will quickly destroy the corpus luteum. This is called **luteolysis,** and it will often cause a new estrous cycle to begin. If the animal is in early pregnancy, luteolysis will terminate the pregnancy. Drugs with $PGF_{2\alpha}$ activity are commonly used to synchronize estrous cycles in livestock species so that groups of animals can be bred together.

TEST YOURSELF

1. Why are kidney failure patients often anemic?
2. How do the actions of gastrin on the stomach differ from those of secretin and cholecystokinin?
3. Why are prostaglandins referred to as "tissue hormones?"
4. Why do hormones used as drugs have such great potential for undesirable side effects?

CHAPTER 15

THE URINARY SYSTEM

Joann Colville

WASTE EXCRETION

An animal's body is a fine-tuned machine that relies on numerous metabolic reactions to keep it alive and well. These reactions are chemical and are of great benefit to the body, but they also result in many byproducts. Some of these byproducts are useful to the body and are recycled. Others are of no further use and actually may be harmful if they are allowed to accumulate. These potentially harmful substances are called *waste products* and must be eliminated from the body.

The following are some examples of metabolic waste products:

1. Carbon dioxide and water from carbohydrate and fat metabolism
2. Nitrogenous wastes (primarily urea) from protein metabolism
3. Bile salts and pigments from red blood cell breakdown
4. Various salts from tissue breakdown and excess intake

The body has several routes by which waste products can be eliminated from the body, such as follows:

1. Respiratory system removes carbon dioxide and water vapor.
2. Sweat glands eliminate water, salts, and a small amount of urea.
3. Digestive system removes bile salts and pigments.
4. Urinary system removes urea, salts, water, and other soluble waste products.

The urinary system is the most important single route of waste product removal in the body. It removes nearly all the soluble waste products from blood and transports them out of the body. The urinary system is also a major route of elimination for excess water in the body.

PARTS OF THE URINARY SYSTEM

The urinary system is made up of the following parts (Figure 15-1):

1. Two kidneys that make urine and carry out other vital functions
2. Two ureters that carry urine to the urinary bladder
3. One urinary bladder that collects, stores, and releases urine
4. One urethra that empties urine from the body

THE KIDNEYS

The combining word forms for "kidney" are *nephr-* or *nephro-* (Greek) and *ren* or *reno-* (Latin). For example, *nephrology* is the study of the kidney, and the artery and vein that supply and drain blood from the kidney are the *renal* artery and vein.

FUNCTIONS

The kidney's most obvious role is production of urine, the fluid that facilitates the elimination of metabolic waste materials from the body. In the process of making urine, the kidney also helps maintain **homeostasis** in the body by manipulating the composition of blood plasma. In this way the kidney can regulate such things as body acid-base and fluid-electrolyte

CLINICAL APPLICATION Urinalysis

Urinalysis is the laboratory examination and evaluation of a urine sample. It involves a gross (unmagnified) examination for color and clarity, a microscopic examination for formed elements (see following text), and a chemical analysis for dissolved substances. A lot of information about how well the kidneys are working and the state of an animal's health can be gleaned from looking at the composition of its urine. A urinalysis is often part of a routine physical examination. Normally urine is about 95% water. Nitrogenous wastes (from protein breakdown), electrolytes (e.g., sodium, potassium, bicarbonate, ammonium), and pigments (from red blood cell breakdown, foods, or drugs) are dissolved in the water. Formed elements (e.g., red blood cells, white blood cells, parasites, and crystals) may be present in abnormal conditions.

balances. The kidney must filter enough water and electrolytes out of blood to equal the amount that is being put into it from other sources. For example, sodium, potassium, chloride, and nitrogenous waste (primarily urea from protein breakdown) levels in plasma must be maintained within specific, narrow concentration limits for health and life to continue. If the kidney fails to remove these substances adequately from plasma, their concentrations can rise to toxic levels and the animal can die.

The kidneys also have close associations with the endocrine system (the system of hormones that help regulate body functions). The kidneys produce hormones, regulate the release of hormones from other organs, and are themselves influenced by hormones. For example, the kidney can influence the rate of release of **antidiuretic hormone (ADH)** from the posterior pituitary gland and aldosterone, which is the mineralocorticoid secreted by the cortex of the adrenal gland. They are also

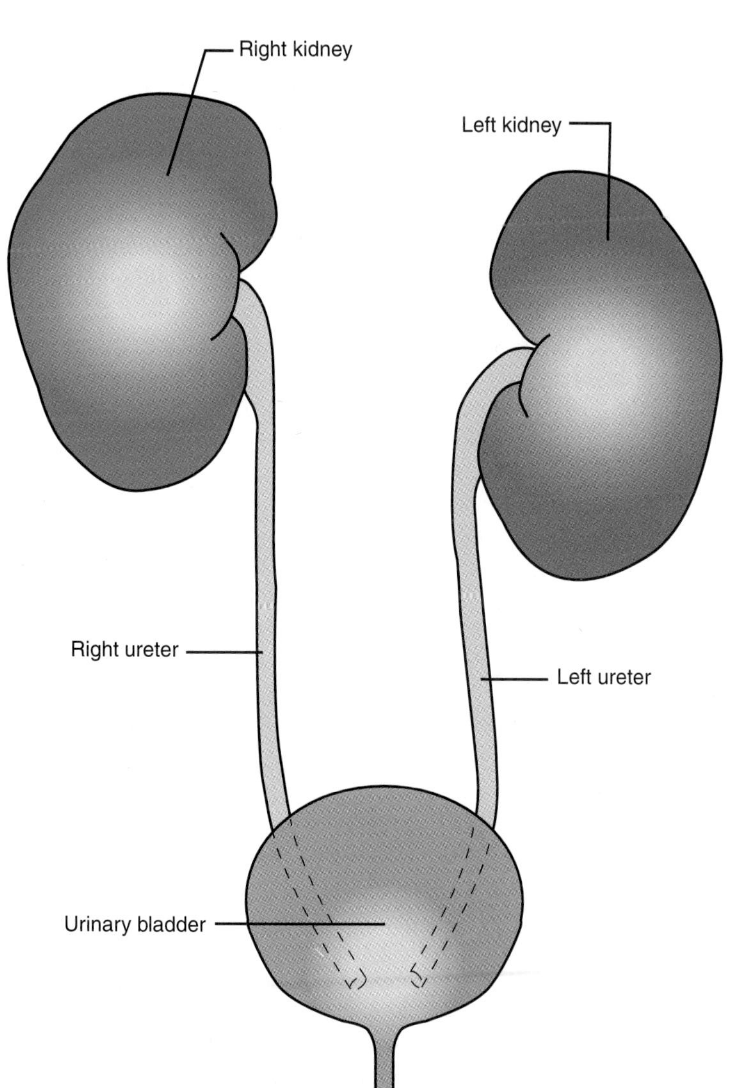

FIGURE **15-1** **Parts of Urinary System.** Urinary system is made up of two kidneys, two ureters, one urinary bladder, and one urethra.

influenced by both of these hormones. The kidneys also produce **erythropoietin,** the hormone necessary for red blood cell production, and some **prostaglandins.** (See Chapter 14 for more information about these and other hormones.)

Maintaining homeostasis in the body is the most important overall function of the kidneys. The main processes by which the kidneys help maintain homeostasis include the following:

1. *Blood filtration, reabsorption, and secretion.* The blood is filtered, useful substances are returned to the circulation, and waste products are secreted from the bloodstream into the fluid that eventually becomes urine. (More details on these processes are discussed later in this chapter.)
2. *Fluid balance regulation.* The amount of urine that is produced helps ensure that the body contains just the right amount of water to maintain a healthy internal environment. If the body has an excess and needs to get rid of water, more urine is formed **(diuresis).** If it needs to conserve water, less urine will be produced and the animal will pass little urine **(oliguria)** or no urine at all **(anuria).** Much of this function is under the control of the hormones ADH and aldosterone.
3. *Acid-base balance regulation.* The kidney helps maintain acid-base homeostasis by removing hydrogen and bicarbonate ions from the blood and excreting them in urine.
4. *Hormone production.* Specialized cells in the kidney produce erythropoietin, the hormone necessary for red blood cell production. Some prostaglandins are also produced in the kidney.

LOCATION

The kidneys are located in the dorsal part of the abdomen, just ventral to and on either side of the first few lumbar vertebrae. In common domestic animals, except the pig, the right kidney is more cranial than the left. A thick layer of fat (called the *perirenal fat*) usually surrounds the kidneys and helps protect them from pressure exerted on them by surrounding organs.

The kidneys are located **retroperitoneal** to the abdominal cavity; that is, they are outside the parietal peritoneum (between the peritoneum and the dorsal abdominal muscles) and are therefore considered officially *outside* the abdominal cavity. To a limited extent, the kidneys move with movements of the diaphragm. As the diaphragm contracts, the kidneys are pushed caudally, sometimes by nearly half the length of a vertebra. In many species the right kidney is less mobile because it fits into a depression in the liver, which helps stabilize it. The left kidney does not have this stabilizer; so it is more mobile. For this reason, abdominal radiographs should be taken when the patient has exhaled completely. The positions of the kidneys and abdominal organs are more standardized that way.

GROSS ANATOMY

The kidneys are covered by a fibrous connective tissue capsule and are "bean" shaped in most animals (Figure 15-2). Look at a kidney bean, and you'll have a good idea where its name came from. The right kidney in horses seems compressed end to end, making it appear somewhat heart shaped. Kidneys are reddish-brown. If you look at that kidney bean again, you'll see that the color is about right. With the exception of cattle, the kidneys of domestic animals have a smooth surface. The surface of cattle kidneys is divided into about 12 lobes, which gives it a lumpy appearance.

The indented area on the medial side of the kidney is called the **hilus.** This is the area where blood and lymph vessels, nerves, and the **ureters** enter and leave the kidney. If you cut the kidney of most animals in half longitudinally through the hilus, you'll find a funnel-shaped area inside the hilus. This area is the **renal pelvis.** It is a urine-collection chamber that forms the beginning of the ureter. The renal pelvis is lined with transitional epithelium—the type of epithelium that can stretch considerably without being damaged. Cattle do not have a distinct collection chamber that can be called a *renal pelvis.*

The outer portion of the kidney is called the renal **cortex.** It is reddish-brown and has a rough, granular appearance. The inner portion around the renal pelvis is the renal **medulla.** It has a smooth appearance with a dark purple outer area that sends rays up into the cortex and a pale gray-red inner area that extends down to the renal pelvis. The shape of the cortex and medulla and how they relate to each other vary among species. In some species such as cattle and pigs, the medulla has numerous pyramid-shaped areas (they look like candy corn) with the apex pointing to the renal pelvis (pigs) or directly to the ureter (cattle). This gives the medulla a scalloped appearance. The cortex fills in around the scallops. Kidneys with this structure are called *multipyramidal* or *multilobar.* In other species such as the dog, horse, and cat, the medullary pyramids fuse to occupy the entire inner area, and the cortex is pushed to the outside area. These kidneys are called *unipyramidal* or *unilobar* (see Figure 15-2). The calyx is a cuplike extension of the renal pelvis into which the medullary pyramids fit. The calyces act as a funnel that directs fluids into the renal pelvis. From there the fluid moves into the ureter. In cattle the calyces empty directly into the ureter. The cortex and medulla each contain specific structures with specific functions, which are discussed later in this chapter.

MICROSCOPIC ANATOMY

A kidney is made up of hundreds of thousands of microscopic filtering, reabsorbing, and secreting systems called **nephrons.** The nephron is the basic functional unit of the kidney. It is the smallest part of the kidney that can carry out its basic functions. The number of nephrons per kidney varies with the size of the animal. For example, a medium-sized cat has about 200,000 nephrons per kidney, and a medium-sized dog has about 700,000. Sheep, pigs, and humans have about 1,000,000 nephrons per kidney, and cattle have about 4,000,000. Each neph-

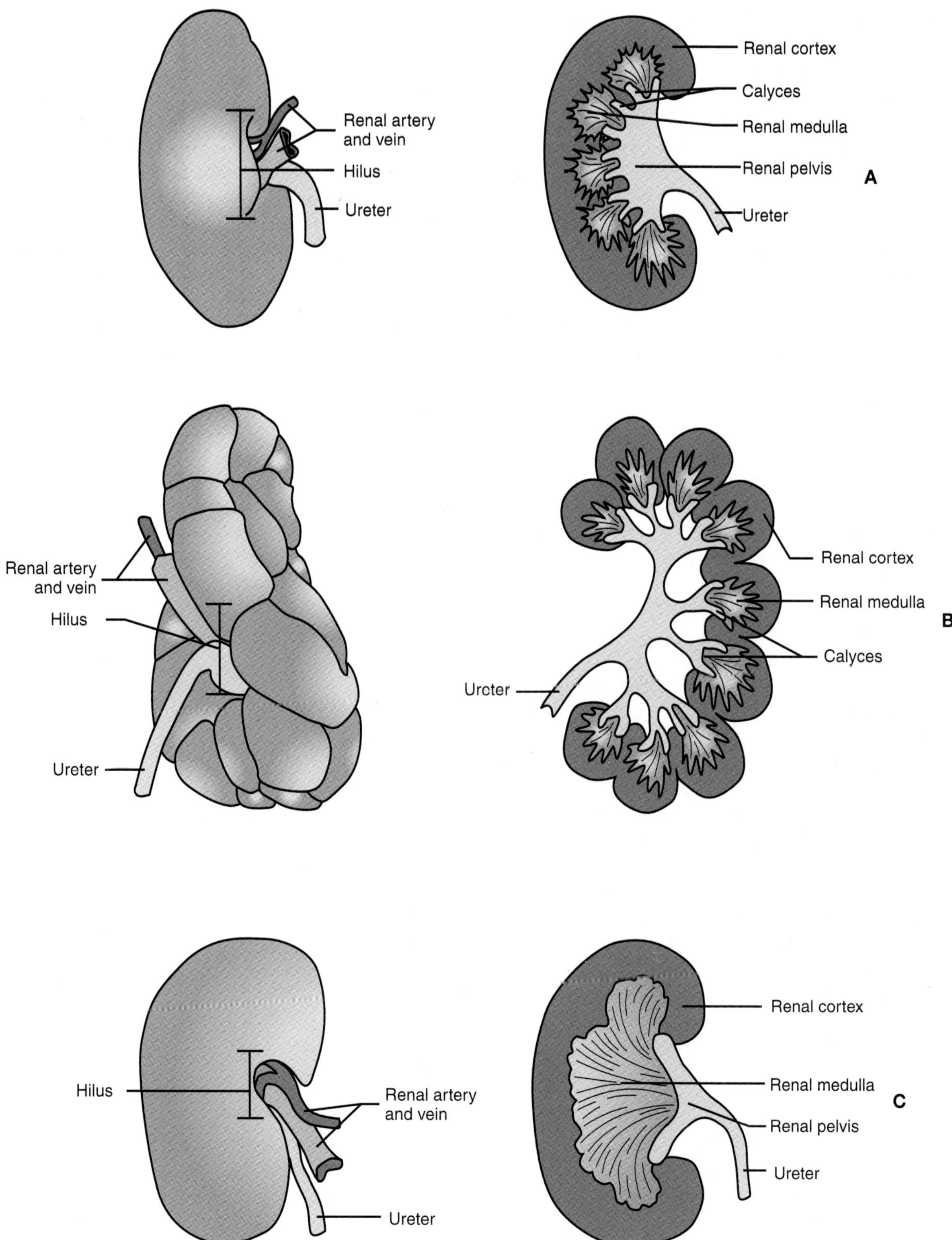

FIGURE **15-2** **Gross Anatomy of Kidney.** Pig **(A)** and cattle **(B)** kidneys are multipyramidal (multilobar). **C,** Cat and dog kidneys are unipyramidal (unilobar).

ron is composed of a renal corpuscle, a proximal convoluted tubule, a loop of Henle, and a distal convoluted tubule (Figure 15-3).

The **renal corpuscle** is located in the cortex of the kidney. It is made up of the **glomerulus** and **Bowman's capsule.** The glomerulus is a "tuft" of capillaries. Bowman's capsule is a double-walled capsule that surrounds the glomerulus. The inner layer of Bowman's capsule is the visceral layer, and it adheres closely to the surfaces of all glomerular capillaries. The outer layer is called the *parietal layer.* The space between the two layers is the **capsular space.** The capsular space is continuous with the proximal convoluted tubule. The function of the renal corpuscle is to filter blood as the first stage of urine production. The fluid that is filtered out of blood is called the **glomerular filtrate.**

The **proximal convoluted tubule (PCT)** is a continuation of the capsular space of Bowman's capsule. It is the longest part of the tubular system of the nephron. The epithelial cells of the PCT are cuboidal in shape with a brush border (thousands of tiny projections of cell membrane) on their lumen side. The brush border increases the cellular surface area exposed to the fluid in the tubule by a factor of about 20. This is especially important to the PCT's reabsorption and secretion functions. The PCT follows a twisting (hence the name *convoluted*) path through the cortex. The glomerular filtrate, now called the **tubular filtrate** (sometimes referred to as

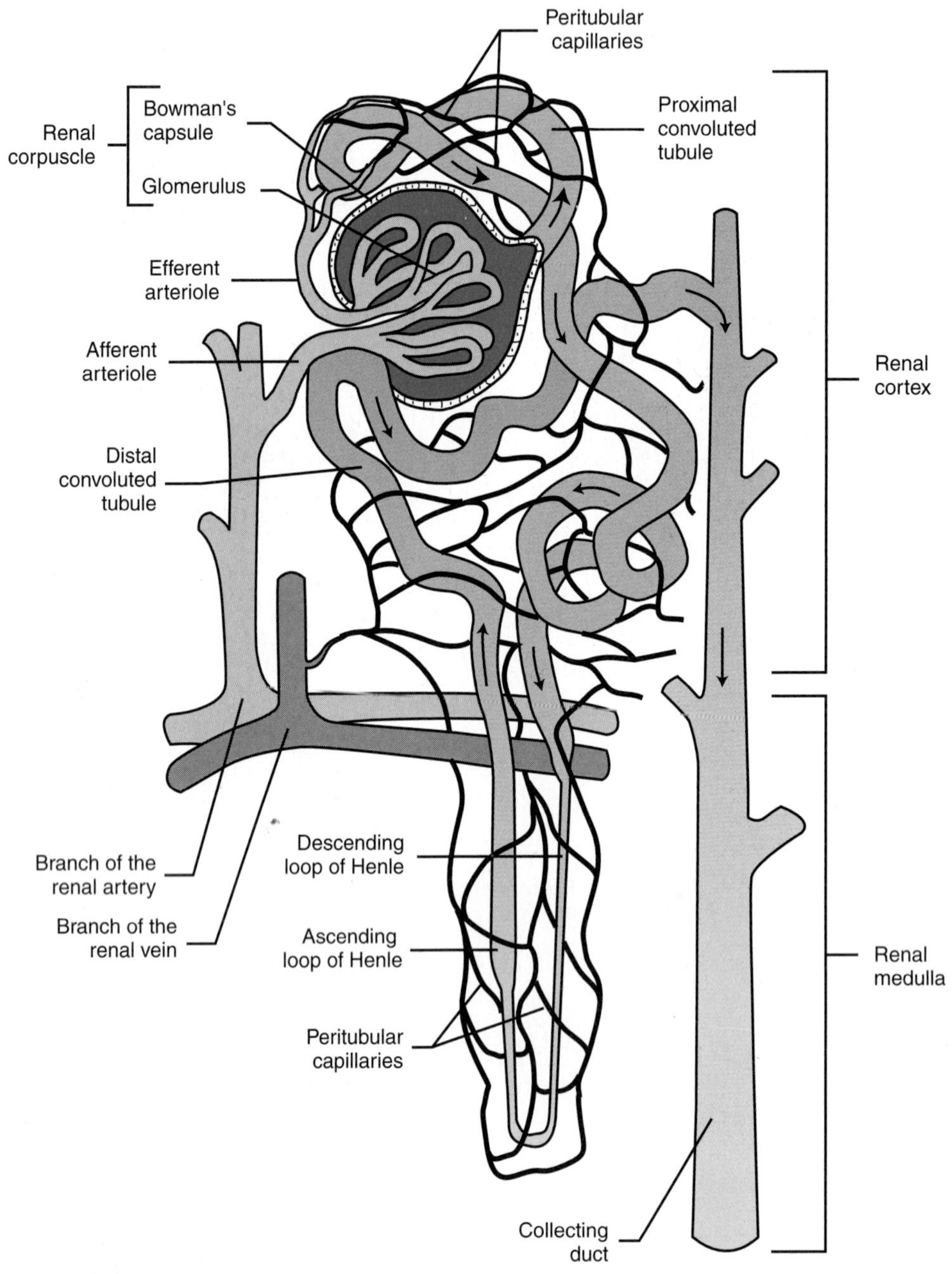

FIGURE **15-3** **Microscopic Anatomy of Nephron.** Arrows indicate direction of fluid flow through the nephron.

primitive urine), begins its journey through the tubular part of the nephron here.

The **loop of Henle** continues from the PCT and descends into the medulla of the kidney, makes a U-turn, and heads back up into the cortex. The descending part of the loop of Henle has epithelial cells similar to the cells of the PCT, including the brush border. As the loop of Henle makes its U-turn, the wall becomes thinner as the epithelial cells flatten down to simple squamous epithelial cells and lose their brush border. The lumen gets narrower here, too. As the loop of Henle ascends back up into the cortex, its wall becomes thicker again but the cells do not regain the brush border. The lumen also expands as the loop of Henle ascends towards the cortex.

The **distal convoluted tubule (DCT)** is a continuation of the ascending part of the loop of Henle. The DCT follows a twisting path through the cortex. Even though it is also called a *convoluted tubule,* the DCT is not as twisted as the PCT.

The DCTs from all the nephrons in the kidney empty into a series of tubules called **collecting ducts.** The collecting ducts carry **tubular filtrate** through the medulla and eventually empty into the renal pelvis that will become the ureter. The collecting ducts also play an important role in urine volume because they are the primary site of action of ADH. Potassium regulation and control of acid-base balance are two other important functions that take place in the collecting ducts.

NERVE SUPPLY

The nerve supply to the kidney is primarily from the sympathetic portion of the autonomic nervous system. It controls the blood flow through the glomerular capillaries but is not essential for the kidney to function. A transplanted kidney can work well even though its sympathetic nerve supply has been disrupted.

BLOOD SUPPLY

Each kidney has a large blood supply (Figure 15-4). This makes sense when you consider that the function of the kidney is to clear waste products from the blood. Up to 25% of the blood pumped by the heart goes to the kidneys. In fact, all the circulating blood in the body passes through the kidneys every 4 to 5 minutes. The main blood vessels that are responsible for this journey through the kidneys are the following:

1. The **renal artery** branches off the abdominal portion of the aorta. It enters the kidney at the hilus and then divides and subdivides into smaller arteries and arterioles until it becomes a series of afferent glomerular arterioles.

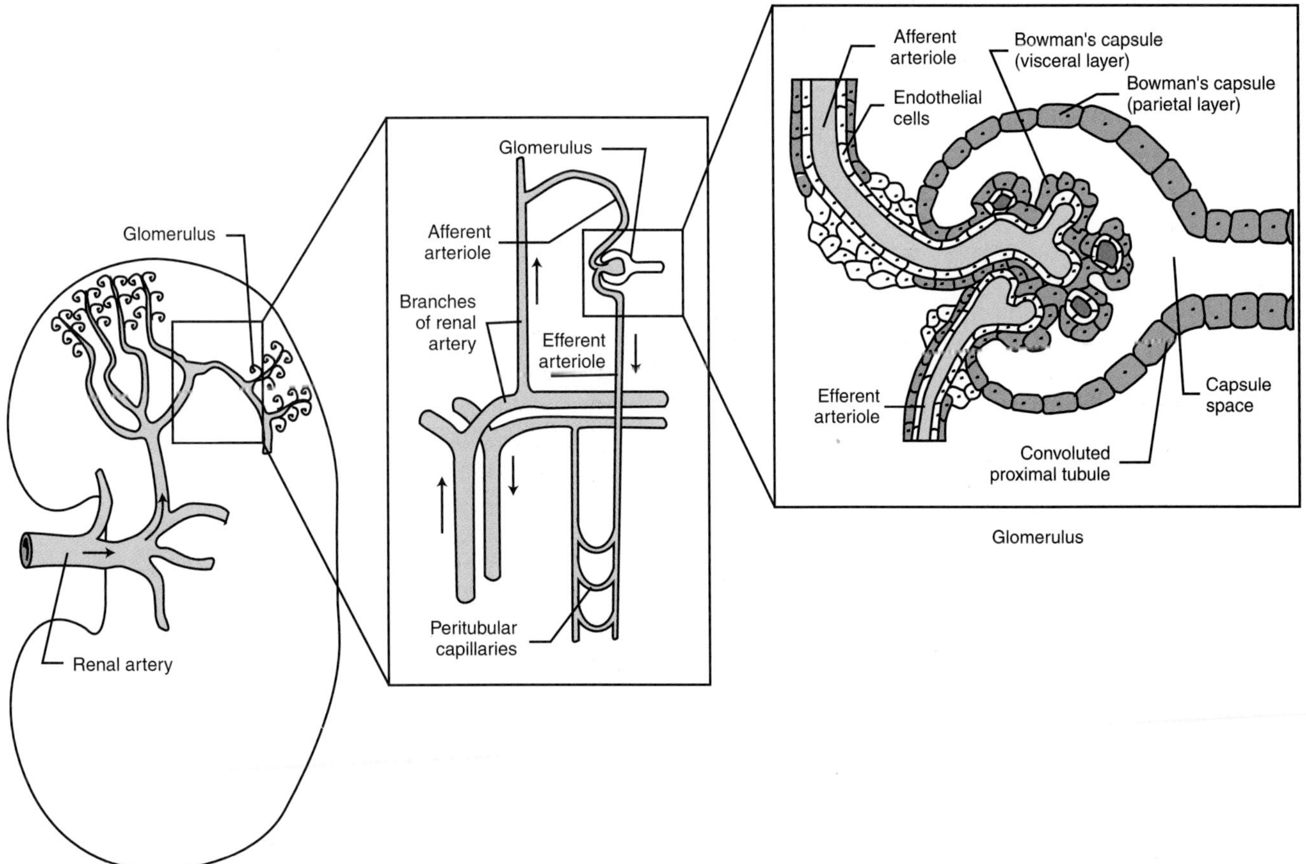

FIGURE **15-4 Arterial Blood Supply to Renal Corpuscle.** Arrows show direction of blood flow.

2. The **afferent glomerular arterioles** carry blood into the **glomerular capillaries** of the renal corpuscle.
3. **Glomerular capillaries** are a continuation of the afferent arterioles. They filter some of the plasma out of blood and put it in the capsular space of Bowman's capsule, where is it known as the *glomerular filtrate*. Not all the plasma is filtered out, or blood flow would come to a screeching halt. The blood in the glomerular capillaries leaves the glomerulus and enters the **efferent glomerular arterioles.** The blood is still arterial blood at this point because oxygen exchange has not taken place yet. This is the only place in the body where blood entering *and* leaving the capillaries is oxygenated blood.
4. The **efferent glomerular arterioles** divide into a network of capillaries that surround the rest of the nephron. These capillaries are known as the *peritubular capillaries* (see Figure 15-3). Oxygen transfer to the cells of the nephron takes place here. Also at this level, substances are taken out of the tubular filtrate and put back into blood. This is known as *tubular reabsorption*. Other substances are secreted from the blood into the tubules at this level. This is called *tubular secretion*. More information on these actions is discussed later.
5. The **peritubular capillaries** that surround the nephron converge to form venules that in turn converge to form larger veins that eventually become the renal vein.
6. The **renal vein** leaves the kidney at the hilus and joins the abdominal portion of the caudal vena cava. From a waste-content standpoint, the blood in the renal veins is the "purest" in the body.

TEST YOURSELF

1. What are the six structures that make up the urinary system?
2. Nitrogenous waste materials from protein breakdown are eliminated from the body primarily as what?
3. Name one hormone whose release is regulated by the kidney, one hormone that directly affects kidney function, and one hormone produced by the kidney.
4. What is the difference between the hilus of the kidney and the renal pelvis?
5. What is meant by the term *retroperitoneal*?
6. List, in order, the parts of the nephron. Indicate if a specific part is found in the cortex or the medulla of the kidney.

MECHANISMS OF RENAL ACTION

The three main mechanisms by which the kidneys carry out their role of waste elimination are filtration of the blood, reabsorption of useful substances back into the bloodstream, and secretion of waste products from the blood into the tubules of the nephron.

Filtration of Blood

Filtration of blood occurs in the renal corpuscle. Normally, capillaries are found between arterioles and venules and have very low blood pressure. The glomerular capillaries are different in that they are found between two arterioles and have a high blood pressure that is only about 30% lower than the blood pressure in the aorta. The high blood pressure in the glomerular capillaries forces plasma out of the capillaries and into the capsular space of Bowman's capsule. The transfer of plasma out of the capillaries is helped by the presence of many **fenestrations,** or pores, in the capillary endothelium. These fenestrations are larger than the fenestrations found in the endothelium of other capillaries and allow more fluid to leave the bloodstream. The fluid is known as the *glomerular filtrate* when it enters the capsular space and is similar to plasma except that it contains virtually no proteins. Most of the plasma protein molecules are too large to pass through the fenestrations. The fenestrations are not large enough to allow any blood cells to leave the capillaries. If the endothelium of the glomerulus is damaged, proteins and blood cells can leak into the glomerular filtrate. Because no mechanism exists to get the proteins back into the bloodstream through tubular reabsorption, they will show up as abnormal constituents of urine. The presence of abnormal amounts of proteins in urine can be used as an indicator of glomerular damage.

The **glomerular filtration rate (GFR)** is the term used to describe how fast plasma is filtered as it passes through the glomerulus. The GFR depends on the rate of blood (and therefore plasma) flow to the kidney. It is expressed in milliliters per minute. In a 25-lb dog, approximately 180 ml of plasma (that's about 300 ml of blood by the time you factor in the cells) flow to the kidney every minute. As blood passes through the kidney, about 45 ml of glomerular filtrate is formed every minute. In other words, about 25% of the plasma (45ml/180ml) is removed from circulation each minute. Over a 24-hour period, that amounts to about 64 L of glomerular filtrate being formed. That's over 16 gallons. If all that glomerular filtrate became urine that had to be eliminated from the body, imagine how often you'd have to take this dog outside to go to the bathroom! Luckily, another mechanism (reabsorption) is used by the kidney to reduce the volume of glomerular filtrate down to about 680 ml of urine produced over a 24-hour period.

Reabsorption

Once plasma leaves the circulation and passes into the capsular space to become the glomerular filtrate, it is considered to be outside the body proper even though physically it is still contained within the boundaries of the body. The glomerular filtrate contains the waste products that must be cleared from the body. This is a good thing. Unfortunately, it also contains substances found in plasma that the body does not want to lose because it needs them to maintain homeostasis. Some of the most important of these substances are sodium, potassium, calcium, magnesium, glucose, amino acids, chloride, bicarbonate, and water. So a mechanism is necessary to get these

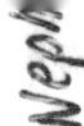

substances back into the body by way of the blood. This mechanism is reabsorption of useful substances from the tubules of the nephron into the blood of the peritubular capillaries.

The glomerular filtrate enters the PCT and becomes tubular filtrate. Changes in its composition begin immediately. Some of those changes involve removal of some of the constituents of the tubular filtrate through reabsorption back into the bloodstream. For any substance to be reabsorbed back into the body, it must pass out of the tubular lumen, through or between the tubular epithelial cells, into the interstitial fluid, and through the endothelium into the peritubular capillaries (Figure 15-5). Some substances move passively through osmosis or diffusion. Others have to be actively transported across cell membranes.

As the glomerular filtrate enters the lumen of the PCT, sodium is actively "pumped" out of the fluid and back into the bloodstream. Sodium in the tubular filtrate attaches to a carrier protein, which carries it into the cytoplasm of the PCT epithelial cell. The transfer of sodium from the tubular lumen into the epithelial cell requires energy. At the same time, glucose and amino acids attach to the same protein as sodium and follow the sodium into the epithelial cell by passive transport. This process is called **sodium cotransport.** No extra energy is expended because the glucose and amino acids are hitching a ride with the sodium by attaching to the same protein. Once the sodium is in the epithelial cell, it must be actively pumped out of the cell into the interstitial fluid, where it will move into the peritubular capillaries. Glucose and amino acids passively diffuse out of the tubular epithelial cell, into the interstitial fluid, and into the peritubular capillaries. Sodium ions are also reabsorbed in the ascending part of the loop of Henle and the DCT, where they are usually exchanged for hydrogen, ammonium, or potassium ions that are secreted into the tubular filtrate. This exchange occurs under the influence of aldosterone (the mineralocorticoid hormone produced in the cortex of the adrenal gland).

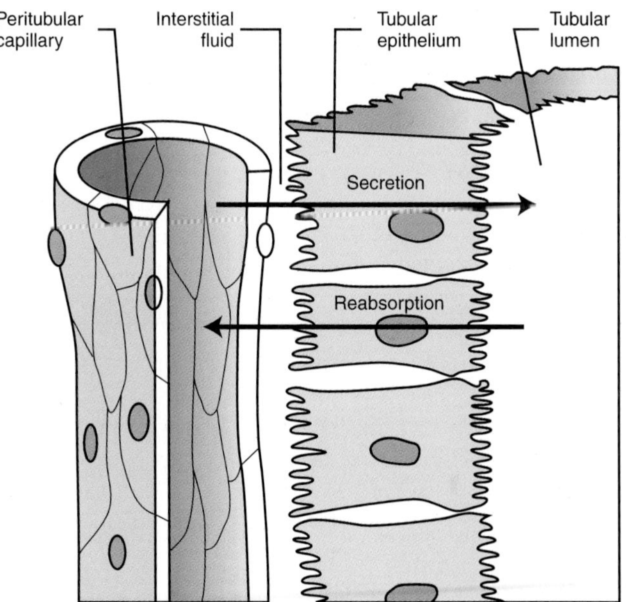

FIGURE **15-5** **Reabsorption and Secretion.** Reabsorption involves movement of substances out of tubular lumen, through tubular epithelium and interstitial fluid, and into peritubular capillary. Secretion involves movement of substances in the opposite direction from peritubular capillary through interstitial space, tubular epithelium, and tubular lumen.

Potassium diffuses out of the tubular filtrate by moving between the epithelial cells, into the interstitial fluid, and into the peritubular capillaries. Potassium reabsorption takes place in the PCT, ascending part of the loop of Henle, and the DCT. Calcium moves through the epithelial cells by a mechanism not yet known but apparently under the influence of vitamin D, parathyroid hormone (PTH), and calcitonin. Calcium reabsorption takes place in the PCT, ascending loop of Henle, and the DCT. Magnesium is reabsorbed from the PCT, ascending loop of Henle, and the collecting duct. PTH release increases the reabsorption of magnesium.

When sodium (Na^+) has been pumped out of the epithelial cell and into the interstitial fluid, an electrical imbalance is created between the tubular lumen, which becomes negatively charged, and the interstitial space, which becomes positively charged. Chloride (Cl^-), which readily diffuses through cell membranes, moves from the tubular filtrate into the epithelial cells and interstitial space to restore electrical neutrality. When sodium, glucose, amino acids, and chloride have left the tubular filtrate, some of the water left behind in the filtrate moves into the interstitial space and peritubular capillaries by osmosis. Once some of the water has left the tubular filtrate, the concentration of other substances in the filtrate increases beyond their concentration in the blood of the peritubular capillaries. This results in these substances passively diffusing through cell membranes, moving through the epithelial cells into the interstitial fluid, and passing into the peritubular capillaries. One of the substances that is passively reabsorbed in this way is urea. Even though urea is one of the waste products that the body wants to get rid of, not all of the urea that is filtered through the glomerulus is eliminated in urine. The body maintains a "normal" level of urea in blood that can be measured as the blood urea nitrogen (BUN).

About 65% of all reabsorption takes place in the PCT, where about 80% of the water, sodium, chloride, and bicarbonate and 100% of the glucose and amino acids in the tubular filtrate are reabsorbed. Additional reabsorption also takes place in the loop of Henle, DCT, and collecting ducts.

Secretion

Many waste products and foreign substances are not filtered from the blood in sufficient amounts from the glomerular capillaries. The body still needs to get rid of these substances; so it transfers them from the peritubular capillaries, to the interstitial fluid, to the tubular epithelial cells, and into the tubular filtrate in the tubules. This is called *secretion* (see Figure 15-5). Most secretion takes place in the DCT. Hydrogen, potassium, and ammonia are some of the more important substances eliminated by secretion. Drugs such as penicillin

Clinical Application: Renal Threshold of Glucose

There is a limit to the amount of glucose that can be reabsorbed by the proximal convoluted tubules. This limit is known as the *renal threshold* of glucose. If the blood glucose level gets too high, the amount of glucose that is filtered through the glomerulus exceeds the amount that can be reabsorbed (the renal threshold) and the excess is lost in urine. In dogs the renal threshold for glucose is approximately 180 mg/dl. This means that if the blood glucose level exceeds 180 mg/dl (normal range, 62 to 108 mg/dl) the PCT cannot reabsorb any more than 180 mg/dl back into the body. So if a dog has a blood glucose level of 500 mg/dl, only 180 mg/dl will be reabsorbed and 320 mg/dl will be lost in the urine. In cats the renal threshold for glucose is 240 mg/dl (normal range, 60 to 124 mg/dl). Fortunately, the renal threshold exceeds the *normal* amount of glucose found in blood; so 100% of the glucose filtered through the glomerulus is reabsorbed back into the body, and no glucose is lost in the urine. However, in pathological conditions such as uncontrolled diabetes mellitus, in which blood glucose levels can be extremely high because of insufficient insulin production, the amount of glucose filtered through the glomerulus exceeds the limit that can be reabsorbed by the PCT. When this occurs, glucose appears in the urine **(glucosuria).** The glucose in urine pulls water out, resulting in an abnormally high urine volume production (polyuria) caused by osmosis **(osmotic diuresis).** The loss of water will cause a water imbalance in the body that the animal will try to correct by drinking increased amounts of water **(polydipsia).** Polyuria and polydipsia (PU/PD) are nonspecific clinical signs associated with many pathological conditions. PU/PD with an accompanying glucosuria can help pinpoint diabetes mellitus.

and some of the sulfonamides are also eliminated from the body by secretion. This can be useful if an animal has a urinary tract infection with microorganisms sensitive to one of these drugs.

Urine Volume Regulation

Urine volume is determined by the amount of water contained in the tubular filtrate when it reaches the renal pelvis. Two hormones—ADH released from the posterior pituitary gland and aldosterone secreted by the adrenal cortex—are responsible for the majority of urine volume regulation.

ADH plays the most important role in regulating urine volume. It acts on the DCT and collecting ducts to promote water reabsorption and thereby prevent water loss from the body. If ADH control is absent, water will not be reabsorbed and will be lost in urine. This results in increased urine volume **(polyuria).**

Aldosterone increases reabsorption of sodium in the DCT and collecting duct back into the bloodstream. This causes an osmotic imbalance that encourages water to follow the sodium out of the tubular filtrate and into the blood. The hitch is that the water cannot move out of the DCT and collecting duct unless sufficient ADH control is present. This is one of those situations in the body where several things have to happen just right for normal function (and therefore health) to be maintained.

The glomerular filtrate moves through the tubules and eventually into the renal pelvis because of the difference in pressure that exists between the fluid in Bowman's capsule and fluid in the renal pelvis. The pressure in Bowman's capsule is higher than the almost nonexistent pressure in the renal pelvis. Like the difference in pressure that forces plasma to leave the afferent capillary and enter the capsular space, the difference in pressure between Bowman's capsule and the renal pelvis forces the fluid to move along through the tubules of the nephron.

Clinical Application: Diabetes Insipidus

Antidiuretic hormone (ADH) released by the posterior pituitary gland plays a major role in controlling urine volume by regulating water reabsorption from the collecting ducts. If the pituitary is not releasing adequate amounts of ADH, the collecting ducts will not reabsorb adequate amounts of water and polyuria develops along with a compensatory polydipsia. This condition is known as *diabetes insipidus,* and it has to be distinguished from diabetes mellitus. Both diseases are associated with polyuria and polydipsia (as are many other diseases). The urine produced in diabetes mellitus contains large amounts of sugar and therefore would taste sweet (if you were inclined to taste it to find out). The word *insipid* means tasteless. The disease *diabetes insipidus* was given its name because clinically it looked similar to diabetes mellitus, but the urine was "tasteless" rather than sweet because it did not contain glucose. Another form of diabetes insipidus results from an inability of the collecting ducts to respond to the presence of adequate amounts of ADH. The clinical signs are the same. Further diagnostic testing would have to be done to reach a definitive diagnosis of diabetes insipidus. Like diabetes mellitus, diabetes insipidus occurs most often in dogs and cats.

Test Yourself

1. What is the difference between glomerular filtrate and tubular filtrate?
2. What is the function of the brush border on the epithelial cells of the PCT?
3. How does the blood in the efferent glomerular arteriole differ from the blood in the afferent glomerular arteriole?
4. What is the difference between tubular reabsorption and tubular secretion?
5. How does ADH affect urine volume?
6. What is the mechanism by which glucose and amino acids are reabsorbed out of the PCT and back into the body?
7. Explain the concept of the renal threshold of glucose.
8. Diabetes insipidus gets its name from what physical characteristic of urine produced by patients with this disease.

Clinical Application: Urine Production Review

Urine is constantly being produced by the kidneys and sent down through the ureters into the urinary bladder for storage until it is eliminated. The kidney takes plasma that contains the waste materials of metabolism and, as it passes through a nephron, converts it into urine that is ready to be eliminated from the body. It accomplishes this through a series of processes designed to eliminate waste materials and preserve substances needed by the body to maintain homeostasis. Urine production can be broken down into the following six basic steps:

1. Blood enters the glomerulus via the afferent glomerular arteriole.
2. High blood pressure in the glomerular capillaries forces some plasma (minus large proteins and the blood cells) out of the capillaries and into the capsular space of Bowman's capsule. The fluid is known as the *glomerular filtrate.* From there it moves into the proximal convoluted tubule, where it becomes known as *tubular filtrate.*
3. The balance of the plasma not forced out of the glomerular capillaries along with the blood cells leaves the glomerulus via the efferent glomerular capillaries and enters a peritubular capillary network around the rest of the nephron.
4. While the tubular filtrate travels through the tubules of the nephron, some of its constituents (useful substances) are reabsorbed back into the peritubular capillaries (Figure 15-6).
5. Other substances (waste products) are secreted from the peritubular capillaries into the tubular filtrate while it travels through the tubules (see Figure 15-6).
6. By the time the tubular filtrate reaches the collecting ducts, it has decreased in volume, has changed chemical composition many times, and is now ready to leave the kidney on its way to being eliminated. When the tubular filtrate enters the renal pelvis, it is considered urine and nothing more will be done to its composition. (One exception here is that mucus may be added to horse urine after it reaches the renal pelvis.)

THE URETERS

Each kidney has a tube called the *ureter* that exits the kidney at the hilus and connects to the urinary bladder near the neck of the bladder at its caudal end.

Anatomy

The ureters are tubes composed of three layers: an outer fibrous layer, a middle muscular layer made up of smooth muscle, and an inner layer lined with transitional epithelium. The ureters are a continuation of the renal pelvis. Each ureter leaves its kidney at the hilus. The transitional epithelium allows the ureters to stretch as urine is passed through them on its way to the urinary bladder.

Function

The ureters continuously move urine from the kidneys to the urinary bladder. The smooth muscle layer propels the urine through the ureter by peristaltic contractions, much like the contractions of the intestines. This enables urine to move down to the urinary bladder regardless of the position of the animal's body.

The ureters enter the urinary bladder at such an oblique angle (Figure 15-7) that when the bladder is full, it collapses the opening of the ureter to prevent urine from backing up into the ureter. It does not prevent more urine from entering the bladder, however, because the strength of the peristaltic contractions is enough to force the urine through the collapsed opening into the urinary bladder.

Test Yourself

1. Why is it important that the ureters have an inner lining of transitional epithelium?
2. What prevents urine from backing up into the ureters when the bladder wall contracts to expel urine?
3. The ureter is continuous with what structure in the kidney (except in cattle)?

URINARY BLADDER

The urinary bladder stores urine as it is produced and releases it periodically from the body.

Anatomy

The urinary bladder has two parts: a muscular sac and a neck. It looks and acts a lot like a balloon. The bladder sac size and position vary depending on the amount of urine it contains. The bladder is lined with transitional epithelium that stretches as the bladder fills with urine. Have you ever made a water balloon? The effect is similar. The wall of the urinary bladder contains smooth muscle bundles that run lengthwise, obliquely, and in a circular direction. When these muscles contract, the bladder is squeezed and urine is expelled (like letting the water out of the water balloon). The neck of the bladder extends caudally from the sac into the pelvic canal and joins the urethra. Around the neck of the urinary bladder are circular "sphincter" muscles composed of skeletal muscle fibers. The contraction and relaxation of these sphincter muscles, which are under voluntary control, open and close the passageway for urine to leave the bladder and enter the urethra. This provides some voluntary control over the process of urination.

When the urinary bladder is empty, it is round and rests on the pubic bones. Structurally, it has a thick wall, is lined with many thick folds of transitional epithelium, and has virtually no lumen when it is empty. In large animals the empty bladder is confined to the pelvic cavity, but in carnivores it extends into the abdominal cavity. As the bladder fills with urine, it becomes pear shaped and extends cranially into the abdominal

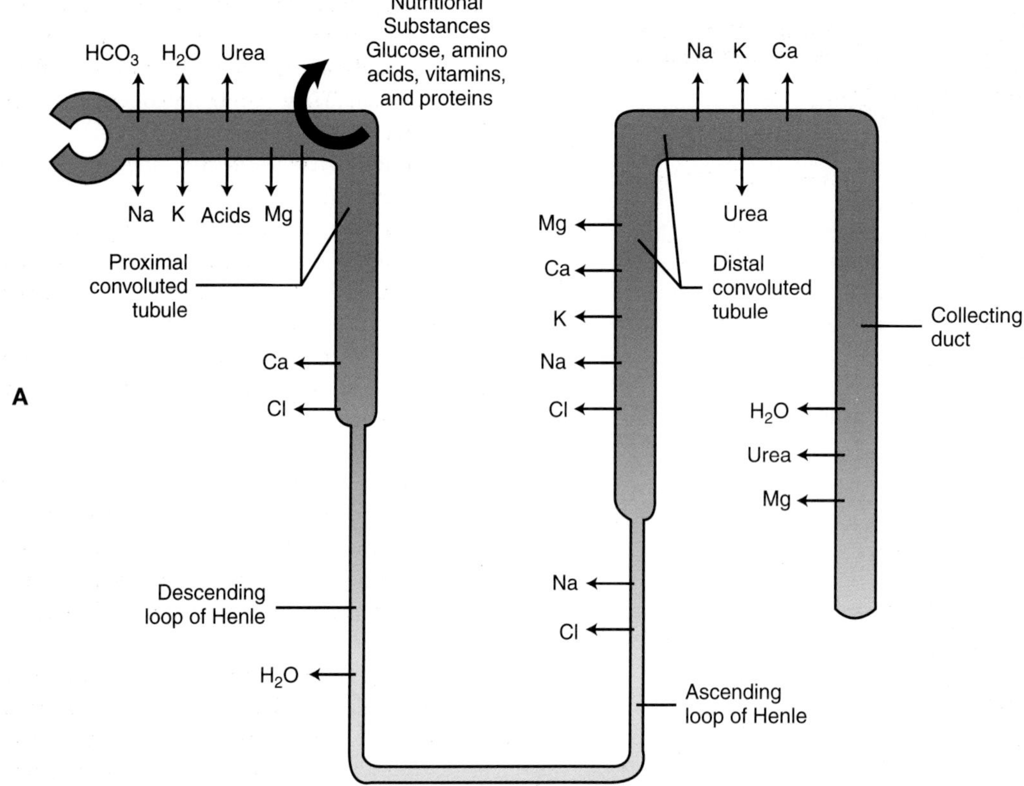

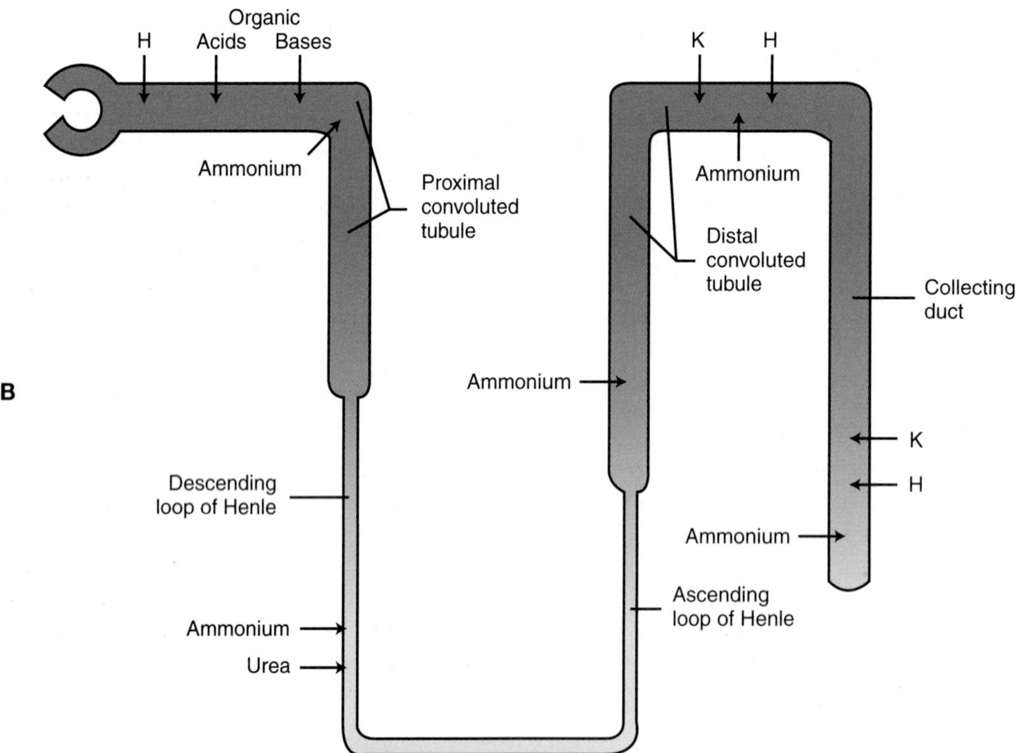

FIGURE **15-6** **Substances Involved in Reabsorption and Secretion. A,** Substances that are recovered from tubular filtrate through reabsorption into peritubular capillaries. **B,** Substances that are eliminated from the body as necessary through secretion into tubular filtrate from peritubular capillaries.

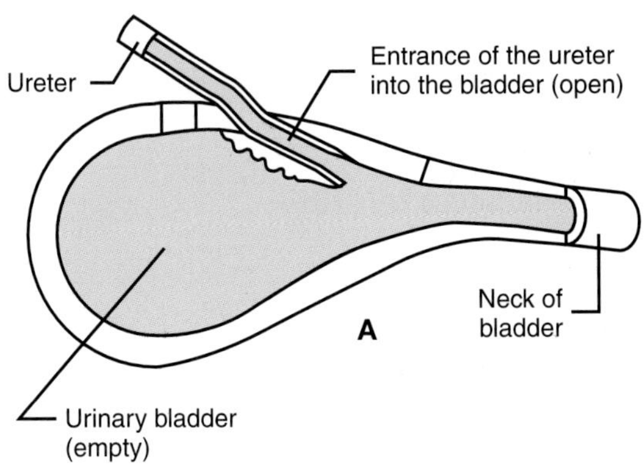

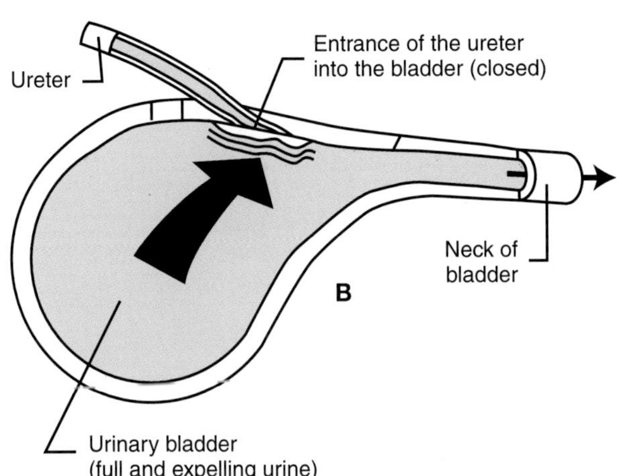

FIGURE **15-7** **Entrance of Ureters Into Urinary Bladder.** **A,** When bladder is empty and while it is filling, entrances remain open and urine flows freely into bladder. **B,** When bladder is full, pressure of the urine present collapses entrances so that when urine is expelled, it does not flow back into ureters.

cavity, the folds smooth out, and the wall becomes thinner (see Figure 15-7).

Function

The function of the urinary bladder is to collect, store, and release urine. The kidneys constantly produce urine; so if it were not for the urinary bladder, animals would constantly drip urine as it was being produced.

Control of Urination

Urination (also known as **micturition** or **uresis**) is the expulsion of urine from the urinary bladder into the urethra for elimination from the body. The process involves the following two to three steps:

1. Urine accumulation: The urinary bladder constantly accumulates urine until the pressure of the filling bladder reaches a certain "trigger" point that activates stretch receptors in the bladder wall.
2. Muscle contraction: When the trigger point is reached, a spinal reflex is activated that returns a motor impulse to the bladder muscles. The muscles of the bladder wall contract. These contractions are responsible for the sensation of having to urinate. In animals that are not "housebroken," emptying of the bladder will occur at this point.
3. Sphincter muscle control: Animals that have been trained can control the reflex release of urine through voluntary control of the muscular sphincter around the neck of the bladder. This results in temporary control of urination. However, a limit exists as to how long an animal can hold urine in its bladder. Urine is constantly being produced; so the bladder just keeps getting fuller because the animal is not urinating. The fuller the bladder gets, the more pressure that is applied to the muscular sphincter, until eventually the sphincter relaxes and urine is released. Something to consider when an animal "has an accident" is how long that animal had been expected to hold its urine.

As the bladder fills with urine, its walls become thinner as the transitional epithelium becomes thinner. This makes the bladder more susceptible to rupture. Remember the water balloon? If you fill the balloon to its stretched capacity and then squeeze it too hard, you can guess what will happen. The same thing happens if a urinary bladder is traumatized when it is too full. Manual palpation of an overextended bladder has been known to cause it to rupture.

TEST YOURSELF

1. How does the bladder know when to empty itself?
2. What part of the urinary bladder is under voluntary control and allows an animal to be "housebroken?"
3. Does urine production stop when the urinary bladder is full?

URETHRA

Anatomy

The urethra is a continuation of the neck of the urinary bladder that runs through the pelvic canal. Like the ureters and urinary bladder, it is lined with transitional epithelium that allows it to expand. The female urethra is shorter and straighter than the long, curved male urethra. In the female the urethra opens on the floor (ventral portion) of the vestibule of the vulva. In the male the urethra runs down the center of the penis (see Chapter 16).

Function

In both females and males, the urethra carries urine from the urinary bladder to the external environment.

In the female the urethra has a strictly urinary function; it carries only urine. In males the urethra also has a reproductive

CLINICAL APPLICATION: Renal Dysfunction and Uremia

Renal dysfunction is the term used to describe any pathological condition that results in inability of the urinary system to remove waste materials adequately from the blood. When this happens the waste materials, especially nitrogenous wastes from protein breakdown, build up in the blood and become toxic to the animal. The resulting condition is described as **uremia** (literally "urine in the blood"). The causes of uremia can be prerenal, renal, or postrenal.

Prerenal uremia is associated with decreased blood flow to the kidneys and may be caused by conditions such as dehydration, congestive heart failure, or shock if these conditions are left untreated. In these cases the kidneys are functioning normally, but not enough blood is reaching the kidney; therefore waste materials cannot be removed adequately.

Renal uremia is associated with an inability of the kidney to regulate urine production adequately because of damage to the nephrons. Toxins, inflammation, or infections that localize in the kidneys and destroy nephrons are some of the causes of uremia associated with kidney dysfunction. Even though adequate blood flow may continue to the kidneys, not enough functional nephrons are present to regulate normal urine production, and the waste materials cannot be removed from the blood. The kidneys have far more nephrons than they need to function properly under normal conditions; so a large reserve of nephrons can take over if some of the nephrons are damaged or destroyed. Two thirds of the total nephrons in both kidneys must be nonfunctional before clinical signs of renal dysfunction become evident.

Postrenal uremia is usually associated with an obstruction that prevents urine from being expelled from the body. Tumors, blood clots, or uroliths (stones) can cause the obstruction. Remember that urine is constantly being produced even if it is prevented from being expelled from the body by the obstruction. Eventually, urine will back up into the kidney pelvis and then into the nephrons. This will result in increased pressure in the nephrons and nephron damage. Now it becomes a case of renal dysfunction, but the underlying cause was a postrenal obstruction.

Uremia is diagnosed by evaluating a blood sample for the presence of increased amounts of waste materials. The easiest waste material to evaluate is urea, which is the nitrogenous waste product of protein breakdown. The amount of blood urea nitrogen (BUN) in plasma indicates how well the blood is being "cleansed." Elevated BUN levels indicate a problem but do not distinguish among prerenal, renal, and postrenal uremia. Further diagnostic testing is necessary to make that distinction.

CLINICAL APPLICATION: Uroliths and Urolithiasis

Urine normally contains body waste products dissolved in water. Some of these waste products are just barely soluble, and under certain conditions they may precipitate out of solution to form crystals. This does not cause problems if the crystals move through the urinary system rapidly. If their transit time through the urinary system is prolonged, they may interact with each other and form aggregates known as **uroliths, urinary stones,** or **urinary calculi.** Uroliths are commonly seen in dogs, cattle, sheep, and goats but are uncommon in horses. They take on a slightly different morphologic feature in cats (see the following Clinical Application on feline lower urinary tract disease).

All uroliths have an organic matrix that stays fairly constant and makes up about 2% to 10% of its structure. The remaining 90% to 98% of the urolith structure is made up of one or more of about 20 different minerals. The chemical names of some of the more common minerals involved are magnesium ammonium phosphate hexahydrate (struvite), calcium oxalate, calcium phosphate, urate, ammonium urate, and cystine. Struvite stones are the most common type found in dogs. Calcium carbonate, struvite, and calcium oxalate stones are some of the more common types found in ruminants. The mechanism of urolith formation is not understood. We know that uroliths form when adequate amounts of the minerals are present in the urine, the transit time of crystals through the urinary system is slowed, and the pH of the urine favors precipitation. Some crystals stay in solution in an acidic urine but precipitate out of solution in alkaline urine (e.g., struvite crystals) and other crystals stay in solution in alkaline urine but precipitate out of solution in acid urine (e.g., urate crystals). Diet, frequency of urination, urinary tract infection, and urine volume can influence these factors. For example, diet and the presence of certain bacteria associated with urinary tract infections can influence the pH of urine. Also, a housebroken animal that must consistently hold its urine for long periods will have a decreased crystal transit time through the lower urinary tract (bladder and urethra).

Urolithiasis (the presence of urinary stones) can occur anywhere in the urinary system (the kidneys, ureters, urinary bladder, or urethra). Clinical signs associated with uroliths depend on where the stones are located. Some stones may cause no noticeable signs. Others may cause inflammation of the bladder (cystitis) or urethra (urethritis) or an obstruction anywhere along the urinary tract. Urethral obstruction is more common in males in general and in male ruminants at the urethral sigmoid flexure (see Chapter 16). If the stone is obstructing the renal pelvis or ureter of one kidney, urine is prevented from leaving the kidney and the pressure in the nephrons from fluid backup will eventually destroy that kidney. As long as the other kidney is functioning normally, no clinical signs may be evident. Remember that two thirds of the total number of nephrons in both kidneys must be nonfunctional before clinical signs of renal dysfunction become evident.

Treatment of urolithiasis is aimed at removing the stones and preventing them from forming again. Some commercially available diets for dogs and cats can dissolve and prevent some types of stones. Some stones will have to be surgically removed. In ruminants, surgical removal of the stones is often necessary. Diets and urinary tract infections must be controlled to prevent urolith recurrence.

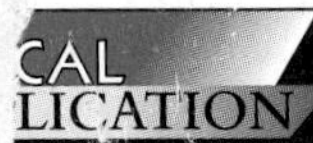

Feline Lower Urinary Tract Disease

elin lower urinary tract disease was previously known as *feline urological syndrome*. It is caused by the presence of uroliths that cause trauma, difficult urination, or obstruction. Feline uroliths differ from uroliths in other species in that they are much smaller and resemble sand rather than large stones. Feline urolithiasis can be very irritating—sort of like having sandpaper in the urine. If the sand contains a lot of the organic matrix, it clumps together to become a gelatinous plug with a gritty, toothpaste consistency. This plug can cause an obstruction, most often at or near the urethral orifice and most often in male cats. Struvite and calcium oxalate uroliths are the most common types of uroliths in cats.

As with uroliths in other species, urine pH, diet, and the presence of a urinary tract infection play important roles in urolith formation. Keeping the urine acidic (sometimes with a special diet and sometimes with medications) will keep the struvite crystals in solution. Struvite crystals are composed of magnesium, ammonium, and phosphate; so a diet low in these substances may help to reduce the chances of the crystals forming.

If a plug has formed, it will have to be manually removed to prevent a urinary bladder rupture or postrenal uremia from developing. One method of removal involves passing a catheter into the urethra and flushing the plug back into the urinary bladder. By manipulating the urine pH to make it more acidic, the plug can be dissolved. If back-flushing does not work, the plug may require surgical removal.

function. The vas deferens and accessory reproductive glands enter the urethra as it passes through the pelvic canal. Spermatozoa and seminal fluid are discharged into the urethra here during ejaculation and are pumped out as semen. At the beginning of ejaculation, the sphincter at the neck of the urinary bladder closes, preventing semen from entering the bladder and mixing with urine (see Chapter 16).

TEST YOURSELF

1. Besides its urinary function, what other function does the urethra serve in a male animal?
2. How much kidney function must be destroyed before clinical signs of renal dysfunction become evident?
3. Explain the difference between prerenal and postrenal uremia.
4. What is a urolith?
5. Name two conditions that can predispose an animal to urolith production.
6. How do uroliths in cats differ from uroliths in other species?
7. What is the chemical composition of a struvite crystal?

CHAPTER 16

THE REPRODUCTIVE SYSTEM

Thomas Colville

The reproductive system is an oddity. The rest of the body's systems work to ensure the survival of the animal they are part of, whereas the reproductive system works to ensure the survival of the *species* of animal. It interacts with other body systems, but purely reproductive structures are not essential to the life of an animal. Think about it. The testes, ovaries, and other reproductive organs of male and female animals are commonly removed surgically to prevent reproduction and influence behavior. If no complications result from the surgery, the rest of the body systems continue to go merrily on their way and the animal is none the worse for its loss. It just cannot reproduce. However, it is a different story with structures that the reproductive system shares with other systems. For example, the urethra in the male has both urinary and reproductive functions. It *is* essential to life and must not be damaged or removed.

Another difference from other body systems is that the reproductive system requires a second animal (of the opposite sex) to fully carry out its function, which is to produce a brand new animal (the offspring). What we refer to as the "reproductive system" in an individual animal is actually only half a system. A complete reproductive system is made up of all the male reproductive organs and structures in one animal *and* all the female reproductive organs and structures in another. Both are necessary for an offspring to be produced.

The basic reproductive process starts with fertilization—the head of a **spermatozoon** penetrating into the cytoplasm of an **ovum.** The fertilized ovum must be provided with a hospitable place to grow and develop until the offspring is born. After birth the offspring must be fed and cared for until it can fend for itself. For these basic processes to occur, the physical characteristics and behavior of two different animals must be synchronized and coordinated with delicate precision. This elegant process of developing and bringing together a male animal and a female animal at the appropriate time and in appropriate states of readiness to produce a viable offspring is the amazing role of the reproductive system.

For simplicity's sake, we discuss the male and female reproductive systems as separate physical entities. Remember, though, that the reproductive system is made up of *both* the male and female systems working in concert with each other.

TEST YOURSELF

1. How does the reproductive system differ from other body systems?
2. Why is the reproductive system of an individual animal considered only half a system?

EIOSIS

...r discussion of reproduction begins at the most basic level, ...at is, the cell. Reproductive cells (ova and spermatozoa) are produced by the unique process of cell division called **meiosis.** This is the first step in the process by which nature "shuffles the genetic cards" each time a new animal is conceived. Meiosis ensures that the genetic makeup of each new animal is unique. Each animal that enters the world has characteristics similar to others of its species and breed, but its precise genetic makeup is completely unique. Short of an identical twin (or a clone), an animal has never been nor ever will be of the same exact genetic makeup as another animal in the world. We should keep this uniqueness in mind when we are examining and treating patients. It can affect things such as behavior, clinical signs of disease, doses of drugs, and responses to treatments. Even though all golden retrievers look a lot alike, a particular animal may respond differently to our drugs and treatments than others of its breed that we have worked with before.

Table 16-1 Diploid Chromosome Numbers of Some Common Species

Species	Diploid Chromosome Number
Cat	38
Cattle	60
Corn	20
Dog	78
Donkey	62
Fox	34
Goat	60
Horse	64
Human	46
Mouse	40
Pig	38
Rabbit	44
Rat	42
Sheep	54
Tomato	24

CHROMOSOMES

Diploid Chromosome Number

The genetic material in the body's cells is contained in the nuclei in the form of coiled masses of DNA called **chromosomes.** This genetic material contains a complete "blueprint" for all of the structures and functions in the animal's body. For the body to function efficiently, each cell must contain the same genetic information. So each of the cells in an animal's body, with the exception of the reproductive cells (spermatozoa or ova), contains identical chromosomes. Another member of the same species has a slightly different genetic code on its chromosomes (the cause of that uniqueness business), but the total *number* of chromosomes in the nucleus of each of its body cells (except for the reproductive cells) is the same. This is called the **diploid chromosome number,** which is always an even number because the chromosomes occur in pairs. (*Di-* means "double," and *ploid* refers to chromosomes.) Therefore all cattle have the same number of chromosomes in the nuclei of their cells. The same goes for all dogs, horses, humans, and even corn and tomato plants. Table 16-1 contains the diploid chromosome numbers of some common species. The diploid chromosome number is sometimes expressed generically with the abbreviation *2n*. The *n* is a mathematical expression that represents a number, and the *2* indicates that the number is doubled (diploid).

Sex Chromosomes

One of the pairs of chromosomes that make up the diploid chromosome number contains the **sex chromosomes.** They determine the basic sex (male or female) of the animal. They are designated as being either "X" chromosomes or "Y" chromosomes. If both of the sex chromosomes are X chromosomes (XX), the individual is genetically female. If one is an X and the other is a Y (XY), the individual is genetically male. (The YY combination is not possible for reasons that we'll talk about shortly.) Many other factors, including the influence of hormones, help determine the overall "maleness" or "femaleness" of an individual, but the makeup of the sex chromosomes is a basic determining factor. So the full diploid chromosome makeup of a female animal is often abbreviated as 2n,XX and that of a male animal as 2n,XY.

Haploid Chromosome Number

Some basic mathematics reveals why the reproductive cells cannot have the diploid number of chromosomes. If the ovum of a goat and the spermatozoon that fertilizes it each contained the full, caprine diploid chromosome number of 60, then the fertilized ovum would contain a total of 120 chromosomes! That is too many. The number of chromosomes in the reproductive cells has to be reduced to half of the diploid number for things to work out. In this way, when the spermatozoon and the ovum come together, the total number of chromosomes in the fertilized ovum gets back to the diploid number.

The reduced number of chromosomes in the reproductive cells is called the haploid number (*hapl-* means "single") and is abbreviated n,X or n,Y, depending on which sex chromosome is present. The **haploid chromosome number** in the reproductive cells results from a "reduction division" of cells called *meiosis.* Meiosis is referred to as a reduction division because as a cell *divides* by this process, the total number of chromosomes in each of the daughter cells is *reduced* to one half the number that the parent cell had. One of each pair of diploid chromosomes from the parent cell goes to each of the daughter cells. Each daughter cell then has the haploid chromosome number.

CLINICAL APPLICATION: Chromosome Combinations

If you want to do some interesting mathematical problems, calculate how many different combinations of chromosomes could result for different species by randomly assigning one of each pair of diploid chromosomes to each daughter cell until you have the haploid number. Hint: because the diploid chromosomes occur in pairs, you can start with the number 2 and multiply it times itself as many times as there are *pairs* of chromosomes. For example, a diploid chromosome number of 8 would have 4 pairs of chromosomes; so the number of possible haploid chromosome combinations would be 2^4, or 16 possible combinations. Try using that calculation for some of the diploid chromosome numbers listed in Table 16-1. (Divide the diploid chromosome number in half and take 2 times itself that many times.) You are going to get some very large numbers. Those large numbers represent the number of possible combinations of chromosomes that could occur in each spermatozoon *or* ovum from an animal of that species.

If you want to calculate the number of chromosome combinations possible in an *offspring* of that species, you need to take the number of possible chromosome combinations for a spermatozoon and multiply it by the number of possible chromosome combinations for an ovum. You're going to come up with some huge numbers.

For a human, for example, the diploid chromosome number is 46; so the number of possible combinations of chromosomes in each spermatozoon or ovum is 2^{23}, or 8,388,608. The number of possible combinations of chromosomes in a human infant would then be $2^{23} \times 2^{23}$, or 70,368,744,177,664. Barring an identical twin, the chances of your parents producing a brother or sister with the exact same chromosome combination as you are 1 in 70,368,744,177,664!

Meiosis vs. Mitosis

You may recall that when most of the body's cells divide, they do it through a process called **mitosis.** When a cell divides by mitosis, each of its chromosomes first produces a duplicate copy of itself. When the two daughter cells pull apart, half the chromosomes go to one cell and half go to the other. Each of them ends up with an identical, full diploid set of chromosomes. The genetic makeup of the two daughter cells is exactly the same as each other and as the parent cell. This ensures that the genetic information in all of the body's cells (except for the reproductive cells) stays exactly the same.

When the reproductive cells are produced by meiosis, the chromosomes do not produce duplicate copies of themselves before the daughter cells pull apart. Half of the total chromosomes (one from each diploid chromosome pair), including one sex chromosome, go to each daughter cell. Which chromosomes go to which daughter cell is entirely random. The chromosomes merely pull apart into their new cells. In this way the genetic material of the reproductive cells gets "shuffled," resulting in a genetically unique offspring.

SPERMATOGENESIS

Spermatozoa, the male sex cells, are produced in the seminiferous tubules of the testes through a process called **spermatogenesis** (*genesis* means to create). They are produced continuously and in very large numbers in an effort to ensure that one spermatozoon will successfully reach and fertilize the ovum when breeding occurs. So the process of spermatogenesis is designed to produce huge numbers of spermatozoa (Figure 16-1).

Spermatogenesis begins at the periphery of the **seminiferous tubule** with a cell called a *primary spermatocyte.* This cell has the normal diploid chromosome number for the species. The chromosome complement of the cell is abbreviated 2n,XY. Keep in mind that the *XY* refers to the sex chromosomes, which, in a male, are always an X and a Y. The primary spermatocyte divides by meiosis into two secondary spermatocytes, which are pushed inward toward the center of the tubule lumen. These now have haploid chromosome numbers. One has an n,X chromosome complement, and the other has an n,Y. The two secondary spermatocytes divide *by mitosis* (so that the chromosome number does not get reduced further) into four spermatids. Two of the spermatids have n,X chromosome complements, and two have n,Y. As a result of the cell divisions that produced them, the spermatids are located near the center of the tubule lumen. They do not undergo any further cell divisions, but they grow tails and undergo other physical changes that convert them to spermatozoa. When the spermatozoa are fully developed, they detach and are carried to an organ called the *epididymis* for storage before ejaculation. (This is discussed in more detail later.)

Half of the spermatozoa produced have an X sex chromosome, and half have a Y sex chromosome. This is the means by which the genetic sex of the offspring will be determined. If an X-bearing spermatozoon fertilizes the ovum (which always contains an X sex chromosome), the offspring will have XX sex chromosomes and be genetically female. If a Y-bearing spermatozoon is successful, the offspring will have XY sex chromosomes and be genetically male. This ensures sexual equality of numbers in that about the same number of females and males will be conceived.

OOGENESIS

Ova, the female sex cells, are produced in follicles in the ovaries through a process called **oogenesis.** They are not produced continuously like spermatozoa. At or soon after birth, a female has a fixed number of primary **oocytes** (the precursor cell to ova) formed in her ovaries. That is the total number available in her lifetime. They remain in a quiet, immature state until they are "recruited" as part of an ovarian cycle. Each ovarian cycle produces one or more mature ova, depending on the species. Because spermatozoa come to the ovum to fertilize it, large numbers

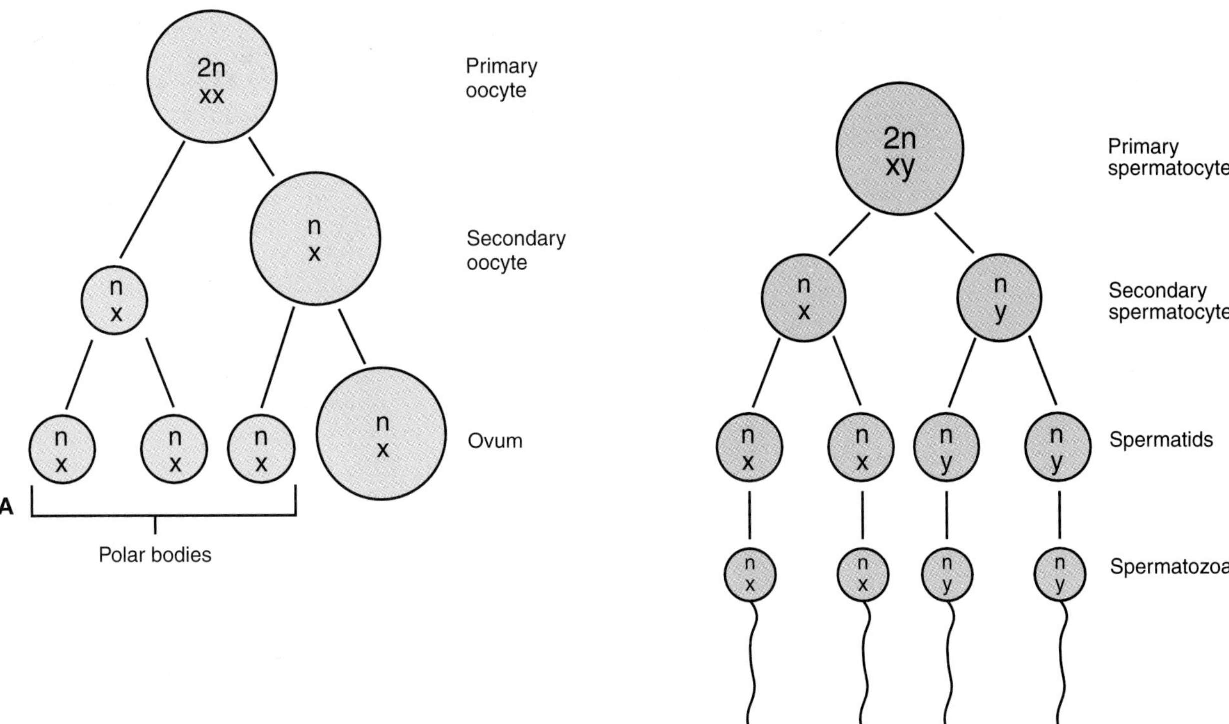

FIGURE **16-1** **Meiosis.** This process reduces the diploid chromosome number to the haploid number in reproductive cells. **A,** Oogenesis. **B,** Spermatogenesis.

of ova are not needed. Therefore the process of oogenesis is designed to produce small numbers of ova at a time (see Figure 16-1).

Oogenesis takes place in the developing **ovarian follicle.** The primary oocyte is the immature cell that waits quietly in the ovary for the signal to start developing. It has the normal diploid chromosome number for the species. The chromosome complement of the cell is abbreviated 2n,XX. When it becomes activated, the primary oocyte divides by meiosis into a large secondary oocyte and a small **"polar body."** Each has the haploid chromosome number n,X. Polar bodies are essentially "garbage cans" for excess chromosomes. They will not develop into ova. The secondary oocyte and the first polar body divide *by mitosis* (to preserve the haploid chromosome number) into an ovum and three polar bodies. So from one primary oocyte, one mature ovum will result.

TEST YOURSELF

1. What is the difference between the diploid chromosome number and the haploid chromosome number? In which body cells is each found?
2. Which reproductive cell, the ovum or the spermatozoon, determines the genetic sex of the offspring when fertilization occurs?
3. How does cell division by meiosis differ from cell division by mitosis?
4. How does spermatogenesis differ from oogenesis? Why are the basic processes so different?

MALE REPRODUCTIVE SYSTEM

The jobs of the male part of the reproductive system sound pretty simple: produce male sex hormones, develop male reproductive cells (spermatozoa), and deliver the spermatozoa to the female system at the appropriate time. However, a rather complicated system of organs, glands, structures, and tubes is required to carry out these jobs. Figure 16-2 illustrates the reproductive system of the bull, and Figure 16-3 illustrates that of the dog. Let's start our examination of the male reproductive system with the basic organs of male reproduction—the testes.

TESTES

Characteristics

The **testes** are the male **gonads**—the organs where the male reproductive cells are formed. They are generally oval, and their size varies considerably among species. In common domestic animals, they are located outside the abdomen in the inguinal (groin) region housed in a sac of skin called the *scrotum*.

Functions

The testes have two main functions: spermatogenesis and hormone production. Spermatogenesis is the process by which spermatozoa, the male reproductive cells, are produced in the seminiferous tubules of the testes. Between the seminiferous tubules, cells called **interstitial cells** (*interstitial* means "between") produce male sex hormones, or **androgens.** The

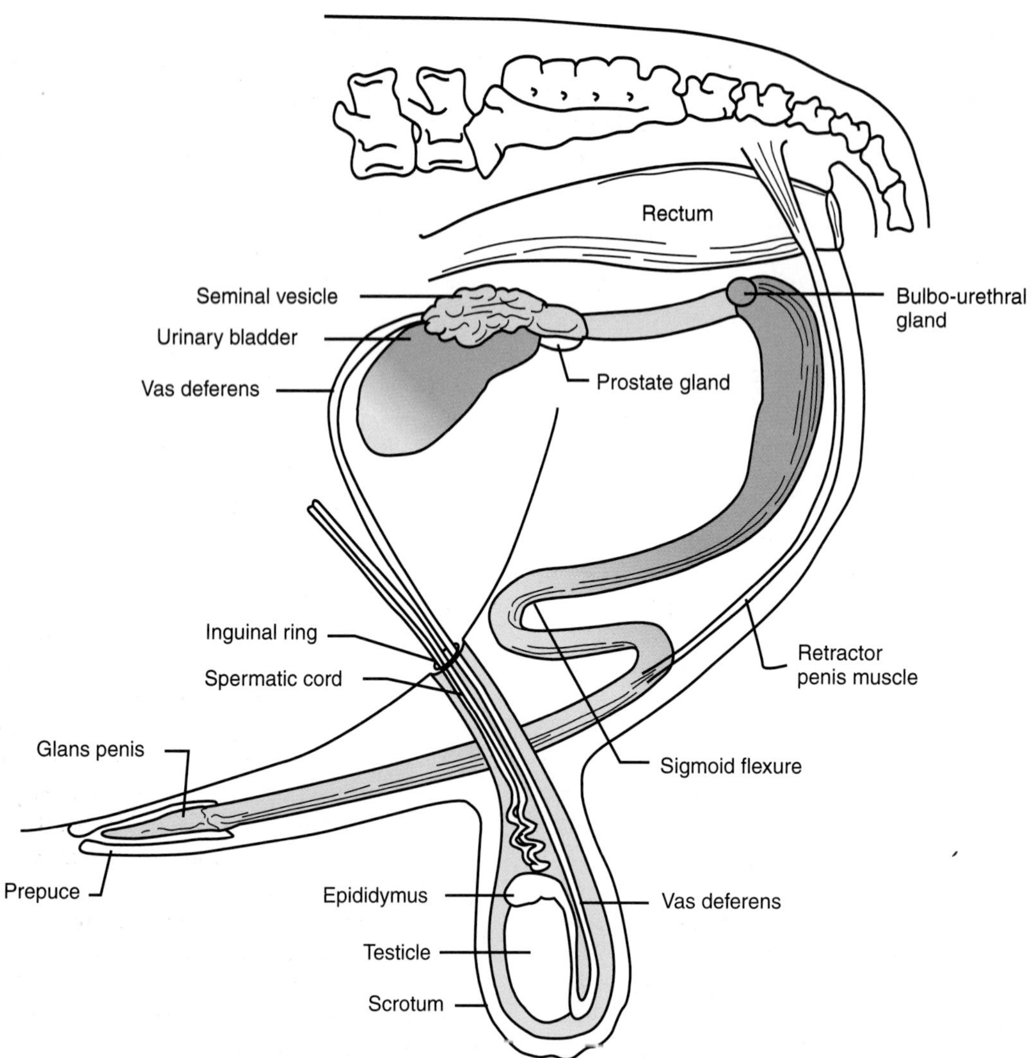

FIGURE **16-2** **Reproductive System of Bull (Lateral View).**

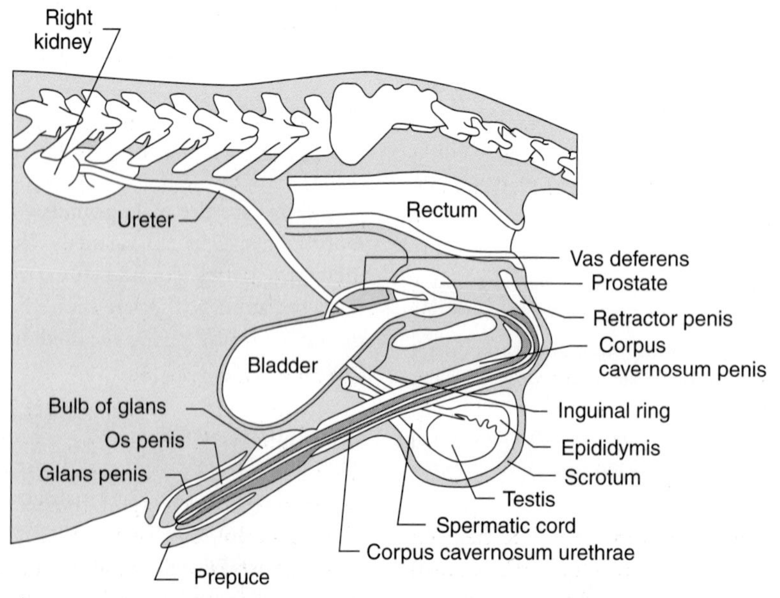

FIGURE **16-3** **Male Urinary and Reproductive Organs of Dog (Lateral View).**

principal androgen they produce is testosterone, which is responsible for the development of male secondary sex characteristics (such as the male body shape) and the male libido (sex drive). It also has a general anabolic (protein-building) effect on the body, which results in the enhanced muscle and bone development that gives male animals their size and bulk.

Spermatozoa

Spermatozoa are long, thin cells with three main parts: an enlarged head, a midpiece, and a long, narrow tail. The head contains the nucleus of the cell and is covered by a caplike structure called the **acrosome.** The acrosome contains digestive enzymes that are released once the spermatozoon is inside the female reproductive tract. They help the spermatozoon reach the ovum and penetrate through the layers surrounding it to accomplish fertilization. The midpiece is the "power plant" of the cell. It contains a large concentration of energy-producing mitochondria arranged in a spiral pattern. The long, thin tail resembles the flagellum that many single-celled organisms use for propulsion. It contains musclelike contractile fibrils that produce a whiplike movement of the tail and propel the cell forward once it is activated.

Development and Location

Before birth the testes begin development in the abdominal cavity near the kidneys. They are attached to their eventual permanent home in the scrotum by a band of connective tissue called the **gubernaculum.** As the tiny embryo grows, the gubernaculum remains fairly constant in length. This results in the testes gradually being pulled caudally and ventrally. What is actually happening is that the fetus is growing longer and larger while the testes are being held in place. At or soon after birth, they are normally pulled down through the **inguinal rings** into the scrotum. The inguinal rings, located in the groin region, are two slitlike openings in the abdominal muscles. This process is referred to as the *descent of the testes* and is illustrated in Figure 16-4.

Scrotum

The **scrotum** is the sac of skin that houses the testes. Besides providing a home for the testes, the scrotum also helps regulate their temperature. The testes have to be kept slightly cooler than body temperature to produce spermatozoa. A bandlike muscle, the **cremaster muscle,** passes down through the inguinal ring and attaches to the scrotum. It can adjust the position of the testes relative to the body. In warm conditions, the cremaster muscle relaxes, and the testes hang down away from the warm body. This position helps to reduce their temperature. In cold conditions, however, the cremaster muscle pulls the testes up tight against the body wall, which helps to warm them.

Spermatic Cord

The **spermatic cords** link the testes with the rest of the body. They are tubelike, connective tissue structures that contain blood vessels, nerves, lymphatic vessels, and the vas deferens. The arrangement of blood vessels in the spermatic cord is particularly interesting. They form a heat-exchange mechanism that helps keep the temperature of the testes slightly lower than the rest of the body. As Figures 16-5 and 16-6 show, the single testicular artery carries blood down to the testis. Surrounding the artery is a structure called the **pampiniform plexus,** which is an intricate meshwork of tiny veins derived from the testicular veins. As body temperature blood passes down to the testis through the testicular artery, it becomes cooled by the blood returning from the testis in the pampiniform plexus. At the same time, the blood in the pampiniform plexus becomes warmed by the blood in the testicular artery. This heat-exchange mechanism helps maintain the testes at a temperature slightly lower than body temperature but keeps the body as a whole from losing heat by warming the blood from the testes back to body temperature before it returns to the abdomen.

Structure

Tunics. Two layers of connective tissue called the **vaginal tunics** surround the testes in the scrotum. They are derived from layers of peritoneum that were pushed ahead of the testes as they descended through the inguinal rings (see Figure 16-4). The very thin inner layer, the **proper vaginal tunic,** is derived from the visceral layer of peritoneum that coated the testes as they developed in the abdomen. It is tightly adherent to the surface of the testes and the structures of the spermatic cords. It is so thin and transparent that it is invisible to the naked eye. The thick outer layer, the **common vaginal tunic,** is derived from the parietal layer of peritoneum that lines the abdominal cavity. It forms a fibrous sac around each testis and spermatic cord. The tunics become significant when an animal is to undergo a castration **(orchiectomy).** An incision into the scrotum will reveal the tunic-covered testis. In one common method of castration, an incision is made in the outer, common vaginal tunic and the testis is everted through the incision in the tunic, thereby exposing the blood vessels in the spermatic cord. The blood vessels can then be **ligated** (tied off) or clamped for a time before the testis is removed.

Capsule. Beneath the tunics, each testis is enclosed by a heavy, fibrous connective tissue capsule called the **tunica albuginea** (Figure 16-7). This capsule protects and supports the soft contents of the testis. Many small partitions, called **septa,** extend into the testis from the capsule. The septa divide each testis into tiny lobules that contain the seminiferous tubules, as well as other cells and structures.

Seminiferous Tubules. The seminiferous tubules are where spermatogenesis takes place. Each tubule is shaped like a long, convoluted U that is attached at both ends to a complex system of ducts called the **rete testis** (a *rete* is a complex network of something in the body). Between the seminiferous tubules are the endocrine cells of the testis known as the *interstitial cells.* The interstitial cells produce androgens, the male sex hormones, under the influence of luteinizing hormone (LH) from

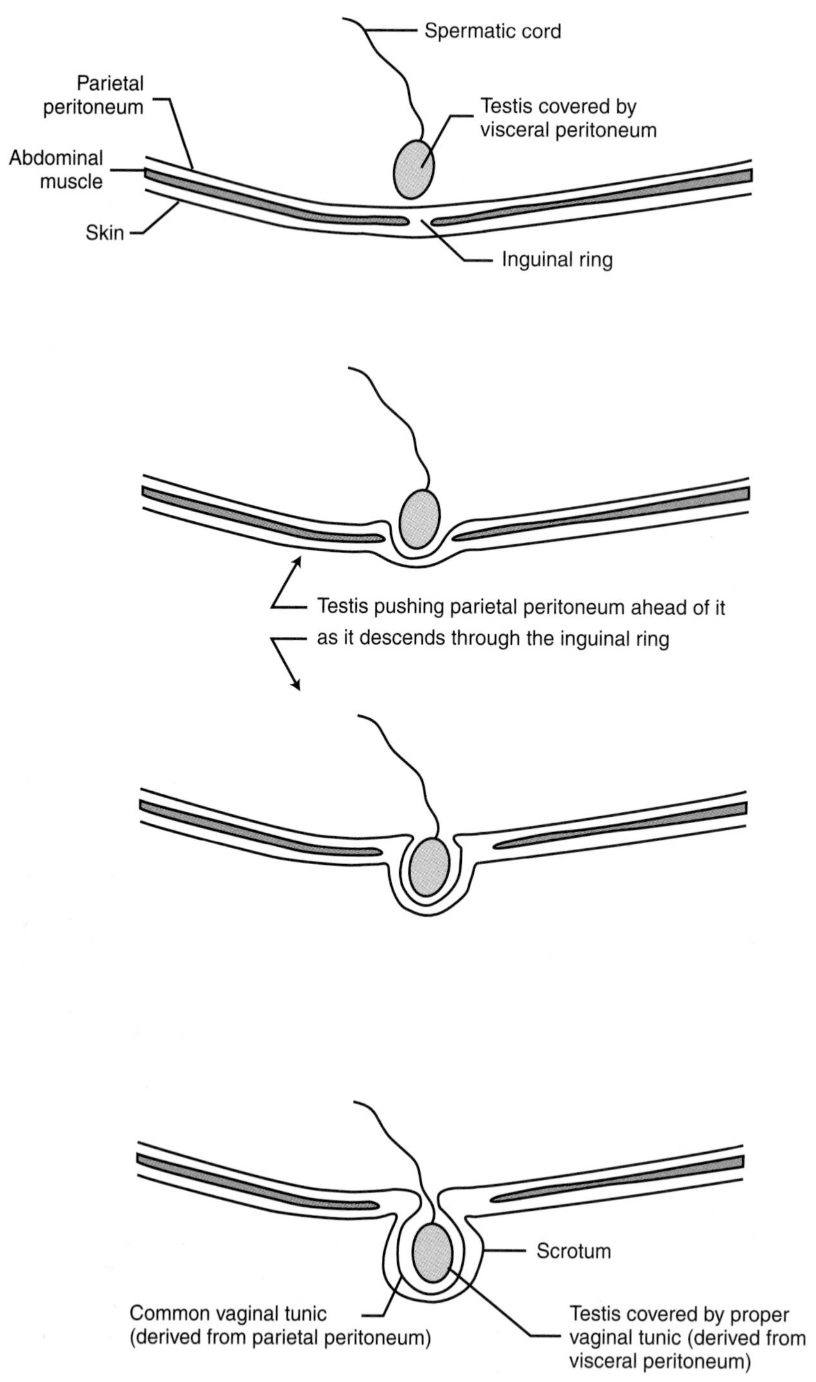

FIGURE **16-4** **Descent of Testes and Derivation of Vaginal Tunics.**

CLINICAL APPLICATION Cryptorchidism

Sometimes one or both of the testes do not descend into the scrotum. This is referred to as **cryptorchidism.** This condition can be either unilateral (one testis failed to descend) or bilateral (both testes failed to descend). An undescended testis can be located anywhere along the normal path of descent, from the region of the kidney to an area just outside the inguinal ring but not completely down in the scrotum (called a "high flanker").

Testes retained in the abdominal cavity are usually sterile (cannot produce spermatozoa) because spermatogenesis requires a temperature slightly lower than body temperature. The interior of the abdomen is too hot for spermatozoa to be produced. Testosterone continues to be produced, however. So a bilaterally cryptorchid animal has all the characteristics of a male animal but cannot reproduce.

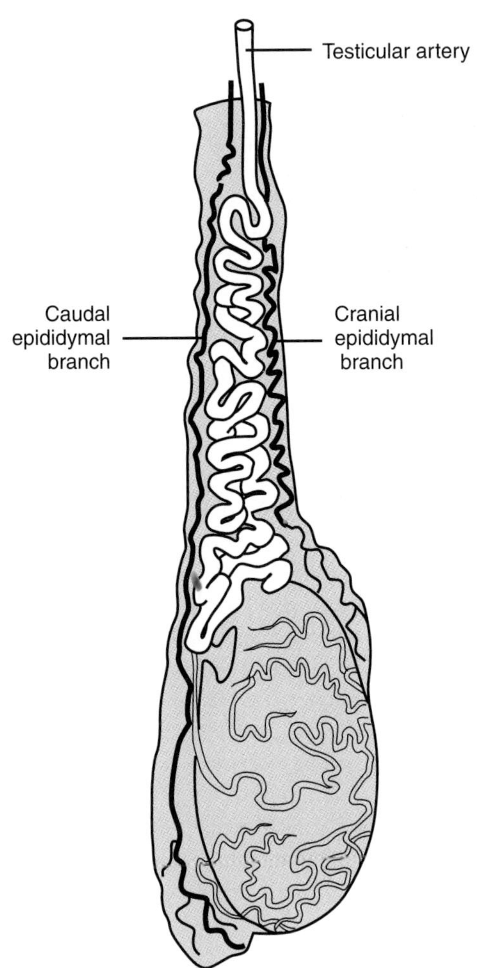

FIGURE **16-5** **Arterial Blood Supply to Testis and Epididymis of Bull.** Testicular artery passes down center of spermatic cord.

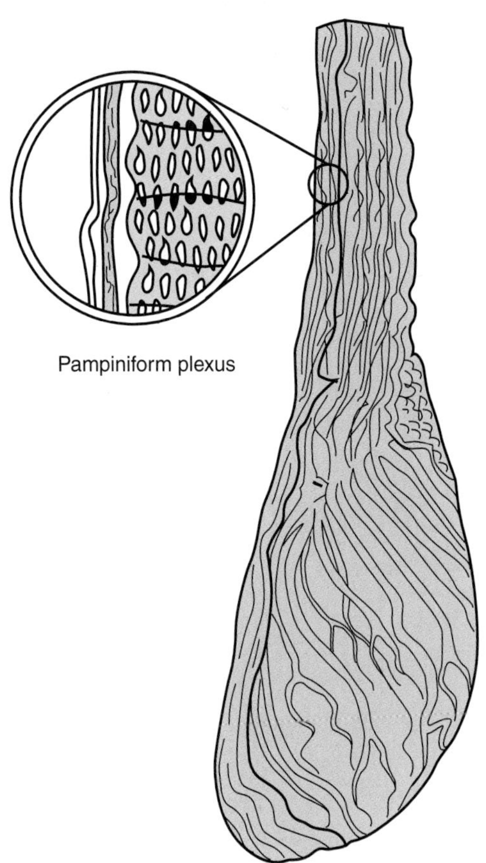

FIGURE **16-6** **Pampiniform plexus is formed from testicular veins visible on the surface of testis. It surrounds the testicular artery and helps cool blood passing down to testis.**

the anterior pituitary gland. LH is sometimes referred to as interstitial cell–stimulating hormone (ICSH) in the male.

Inside the seminiferous tubules, spermatozoa are produced by the process of meiosis (see Figure 16-1). The "parent" cells stay out toward the periphery of the tubule and push the "daughter" cells toward the center of the tubule as they divide. Primary spermatocytes divide to produce secondary spermatocytes, which divide to produce spermatids. The spermatids undergo physical changes to become spermatozoa. While they are undergoing these transformations, the spermatids are attached to large "nurse" cells called **Sertoli cells.** In addition to providing mechanical and nutritional support, the Sertoli cells also help shield the developing spermatozoa from the body's immune system. Proteins on the surfaces of the genetically unique spermatozoa would stimulate the immune system to produce antibodies against them if they were not shielded. This would cause an autoimmune reaction, meaning the immune system would attack part of its own body—the spermatozoa. The Sertoli cells are also known to produce small amounts of estrogens under stimulation of follicle-stimulating hormone (FSH) from the anterior pituitary gland.

Duct System. When spermatozoa complete their physical development in the seminiferous tubules, they are transported to a storage site where they will be prepared for ejaculation. After they detach from their protective Sertoli cells, the spermatozoa enter the complex of ducts that make up the rete testis. From there they flow through the **efferent ducts** to their storage site—the **epididymis.**

Grossly, the epididymis is a flat, ribbonlike structure that lies along the surface of the testis. It is actually a single, long, very convoluted tube that connects the efferent ducts of the testis with the vas deferens. If the tube that makes up the human epididymis were stretched out, it would be about 6 meters (20 feet) in length. The epididymis is divided into three regions: (1) the "head" of the epididymis is where the spermatozoa enter from the efferent ducts, (2) the "body" is the main portion that lies along the surface of the testis, and (3) the "tail" continues on as the vas deferens.

The epididymis functions as a storage site for spermatozoa before they are expelled by ejaculation and as a place for them to mature. Spermatozoa are immature when they leave the

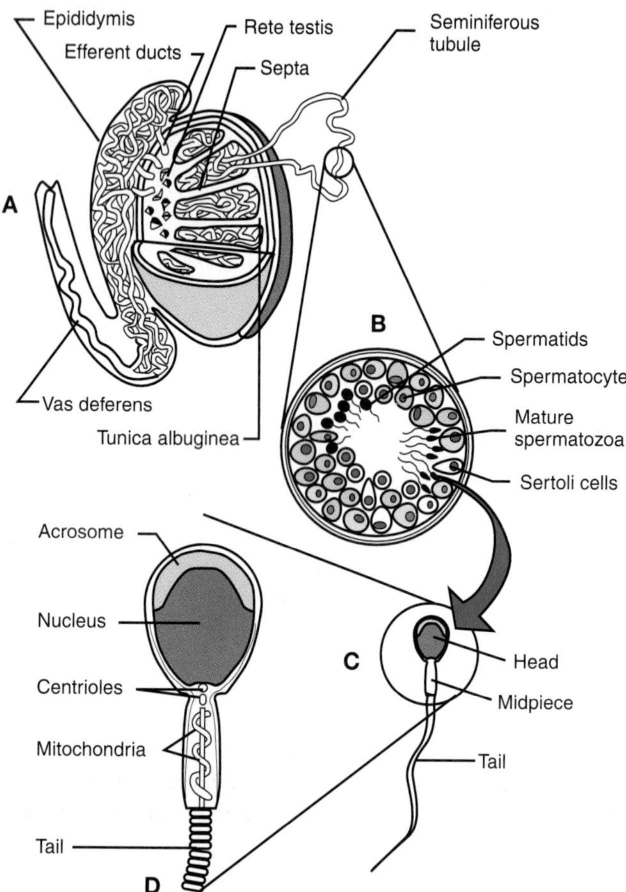

FIGURE **16-7** **Structure of Testis.** **A,** Testis and epididymis. **B,** Enlarged cross section of seminiferous tubule. **C,** Mature spermatozoon. **D,** Head area detail of mature spermatozoon.

CLINICAL APPLICATION **Sertoli Cell Tumor**

On occasion, Sertoli cells can multiply out of control, particularly in dogs. This produces what is termed a *Sertoli cell tumor* in the testis. Because normal Sertoli cells produce small amounts of estrogens, this action can become exaggerated as the cells multiply out of control. The level of estrogens in the animal's bloodstream rises rapidly, producing feminization of the male dog. The prepuce often becomes pendulous, and the mammary glands may become enlarged (gynecomastia) and can even produce milk. The penis and the opposite testis atrophy, and other male dogs may be attracted to the affected animal as if he were a female in heat. The signs of feminization are often the primary complaints when affected animals are presented to the veterinary clinic. The primary treatment for a Sertoli cell tumor is usually castration of the animal.

seminiferous tubules. They must mature in the epididymis for a week or more before they can fertilize ova. If the spermatozoa are never ejaculated (e.g., in an individual that has had a vasectomy), they live out their lives in the epididymis, die, and are broken down and absorbed by the tubular lining cells.

TEST YOURSELF

1. What are the two main functions of the testes? Where in the organ does each take place?
2. What are the three main parts of a spermatozoon? What is the main purpose or function of each?
3. Why is a bilaterally cryptorchid animal usually sterile?
4. What is important about the scrotum's ability to adjust the position of the testes relative to the body?
5. What are the main components of the spermatic cord?
6. From what are the proper and common vaginal tunics that cover the testes derived?
7. Where are spermatozoa stored before ejaculation?

VAS DEFERENS

Something has to move the spermatozoa from the epididymis (located way down in the scrotum) up to the urethra (within the pelvic cavity) when ejaculation occurs. This is the job of the **vas deferens.** Also known as the *ductus deferens,* the vas deferens is a muscular tube that connects the tail of the epididymis with the pelvic portion of the urethra. Thick layers of smooth muscle in its wall give it a very solid and cordlike texture. The vas deferens passes up through the inguinal ring as a part of the spermatic cord. Once inside the abdomen, each vas deferens separates from the rest of the spermatic cord, loops back caudally, and connects with the urethra just caudal to the neck of the urinary bladder (see Figures 16-2, 16-3, and 16-8). In many species the vas deferens enlarges just before joining the urethra. This enlargement, if present, is called the **ampulla.** The ampulla may contain glands that contribute material to semen.

The job of the vas deferens is to propel spermatozoa and the fluid they are suspended in quickly from the epididymis to the urethra when ejaculation occurs. Once they are in the urethra, the spermatozoa are mixed with secretions from accessory reproductive glands to form semen, which is pumped out into the female reproductive tract.

URETHRA

The **urethra** of the male has two functions. Most of the time it carries urine from the urinary bladder outside the body. This is its urinary function. However, when ejaculation occurs, urine flow is temporarily blocked. Spermatozoa from the vas deferens and secretions from the accessory reproductive glands enter the urethra and are pumped out as semen. Ejaculation is its reproductive function.

The urethra is spoken of as having two portions. The *pelvic portion,* within the pelvic cavity, is where the vas deferens and accessory reproductive glands enter the urethra. The remainder of the urethra, which runs down the length of the penis, is known as the *penile portion* of the urethra.

ACCESSORY REPRODUCTIVE GLANDS

Spermatozoa make up only a very small portion of the total volume of semen. The majority is made up of secretions from the various accessory reproductive glands. The ducts of all the

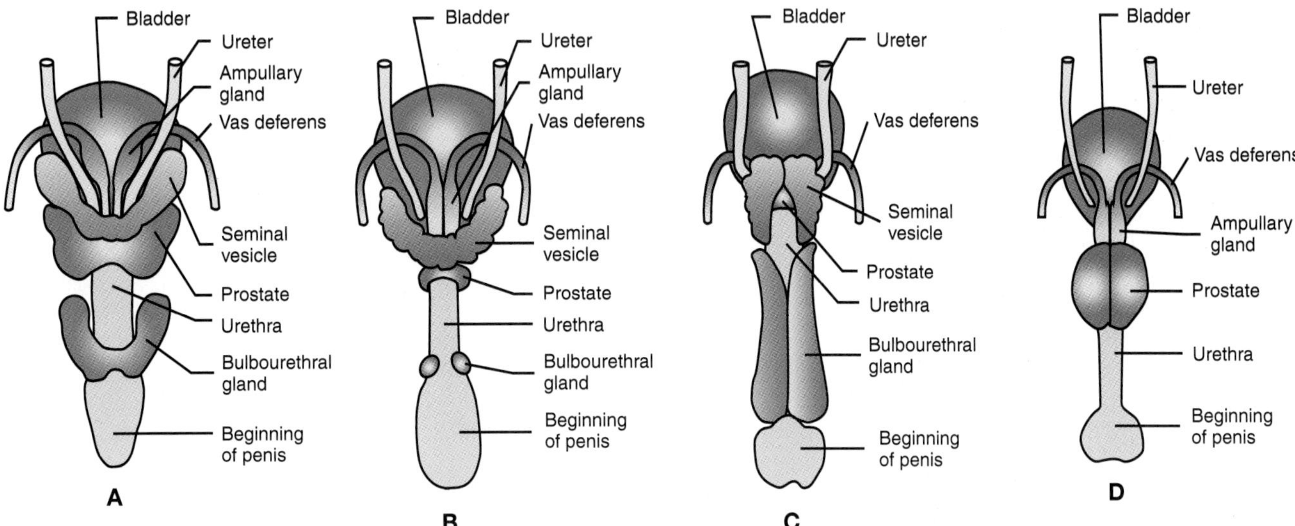

FIGURE **16-8** **Accessory Reproductive Gland.** Comparisons among some common domestic species (dorsal views). **A,** Stallion. **B,** Bull. **C,** Boar. **D,** Dog.

> **CLINICAL APPLICATION — Vasectomy**
>
> If a section of each vas deferens is removed surgically from an animal, the animal is rendered sterile (it cannot reproduce). This procedure is known as a *vasectomy.* It prevents spermatozoa from reaching the urethra during ejaculation. The other components of semen are ejaculated, but no spermatozoa are included. The individual is "firing blanks," so to speak. The spermatozoa live out their lives in the epididymis, die, and are absorbed by the lining cells.
>
> Vasectomy is a common contraceptive (done to prevent pregnancy) surgery in humans. It is performed less commonly for that reason in nonhuman animals but is sometimes performed on bulls to create "teaser" animals. Teaser bulls are used to help identify cows in heat so that they can be bred, often by artificial insemination, to other males.

accessory reproductive glands enter the pelvic portion of the urethra (see Figure 16-8). Different species have different combinations of accessory reproductive glands. Table 16-2 provides a summary of which animals have which glands.

The accessory reproductive glands produce alkaline fluid containing things like electrolytes, fructose, and prostaglandins. The alkalinity of the fluid helps counteract the acidity of the female reproductive tract. This helps more spermatozoa survive to reach the oviducts, where they hope to meet up with an ovum. Fructose is a simple sugar that acts as an energy source for the very active spermatozoa. Some of the prostaglandins are thought to stimulate the contractions of the female reproductive tract that help move the spermatozoa up to the oviducts.

Seminal Vesicles

Ducts from the two **seminal vesicles,** sometimes called *vesicular glands,* enter the pelvic urethra in the same area as the vas deferens. They are present in all common domestic animals except for the cat and dog.

Prostate Gland

The **prostate gland** is a single structure that more or less completely surrounds the urethra. Multiple ducts carry its secretions into the urethra. It is present in all common domestic animals. In dogs, it is particularly large because it is the only accessory reproductive gland they have.

Bulbourethral Glands

The two **bulbourethral glands,** also known as the *Cowper's glands,* are located further caudally than the other accessory reproductive glands. Their ducts enter the urethra back near the caudal border of the pelvis. All common domestic animals have bulbourethral glands except for the dog. They secrete a mucinous (mucus-containing) fluid just before ejaculation that clears and lubricates the urethra for the passage of semen.

PENIS

The **penis** is the male breeding organ. It is made up mainly of muscle, erectile tissue, and connective tissue, with the urethra running down its center. It has a very large blood supply and many sensory nerve endings. When the male is sufficiently aroused and stimulated, the erectile tissue becomes engorged with blood, causing the penis to enlarge and stiffen. This allows it to be inserted into the vagina of the female for breeding.

The three main parts of the penis are the roots, the body, and the glans.

Roots

The **roots of the penis** attach it to the brim of the pelvis. They consist primarily of two bands of connective tissue, called the **crura,** covered by the ischiocavernosus muscles.

Body

The **body of the penis** is its largest part. It is mainly made up of two bundles of **erectile tissue.** Erectile tissue is composed of a spongy network of fibrous connective tissue and many tiny, blood-filled spaces called *sinuses.* In the nonerect state, the amount of blood flowing into the erectile tissue is the same as the amount flowing out. When more blood flows into erectile tissue than leaves it, however, the sinuses engorge with blood and try to enlarge. The network of connective tissue surrounding the engorged sinuses prevents them from swelling up like a bunch of water balloons. Instead, the relatively inelastic connective tissue around the blood sinuses causes enough **hydraulic pressure** to be generated in the engorged erectile tissue to cause the penis to become a little larger and a lot stiffer. This is called *erection* of the penis.

The two erectile tissue structures that make up the body of the penis are the smaller **corpus cavernosum urethrae** and the larger **corpus cavernosum penis.** The corpus cavernosum urethrae, also called the *corpus spongiosum,* forms a "sleeve" around the urethra as it passes through the body of the penis. The larger body of erectile tissue dorsal to the urethra is the corpus cavernosum penis.

Table 16-2 Male Accessory Reproductive Glands

Animal	Seminal Vesicles	Prostate Gland	Bulbourethral Glands
Boar	+	+	+
Bull	+	+	+
Cat	–	+	+
Dog	–	+	–
Human	+	+	+
Ram	+	+	+
Stallion	+	+	+

+ indicates the presence of a gland; - indicates the gland is absent.

CLINICAL APPLICATION — Canine Prostate Problems

The prostate gland of the dog is very large—about the size of a walnut in a medium-size dog. Many conditions can cause it to become even larger, such as infection, tumors, or just normal aging. Because the urethra runs through the center of the gland, significant enlargement of the prostate squeezes the urethra. This can partially or completely block the passage of urine, leading to difficulty urinating. Instead of urine passing in a large stream, it dribbles out or may stop entirely. The cause of prostate gland enlargement must be determined to formulate an effective treatment strategy. Some conditions can be managed with medication, but others require surgery.

Glans

The **glans of the penis** is its tip, or the distal, free end of the organ. Its structure and appearance vary considerably among species. Horses have a very well-defined glans that contains a considerable amount of erectile tissue. In ruminants the glans is small and not well defined. Cats have short spines covering their glans. The penis of the dog is a special case that is described more completely below. Regardless of the species, the surface of the glans has a rich supply of sensory nerve endings that make it very sensitive to physical stimulation.

Prepuce

The **prepuce** is the sheath of skin that encloses the penis when it is not erect. The outer part of the prepuce is normal skin, but the inner portion that is in contact with the penis is a smooth, moist mucous membrane. The prepuce of the boar also contains a small preputial pouch in which urine and cellular debris accumulate. Decomposition of the material in this pouch gives boars their typical "ripe" odor. (This is considered very sexy to sows—a clear case of different strokes for different folks!)

Penis of the Dog

The penis of the dog and other canine species is somewhat unique (see Figure 16-3). It includes a bone and an erectile structure that causes the male and female to get stuck together for awhile after breeding is completed. The bone in the penis of the dog is called the **os penis.** The urethra runs through a groove in the ventral surface of this bone. No other domestic animals have a similar bone, but several wildlife species, including raccoons, beaver, and walruses, have one as well. It is rarely of clinical significance unless it is fractured (very rare) or unless urinary stones (calculi) lodge in the urethra where it enters the groove in the os penis and obstruct urine flow.

The other unique structure in the penis of the dog is an enlargement toward the rear of the glans called the **bulb of the glans.** It is made up of erectile tissue that is derived from the corpus cavernosum urethrae. During breeding the bulb becomes engorged with blood more slowly than the other erectile structures. It usually does not reach full size until after ejaculation has taken place. Once it enlarges, however, the swollen bulb is tightly clamped in place by contractions of the muscles surrounding the vagina and vulva of the female. This makes it impossible for the male to withdraw the penis. The male then typically dismounts from the female and turns so that he faces the opposite direction from her. The two stand in a tail-to-tail position looking for all the world like the fictional "Pushme-Pullyou" from the Dr. Doolittle story. This is known as the **"tie"** and seems to be important for conception to occur in the dog. The tie typically lasts 15 to 20 minutes and does not seem to be uncomfortable for either animal. Once the erection of the bulb subsides, the animals can separate. Forcing the animals apart prematurely can cause injury. So tell well-meaning people *not* to throw cold water on a pair of tied dogs in an effort to separate them. Just let nature take its course.

Sigmoid Flexure

The nonerect penis of the bull, ram, and boar is normally bent into an S shape. This is called the **sigmoid** (S-shaped) **flexure** (see Figure 16-2). The penises of these animals also have a higher proportion of connective tissue to erectile tissue than other species, and so the penis does not enlarge much when erection occurs. Rather, the main mechanism of erection in these species is straightening of the sigmoid flexure from internal hydraulic pressure. The basic principle is the same as a garden hose that wants to straighten out when the water is turned on. This causes the penis to protrude from the prepuce for breeding. A long, thin, cordlike muscle, the **retractor penis muscle,** originates up near the base of the tail and attaches to the bend of the sigmoid flexure. It functions like a big elastic band. When erection straightens out the sigmoid flexure, the retractor penis muscle stretches. When the erection subsides, the retractor penis muscle pulls the penis back into its nonerect S shape.

Reproductive Functions

Erection. Erection is the enlargement and stiffening of the penis that prepares it for breeding. It results from a parasympathetic reflex triggered by sexual stimuli. In most species the important stimuli are probably olfactory cues (smells) and behavioral changes that signal the male that the female is in "heat" and receptive.

Erection occurs when more blood enters the penis via the arteries than leaves it via the veins. The connective tissue–enclosed erectile tissue becomes engorged with blood, causing the penis to become enlarged and rigid. Mechanically what happens is that the arteries supplying blood to the penis dilate, increasing the blood flow into the organ. At the same time, the veins carrying blood away from the penis are compressed against the brim of the pelvis by contractions of the ischiocavernosus muscles (part of the roots of the penis). This acts like a tourniquet and decreases the flow of blood out of the penis. The net effect is that more blood enters the penis than leaves it. This generates hydraulic pressure in the erectile tissue, producing the enlargement and stiffening of the penis that we call *erection*.

Ejaculation. Ejaculation is the reflex expulsion of semen from the penis. It is produced by a continuation of the stimuli that produced erection, plus the physical actions and sensations of breeding. The process consists of two stages. The first involves the movement of spermatozoa and fluids from the accessory reproductive glands into the pelvic portion of the urethra. At the same time, the sphincter muscle around the neck of the urinary bladder tightly closes to prevent the movement of semen into the bladder. This is quickly followed by the second stage of ejaculation—rhythmic contractions of the urethra that pump the semen out into the female reproductive tract.

TEST YOURSELF

1. Will the volume or gross appearance of the semen of an animal that has had a vasectomy be significantly different from that of a normal animal? Why or why not?
2. How does the function of the bulbourethral glands differ from that of the other accessory reproductive glands?
3. What are the three main parts of the penis?
4. How does the mechanism of erection in animals with a sigmoid flexure in their penis differ from that of other animals?
5. What structures do spermatozoa pass through from their site of production to their eventual deposition in the female reproductive tract?

FEMALE REPRODUCTIVE SYSTEM

The female part of the reproductive system is a bit more complex than the male part because it has more jobs to do. Some are similar to those of the male, such as production of female sex hormones and development of female reproductive cells (ova). In addition, however, the female system receives the male reproductive cells, furnishes a site for them to fertilize the ovum (the oviduct), provides a hospitable environment for the embryo to grow and develop, carries it for the entire period of pregnancy, and then pushes the offspring out into the cold, cruel world when it is fully developed. Things do not stop at birth though. In the period immediately after birth, the mammary glands provide nutrition to the newborn. This is a lot of work for one system to do.

Nearly all of the female reproductive system is internal, that is, located within the abdominal and pelvic cavities. Figures 16-9 and 16-10 illustrate the female reproductive system of the bitch, and Figure 16-11 compares the female reproductive systems of several species. The main reproductive organs—the

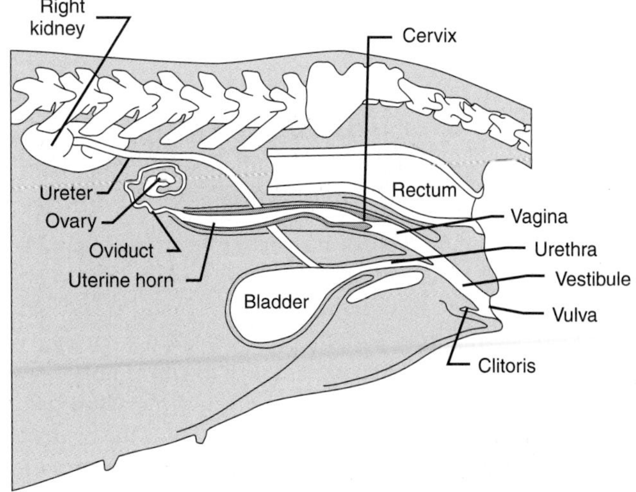

FIGURE **16-9** **Female Urinary and Reproductive Organs of Bitch (Lateral View).**

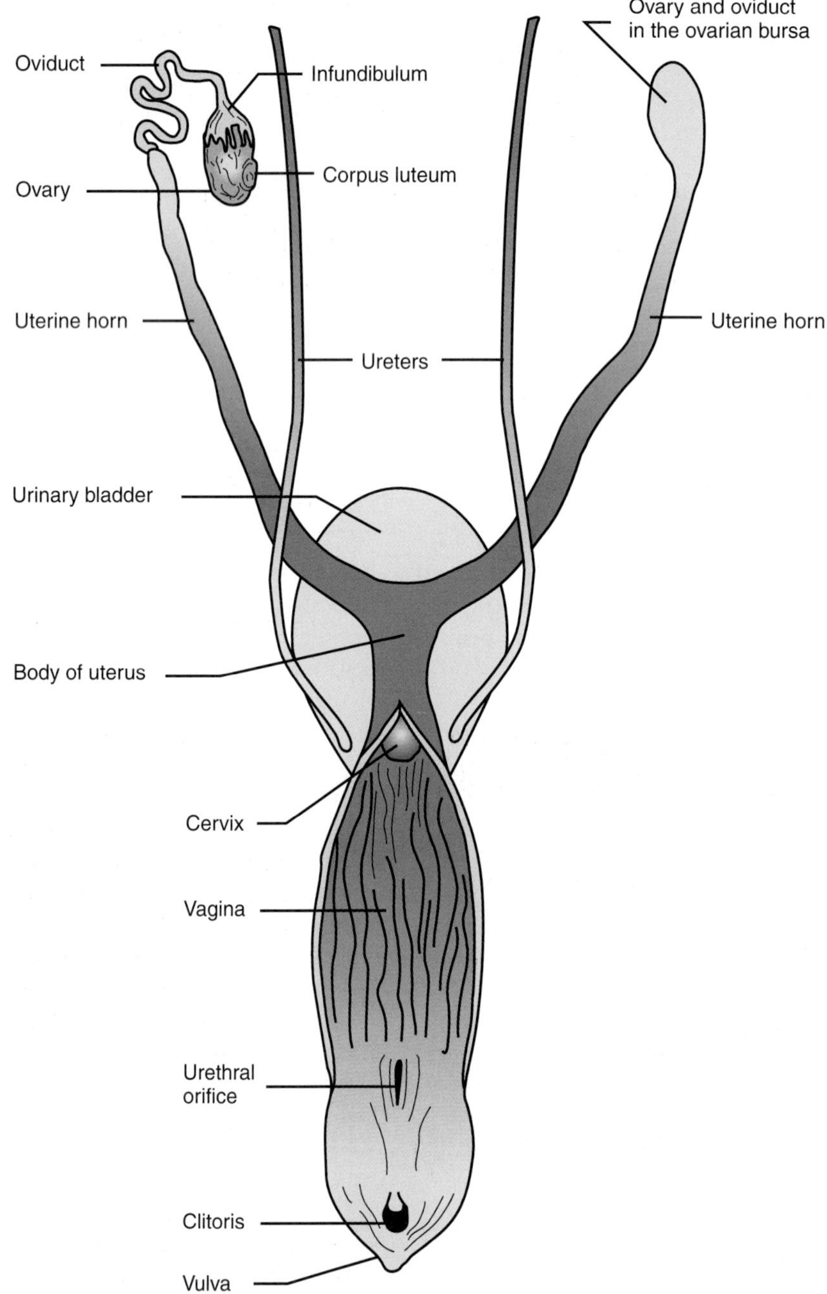

FIGURE **16-10** **Reproductive System of Bitch (Dorsal View).**

ovaries, oviducts and uterus—hang by broad sheets of peritoneum from the dorsal part of the abdominal cavity. The sheets of peritoneum are called the left and right **broad ligaments.** Each broad ligament has segments that are named according to the organ they directly support, although the divisions are not clearly apparent at a quick glance. The mesovarium is the part that supports the ovary, the mesosalpinx supports the oviduct, and the mesometrium supports the uterus. (The term *meso* refers to a sheet of tissue that attaches an organ to the body wall.) The broad ligaments also contain the blood vessels and nerve fibers that supply the ovaries, oviducts, and uterus.

Ovaries

Characteristics

The **ovaries** are the female gonads—the female equivalent of the male testes. They are located in the dorsal part of the abdominal cavity near the kidneys. Their shape varies among species. They are somewhat almond shaped in most species, but the ovaries of the horse are indented, making them bean-like in appearance. The ovaries of sows, because their large litter sizes require large numbers of follicles, often look like clusters of grapes.

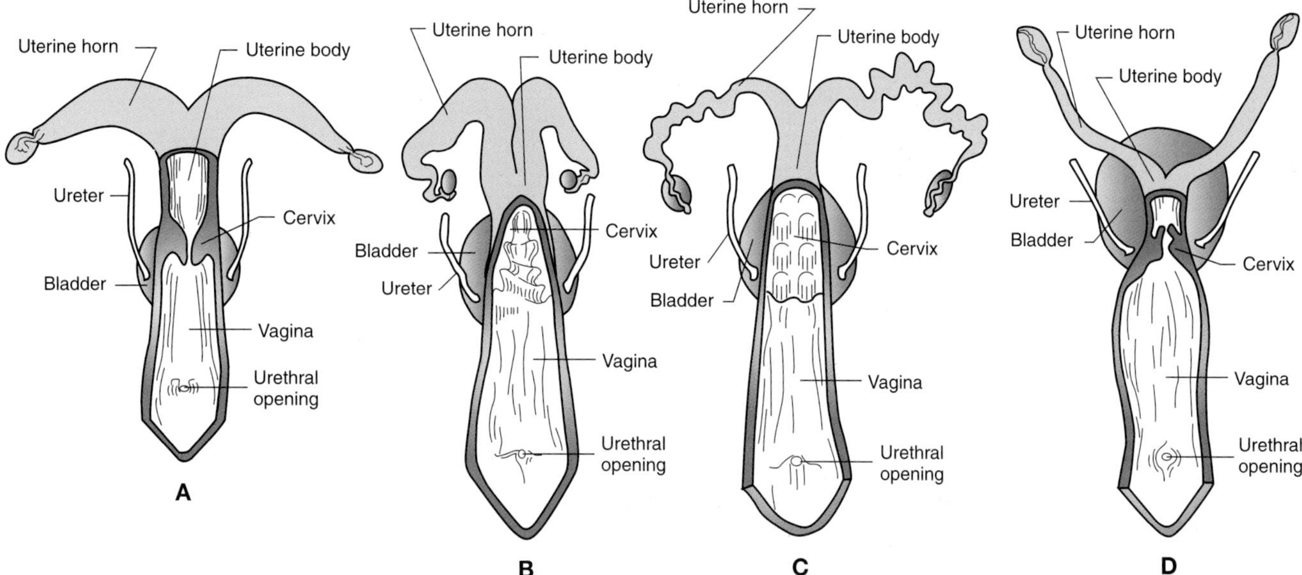

FIGURE **16-11** **Female Reproductive Tract.** Comparisons among some common domestic species (dorsal views). **A,** Mare. **B,** Cow. **C,** Sow. **D,** Bitch.

Clinical Application: Ovariohysterectomy

Ovariohysterectomy is a surgical procedure in which the ovaries, oviducts, and uterus are removed from an animal. It is commonly known as *spaying* an animal. Despite the frequency with which it is performed, an ovariohysterectomy is a major surgical procedure that involves opening the abdominal cavity. To safely remove the reproductive organs, the blood vessels supplying them first must be tied off (ligated). The blood vessels to each ovary are usually ligated along with the portion of the broad ligament (mesovarium) that contains them. This portion is referred to surgically as the *ovarian pedicle* or *ovarian stump.* The ovaries then can be severed safely from their ligated blood vessels. The remainder of the broad ligament is usually either ligated en masse or cut back toward the body of the uterus. The blood vessels in this part of the broad ligament are usually small. The body of the uterus and its accompanying blood vessels are ligated and transected. The reproductive organs then can be removed safely from the abdominal cavity and the incision sutured closed.

Functions

Like the testes, the ovaries have two main functions: the production of reproductive cells and hormones. Oogenesis is the process by which ova, the female reproductive cells, are produced in **follicles** in the ovaries. Unlike spermatozoa, ova are not constantly produced during the reproductive life of the animal. At or soon after birth the ovaries are seeded with tens of thousands of immature reproductive cells called *oocytes.* Some of these oocytes will mature into ova (the mature female reproductive cells) through the activities of the ovarian cycle. The rest will either degenerate or never begin development. No more oocytes are produced during the animal's life, however. The number of oocytes in the ovaries soon after birth is the maximum number that will be available to that animal during her lifetime.

The hormones produced in the ovaries fall into two categories: **estrogens** and **progestins.** Estrogens are produced by the cells of the developing ovarian follicles and are responsible for the physical and behavioral changes that prepare the animal for breeding and pregnancy. Progestins, principally progesterone, are produced by the corpus luteum that develops from the empty follicle after ovulation. Progestins help prepare the uterus for implantation of a fertilized ovum. They are also necessary for pregnancy to be maintained once implantation occurs.

Ovarian Cycle

Ova are not constantly produced in the ovaries. Their production involves a complex sequence of events carried out in a repeating (cyclical) fashion under the influence of two hormones—FSH and LH—from the anterior pituitary gland. Each cycle includes the development of an ovum within a follicle, its release from the follicle (ovulation), formation of a **corpus luteum,** and the degeneration of unripened follicles and, eventually, the corpus luteum. Figure 16-12 illustrates the main sequence of events in this process. The number of follicles involved in each cycle depends on the species. **Uniparous** species, such as the horse, cow, and human, normally give birth to only one offspring at a time. Their ovaries produce one mature ovum per cycle. **Multiparous** species, such as the cat, dog, and sow, give birth to litters of young. Their ovaries produce multiple ova per cycle.

The beginning stage of follicle development in the ovary is the primordial (sometimes called the *primary*) follicle. The thousands of immature oocytes in the ovaries of newborn

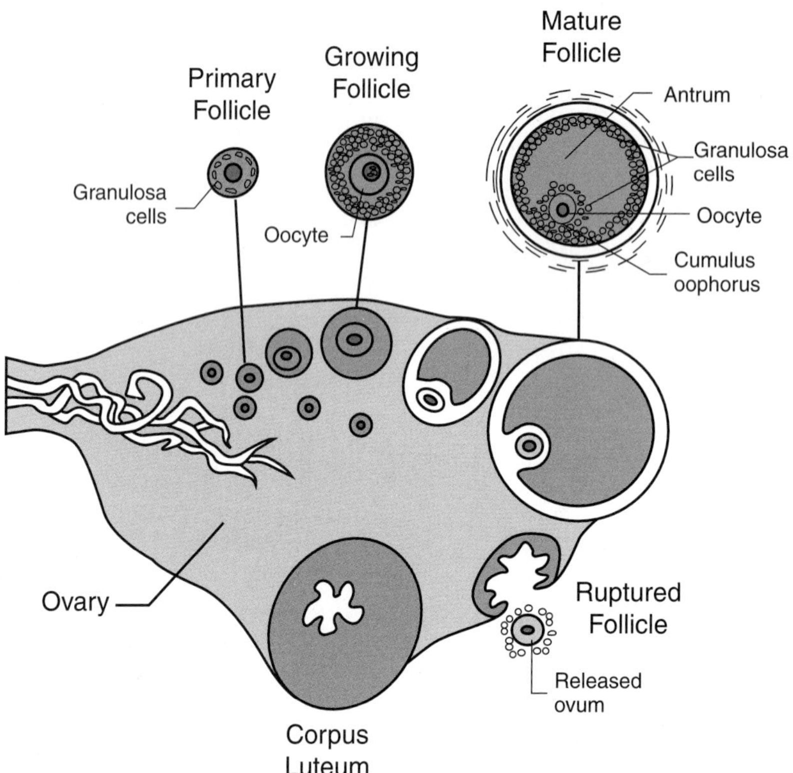

FIGURE **16-12** **Ovarian Cycle.** Schematic representation of sequence of events of ovarian cycle, starting with primary follicle and proceeding *(clockwise)* to mature follicle, ovulation, and formation of corpus luteum. These stages would not all be present at one time in an ovary.

animals reside in this stage until they become activated later in life and begin to develop further. The primordial follicle consists of the immature reproductive cell (the oocyte) surrounded by a single layer of flattened follicular cells. When FSH is released from the anterior pituitary, the whole ovary is bathed in it. Something, however, causes just a few of the thousands of primordial follicles to begin developing. This is known as *follicular recruitment* or *follicular activation*.

Once a primordial follicle has become activated, it is referred to as a *growing follicle.* The follicular cells become thickened into cuboidal shapes and begin to multiply. Multiple layers of follicular cells form around the developing oocyte. At this stage the follicular cells are called **granulosa cells.** As the granulosa cells multiply, the follicle starts to grow rapidly in size. The granulosa cells do more than just physically surround the developing oocyte. They also produce estrogen hormones that begin preparing the animal for breeding and pregnancy. The larger the follicle(s) become(s), the greater the amount of estrogens produced. As the follicle continues to grow, fluid-filled spaces begin to form between the granulosa cells. The spaces gradually become confluent (join together), forming one large, fluid-filled space called the **antrum.**

When the follicle has reached its maximum size, it looks like a large, blisterlike structure on the surface of the ovary. At this stage it is called a **mature follicle.** Alternative names for the mature follicle include *graafian follicle* and *vesicular ovarian follicle.* Inside the mature follicle, the oocyte sits on a little mound of granulosa cells called the **cumulus oophorus** and is surrounded by a thin layer of granulosa cells called the **corona radiata.** Most of the volume of the mature follicle is made up of the fluid-filled antrum. At this stage, estrogen production from the follicle(s) is at a maximum level, and the animal is ready for breeding to take place. In most animal species, **ovulation** (rupture of the mature follicle with release of the reproductive cell into the oviduct) occurs spontaneously as a result of the rising level of LH. This generally occurs regardless of whether breeding has taken place. In some species, however, such as the cat, rabbit, and ferret, breeding must take place before ovulation can occur. For this reason the cat, rabbit, and ferret are called *induced ovulators.* (This is the reason why the heat periods of cats can be so prolonged if they are not bred.) Once the mature reproductive cell is released from the follicle, its name changes. It is now called an *ovum*.

Ovulation is a traumatic and somewhat explosive event. The surface of the mature follicle weakens and physically ruptures, suddenly releasing the fluid from the antrum. The rush of fluid out of the follicle carries the ovum with it, still surrounded by its halo of granulosa cells—the corona radiata. The empty follicle fills with blood that rapidly clots, forming the **corpus hemorrhagicum.**

Under continued stimulation by the high LH level, the granulosa cells that line the blood-filled follicle begin to multiply again. This time they form a solid structure, the corpus luteum, that gets about as large as the mature follicle was just before ovulation. The term *corpus luteum* literally means "yellow body" because it has a pale yellow color grossly. The corpus luteum produces hormones called *progestins.* The principal progestin is progesterone, which is necessary for pregnancy to be maintained if the ovum is fertilized. If the ovum has been fertilized and implants in the uterus, it sends an endocrine signal to the ovary that causes the corpus luteum to be maintained. If the ovum has not been fertilized, no endocrine signal is sent and the corpus luteum degenerates after a short period.

Not all follicles that were activated in a particular ovarian cycle fully develop and ovulate. It is as if the ovary "auditions" follicles and chooses particular ones to fully develop. The rest may degenerate at any stage of their development. This is called **follicular atresia** and is a normal part of each ovarian cycle.

TEST YOURSELF

1. What two main types of hormones are produced in the ovary? Where is each produced?
2. What changes does an ovarian follicle undergo as it develops from a primordial follicle to a mature follicle?
3. After ovulation has occurred, what cells in the ovary multiply to form the corpus luteum?

Oviducts

The two **oviducts** also are known as the *fallopian tubes* and *uterine tubes.* Physically, they are small, convoluted tubes that extend from the tips of the uterine horns. Their roles are to guide ova from the ovary to the uterus and serve as the usual site for fertilization of ova by spermatozoa. The oviducts are not attached to the ovaries at all. When ovulation takes place, they have to "catch" the ova in the funnel-like **infundibulum.** The infundibulum is the enlarged opening at the ovarian end of each oviduct. At the time of ovulation, it more or less surrounds the area of the ovary where follicles have formed. Muscular, fingerlike projections called **fimbriae** form the margin of the infundibulum. They "feel" along the surface of the ovary and position the infundibulum where the follicle(s) is(are) located. This helps ensure that the infundibulum is properly positioned to catch the ovum or ova when ovulation occurs. If ova miss the opening of the oviduct, they fall into the abdominal cavity, where they usually just disintegrate after a time.

When examined closely, the complex physical structure of the oviducts becomes apparent. They contain a lot of smooth muscle fibers in their walls. Their linings are very intricate and folded, and the lining cells are covered with countless, movable cilia. When an ovum enters the oviduct after ovulation, delicate muscle contractions and gentle movements of the cilia begin slowly and gently moving it toward the uterus. The greatly folded lining of the oviduct keeps it in continuous, gentle contact with the ovum. If breeding has taken place, spermatozoa are already up in the oviducts when ovulation occurs. The oviducts are the usual place where the ovum and some lucky spermatozoon come together. This is called *fertilization* of the ovum. Once fertilization has taken place, the oviducts gently conduct the fertilized ovum down to the uterus for implantation.

Uterus

The **uterus** is the womb, where the fertilized ovum implants and lives while it grows and develops into a new animal. When fully developed, the uterus helps push the newborn out through the birth canal into the outside world. Although it seems like a simple receptacle in which the fetus can develop, the roles of the uterus are actually quite complex. It has to grow along with the developing offspring and then return to its original size after birth. It forms part of the placenta, which is the life-support system that keeps the fetus alive while it develops during pregnancy. The uterus has to remain quiet during the pregnancy and contract powerfully at the time of birth. After it has delivered the newborn and the placenta (the **afterbirth**), it has to contract quickly to stop bleeding from the site(s) where the placenta was attached to its lining. It does not have the complex, cyclical functions of the ovaries or the intricate structure of the oviducts, but the uterus is vital to the success of reproduction.

Physically, the uterus is a hollow, muscular organ. In common domestic animals, it is somewhat Y shaped, with the uterine body forming the base of the Y and the two uterine horns forming the arms. The body of the uterus extends in a caudal direction, eventually joining with the cervix at its caudal end. The two uterine horns project cranially. The oviducts extend from the tips of the uterine horns. The whole organ is suspended from the dorsal part of the abdomen by the mesometrium portion of the broad ligament.

The thick wall of the uterus is made up of three layers: (1) the lining endometrium is composed mainly of simple columnar epithelium and simple tubular glands that secrete mucus and other substances; (2) the thickest layer of the wall is the myometrium, which is made up of thick layers of smooth muscle that give the uterus the strength to push the fetus out at parturition (the birth process); and (3) the outermost layer is the perimetrium, which is covered by the visceral layer of peritoneum.

The fertilized ovum implants in the uterus and begins development. As the offspring develops, the placenta forms around it and attaches to the lining of the uterus so that nutrients, wastes, and respiratory gases can be exchanged between the fetal bloodstream and the maternal bloodstream (this is explained more fully in the section on fertilization and pregnancy). When the time comes for the offspring to be delivered, the muscular uterus provides most of the force necessary to open (dilate) the cervix so that the fetus can pass through it on its way to the outside world.

Cervix

The **cervix** is a muscular valve that seals off the uterus from the outside world most of the time. It is a powerful, smooth muscle sphincter located between the body of the uterus and the vagina. It functions to control access to the lumen of the uterus from the vagina. The cervix is normally tightly closed, except at the two ends of pregnancy: estrus (the heat period) and parturition (the birth process). The cervix opens at estrus to admit spermatozoa during breeding. It then tightly closes again during pregnancy and does not open again until birthing time. Uterine contractions during the first stage of labor push the newborn against the cervix and gradually pry it open (called *dilation* of the cervix) so that "junior" can slide down the birth canal and out into the world.

VAGINA

The **vagina** is the tube that receives the penis at breeding time and acts as the birth canal at birthing time. Structurally, it is a muscular tube that extends caudally from the cervix and connects it with the vulva. Although the lumen of the vagina is closed most of the time, it can stretch considerably to accommodate the penis at breeding and the newborn during the birth process. Mucous glands lining the vagina lubricate it at the time of breeding.

VULVA

The **vulva** is the only portion of the female reproductive system that is visible from the outside. Its main parts are the **vestibule,** the **clitoris,** and the **labia.** The word *vestibule,* in anatomical terms, means the entrance into a canal of some sort. In this case the vestibule of the vulva is the entrance into the vagina from the outside world. It is the short space between the labia and the opening of the vagina. The urethra, the tube that carries urine out from the urinary bladder, opens on the floor (ventral portion) of the vestibule. The clitoris is also located on the floor of the vestibule a little farther to the exterior than the urethral opening. The clitoris is the female equivalent of the penis of the male. It is **homologous** (equivalent in embryological origin) to the penis and has a similar basic structure. It is attached by two roots and has a body composed of erectile tissue and a glans that is extensively supplied with sensory nerve endings. The labia (lips) form the external boundary of the vulva.

TEST YOURSELF

1. When ovulation occurs, what causes the ovum to enter the oviduct?
2. Describe the functions of the uterus relating to pregnancy and parturition.
3. Where is the urethral opening located in the female?

THE ESTROUS CYCLE

To get the ovum and some lucky spermatozoon together at the right time (when both are mature) in the right place (the oviduct), some intricate coordination has to take place with two different animals. The situation in the male is pretty straightforward. Spermatozoa are constantly produced in the testes, and the testosterone level stays pretty level. So the male is basically always ready for breeding. He just needs the appropriate signals from the female to get the process underway. Because ovum production in the ovary of the female is not continuous but occurs in a cyclical manner, the timing of breeding is controlled by the ovarian cycle of the female.

In all common domestic animals, breeding takes place only during a definite period in each reproductive cycle when the chance of a successful pregnancy is the highest. This period when the female is receptive to the advances of the male is known as the heat period, or estrus. It is characterized by physical and behavioral changes that communicate the "window of opportunity" for breeding to the male. The timing of breeding is critical if pregnancy is going to result. The spermatozoa and the ovum must enter the oviduct at just the right times with respect to each other.

The **estrous cycle** is defined as the time from the beginning of one heat period to the beginning of the next. It is controlled by two hormones from the anterior pituitary gland: FSH and LH. FSH and LH stimulate activity in the ovaries that causes one or more reproductive cells (ova) to mature and be released. They also stimulate the production of hormones by the developing follicle (estrogens) and the corpus luteum (progestins) after ovulation. The estrogens and progestins are directly responsible for the physical and behavioral changes in the female that are associated with the estrous cycle. Different animal species have different patterns of estrous cycles although all go through the same basic stages.

Estrous Cycle Intervals

Animals can be classified according to how and when their estrous cycles occur during the year. **Polyestrous** animals, such as cattle and swine, cycle continuously throughout the year if they are not pregnant. As soon as one cycle ends, another begins. Some polyestrous animals show seasonal variations in their estrous cycles. They cycle continuously at certain times of the year and not at all at others. These animals, such as the horse, sheep, and cat, are called **seasonally polyestrous** animals. **Diestrous** animals, such as the dog, have two cycles per year, usually in the spring and fall. **Monoestrous** animals, such as the fox and mink, usually have only one cycle each year.

Stages of the Estrous Cycle

Although it is a continuous process, the estrous cycle can be divided into a series of characteristic stages. These stages reflect what is going on in the ovary as follicles develop, mature, rupture, and are replaced by corpora lutea. Keeping the events of the ovarian cycle in mind makes it easier to correlate what is going on in the ovary with the stages of the estrous cycle. The estrous cycle stages are proestrus, estrus, metestrus, and diestrus. (Another stage, anestrus, occurs in some animals between breeding seasons.)

Proestrus is the period of follicular development in the ovary. During this stage, follicles begin developing and growing. As they increase in size, the follicles' output of estrogen increases accordingly, causing many physical changes that prepare the rest of the reproductive tract for ovulation and breeding. These include thickening and development of the linings of the oviduct, uterus, and vagina. The epithelial lining of the vagina also begins cornifying, that is, forming a layer of tough keratin on its surface to help protect against the physical trauma of breeding that is about to come.

Estrus is the heat period, or the period of sexual receptivity in the female. It occurs when the estrogen level from the mature follicles reaches its peak. This high estrogen level causes physical and behavioral changes that signal the female's willingness to breed to the male. In most species, ovulation occurs near the end of estrus. In some species however, such as the cat, ferret, and rabbit, ovulation does not occur until the animal is bred. These species, called *induced ovulators*, remain in a prolonged state of estrus if they are not bred. The behavioral signs of estrus in the cat—particularly the vocalizing, rolling, and rubbing—can be very annoying to owners. They may even be misinterpreted as signs of illness by novice owners.

Metestrus is the period after ovulation when the corpus luteum develops. The granulosa cells left in the now-empty follicle begin to multiply under continued stimulation from LH. They soon produce a solid structure, the corpus luteum (yellow body), which is about the same size as the former mature follicle. The hormone progesterone, which is produced by the corpus luteum, temporarily inhibits follicular development in the ovary, causes the lining of the uterus to get very thick and "juicy" in preparation for implantation of a fertilized ovum and causes loss of the cornified epithelial lining that developed in the vagina during proestrus and estrus.

Diestrus is the active luteal stage when the corpus luteum has reached maximum size and exerts its maximum effect. If the animal is bred and becomes pregnant, the corpus luteum receives an endocrine signal from the developing embryo and is retained well into the pregnancy. If the animal is not pregnant, the corpus luteum degenerates at the end of diestrus. The animal either goes back into proestrus; or the ovary shuts down, and the animal goes into anestrus. Some animal species, particularly the dog, can have an exaggerated diestrus period, resulting in **pseudocyesis,** or what is commonly called **pseudopregnancy** (false pregnancy). Affected animals may act and look pregnant. The mammary glands often enlarge; the pelvis may relax; and the animal often shows maternal behavior patterns, such as nest building. In extreme cases, lactation and signs of labor may occur. Most cases of pseudopregnancy resolve spontaneously, but hormonal therapy may be required in some severe cases.

Anestrus is a period of temporary ovarian inactivity seen in seasonally polyestrus animals, as well as diestrous and monoestrous animals. It is the period between breeding cycles when the ovary essentially shuts down temporarily. The anestrus period can be cited to dog and cat owners who are reluctant to spay their animals because they are afraid the animals will become fat and lazy after the procedure. In reality, dogs and cats are functionally "spayed" for a good portion of each year while they are in anestrus. Animals become fat and lazy if they are fed too much and exercised too little regardless of whether they have been spayed.

TEST YOURSELF

1. What is the difference in the estrous cycle intervals of polyestrous animals, seasonally polyestrous animals, diestrous animals, and monoestrous animals?
2. How do the stages of the estrous cycle relate to the events of the ovarian cycle?

FERTILIZATION AND PREGNANCY

COPULATION

Copulation, or the act of breeding, is allowed by the female during the estrus (heat) period. In most animals, it is done in a standing position with the male mounting the female from behind. (An exception to this is the camel, which breeds in a kneeling position. Most of us do not have occasion to treat or breed camels, but who knows what piece of obscure information might come in handy for a trivia game!) Mounting is followed by **intromission** (insertion of the penis into the vagina), thrusting, and ejaculation.

When ejaculation occurs, the semen is usually deposited in the upper portion of the vagina. Exceptions to this are the horse and pig, in which semen is usually deposited directly into the uterus.

TRANSPORT OF SPERMATOZOA

The spermatozoa have to cover a lot of territory to travel from where they are deposited up to the oviducts, where they can seek out the ovum. The distance is huge on the microscopic scale of these tiny cells. They start actively swimming as soon as they are deposited in the female reproductive tract, but if they were to cover the whole distance under their own power, it would take over an hour for them to arrive in the oviducts. In actuality, they begin arriving within a couple of minutes after ejaculation. How do they make the trip so quickly? The answer is that they are transported ("Beam us up, Scotty!") by contractions of the uterus and oviducts and the action of cilia in the oviducts. Copulation causes the hormone oxytocin to be released from the posterior pituitary gland of the female. Oxytocin causes the smooth muscle of the estrogen-primed female reproductive tract to contract, giving the spermatozoa a free ride.

The reason for the rush to get the spermatozoa up to the oviducts so quickly is that timing is everything at this point. The spermatozoa must arrive at the oviducts before the ovum does to undergo **capacitation**, which is a process that enhances their fertility. Nature has an exquisite method for timing this whole process. Breeding is only allowed by the female during the estrous, or heat, period. So spermatozoa enter the female reproductive tract when the oocyte in the follicle is fully developed but has not yet been released. Release of the ovum (ovulation) is delayed until near the end of the estrous period in most species. This nifty little bit of traffic control helps ensure that the spermatozoa arrive at the oviducts first and have time to undergo capacitation before the ovum shows up ready to be fertilized.

CAPACITATION

Capacitation describes a series of changes that spermatozoa undergo in the female reproductive tract to increase their chances of successfully fertilizing an ovum. Many of the changes are subtle, involving changes in ion movement through the cell membranes, an increase in the cells' metabolic rates, and an increase in the rate at which simple sugars are used for energy production. A more dramatic change is in the acrosome, the digestive enzyme-containing caplike structure that covers the head of the spermatozoa. Capacitation causes the release of the enzymes that, up until now, have been sealed off. The digestive enzymes help the spermatozoa penetrate through the layers surrounding the ovum to accomplish fertilization.

FERTILIZATION OF THE OVUM

Spermatozoa are "preprogrammed" to seek out anything large and round and attempt to penetrate into it. Many go astray and attempt to fertilize things other than ova, such as epithelial cells in the oviducts. This is one of the reasons why such a large number of spermatozoa must be introduced into the female reproductive tract in the first place—to increase the odds that one will reach and fertilize the ovum. A significant number of spermatozoa find and swarm around the ovum once it moves down into the oviduct. Many begin tunneling through the layers surrounding the ovum aided by the digestive enzymes of their acrosomes. Only one spermatozoon, however, will physically penetrate through the cell membrane of the ovum and deliver its genetic material into the cell. Once a single spermatozoon has entered the ovum, a change takes place in the cell membrane that blocks other spermatozoa from entering.

THE ZYGOTE

Once an ovum is fertilized, it gets another name change. It is now called a **zygote.** Immediately after fertilization, the nucleus of the spermatozoon is called the *male pronucleus,* and the nucleus of the ovum is called the *female pronucleus*. Each carries the haploid chromosome number, that is, one half the number in the rest of the body's cells. The male and female pronuclei quickly join together to restore the diploid chromosome number and determine the unique genetic makeup of the offspring. The full genetic map for the new animal has been established, but it is only a map at this point.

CLEAVAGE

As soon as the two pronuclei join to form a single nucleus, the zygote begins to divide rapidly by the normal process of mitosis. This rapid division is called **cleavage.** The single cell divides into two cells, which quickly divide into four, then eight, then sixteen, and so forth. Cleavage occurs so rapidly that the cells of the zygote do not have time to grow between divisions. The number of cells making up the zygote is increasing dramatically, but its overall size is still about the same as the original ovum, even after several days.

While cleavage is taking place, the zygote is slowly moving down the oviduct toward the uterus (Figure 16-13). Delicate, muscular contractions and the movements of cilia are gently propelling it along. After a few days the zygote is a solid mass of cells that looks like a tiny raspberry; this is known as the **morula** stage. The cells of the morula continue to divide and gradually form a hollow cavity in the center. By the time it reaches the uterus a few days later, it is formed into a hollow ball of cells with a "bump" on one side that eventually forms into the embryo (Figure 16-14). It is now called a **blastocyst,** and it is ready to implant itself in the lining of the uterus.

IMPLANTATION

Implantation is the means by which the blastocyst makes itself a home by attaching itself to the lining of the uterus (the endometrium). When it comes to rest against the uterine lining, enzymes produced by the blastocyst dissolve away a small pit. The blastocyst implants itself in the pit. In multiparous species, such as swine, the multiple blastocysts randomly space themselves along the horns and body of the uterus as they implant.

During the early part of pregnancy, the developing offspring is called an **embryo.** Later it is referred to as a **fetus.**

Up until now the dividing zygote has obtained its nourishment by diffusion from the fluid of the oviduct and uterus. By the time of implantation, it has become too large and metabolically active for its needs to be met by this mechanism. A more effective method of supplying oxygen and nutrients and carrying wastes away must be developed. This role is carried out by the **placenta,** a complex structure that begins to form as soon as the blastocyst implants in the uterus.

TEST YOURSELF

1. Why is the timing of copulation so important? How is the precise timing accomplished?
2. Describe what happens to a zygote between fertilization and implantation.

THE PLACENTA

The placenta is a life-support system for the developing fetus. During gestation (pregnancy) the fetus leads a "parasitic" existence as it grows and develops; that is, it receives all the nutrients and other substances it needs to grow and develop from its mother. It also depends on her to dispose of the waste products it produces. Remember that during the period of pregnancy, the fetus is undergoing incredibly rapid growth and its cells are differentiating into all of the tissues, organs, and systems needed to support independent life after it is born. Its need for nutrients and waste elimination is huge and grows minute by minute along with its body. Fortunately, the pla-

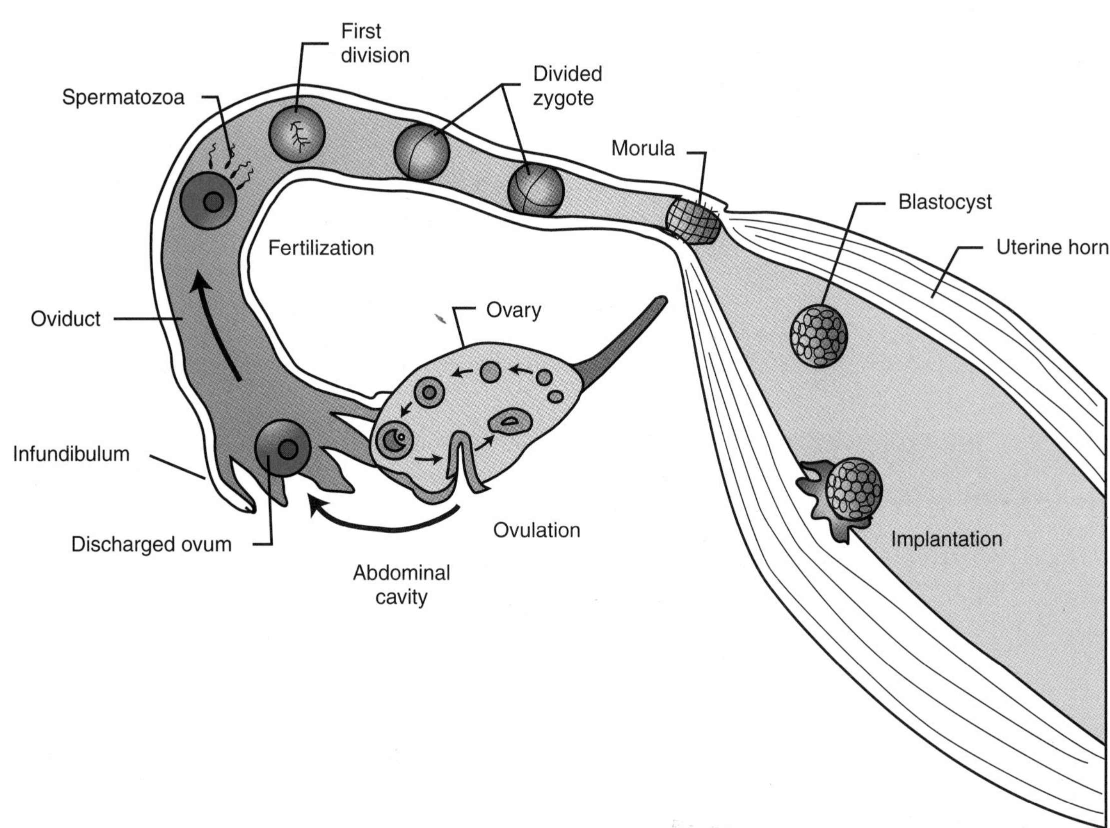

FIGURE **16-13** **Fertilization and Implantation.** After ovulation, ovum starts moving slowly down oviduct toward the uterus. Spermatozoon in oviduct fertilizes the ovum, forming single-celled zygote. Cleavage of zygote begins almost immediately as single cell divides into two cells, two cells divide into four, and so on. After a day or two, zygote has formed into solid mass of cells (morula). Morula continues to develop into hollow ball of cells (blastocyst), which enters the uterus and implants in its wall.

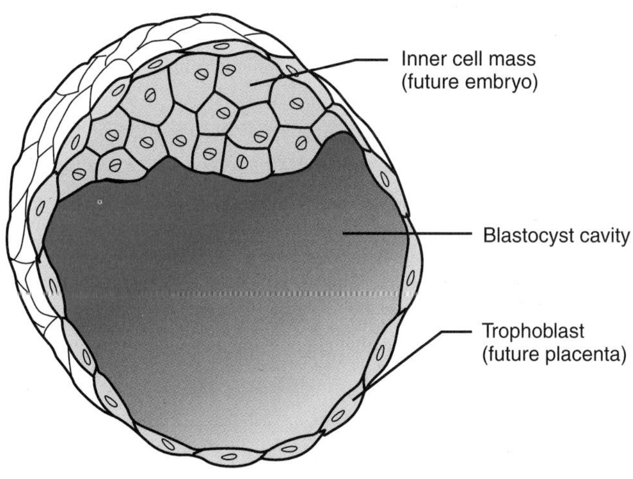

FIGURE **16-14** **Blastocyst.**

centa grows right along with the fetus and meets its needs every step of the way.

Structure

The placenta is a multilayered, fluid-filled, membranous sac that develops around the embryo and is connected to it by the umbilical cord (see Figure 16-16). In some area(s) the outermost layer of the placenta attaches to the lining of the uterus. It is at this (these) area(s) of attachment that the actual exchange of nutrients and wastes takes place between the fetal circulation and the maternal circulation. The fetal and maternal blood vessels are separate but in close proximity to each other in this area. Normally no direct mixing of fetal and maternal blood occurs. The nutrients and wastes are exchanged across the very thin layers that separate the two sets of blood vessels.

Grossly, the placenta consists of layers of soft membranes that form two fluid filled sacs around the developing fetus. The layer immediately around the fetus is called the **amnion.** It forms a sac around the fetus called the **amniotic sac.** The fetus floats in amniotic fluid inside this sac. Surrounding the amniotic sac is another layer called the **allantois,** which forms the fluid-filled **allantoic sac.** The outside of the allantoic sac is covered by the **chorion,** which attaches to the uterine lining. The chorion is linked to the fetus by the umbilical cord.

The **umbilical cord** is the link between the fetus and the nutrient and waste exchange structures of the placenta. As its name implies, it is a cordlike structure that contains blood vessels (the umbilical arteries and vein) and a drainage tube from the fetus' urinary bladder (the urachus). The two **umbilical arteries** carry unoxygenated, waste-filled blood from the fetus to the placenta. The single **umbilical vein** carries nutrient- and oxygen-rich blood back from the placenta to the fetus. The **urachus** is a tube that runs from the cranial tip of the

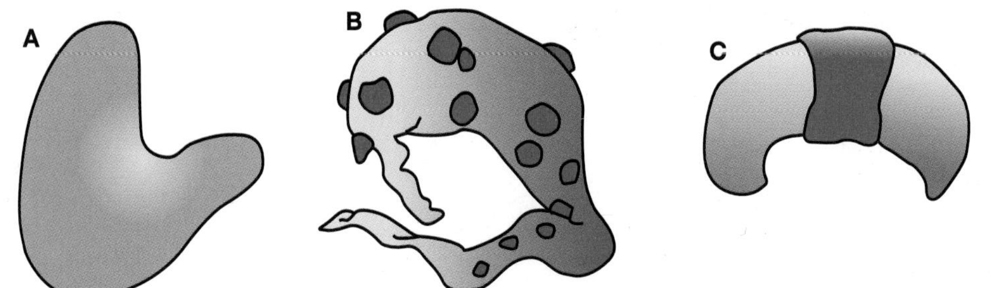

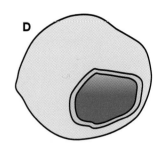

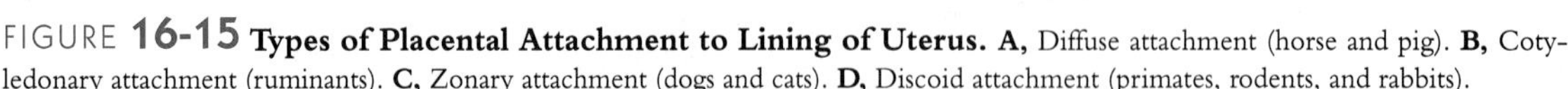
FIGURE 16-15 **Types of Placental Attachment to Lining of Uterus. A,** Diffuse attachment (horse and pig). **B,** Cotyledonary attachment (ruminants). **C,** Zonary attachment (dogs and cats). **D,** Discoid attachment (primates, rodents, and rabbits).

CLINICAL APPLICATION — The Afterbirth

At birth the placenta is often referred to as the *afterbirth* because it is delivered after the offspring. What actually happens is that the fetus is delivered *through* the placenta. The powerful contractions of uterine and abdominal muscles during labor cause the membranes of the placenta to rupture and release their fluid. This is called the "water breaking." Often the amnion still partially covers the newborn after it is delivered. The dam will usually lick this off, starting at the face so that the newborn can draw those important first breaths. If she does not carry out this important activity, humans must intervene if they are present. The membrane is very soft and is easily broken and pulled away from the newborn's face. Few things in veterinary medicine are more rewarding than removing the membrane from the face of a newborn animal and watching it take its first breaths.

fetus' urinary bladder through the umbilical cord to the allantoic sac. The kidneys of the developing fetus are not fully functional through most of the pregnancy; therefore they do not produce urine as we know it. They do, however, produce a watery fluid that must be removed from the urinary bladder. The urachus drains this fluid out into the allantoic sac.

Attachment to the Uterus

The area where the chorion attaches to the lining of the uterus is where the fetal and maternal blood vessels intertwine with each other. The exchange of nutrients and wastes takes place here between the fetal and maternal bloodstreams. The type of attachment varies among species but can be categorized into one of four general types: diffuse, cotyledonary, zonary, or discoid (Figure 16-15).

Diffuse Attachment. **Diffuse attachment** means that the attachment sites are spread diffusely over the whole surface of the placenta and the whole lining of the uterus. There are no small limited areas of attachment. This type of placenta is found in pigs and horses (Figure 16-16). Because the attachment sites are so diffuse and loosely attached, this type of placenta usually detaches easily from the uterine lining and is passed after the delivery of the newborn.

Cotyledonary Attachment. **Cotyledonary attachment** is the most complicated type and is somewhat the opposite of the diffuse placental attachment. The areas of attachment are small, separate, and numerous. Each of the dozens or hundreds of attachment sites is called a **placentome.** Each placentome consists of an area on the surface of the placenta called a **cotyledon** that joins with a mushroomlike **caruncle** in the lining of the uterus. The cotyledon and caruncle tightly interdigitate with each other. This type of placenta is found in ruminants, such as cattle, sheep, and goats.

For a cotyledonary placenta to pass after the birth of the offspring, each of the individual placentomes must separate completely. Sometimes this does not occur, and part or all of the placenta is retained in the uterus after the birth process. This retained portion of placenta dies and degenerates within the uterus, creating a potentially dangerous situation for the already stressed dam. It can lead to a serious postpartum (after birth) metritis (infection of the uterus) because bacteria can live and multiply in the dead placental tissue. Ensuring that the placenta is delivered by ruminant animals is important, and appropriate treatment must be given if it is not.

Zonary Attachment. With **zonary attachment,** the placenta attaches to the uterus in a belt-shaped area that encircles the placenta. Found in dogs and cats, this type of attachment also detaches fairly easily after delivery of the newborn. Retained placentas are not common in dogs and cats.

Discoid Attachment. The pattern of **discoid attachment** is fairly self-descriptive. The area of attachment between the placenta and uterus is a single disk-shaped area. This type of attachment is found in humans and other primates, as well as rabbits and many rodents.

TEST YOURSELF

1. Why is the placenta so important to a successful pregnancy?
2. Describe the relationship between the fetus and the amniotic and allantoic sacs of the placenta.
3. Describe the main structures that make up the umbilical cord and the function of each.
4. Which type of placental attachment to the uterus is the simplest and detaches most easily after parturition? Which is most complicated and often results in retention of the placenta?

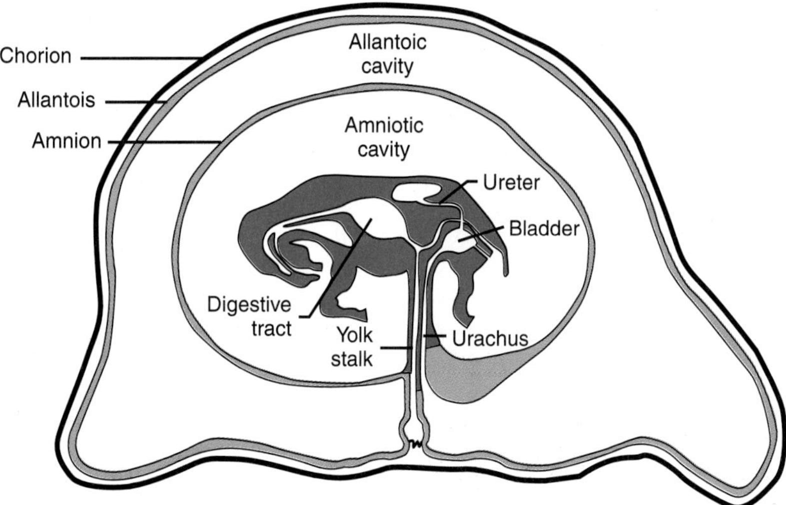

FIGURE **16-16** **Fetus and Placenta of the Horse.**

PREGNANCY

The period of pregnancy is called the **gestation period.** It is the time from fertilization of the ovum to delivery of the newborn. It is often convenient to divide it into three often unequal segments, called **trimesters.** The first trimester is the period of the *embryo* when the newly implanted zygote is getting itself organized and developing its life-supporting placenta. During this period, the developing offspring is often referred to as an *embryo.* Starting with the second trimester, the developing offspring is usually called a *fetus.* The second trimester is the *fetal development* period when all the various parts of the fetus are taking shape and differentiating from each other. All the body tissues, organs, and systems develop during this period. The third trimester is the period of *fetal growth.* All parts of the fetus grow dramatically during this last period of development, preparing it to transition from a parasitic to a free-living existence after birth. The lengths of the gestation period in some common species are listed in Table 16-3.

Table 16-3 Gestation Periods of Some Common Species

Species	Range	Approximate
Cats	56-69 days	2 months
Cattle	271-291 days	9 months
Dogs	59-68 days	2 months
Elephants	615-650 days	21 months
Ferrets	42 days	6 weeks
Goats	146-155 days	5 months
Hamsters	19-20 days	3 weeks
Horses	321-346 days	11 months
Humans	280 days	9 months
Pigs	110-116 days	3 months, 3 weeks, and 3 days
Rabbits	30-32 days	1 month
Sheep	143-151 days	5 months

PARTURITION

The whole, grand purpose of the male and female reproductive systems is fulfilled when **parturition,** the birth process, successfully takes place. At birth the fetus, which has led a parasitic existence up until now, is pushed out of the warm, dark, moist environment of the uterus into the cold, cruel outside world as a free-living, independent animal. In a very short time the body of the fetus has to undergo some pretty dramatic changes. Its lungs, which have been nonfunctional until now, must suddenly expand and start functioning to supply the newborn with the oxygen it needs and eliminate the carbon dioxide its cells are producing as a waste product. Contributing to this process are some dramatic changes in blood flow in and around the heart and lungs. The foramen ovale and ductus arteriosus, which shunted most of the blood from the right side of the fetal heart around, rather than through, the lungs, must both close fairly quickly. (See Chapter 8 for a complete description of these two fetal structures.) The lungs now need their full blood supply to properly oxygenate the blood and eliminate carbon dioxide.

Precisely what triggers parturition is not known. Many factors seem to be involved, including the size and weight of the uterus and fetus and changing hormone levels in the fetus and dam. The hormonal changes form a chain of events that leads to the onset of labor. Around the time of parturition the progesterone level in the bloodstream of the dam declines. Up until now the high progesterone level has kept the muscle of the uterus (the myometrium) quiet, preventing it from prematurely expelling the fetus. At the same time, increased levels of glucocorticoid hormones from the adrenal glands of the fetus stimulate a rise in the dam's estrogen level and the release of prostaglandin $F_{2\alpha}$ from the uterine wall. The estrogen and prostaglandin increase the myometrium's sensitivity to oxytocin, which is released from the dam's posterior pituitary gland.

CLINICAL APPLICATION Dystocia

Usually parturition comes off without a hitch. After all, animals have been giving birth for millions of years without any help. However, sometimes problems develop that interfere with the birth process, causing a **dystocia,** or a difficult birth. The most common causes of dystocia include a fetus that is too large for the dam to pass and a fetus that is in the wrong orientation for delivery, which is called an *abnormal presentation*. Abnormal presentations may involve deviations in the position of the head, one or more legs, or the overall orientation of the fetus from the normal snout-first or rear-legs first position. Sometimes the fetus can be pushed back (called *repelling* the fetus) far enough to allow it to be repositioned for delivery. At times this is not possible, and the fetus must be removed surgically by an operation called a *cesarean section*. In some cases, particularly in cattle, when the fetus is dead, it may have to be cut up (called an *embryotomy*) into small enough segments to be removed through the birth canal to save the life of the dam.

Oxytocin stimulates the myometrium to contract, which starts the labor process.

The three distinct stages to parturition are often referred to as the *three stages of labor.* The first stage of labor consists of *uterine contractions*. The muscle of the uterus (the myometrium) contracts, pressing the membrane-covered fetus down against the cervix. This causes the cervix to gradually dilate. Externally, the dam appears restless and uncomfortable as a result of these uterine contractions. She may repeatedly lie down and get up and may urinate frequently. Some species, such as the dog and pig, may attempt to build a nest into which they will deliver their young.

The second stage of labor consists of the *delivery of the newborn*. This is accomplished by a combination of strong uterine and abdominal muscle contractions. The dam typically lies down and strains in a rhythmic pattern of contractions that gradually become stronger and closer together. Rupture of the "water bags," the amniotic and allantoic sacs of the placenta, usually precedes the actual delivery of the newborn.

The third stage of labor consists of *delivery of the placenta* (afterbirth). The placenta separates from the wall of the uterus and is expelled by weaker uterine contractions. The dam often eats the placenta(s).

In multiparous species, such as the dog, cat, and pig, the second and third stages of parturition intermix with one another. Typically newborns and placentas are delivered alternately; that is, after a newborn is delivered, its placenta is usually expelled before the next newborn is delivered.

INVOLUTION OF THE UTERUS

After parturition is complete, the uterus gradually returns to its nonpregnant size through a process called **involution.** At the site(s) where the placenta(s) was(were) attached, the endometrium sloughs (dies and detaches) into the lumen of the uterus, and the exposed areas heal over. The myometrium slowly continues to contract, squeezing the contents of the uterus out through the birth canal as the organ returns to its nonpregnant size. Initially the discharge contains fresh blood resulting from separation of the placenta from its attachment site(s). Pressure from the continued uterine contractions usually stops the bleeding relatively quickly. The discharge gradually turns darker as dead tissue is liquefied and sloughed from the uterine wall. It generally takes from a few weeks to a month or more for involution to be completed.

TEST YOURSELF

1. What are the basic events of the three trimesters of pregnancy?
2. Describe the three stages of labor.
3. Why is it important that uterine contractions continue after the fetus and placenta are delivered?

MAMMARY GLANDS AND LACTATION

Once parturition is completed, the newborn animal must be nourished and cared for during the **neonatal period.** At this time the mammary glands become very important.

CHARACTERISTICS

The mammary (milk) glands are specialized skin glands. They produce colostrum and milk, which are needed by the newly born animal during the crucial first few hours, days, and weeks of its life. Although, strictly speaking, they are not part of the reproductive system, their function is vital to the survival of the newborn; therefore we discuss them as an extension of the reproductive system.

Mammary glands are present in both male and female animals. They normally only function in females because males do not secrete the proper blend of hormones to make them work. (It is theoretically possible to make a bull give milk with administration of the proper combination of hormones, but who would want to be the one to milk him?)

SPECIES DIFFERENCES

Mammary glands look very different among common species of animals. Their number varies from a low of 2 in horses to a high of 14 in swine, and their locations range from the inguinal (groin) region alone in cattle and horses to locations that span the inguinal, abdominal, and thoracic regions in dogs, cats, and swine. Also, considerable variety is found in the numbers of openings from which milk emerges in the teats or nipples. Cattle, sheep, and goats only have one opening per teat, whereas dogs can have up to 20 openings per nipple. (Humans can have up to 24 openings per nipple!) The mammary gland characteristics of some common species are listed in Table 16-4.

Table 16-4 Mammary Gland Characteristics of Some Common Species

Species	Usual Number of Glands	Location of Glands	Number of Openings in Teats or Nipples
Cat	10	Inguinal, abdominal, and thoracic regions	3-7
Cattle	4	Inguinal	1
Dog	10	Inguinal, abdominal, and thoracic regions	8-20
Goat	2	Inguinal region	1
Horse	2	Inguinal region	2-4
Human	2	Thoracic region	15-24
Pig	14	Inguinal, abdominal, and thoracic regions	2-3
Sheep	2	Inguinal region	1

UDDER OF THE COW

Because they are so large and specialized, the mammary glands of the cow, commonly known as the *udder,* seem like exaggerated caricatures of mammary glands. Their general makeup, however, is just a large version of other animals' mammary glands. For this reason, we use them as our model mammary system (Figure 16-17).

Characteristics

The udder of the cow consists of four mammary glands that are called "quarters." Each quarter is a completely separate unit from the other three. They each have their own milk-secreting systems and ducts leading down to their own teats. This has important clinical significance if infection of the mammary gland(s), a condition called **mastitis,** develops. Infection does not directly spread from one quarter to another. It has to spread down through the teat and duct system of one quarter and up another. The spread of mastitis between quarters can be prevented through good milking hygiene and milking an infected quarter last.

The udder of a high-producing dairy cow can weigh more than 100 lb at milking time. It needs a strong suspensory system to support the heavy weight and attach the udder to the body wall. This suspensory system consists of a slinglike arrangement of ligaments that run down the center and around the sides of the udder. The medial suspensory ligament contains many elastic fibers so that it can stretch. It passes down the center between the left and right halves of the udder. The lateral suspensory ligaments are composed largely of strong but inelastic collagen fibers. They pass down and around the lateral sides of each half of the udder. The strong lateral ligaments provide firm support for the udder, and the elastic medial ligament acts as a "shock absorber" for the udder as the animal moves around.

Alveoli and Duct System

The milk-secreting units of the mammary gland are small structures called *alveoli*. Each alveolus is a tiny, saclike arrangement of cells that secretes milk into a tiny tube called the *alveolar duct*. The alveoli are arranged like clusters of grapes around the alveolar ducts. The tiny alveolar ducts join to form larger ducts, which join to form even larger ducts, and so on. The duct system of the mammary gland is similar to the arrangement of branches in a tree. The clusters of alveoli would be similar to the leaves, and the duct system would be like the small tree branches joining to form larger branches. The largest ducts (similar to the trunks of trees) empty into a large space called the **gland sinus** located just above (dorsal to) the teat. The gland sinus is continuous with the **teat sinus** inside the teat. The two large sinuses form a space shaped like an upside-down pear. They are the spaces where milk accumulates when milk letdown has occurred. The milk can be readily extracted from these large spaces by the suckling of a nursing newborn or the vacuum of a milking machine.

At the tip of the teat is the **streak canal,** which is the passageway from the teat sinus to the outside. It is surrounded by elastic fibers and a ringlike sphincter muscle that keeps it closed most of the time. This helps minimize milk leakage.

MAMMARY GLAND DEVELOPMENT

The mammary glands stay small and undeveloped until puberty (the time of sexual maturity). Up until that time, the proper mix of hormones has not occurred to stimulate their growth and development. Once the estrous cycles begin at puberty, however, the mammary glands respond to the new hormones flowing through the body by enlarging and gearing up to produce milk.

A complex balance of hormones stimulates the mammary glands to develop. Most of the anterior pituitary hormones are involved in the process either directly or indirectly. Prolactin and growth hormone directly encourage mammary gland development. FSH and LH stimulate the ovaries to produce estrogen and progesterone during each heat cycle. The estrogen and progesterone encourage the alveoli and duct systems of the mammary glands to develop. Thyroid-stimulating hormone and adrenocorticotropic hormone influence the process indirectly through their target organs. The levels of these various hormones must be balanced precisely for complete mammary gland development to take place. Abnormally high levels of any, such as might occur when thyroid hormone or corticosteroid drugs are administered to a young animal, can actually inhibit normal mammary gland development.

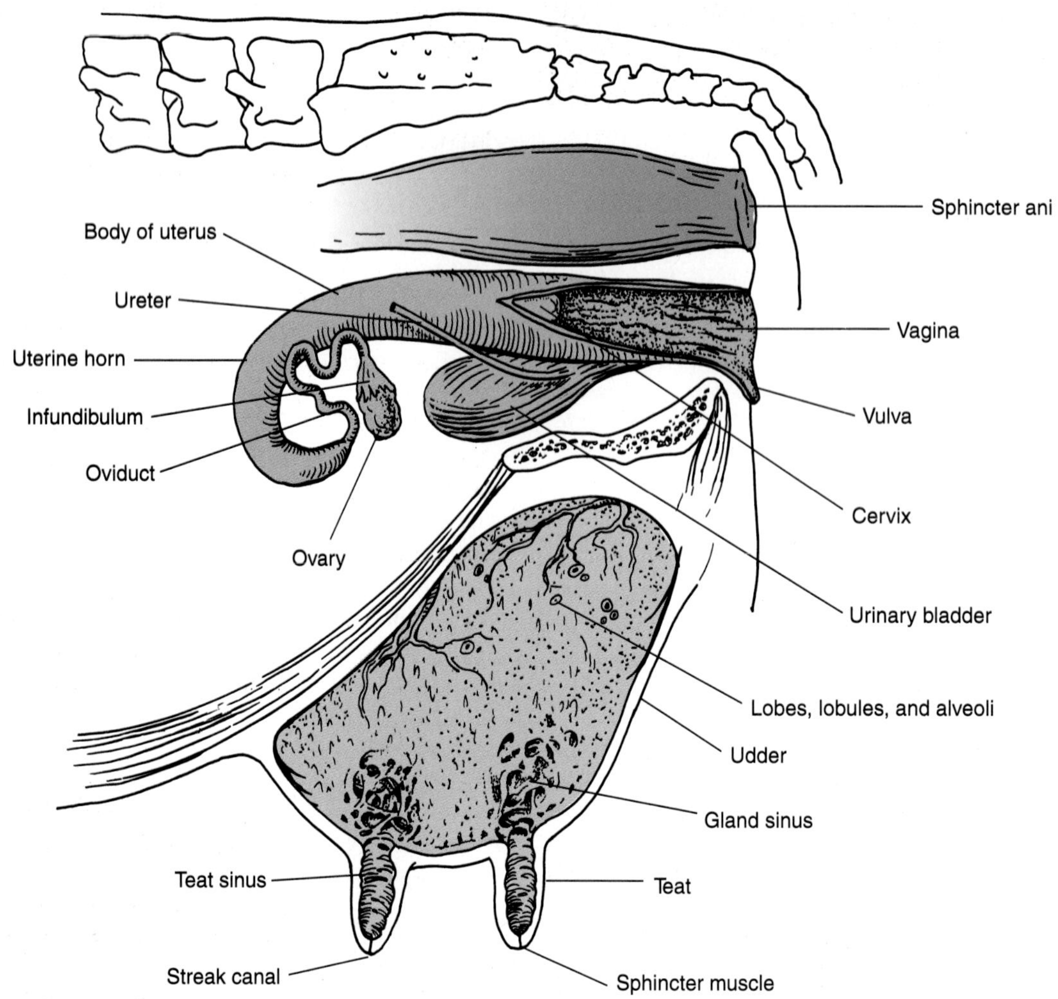

FIGURE **16-17** **Reproductive System and Udder of Cow.** (From McBride DF: *Learning veterinary terminology,* ed 2, St Louis, 2002, Mosby.)

Lactation

The physical growth and development of the mammary glands are the first steps in making them able to produce milk. The rest takes place during pregnancy.

Lactation is the process of milk production. It begins toward the end of pregnancy and is obvious at the time of parturition. Hormones, such as prolactin and growth hormone, from the anterior pituitary gland and hormones from the adrenal cortex are involved in getting it started.

Colostrum

Before it starts to produce milk, the mammary gland produces a sort of premilk secretion called **colostrum.** Colostrum has a different appearance and a different composition from normal milk. It contains larger amounts of proteins, lipids, and amino acids than milk and also contains high levels of various essential vitamins. It supplies important nutrients to the newborn and has a laxative effect that helps clear the dark, sticky **meconium** from the newborn's intestinal tract.

Probably the most critical of colostrum's roles is the transfer of what is called **"passive immunity"** from the dam to the newborn. Among the proteins in colostrum are high levels of immunoglobulins, also called *antibodies,* that form an important part of the body's defense against infection. The antibodies in the colostrum are specific for disease-causing organisms that the dam has been exposed to or vaccinated against. If the newborn drinks sufficient colostrum during the first few hours after birth, the large antibody molecules will be absorbed intact into its bloodstream. This provides it with important passive immunity, that is, complete, preformed antibodies that help protect it against disease-causing microorganisms until its own immune system matures sufficiently to protect it. If colostrum is not consumed within the first few hours, the lining of the newborn's intestine can no longer absorb the large antibody molecules intact. They will be broken down by the digestive process, and passive immunity will not be transmitted. Youngsters that do not get sufficient colostrum in that critical early neonatal period are much more prone to diseases. Even if they do not die of early infections, they are typically weaker and do not grow as rapidly as animals that consumed colostrum at the appropriate time.

CLINICAL APPLICATION Passive Immunity and Vaccinations

The passive immunity that newborns acquire from drinking colostrum is important to their early survival. However, it can interfere with early vaccinations, particularly in puppies and kittens. If a puppy or kitten is vaccinated while it still has a high level of antibodies from its mother in its bloodstream, the vaccine will be inactivated and will not stimulate the animal's immune system to manufacture new antibodies. So why not just wait until the passive immunity from mom wears off? The difficulty is that passive immunity lasts differing lengths of time in different animals. If you vaccinate too early, the vaccine is wasted. If you wait too long to vaccinate, the passive immunity may have worn off, leaving the animal susceptible to infection. The level of passive antibodies in the young animal's bloodstream can be tested, but it is expensive. The most practical solution is to give the young animal a series of vaccinations spread out over the period when protection from passive immunity is most likely to end. Specific vaccination protocols differ, but the first vaccination is usually given somewhere around 6 to 8 of weeks of age, with subsequent vaccinations given every 2 to 3 weeks until the animal is 14 to 16 weeks old.

Maintenance of Lactation

Once it has begun, lactation will continue as long as the mammary gland is emptied regularly by nursing or milking. The key is continued physical stimulation of the teat or nipple, combined with regular removal of milk from the gland. These activities send sensory nerve impulses to the brain. From there nerve pathways lead to the hypothalamus, which stimulates the anterior pituitary gland to continue its production of the hormones that keep lactation going. When nursing or milking stops, the flow of essential hormones stop also. Without hormonal stimulation, lactation gradually ceases, and the mammary gland "dries up." This is called **involution of the mammary gland.**

Milk Letdown

Milk letdown is the immediate effect of nursing or milking. When milk is produced, it accumulates up high in the mammary gland in the alveoli and small ducts. It does not move down into the larger ducts and sinuses, where it is accessible for nursing or milking, until milk letdown occurs. When nursing or milking begins, sensory nerve impulses are sent to the brain. As we've seen, this causes the hypothalamus to stimulate the anterior pituitary gland to produce the hormones necessary to maintain lactation. However, it has another major effect. It also causes the hypothalamus to release the hormone oxytocin from the posterior pituitary gland. The oxytocin travels to the mammary gland and causes musclelike **myoepithelial cells** around the alveoli and small ducts to contract. This squeezes milk down into the large ducts and sinuses, where it can be removed by nursing or milking. The process of milk letdown takes from a few seconds to a minute or more to produce results; so there is often a slight delay from the time a newborn starts to nurse to when the milk starts to flow freely.

TEST YOURSELF

1. Why does mastitis in one quarter of a dairy cow's udder not necessarily spread to the other three quarters?
2. Describe the suspensory apparatus of the udder.
3. Why don't the mammary glands of male animals usually develop and secrete milk?
4. Describe the importance of colostrum to the health of a newborn animal.
5. Describe how nursing or milking causes milk letdown and also helps sustain lactation.

CHAPTER 17

AVIAN ANATOMY AND PHYSIOLOGY

Lori R. Arent

A bird is a unique creature not only in form but also in function. Over time, a body containing specialized structures and organ systems evolved to fill a niche not occupied by any other animal species: the sky. From its outer protective layers to the inner workings of its reproductive system, a bird is designed to fly. Let's take a look at this unique design and explore the wonders of the avian body.

INTEGUMENT

A bird's body is covered by skin and its derivatives: the beak, claws, and feathers. These structures cover and protect the internal organs and block the entrance of disease-causing organisms.

SKIN

The skin of birds consists of two layers: an outer layer called the **epidermis** and an inner layer called the **dermis** (Figure 17-1). The epidermis is relatively thin and consists of flattened epithelial cells that produce **keratin,** a tough fibrous protein necessary for the production of scales, feathers, and the outer sheath of beaks and claws. The inner layer of skin (dermis) is thicker and consists of a tough, fibrous connective tissue. It stores fat for heat insulation and nutrition and supplies a pathway for nerves, blood vessels, and muscles to reach the epidermis. Smooth muscles in the dermis innervate feather follicles to help in the regulation of heat. During hot weather, these depressor muscles press the feathers against the body to promote heat loss. When a bird gets cold or does not feel well, it looks "fluffed" because erector muscles in the dermis elevate the body feathers to trap warm air near the body.

GLANDS

Unlike mammals, birds do not possess sweat glands. Feathers cover such a large portion of a bird's body that sweat glands would not be effective. The one major skin gland that most birds possess is called the **uropygial,** or **preen,** gland. It is located on the dorsal surface at the upper base of the tail. The act of preening stimulates this gland to secrete an oily, fatty substance. A bird uses its beak to spread this oil throughout its feathers to clean and waterproof them. The gland varies in size and structure and is relatively large in aquatic species, such as waterfowl and osprey. The gland is completely lacking in ostriches, some parrots, and in a few other species.

BEAKS

One derivative of a bird's skin is its beak, or bill. It consists of two parts—an upper and lower mandible—and is made of a tough, horny epidermal covering that continually grows. Beaks vary in their hardness and flexibility, depending on their function. Some birds use their beak to tear food into bite-sized

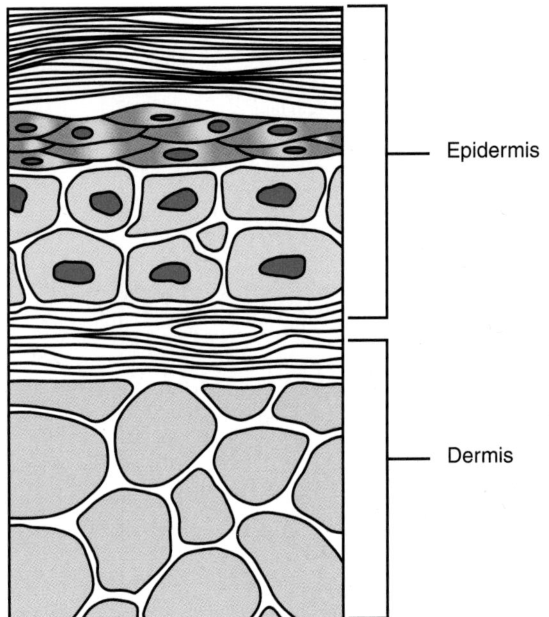

FIGURE **17-1** **Layers of cells in avian skin.**

pieces (hawks), to capture food (herons and woodpeckers), to preen their feathers or those of a mate (parrots and pigeons), to climb (parrots), to pick up and hold things such as food and nesting material as they fly, and sometimes to protect themselves.

CLAWS

Claws possess a horny sheath derived from specialized scales at the end of each toe. Like beaks, they also grow continuously. Species differ in the type of claws they possess, based on their perching habits and method of procuring food. For example, birds of prey have claws called **talons** that are long, sharp, and rounded to catch and kill their prey; vultures, which are scavengers, have short, blunt claws; chickens, pheasants, and other ground feeders have short, sharp claws that are used to scratch the ground for food; and climbing birds, such as woodpeckers and nuthatches, have strongly curved claws for gripping.

TEST YOURSELF

1. What structures are derivatives of a bird's skin and what are they made of?
2. Define the function of the uropygial gland. Do all birds possess this gland?
3. Describe the basic anatomy of a bird's beak and claws. When trimming these structures, what should you be careful to avoid?

FEATHERS

Birds are unique in the animal kingdom in that they possess feathers. Feathers are outgrowths of skin that are made of protein and, once completely developed, are nonliving structures that have sensation only at the base where they originate from a follicle.

CLINICAL APPLICATION: Coping Beaks and Nails

In the wild, the shape and length of a bird's beak and claws are maintained by daily activities that provide natural wear. For example, after completing a meal, birds often **feak** (rub) their beak on a rough surface to clean it and maintain its shape. In captivity, birds are provided with limited wearing surfaces, and their beaks and nails frequently require **coping** (trimming and reshaping). This process must be done with care because both of these structures have a blood and nerve supply that can be hit if they are trimmed excessively. Beaks can be coped using a fingernail file for small birds and a rotary tool for large birds. Claws can be trimmed using a cat or dog nail trimmer, depending on the size of the bird. If bleeding occurs, hemostasis can be achieved by applying topical cauterizing agents, such as silver nitrate or Quick-stop. In parrots, nails are often trimmed with a rotary tool, which immediately cauterizes a blood vessel if it is hit.

Functions

Feathers serve several important functions. First, they are necessary for flight. A bird without a proper complement of flight feathers cannot become airborne. Second, feathers protect the thin skin from trauma, rain, and excessive radiation from sunlight. They also assist in thermoregulation and camouflage and are used in many communication behaviors, such as courtship, defense, and recognition.

Structure

Six types of feathers cover a bird's body. The feather most visibly seen that gives shape to a bird is called a **contour** feather. Contour feathers are the most compact feathers and consist of several components (Figure 17-2).

Inferior Umbilicus. This structure is a tiny opening at the base of the feather where it inserts into the skin. When a new feather is developing, it receives nourishment from blood vessels that pass through this opening.

Superior Umbilicus. This structure is a tiny opening on the feather shaft where the webbed part of the feather begins. In some birds, including several species of herons, hawks, parrots, and grouse, it gives rise to an **afterfeather.** An afterfeather is an accessory feather that is thought to provide additional insulation to retain a bird's body heat.

Calamus. Also called the *quill,* the calamus is the round, hollow, semitransparent portion of a feather that extends from the inferior umbilicus to the superior umbilicus.

Rachis. The rachis is the main feather shaft.

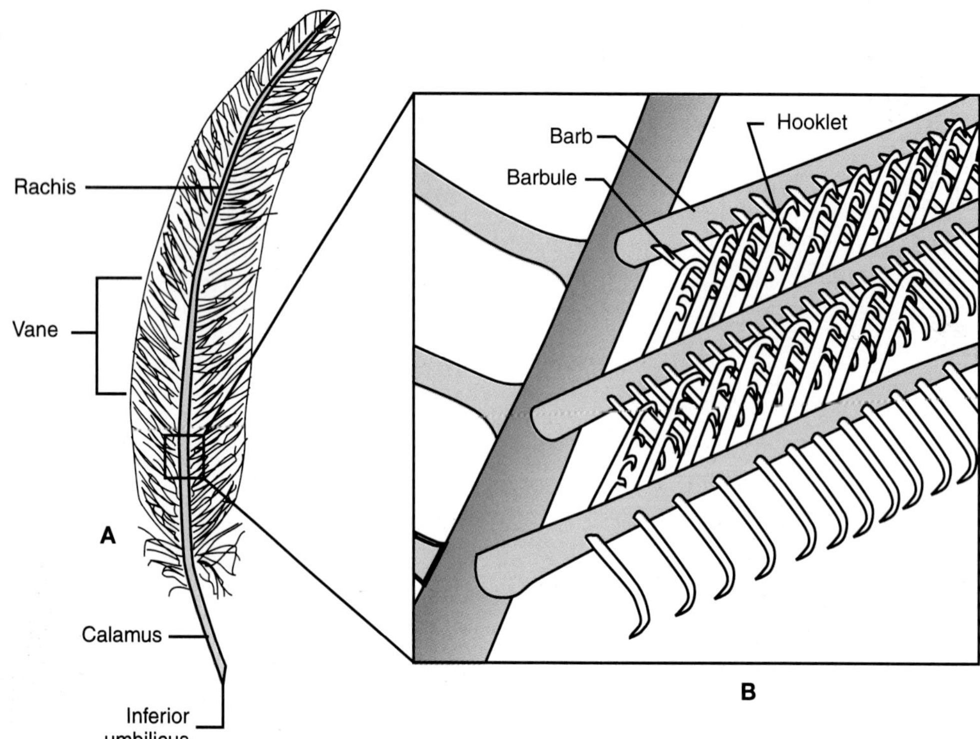

FIGURE 17-2 **Contour Feather. A,** General structure; **B,** microstructure of vane.

Vane. The vane is the flattened part of a feather that appears weblike on each side of the rachis. It consists of numerous slender, closely spaced **barbs.** The barbs give rise to barbules, which have rolled edges and tiny hooklets **(hamuli).** These hooklets interlock each barb with an adjacent one, forming a tightly linked, flexible web (see Figure 17-2, *B*). The degree of tightness varies with the species. For example, the contour feathers of owls have fewer barbules than do those of hawks. The result is a looser feather weave that feels softer and allows air to pass through, creating silent flight.

Types of Feathers

Contour Feathers. Contour feathers typically cover a bird's body and constitute the flight feathers of the wings and tail (Figure 17-3, *A*). The flight feathers in the wing are commonly called **remiges,** and the tail feathers are called **retrices.** Small contour feathers, called **auriculars,** are also found around the external ear openings and apparently improve a bird's hearing ability. They are especially numerous in owls and some species of parrots and hawks. Contour feathers are moved by muscles attached to the walls of the follicles.

Semiplume Feathers. Semiplume feathers possess a main rachis with barbs that lack barbules and hooklets (see Figure 17-3, *B*). They are commonly found under contour feathers, especially on the sides of the abdomen and along the neck and back. Like down feathers, semiplumes provide insulation. They also provide flexibility for the movement of the contour feathers and help with buoyancy in water birds.

Down Feathers. Down feathers are soft, fluffy feathers that lack both a true shaft and barbules and hooklets on their barbs (see Figure 17-3, *C*). They are located next to the skin under contour feathers and function primarily in insulation.

Filoplume Feathers. Filoplume feathers have a bare shaft that lacks barbs on the majority of its length, except at the tip (see Figure 17-3, *D*). They are located on the nape and upper back near contour feathers, and their follicles contain sensitive nerve endings that may play a sensory role in controlling feather movement. Slight movements of the contour feathers are transmitted to pressure and vibration receptors in the skin via the filoplume feathers.

Bristles. Bristles are modified contour feathers with a stiff rachis and few barbs at the base (see Figure 17-3, *E*). They are thought to serve as a sense of touch. Depending on the species, they may be found around the eyes, nostrils (crows, ravens, woodpeckers), mouth (owls), and toes (grouse, some owl species).

Powder Down Feathers. Powder down feathers are unusual feathers that never stop growing. They grow continuously at the base and disintegrate at their tip, creating a waxy powder that is spread throughout the rest of the plumage to clean it and provide waterproofing. They are most highly developed in herons and bitterns, especially on the breast, belly, and back, and can be found more diffusely scattered in hawks and parrots. Birds without a uropygial gland have abundant powder down feathers.

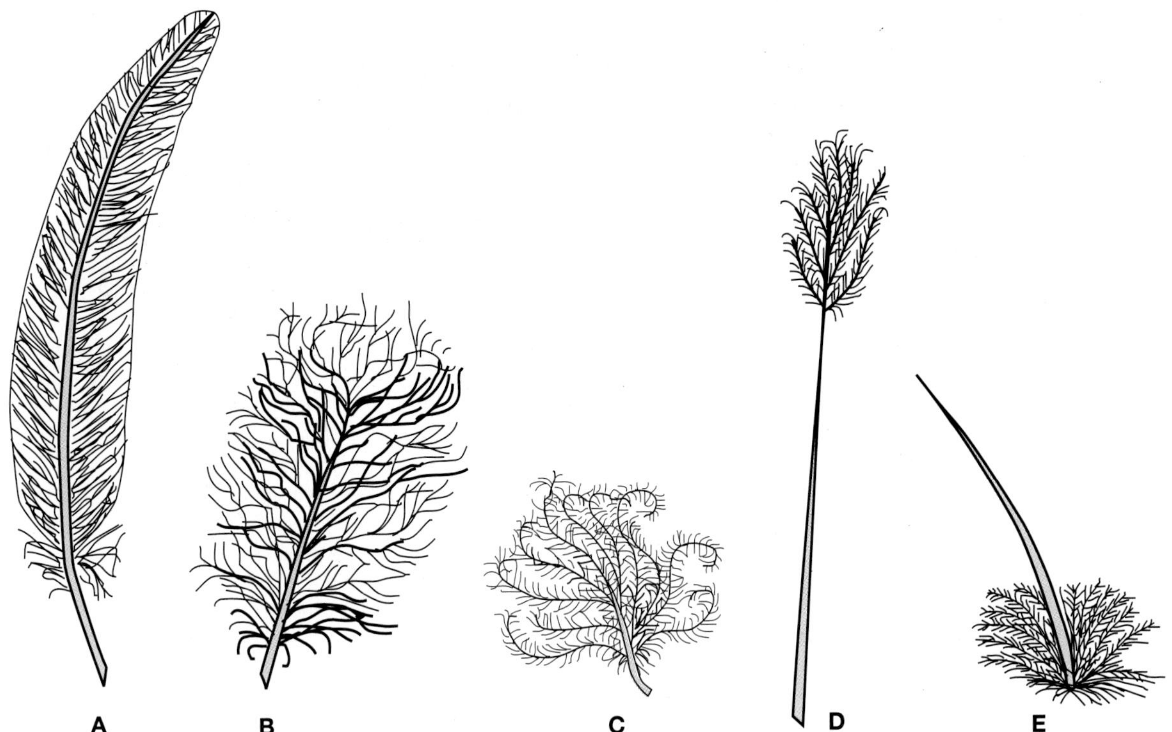

FIGURE **17-3** **Types of Feathers. A,** Contour; **B,** semiplume; **C,** down; **D,** filoplume; **E,** bristle.

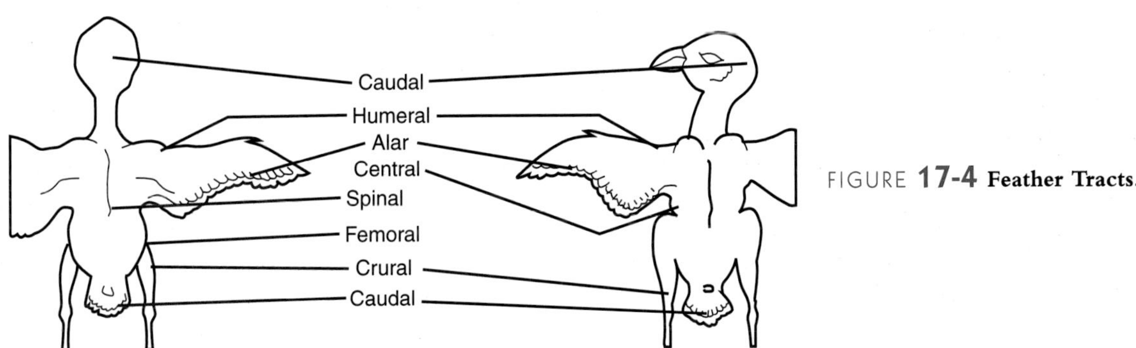

FIGURE **17-4** **Feather Tracts.**

Location

Contrary to their appearance, feathers do not originate from the entire body. They are located in seven tracts, called **pterylae,** which are separated by bare areas of skin called **apteria** (Figure 17-4). However, the feathers in these tracts overlap one another to create the fully feathered look.

Feather Damage

Feathers are durable structures but still can be damaged. External parasites, such as some species of feather mites, can chew and consume parts of the feather vanes, creating weak points (Figure 17-5). Damage also can occur from daily wear and tear. Often, the lighter tips of a bird's flight and tail feathers are worn off by the roughness of daily activities, giving a bird's feathers a more iridescent appearance. In some species, such as mallard ducks and starlings, this is most noticeable in the spring, when males of many species have lost their light feather tips and look more colorful before the breeding season.

Another cause of feather damage occurs during a feather's growth phase. If a feather is stressed during its growth, even for a day, the rachis is pinched off, deleting its blood supply. What develops is called a **fault bar** (stress bar), which is characterized by a weakened area on the feather vane where the barbs lack barbules. When the stressor is removed, the blood supply is returned and normal development continues. The most common stressor is a poor diet. An insufficient food supply or a food supply deficient in essential nutrients often creates fault bars on developing feathers. This can have a severe effect on the plumage of nestling birds because all of their flight feathers grow in at the same time. Any stressor that temporarily deletes the blood supply to these feathers creates fault bars on all of them.

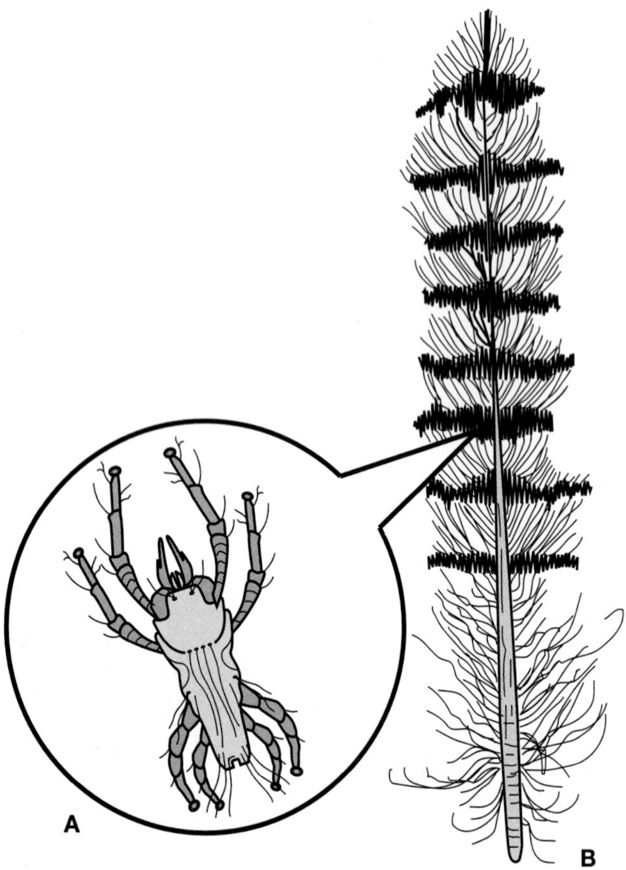

FIGURE **17-5** **A,** Feather mite (not drawn to scale). **B,** Damaged feather.

CLINICAL APPLICATION — Feather-Picking Disorder

One condition seen in many species of psittacines and some human-imprinted raptors is feather picking. Birds with this disorder preen excessively, removing most to all of their body feathers, especially on their chest and legs. Also, in severe cases, the skin surrounding the feathers is self-mutilated.

Causes of this disorder are either pathological or psychological. In the first category, toxins, bacteria, viruses, fungi, parasites, and malnutrition all can lead to feather picking. To determine the cause, a thorough physical examination must be conducted. Radiographs, blood samples for complete blood count and serum chemistry, cytology of feather pulp or of a local skin scraping, feather biopsy, and endoscopy are all diagnostic tools that can be used. If the problem does not appear to be physiological, then attention must be turned to psychological causes. These may include changes in the environment, diet, human exposure, boredom, sexual frustration, anxiety, or exposure to new pets. Many species of parrots, especially African Greys, are very sensitive to these types of conditions.

Treatments for the disorder vary with the cause. Bacterial, viral, parasitic, and fungal infections can be treated with established protocols, and diet can be improved and varied. However, treatment for psychological causes is more difficult, especially if the disorder cannot be attributed to a specific event or situation. Most often, changing components of the care and management of the bird is required, with no guarantee of inhibiting the feather-picking behavior.

TEST YOURSELF

1. List three major functions of feathers.
2. What type of feathers are the flight and tail feathers? Describe their microstructure.
3. Define a fault bar. What causes it?

Molting

The process of feather replacement is called **molting,** and it occurs once to several times a year depending on the species. Molting occurs in a species-specific pattern that allows a bird to continue normal activities, such as procuring food, escaping from predators, reproducing, and finding safe roosting sites. In most species, feather replacement is symmetrical with one or two pairs of flight feathers molted at a time so that a bird still can fly adequately. One major exception is found in many species of waterfowl, which molt their flight feathers all at once after the breeding season. They are flightless during this time but can forage by grazing on land or in the water.

Between 4% and 12% of a bird's body weight is made up of feathers (Pettingill, 1972). Replacing them is a very energy-demanding process that requires a well-balanced diet. In many North American species, the major annual molt is timed so that it occurs between the end of the breeding season and the beginning of migration. Food is usually abundant during this time, and a bird's energy can be directed to its growing feathers.

Feathers develop from papillae in the dermis layer of the skin (Figure 17-6, *A*). These papillae are located in the feather tracts and contain germ cells with the genetic information that dictates the type, size, and color of feathers. These cells are "activated" by physiological and environmental factors. Increasing day length stimulates the pituitary and thyroid glands to produce hormones that stimulate molting, and sex hormones also may play a concurrent role.

Molting begins when a newly developing feather pushes an old one out (Figure 17-6, *B*). It then emerges from the skin and is covered by an epidermal covering called the **periderm.** As a bird begins to preen a growing feather, it gently removes the periderm, which can be seen as small, white flakes in the plumage. Blood vessels from the dermis reach into the new feather to provide nourishment. When a feather is fully grown, the blood dries up and the rachis is pinched closed under the skin.

During feather development, a growing feather is called a **blood feather.** Blood can be seen in the proximal part of the feather shaft during the entire growth phase. Injury to a blood feather not only results in bleeding but can prevent a feather from developing normally until molted again.

A

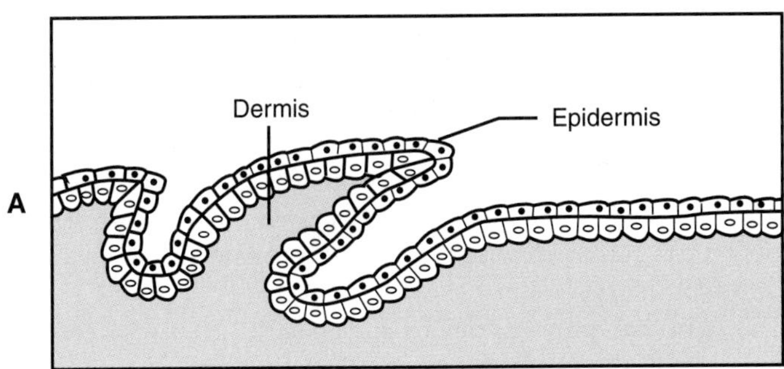

B

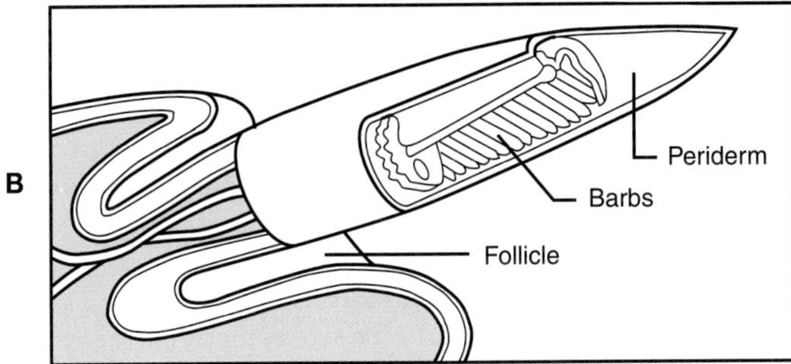

FIGURE **17-6** **Stages of Feather Growth. A,** Feather papilla. **B,** Newly developing feather.

MUSCULOSKELETAL SYSTEM

Feathers are not the only components of a bird that make it unique. A mammal or reptile with feathers still could not fly. Specially designed body systems that complement the feathers are necessary to create a structure that can support aerial locomotion. The first two systems we are going to look at are the musculature and skeleton.

MUSCLES

The average bird has anywhere from 175 to 200 muscles, most of which are paired, located on each side of the body. To allow for flight, many of these muscles have been placed ventrally, near the center of gravity. Reptiles, the avian predecessor, have muscles on their dorsal surface. In birds, these have been replaced with strong "plates" of fused vertebrae, which protect the skeleton during contraction of the powerful flight muscles.

Classification

As in other animals, the muscles of birds are classified as smooth or striated and voluntary or involuntary. Many of the muscles that contain smooth muscle fibers are also involuntary, stimulating the movement of the internal organs. Many muscles with striated fibers are skeletal (associated with bone movement) and are under voluntary control. Cardiac muscle is also striated but has its own intrinsic rhythm that does not require external innervation.

The skeletal muscles of birds can have white or red muscle fibers. Some muscles consist primarily of one type or the other, but many have a mixture of both. People celebrating the Thanksgiving holiday with a traditional turkey dinner are familiar with these fibers as they are often referred to as the "light meat" and "dark meat," respectively. White fibers are thick in diameter, have a low blood supply and little myoglobin (for carrying oxygen), and use stores of glycogen to sustain muscle contraction. They predominate in the flight muscles of short-distance fliers, such as chickens, quail, grouse, and many

CLINICAL APPLICATION — Clipping Wing Feathers

Many pet bird owners desire to have their bird's flight feathers clipped so that it cannot fly. This prevents a bird from injuring itself when out of its cage and prevents accidental escape. Numerous pet birds are lost every year because they fly out open doors and windows.

Two major patterns can be used to clip a bird's wings. The one chosen depends on the owner's wishes and the personal preference of the clinician. The first technique leaves the outer two to four primary flight feathers intact and then trims the next four to six flight feathers underneath the overlying covert feathers. This method hides the trimmed ends and provides a smooth look to the wing. The second technique trims the outermost five to seven flight feathers, again under the overlying coverts. This approach also provides a smooth appearance to the wing and does not leave the outer primaries long, which leaves them vulnerable to breakage. Whichever technique is used, the clipping should be done symmetrically on both wings.

Another consideration in feather clipping involves the presence of blood feathers. If blood feathers are present, it is advisable to wait until those feathers are completely developed before any are trimmed. If blood feathers are cut or damaged, a significant amount of bleeding often occurs. If waiting is not an option, completely developed feathers can be trimmed such that one feather remains intact on each side of every blood feather. Intact feathers on each side are needed to protect a growing feather from injury.

CLINICAL APPLICATION — Treating a Damaged Blood Feather

If a developing feather is cut, nicked, or otherwise damaged, it will often bleed profusely. To treat minor nicks or cuts, pressure can be applied to the affected area and, when dry, Quick-stop applied to ensure coagulation. In *pet birds,* if more severe injury to a feather occurs, the best way to treat it is often to gently pull out the feather and pack the skin opening with Quick-stop. However, because developing feathers have a good nerve supply, anesthetizing the patient may be appropriate before pulling a large feather to prevent pain or discomfort. If bleeding is persistent after a feather is pulled, the skin opening can be sutured closed for a few days to promote hemostasis, but it should be reopened to allow normal healing and new feather growth to begin. In some *wild bird* species, such as birds of prey, pulling a flight or tail feather can result in permanent follicle damage, preventing a new feather from ever growing in. In these species, the proper approach is to stop the bleeding and allow a damaged feather to be removed naturally by the bird or during its normal molt cycle.

other gallinaceous birds that have rapid takeoffs but are capable of only short flights. If these birds are forced to fly repetitively, they quickly become fatigued and cannot fly at all until they recover. In contrast, red fibers are thinner and have a rich supply of blood, fat, myoglobin, and mitochondria. Using these components, they can produce enough energy to sustain muscle contractions for long periods. Red fibers are found in the flight muscles of long-distance fliers, including many species of songbirds, waterbirds, pigeons, and birds of prey.

Wing Muscles

Wings possess several pairs of muscles that are each responsible for a specific action or counteraction: raising or depressing the leading edge of the wing, pulling the wing forward or backward, extending or flexing the wing, or controlling movements of the alula bone (thumb) (Figure 17-7). However, the two most prominent muscle pairs are those responsible for depressing and elevating the wing. Both pairs originate on the sternum but differ in where they insert (Figure 17-8). The larger, more superficial muscle is called the **pectoralis,** and it inserts on the underside of the humerus. When it contracts, it depresses the wing, causing the downstroke. This stroke requires a large muscle because it works against two resistant forces: gravity and a tight wing structure formed when the leading edge of each flight feather touches the adjacent feather. Because of its relatively large size and accessibility, the pectoralis is the muscle of choice for administering intramuscular injections (such as vitamins and antibiotics).

The smaller, deeper flight muscle is called the **supracoracoideus;** it turns into a tendon that passes through a cavity formed by the shoulder girdle and inserts on top of the humerus. When it contracts, it causes the counteraction, that is, elevation of the wing (upstroke). During this stroke, the flight feathers slightly separate from each other, allowing air to pass through. This creates less resistance and allows the wing to move more easily. In strong, long-distance fliers, the two pairs of flight muscles constitute between 20% and 25% of a bird's weight.

Leg Muscles

Like the wing muscles, the leg muscles also have been moved close to the center of gravity. The majority are located in the thigh region over the femur, a smaller number are located over the tibiotarsus, and very few are found over the tarsometatarsus (Figure 17-9). The large group of muscles over the femur can control movements in the distal leg and toes via strong tendons. For example, in perching species, tendons that control movement of the toes originate from flexor muscles in the thigh and extend over the heel joint into the digits. Extensor tendons run down the front of the tibiotarsus and metatarsus, whereas the flexor tendons run along the back. The flexor tendons sit in a grove at the top of the metatarsus. When a bird bends its legs to perch, the tendons also bend and pull the toes closed around the perch. This is called the **perching reflex** and allows a bird to firmly grip its perch while sleeping.

Muscles of the Head and Neck

The most pronounced muscles of the head are the jaw muscles, which control the beak. The extent of this musculature varies among species and is generally correlated with a bird's diet. For example, species that use their beaks to crack open large, coarse seeds and nuts (parrots) have relatively large and strong jaw muscles compared with species that consume smaller seeds (doves) or insects.

A bird has great flexibility in its neck. It has several thin, stringy muscles, some of which are subdivided, weave through each other, and allow movement in different directions. Others are attached to the connective tissue (fascia) of adjacent neck muscles. When one muscle is stimulated, neighboring muscles contract, making a variety of movements possible. For example, young raptors often turn their heads upside down to get a better view of their subject, and parrots move theirs up and down, left and right, and many combinations thereof.

One highly specialized neck muscle in birds is referred to as a "hatching muscle." This muscle, located on the dorsal side of a chick's head, develops during the embryonic stage and is needed to help a chick break out of its shell. It is largest a day or two before hatching, and once a chick reaches the outside world, it rapidly atrophies.

Skeleton

Although muscles do the work to create specific movements, they must be supported by a sturdy framework (Figure 17-10). In birds, this framework is highly specialized because it must support two very different modes of locomotion: walking and flying. As we will see, the special design of the avian skeleton includes many unique features that all contribute to the creation of a remarkably lightweight but sturdy structure. The lightweight nature of the skeleton was a key component in the evolution of flight and can be explained by several general modifications:

1. Reduction in the number of bones
2. Fusion of bones to form plates that provide strength and simplify movements
3. Reduction in the density of bones, which are relatively thin but strengthened by a network of internal bony braces
4. Loss of internal bone matrix (bones are generally hollow and filled with air spaces)

Additional features of the avian skeleton that contribute to its light weight can be seen throughout its structure. To study these, we can divide the skeletal components into two major sections, the axial skeleton and the appendicular skeleton. The bones that provide the general framework of the avian body include the skull, vertebral column, and sternum and are collectively called the **axial skeleton.** The wings, shoulder bones, legs, and pelvic bones support locomotion and are collectively called the **appendicular skeleton.**

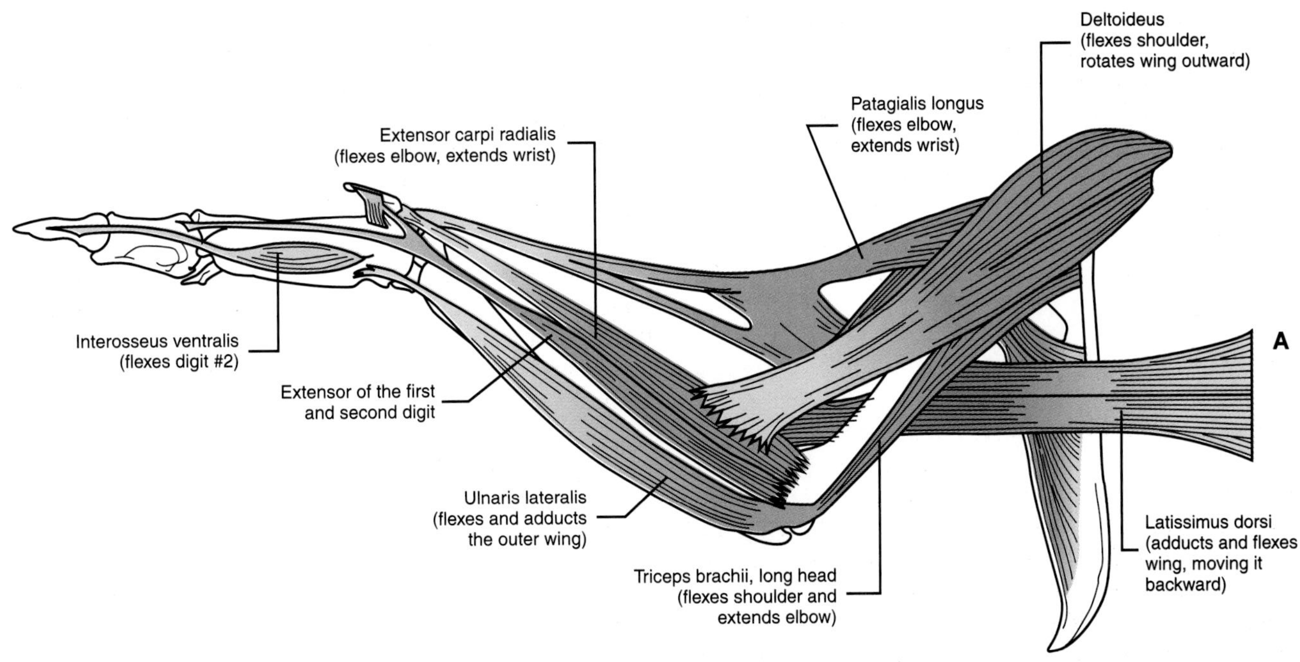
Deltoideus
(flexes shoulder,
rotates wing outward)
Patagialis longus
(flexes elbow,
extends wrist)
Extensor carpi radialis
(flexes elbow, extends wrist)
Interosseus ventralis
(flexes digit #2)
Extensor of the first
and second digit
A
Ulnaris lateralis
(flexes and adducts
the outer wing)
Triceps brachii, long head
(flexes shoulder and
extends elbow)
Latissimus dorsi
(adducts and flexes
wing, moving it
backward)

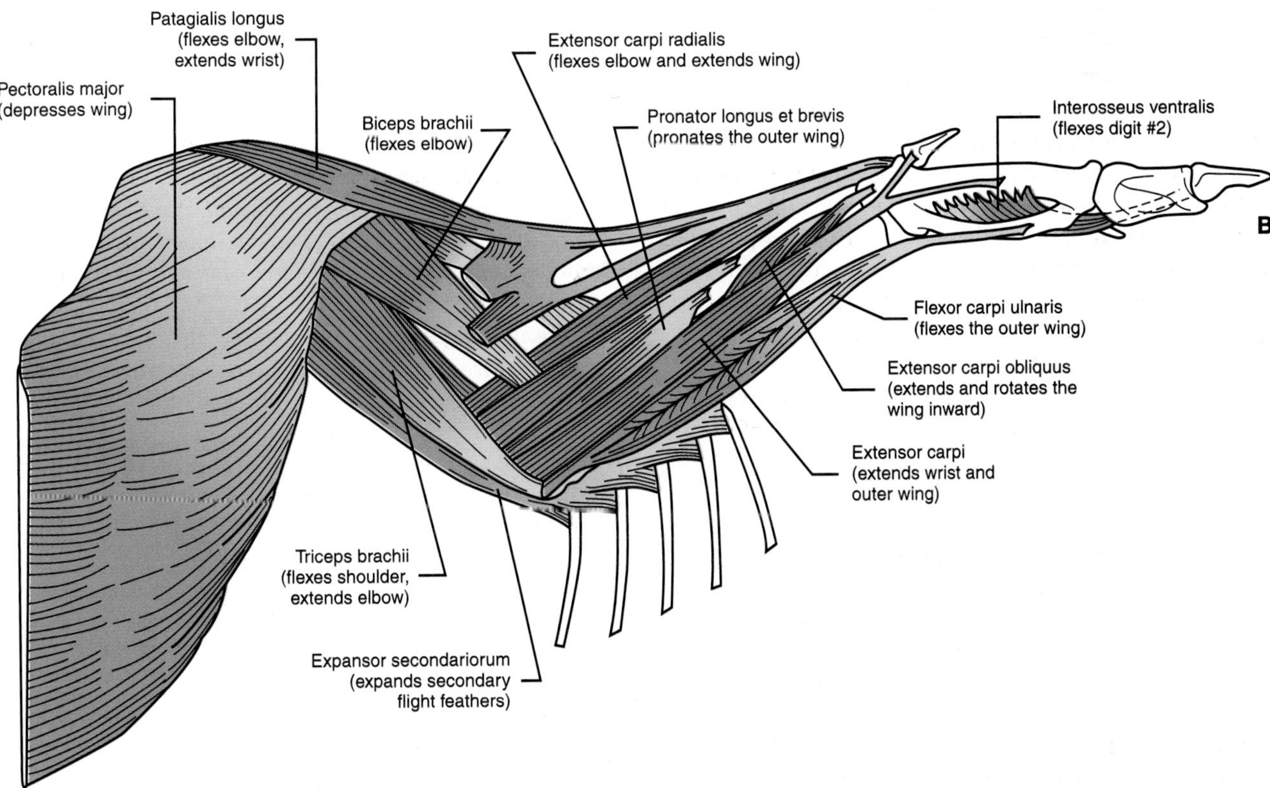
Patagialis longus
(flexes elbow,
extends wrist)
Pectoralis major
(depresses wing)
Extensor carpi radialis
(flexes elbow and extends wing)
Biceps brachii
(flexes elbow)
Pronator longus et brevis
(pronates the outer wing)
Interosseus ventralis
(flexes digit #2)
B
Flexor carpi ulnaris
(flexes the outer wing)
Extensor carpi obliquus
(extends and rotates the
wing inward)
Extensor carpi
(extends wrist and
outer wing)
Triceps brachii
(flexes shoulder,
extends elbow)
Expansor secondariorum
(expands secondary
flight feathers)

FIGURE **17-7** **Wing Muscles and Their Function. A,** Dorsal view; **B,** ventral view.

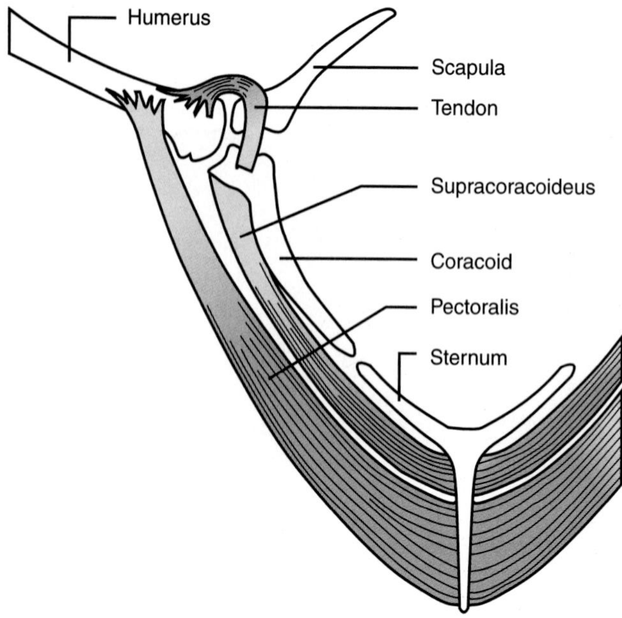

FIGURE **17-8** **Cross Section Through Bird's Flight Muscles.** Shows points of origin and insertion.

Axial Skeleton

Skull. The bird skull possesses several adaptations for lightness (Figure 17-11). Instead of supporting heavy teeth, the jaws extend into a keratinized bill, and the bones of the skull are thinner than in other animals. The shape of the bill varies with the species, and it consists of a lower and upper component. The lower bill hinges on two small, movable bones called the **quadrates.** The upper bill has a somewhat flexible attachment to the skull and can move although slightly. Thus birds actually can move their upper and lower bills independently, which gives them greater control in manipulating food and increases the size of their gape.

Another prominent feature of the skull is the eye sockets. Good vision is important for an aerial creature, and thus a large portion of a bird's skull is devoted to supporting and protecting the eyes. The avian skull has large eye sockets that are bordered by a ring of protective bony plates called the **sclerotic ring.** In most species, a relatively small portion of the skull is devoted to the olfactory system, and as we will later see, the size of the ear canal varies with the species and its lifestyle.

Vertebral Column. The vertebral column of birds is similar to that of other animals in that it consists of five general groups of vertebrae: cervical, thoracic, lumbar, sacral, and coccygeal. Birds have fewer vertebrae than other animals in the three central regions but more vertebrae in the cervical and coccygeal areas, allowing greater mobility of their neck and tail, respectively.

Cervical Vertebrae. The first cervical vertebrae, the **atlas,** contains a single **condyle** (ball and socket type of structure) for attachment of the skull. This allows a greater range of head movements as compared with mammals, which have two condyles attaching the skull to the vertebral column. In addition, birds have more cervical vertebrae than mammals, ranging from 11 (parakeets) to 25 (swans), whereas all mammals have 7. In birds, these vertebrae have special connecting surfaces that allow movement, thus contributing to the flexibility of their necks.

Thoracic Vertebrae. The thoracic vertebrae are rigid and provide a strong support for the rib cage. In birds, the first few ribs are relatively short and incomplete. The other ribs are complete, attach to the underside of the sternum, and possess a projection called the **uncinate process** that overlaps the adjoining rear rib to strengthen the rib cage (see Figure 17-10). One exception to the rigidity of these vertebrae is found in penguins, which swim like fish and require a great degree of flexibility in their backs.

Lumbar and Sacral Vertebrae. These two groups of vertebrae are also rigid. Several of the distal lumbar vertebrae fuse with the sacral vertebrae and first few coccygeal vertebrae to form a light, strong, bony plate called the **synsacrum.** This plate in turn fuses with the pelvis to provide a stiff framework for support of the legs. When a bird lands, the synsacrum acts as a shock absorber to protect the legs and backbone from injury.

Coccygeal Vertebrae. Birds have an average of 12 coccygeal vertebrae. The first few are mobile to allow movement of the tail feathers during flight. The rest are fused into a bony structure called the **pygostyle** that supports the tail feathers.

Sternum. In most species of birds, the sternum is large and concave. It not only protects the chest from traumatic injuries but also acts as the place of origin of the flight muscles. In strong fliers, the sternum has a large bony ridge, or **keel,** to which the muscles attach. In flightless birds, such as the ostrich, the sternum lacks a keel entirely.

Appendicular Skeleton

Pectoral Girdle. The pectoral (shoulder) girdle consists of three pairs of bones: the coracoids, scapulas, and clavicles (Figure 17-12). On each side, the coracoid and scapula are joined, forming a depression called the **glenoid cavity.** The wing attaches to the body by forming a joint in this cavity. During contraction of the powerful flight muscles, the strong, broad coracoids help to protect the sternum, and the scapulas, positioned along the backbone, help protect the rib cage. The clavicles, also known as the *wishbone,* are positioned outward and forward from the body and keep a bird's shoulders separated.

Wings. The wings are connected to the body by forming a joint with the shoulder girdle (Figure 17-13). This joint is highly flexible, allowing rotation of the wing in several planes. The **humerus** extends from the shoulder to the elbow joint

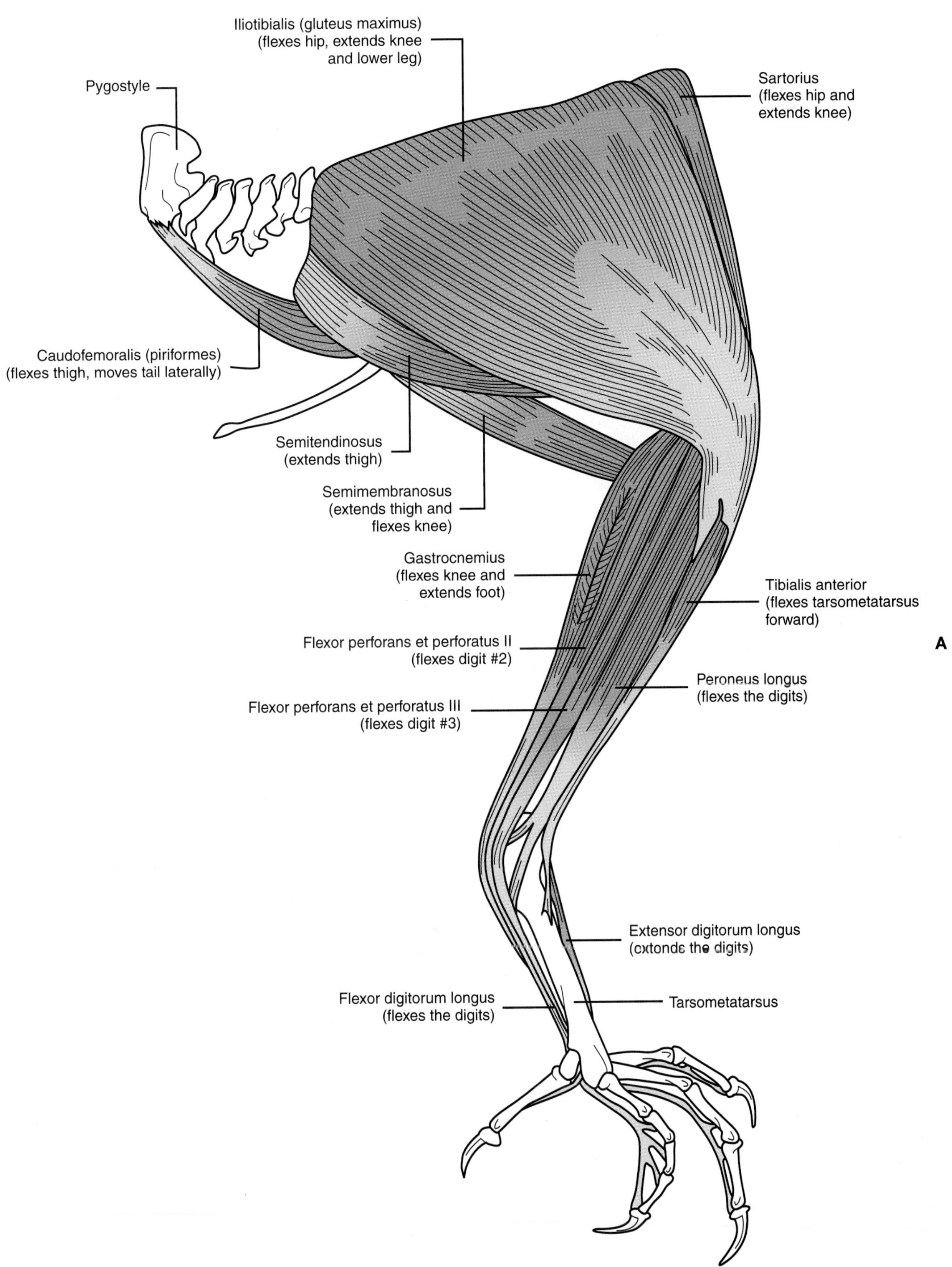

FIGURE **17-9 Leg Muscles and Their Function. A,** Lateral view.

Continued

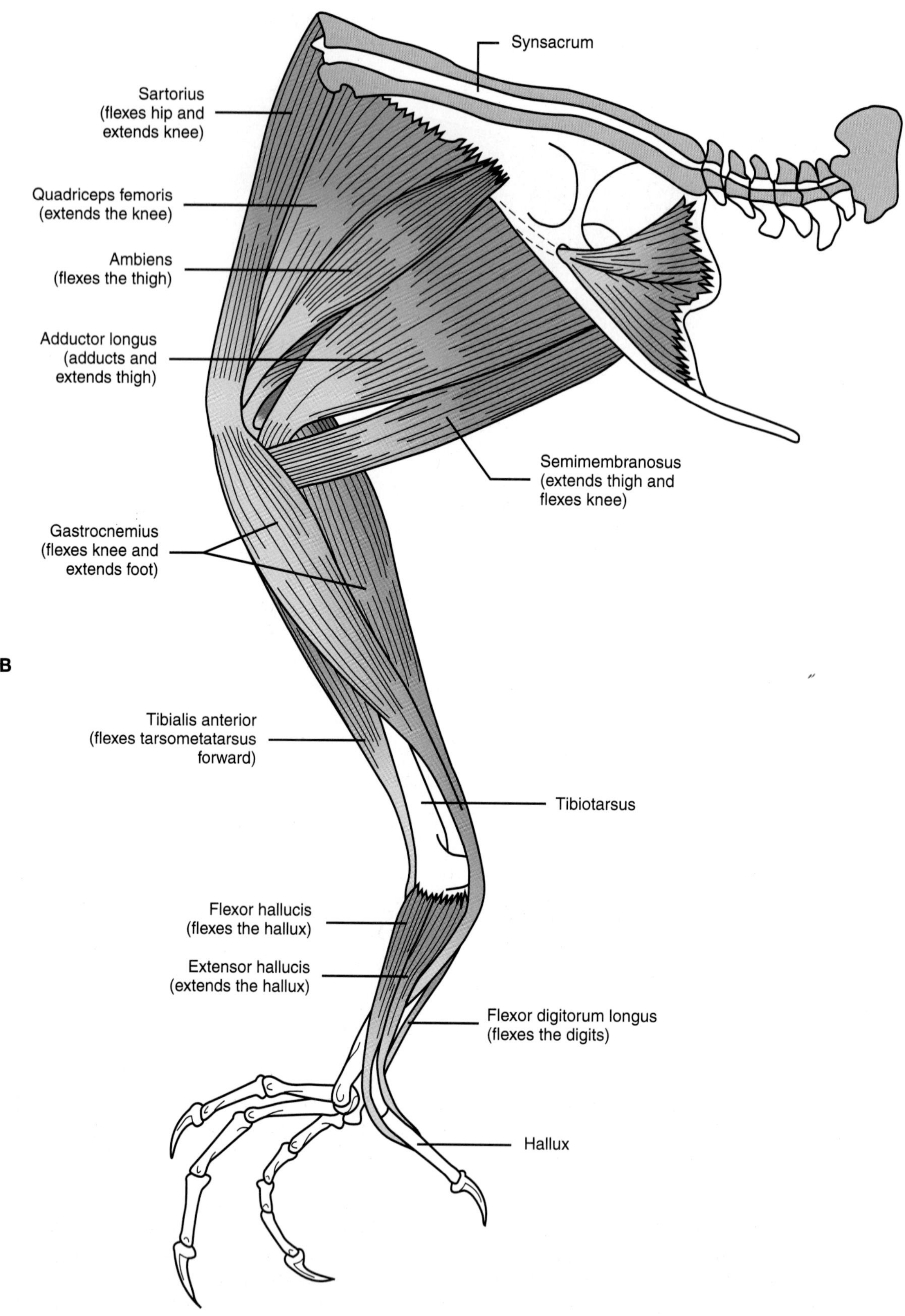
Synsacrum
Sartorius
(flexes hip and
extends knee)
Quadriceps femoris
(extends the knee)
Ambiens
(flexes the thigh)
Adductor longus
(adducts and
extends thigh)
Semimembranosus
(extends thigh and
flexes knee)
Gastrocnemius
(flexes knee and
extends foot)
B
Tibialis anterior
(flexes tarsometatarsus
forward)
Tibiotarsus
Flexor hallucis
(flexes the hallux)
Extensor hallucis
(extends the hallux)
Flexor digitorum longus
(flexes the digits)
Hallux

FIGURE **17-9, cont'd** **B,** Medial view.

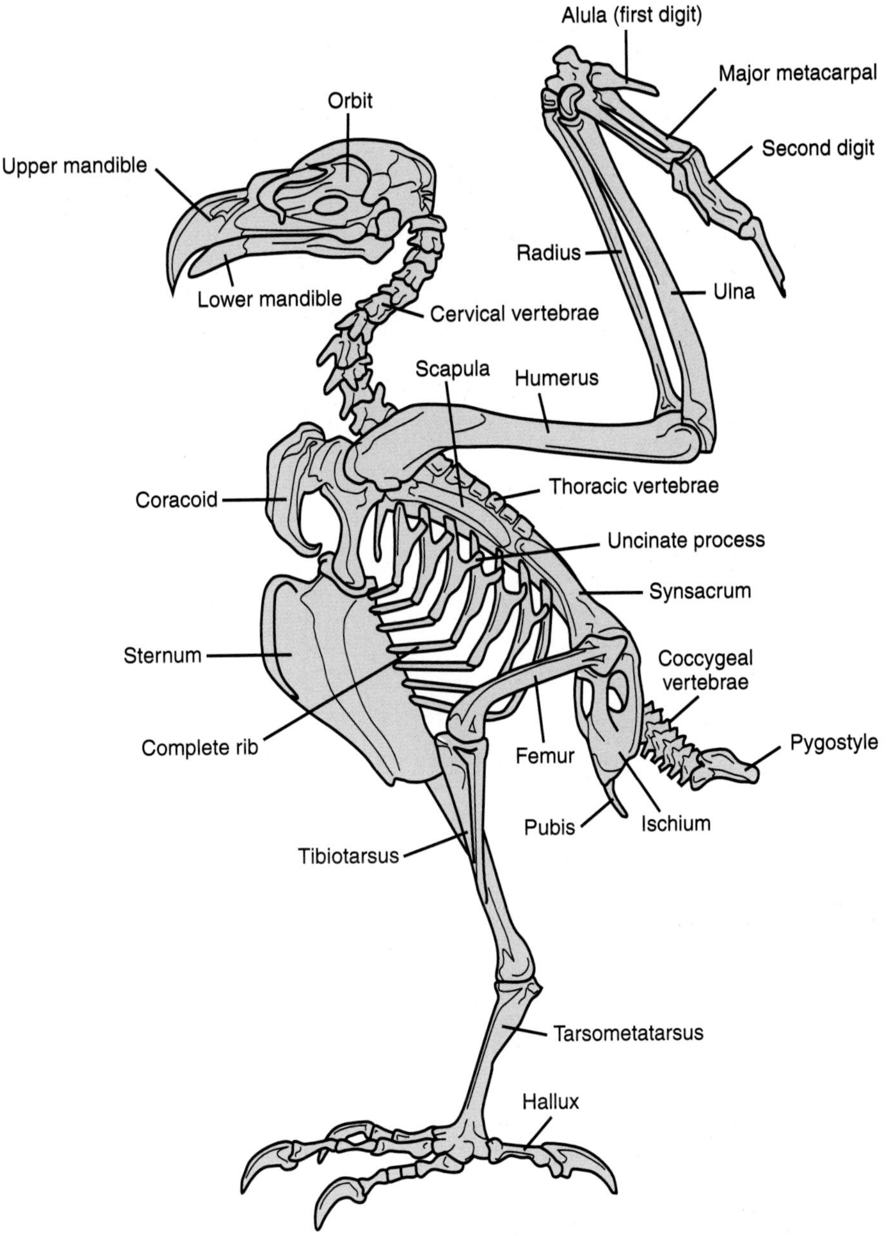

FIGURE **17-10 Skeleton of Hawk.**

and possesses a **deltoid crest** for attachment of wing muscles. Its length varies among species, being relatively short in birds that depend primarily on flapping flight and relatively long in birds that glide and soar.

The elbow joint is less flexible than the shoulder, allowing wing movement only parallel to the wing. The **radius** and **ulna** extend from this joint to the wrist. In birds, the ulna has a larger diameter than the radius and acts as an attachment point for the secondary flight feathers. These two bones create the forearm of the wing and slide past each other slightly during flight.

Extending from the shoulder to the wrist is a web of skin called the **patagium.** This skin is lightly vascularized and possesses a tendon that runs along its cranial edge. It provides elasticity to the wing and assists in the aerodynamics of flight. If a bird damages it patagium, it may be grounded permanently.

The wrist joint consists of two bones and, like the elbow, allows movement only in the plane of the wing. The first finger, called the **alula** bone, originates from the wrist and carries the alula feathers, which are important for steering. The **major** and **minor metacarpal** bones extend from the wrist and join with the second and third fingers near the distal end of the wing. These two fingers, along with the metacarpal bones, support the primary flight feathers.

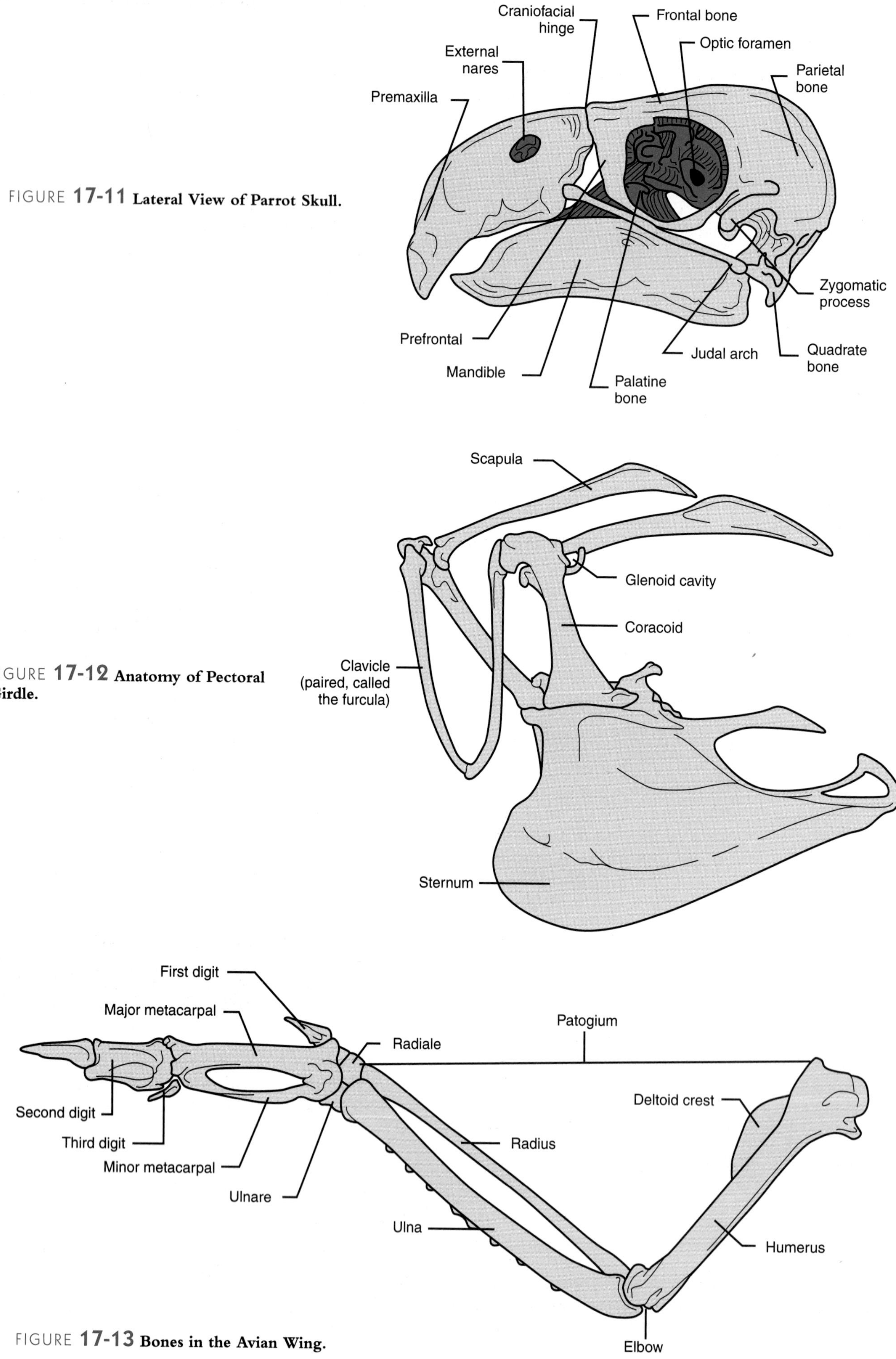

FIGURE **17-11** **Lateral View of Parrot Skull.**

FIGURE **17-12** **Anatomy of Pectoral Girdle.**

FIGURE **17-13** **Bones in the Avian Wing.**

Pelvic Girdle. The pelvic girdle provides a rigid framework for support of the legs (Figure 17-14). Each side is made up of three bones that join where the leg attaches to the body. The **ileum** is relatively broad and fused to the synsacrum. The **ischium** and **pubis** are thin and long, are fused to the ileum anteriorly, and are directed rearward, parallel to the backbone. The distal ends of these three bones are not fused, leaving the lower part of the pelvis open. This provides room for the abdomen and facilitates egg laying in hens.

Legs. The hip joint in birds is well hidden by thigh muscles and is the place where the **femur** attaches to the pelvis (see Figure 17-14). The femur is often referred to as the *drumstick* and is relatively short but wide. It ends at the knee joint, where it is directed a little forward so that the lower part of a bird's leg is placed under its center of gravity. Similar to the deltoid crest of the humerus, the femur possesses two crests called the **greater** and **lesser trochanters**, where leg muscles attach. Two bones are located in the middle section of the leg and are called the **tibiotarsus** and **fibula.** The fibula is relatively small in diameter and acts as a splint. These two bones end at the **ankle** or **hock** joint, and the ankle itself consists of a single, elongated bone called the **tarsometatarsus.**

Feet. The bottom of a bird's foot is called the **metatarsal pad.** It is surrounded by two, three, or four toes, with the majority of species possessing four. Often, one toe faces the rear, and the other three face forward **(anisodactyl).** However, in some species, such as parrots and woodpeckers, the second and third toes face forward, and the first and fourth are directed backward **(zygodactyl).** Owls, osprey, and cuckoos also have this arrangement, but the fourth toe is opposable and can face either forward or backward.

The digits are referred to by a numbering system based on the number of joints they have. The rear toe is digit number one and has one joint. Digit two is the innermost (medial) digit and possesses two joints. The middle toe is digit three with three joints, and the outer (lateral) toe with four joints is digit four.

TEST YOURSELF

1. Name a feather disorder commonly seen in captive parrots. What are two possible causes of this disease?
2. List the two types of skeletal muscle fibers and describe their energy use.
3. Why can a bird perch while sleeping?
4. Describe the attachment of the skull to the vertebral column. What does this type of attachment provide?
5. List the bones in the avian wing from the shoulder to the wing tip.
6. List the bones in the avian leg beginning at the hip and extending down to the toes.

From the tip of a bird's bill all the way down to the tips of its toes, a bird's bone and muscle structures are designed to provide a framework that can support an aerial creature. Now, let's take a peek at the organ systems that actually drive this incredible flying machine.

SENSE ORGANS

The phrase "bird brain" has been used in reference to a lack of intelligence and therefore a small brain. This is very misleading because, in fact, the avian brain is proportionately large to its body, compared with the brains of all other vertebrates, with the exception of mammals. The location of the brain and control centers within the brain that receive nervous stimuli from the senses are similar to mammals (see Chapter 7). In birds, the control centers for vision and hearing are relatively large, whereas those for taste, touch, and smell are relatively small (Figure 17-15).

VISION

The phrase "I'm going to watch you like a hawk" alludes to the fact that the sense of vision is highly developed in birds. An aerial creature needs good vision to fly at variable speeds, find food, escape predators, identify individuals, and participate in courtship rituals. The optic lobes take up the majority of the midbrain, and a large part of the avian skull is devoted to housing and protecting the eyes. The shape of the eye is determined by the orbits. Unlike mammals, which all have round eyes, bird eyes can be round, flat, or tubular, depending on the species. Generally, diurnal birds have round or relatively flat eyes (hawks and swans, respectively), whereas nocturnal species (owls) have tubular eyes (Figure 17-16). In tubular eyes, the diameter of the pupil is larger relative to the size of the retina, and thus more light can be gathered. The eyes fill the eye sockets, leaving little room for muscles or movement.

In birds, the position of the eyes on the head differs among species and appears to depend on their feeding habits. For example, seedeaters and grain eaters have eyes placed laterally

CLINICAL APPLICATION **Diagnosing a Coracoid Fracture**

A cockatiel is presented to the clinic after it flew into a kitchen window. The problem is that now the bird only can fly short distances. It has full extension of its wings but a slight wing droop at rest on its left side. Its flight feathers are intact, and it has a good amount of muscle on its keel. Palpation of the wings reveals no bruising or fractures. Now what? A radiograph is the next logical next step. Often, when birds have head-on collisions, they fracture one of their coracoid bones and only can fly short distances. Wing extension is normal; however, a slight wing droop often occurs, and blood is often found in the back of the mouth. Extremely displaced bone ends may require surgical repair, but most often, immobilizing the wing on the injured side for about 3 weeks, followed by another week of cage rest, allows the bone to heal adequately.

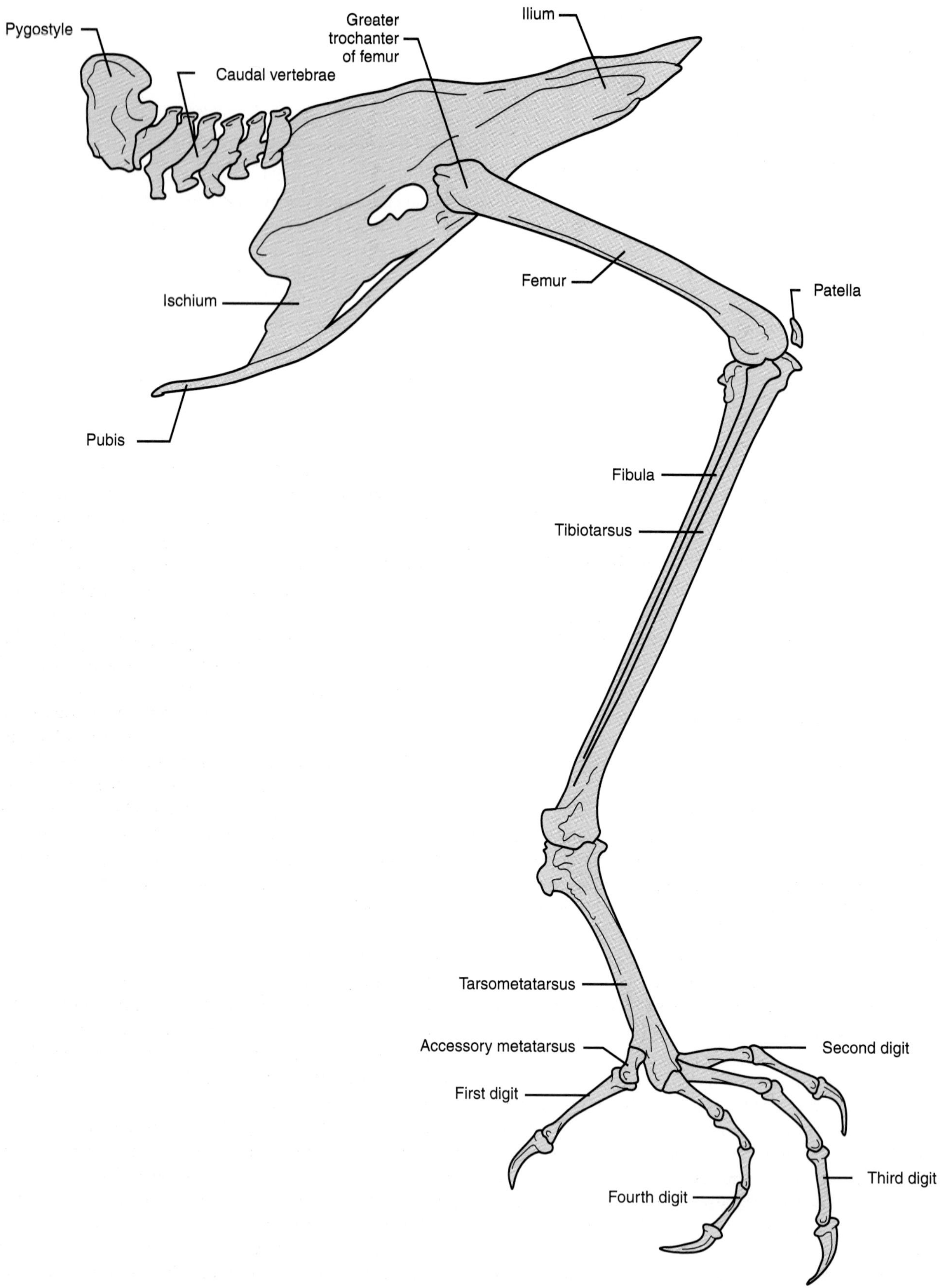

FIGURE **17-14** **Anatomy of the Pelvic Girdle and Leg Bones.** Lateral view.

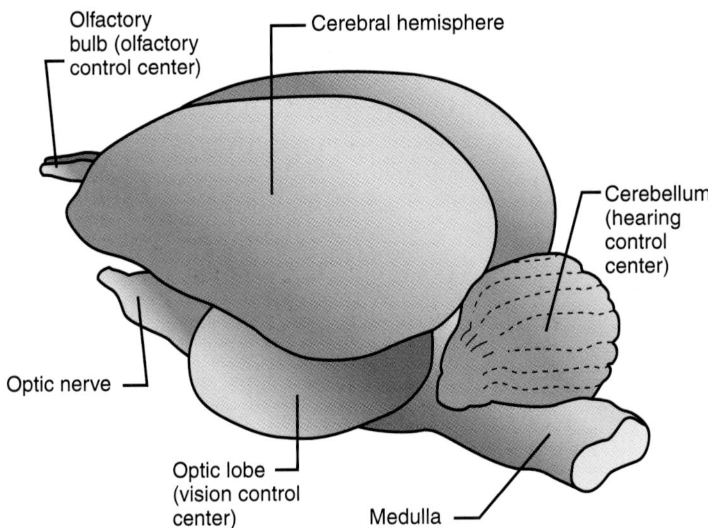

FIGURE **17-15** **Side View of a Bird's Brain.**

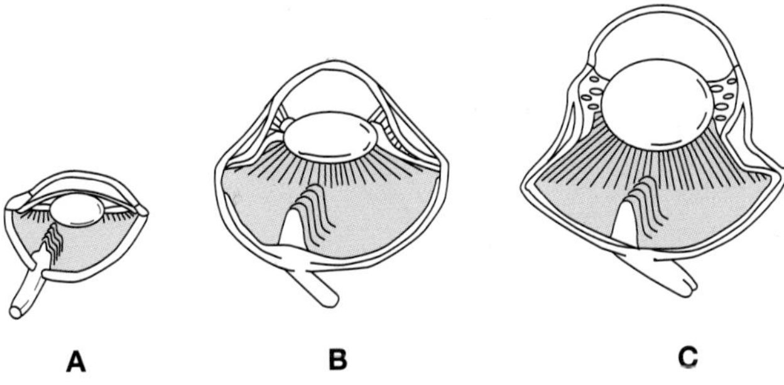

FIGURE **17-16** **Shapes of the Avian Eye. A,** Flat; **B,** round; **C,** tubular.

to allow them to view potential predators from many angles. Owls have eyes that primarily face forward, thereby increasing their binocular vision but reducing their overall field of vision. Perhaps the most unusual placement occurs in bitterns, which have eyes placed low on their heads. These heronlike birds feed in shallow water and may use the low eye placement to get a better view of the water. Also, when an intruder approaches a bittern, it goes into a protective posture in which it freezes in an erect position with its bill tip facing directly up. This puts its eyes in direct view of the intruder.

Anatomy of the Eye

The general structure of the avian eye is similar to that of mammals, with a few exceptions (Figure 17-17, *A*). It consists of three layers of tissue. The outermost layer is called the **sclera.** This tough coat protects the eye and toward the front becomes the transparent **cornea.** At this transition point, the sclera is reinforced by a ring of small bones called the **sclerotic ring.**

The cornea is protected by three eyelids: an upper lid, a lower lid, and a third lid called the **nictitating membrane.** This membrane is thin and transparent and consists of specialized epithelial cells that brush moisture over the eye from the nasal corner laterally (Figure 17-18). It possesses striated muscles that allow a bird to voluntarily control its movement. In many species of diving birds (loons, some ducks), the nictitating membrane has a clear window in its center to act as a contact lens under water. The vascular layer, lens, retina, and anterior chamber are similar to those of mammals. The major difference is that the iris, which functions to control the size of the pupil, contains striated muscles that allow a bird to voluntarily control the size of its pupils. Thus a pupillary light response is not a good diagnostic indicator in birds.

The vitreous in birds is also similar to that in mammals, with the exception of the presence of the pecten, which is a ribbonlike structure attached to the retina (see Figure 17-17, *B* and *C*). This highly vascular structure floats in the vitreous humor in the direction of the lens and is believed to distribute nutrition to the eye. More than 30% of traumatized wild birds suffer from hemorrhages arising from the pecten. These are only detected when the intraocular eye structures are examined (Korbel, 2001).

Photoreception

Birds possess rods and cones that are similar in function to those in mammals (see Chapter 13). Nocturnal birds, such as many species of owls, have more rods than cones on their retina. These rods are specialized in having more **rhodopsin** (the night vision pigment that aids in absorbing light) than do the rods of diurnal birds.

Birds have a relatively high level of visual acuity that results from several anatomical factors. First, a bird's retina is only lightly vascularized. A reduced number of blood vessels decreases interruption of an image as it reaches the back of the eye. Second, a bird's retina is packed with photoreceptor cells (1.5 to 2 times as thick as in other vertebrates) and can be compared to a computer printer. The resolving power of a printer is measured in dots per square inch (dpi). The more dots a printer puts on paper to represent the picture, the less grainy the picture. This is similar to the avian eye. It has more cells that receive and transmit information, thus resulting in a clearer image in the brain. A third factor that contributes to the superior visual acuity of birds is the connection between the photosensitive cells and nerve fibers. In many species, each cone has a single connection with a bipolar nerve cell. This means that each cone has individual representation in the brain. In mammals, multiple cones converge on a bipolar cell, and thus their information is pooled, leading to a lower level of visual acuity.

Like the eyes of other vertebrates, the avian eye possesses a central funnel-shaped area highly concentrated in cones. This area is called the central **fovea** and is the area of sharpest vision. However, many diurnal birds, such as hawks, parrots, and hummingbirds, also have a second fovea placed temporally.

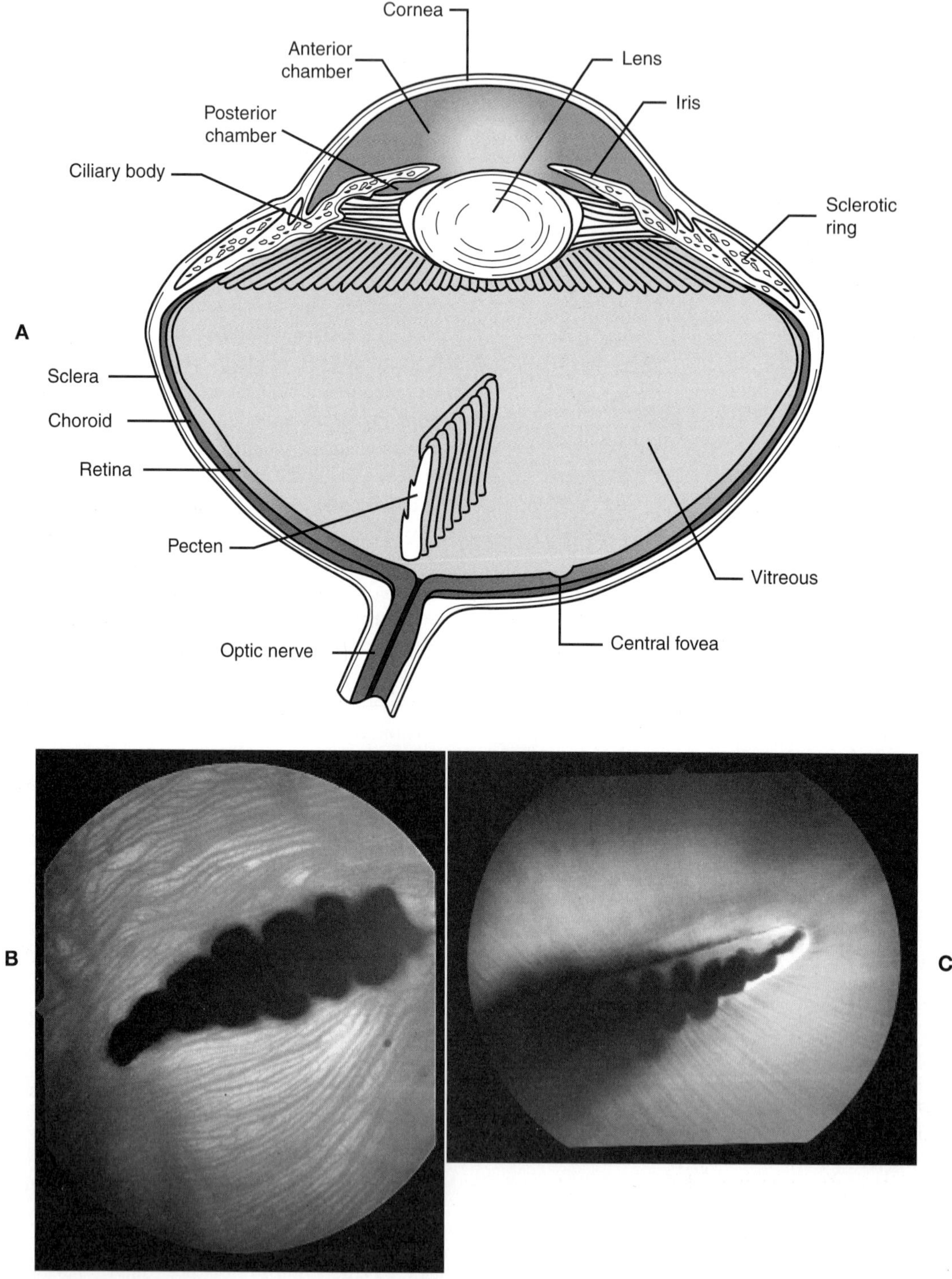

FIGURE **17-17** **The Avian Eye. A,** Diagram of transverse section. **B,** Ophthalmoscopic view through the pupil of intraocular structures in great horned owl (nocturnal bird). **C,** Ophthalmoscopic view through the pupil of red-tailed hawk (diurnal bird). (**B** and **C,** Courtesy R. Korbel.)

This provides another highly sensitive area and helps in binocular vision.

Color Vision

Cone cells in the retina are responsible for processing colored images. Each cone contains one colored oil droplet. Diurnal birds typically have yellow, red, green, and orange droplets, whereas nocturnal birds have pale or transparent droplets. How these droplets function is not completely understood, but they have a role in increasing the receptive ability of visual pigments.

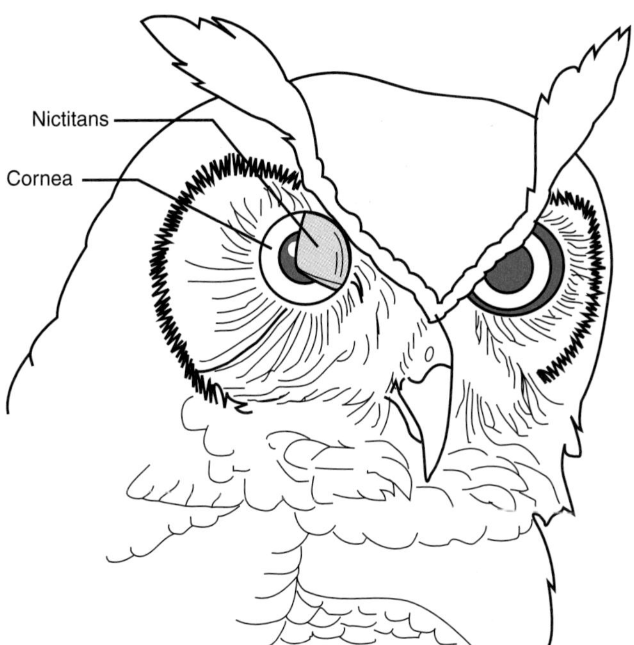

FIGURE **17-18** **Nictitating Membrane.**

Visual Spectrum

Birds can see a wide spectrum of light wavelengths. Although they cannot see infrared light, many diurnal species can see ultraviolet (UV) light. For example, American kestrels *(Falco sparverius)* can find mice by seeing the UV light reflected off the mice's urine. The ability to detect differences in the reflection of UV light is important in other species as well. Some use this ability for distinguishing between ripe and unripe fruit, and others use it to identify males versus females in species that to us have similar plumages. Ostriches and nocturnal species, such as owls and kiwis, cannot detect UV light.

Hearing and Equilibrium

Hearing is another extremely important sense for birds. It is critical for daily activities such as finding food, hiding from predators, defending territories, and communicating with other members of a family or flock. Although the structure of the avian ear is simpler than that of mammals, it has exceptional acoustical ability.

Anatomy of the Ear

A bird's ears are located on the sides of its head, behind and slightly below its eyes. They consist of three chambers: an external, middle, and inner ear (Figure 17-19). The **external ear** is an opening that funnels sound into the eardrum. It is often bordered with special auricular feathers that protect the ear during turbulent flight and yet still allow sound to pass through.

The **middle ear** consists of a single bone, the **columella,**

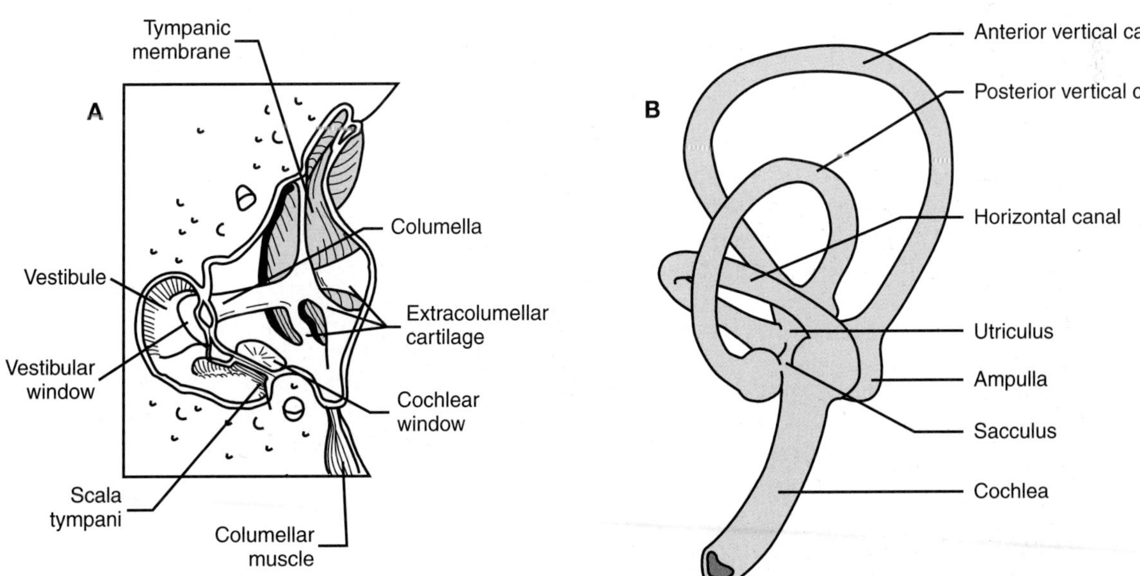

FIGURE **17-19** **Anatomy of Avian Ear. A,** Middle ear. **B,** Inner ear.

which connects to the inner ear and acts as a funnel to transmit sound. This contrasts with mammals, which possess three middle ear bones. The **cochlear window** is located adjacent to where the columella connects with the inner ear. It has a flexible membrane that protects the inner ear from pressure damage.

The **inner ear** is similar to that in mammals. It consists of a membranous labyrinth that functions to maintain balance and equilibrium and the cochlea, which converts sound waves into nervous impulses that are sent to the brain for processing.

Hearing in the Common Barn Owl *(Tyto alba)*

Hearing in birds reaches its highest level of development in nocturnal species, such as the common barn owl. This species can hunt mice and voles in complete darkness, relying on its incredible hearing ability to capture prey. Barn owls have a fleshy flap of skin, called the **operculum,** at each external ear opening that helps to funnel the sound into the ears. In addition, its ear openings are asymmetrical, with one slightly above the midpoint of the eye and the other slightly below it. This feature helps with the vertical location of sound. Barn owls also have large eardrums, columellae, cochleae, and a well-developed acoustic center in the hindbrain. The number of auditory neurons this center receives is about 95,000, compared with 27,000 in the carrion crow (Welty, 1982).

Taste

Birds have a relatively poor sense of taste. They possess taste buds, but these are few in number and scattered on the sides of their tongue and soft palate. Compared with humans, which have about 10,000 taste buds, adult domestic pigeons *(Columba livia)* only have about 50 to 60, and some parrots may have up to 400 (Terres, 1980). Based on experiments with pigeons and chickens, sensitivities and thresholds for bitter, salty, and sour tastes appear to be species specific.

Touch

The skin of birds contains two types of sensory nerve endings that respond to pain, heat, cold, and touch. For many species, the sense of touch is important for finding food. Therefore the nerve endings responsible for touch are often prevalent in the tongues, palates, and bills of birds. The first type of nerve ending is called a **Grandry's corpuscle,** and groups of these are located in the tongue and palate of many species that dig for food, such as woodcock and sandpipers (Figure 17-20, *A*). The second type of nerve ending is called a **Herbst corpuscle** (Figure 17-20, *B*). These are also often located in areas of the mouth such as the tongues of woodpeckers, the palates and beaks of ducks, and the mouth folds of young birds. In addition, Herbst corpuscles are located in the cloaca, legs, wings, uropygial gland, and the bases of many feathers, including the primary flight feathers. These corpuscles are very responsive to even the slightest feather movement. This characteristic explains why birds are sensitive when just the tips of their feathers are touched.

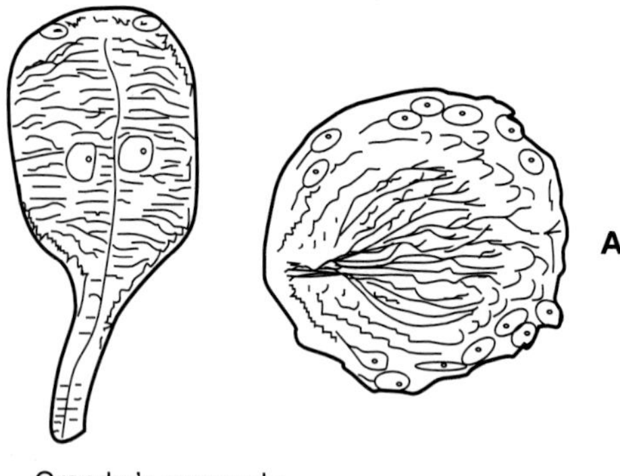

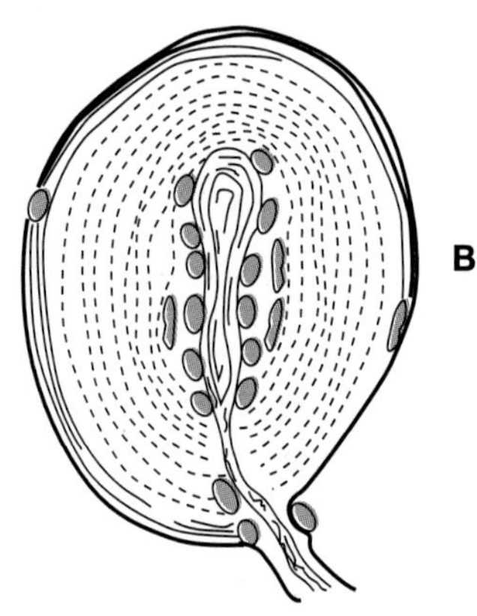

FIGURE **17-20** **Touch Corpuscles. A,** Grandry's. **B,** Herbst.

Smell

The sense of smell varies widely in birds. In a few species, such as the turkey vulture *(Cathartes aura),* Northern bobwhite quail *(Colinus virginianus),* and albatrosses, the sense of smell appears to be well developed and important for locating food. Waterbirds have a less developed but adequate sense of smell. Goslings learn to accept or reject food by smell at an early age, and hen mallards emit a breeding odor that stimulates drakes. The sense of smell in passerines and raptors is thought to be poor, but additional research needs to be conducted.

TEST YOURSELF

1. What are the two most important senses in birds?
2. Which eye structures are found in birds but not in mammals?
3. Where are the bird's ears located?
4. Name the two types of sensory nerve endings in the skin and where they are located.

ENDOCRINE SYSTEM

The function of the endocrine system in birds is similar to that in mammals (see Chapter 14). The hormones produced by the

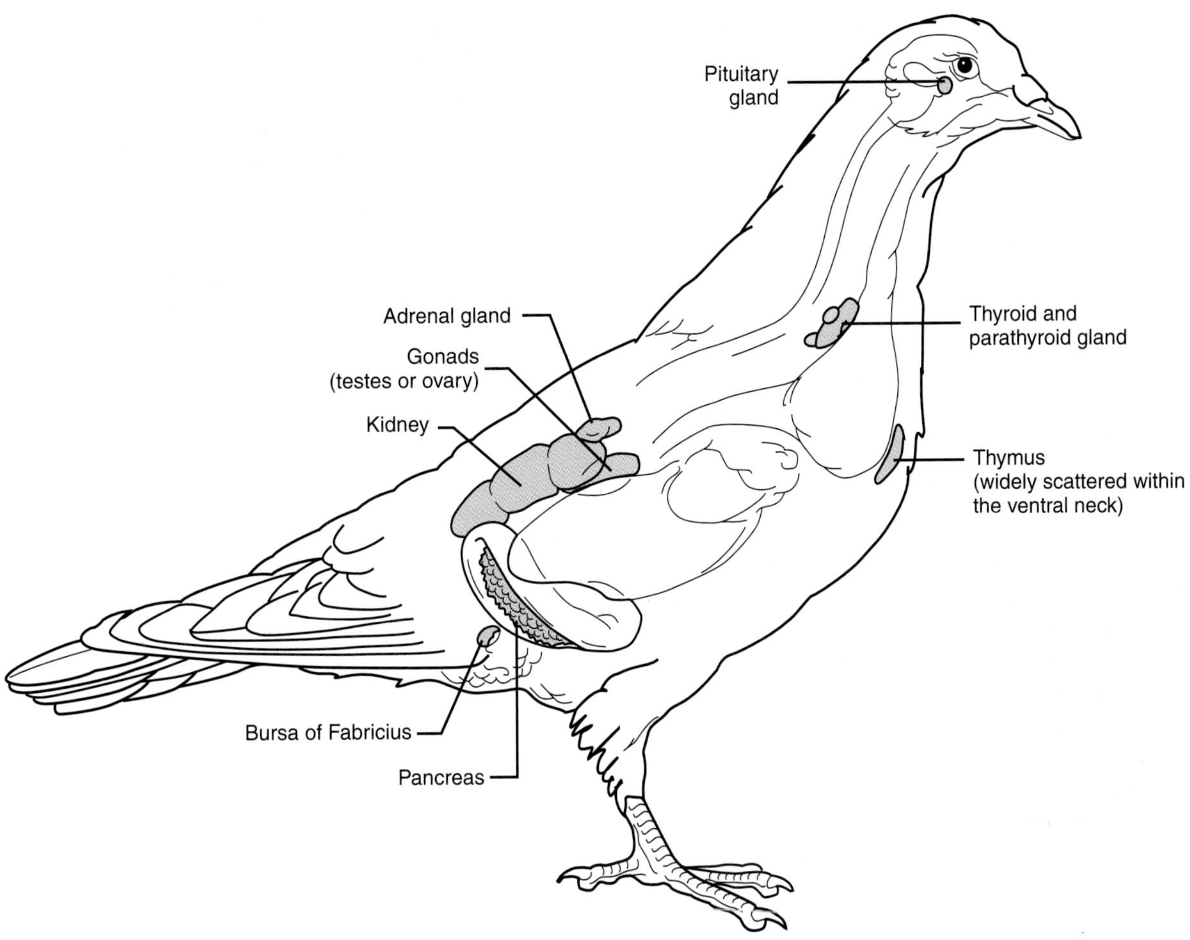

FIGURE **17-21** **Major Endocrine Glands in Rock Dove.**

glands influence many body systems and control such things as the stress response, courtship and reproduction, body growth, and, in birds, the process of molting. There are seven major endocrine glands, and the pancreas, in addition to having a digestive function, also has an endocrine component (Figure 17 21). As we continue our study of the avian body, we touch on the function of some of these glands and the substances they produce (Box 17-1).

DIGESTIVE SYSTEM

Birds have a fast metabolism and a high energy demand. To meet this need, they have a digestive system that can absorb energy from foods in a rapid and efficient manner with relatively little waste. Depending on the species, birds assimilate between 60% and 99% of the energy in the food they consume.

ANATOMY

The basic anatomy of a bird's digestive system is similar to that of reptiles and mammals. However, it has been refined and adapted to meet the high and variable energy demands of different bird species (Figure 17-22).

Beak (Bill)

The beaks of birds vary with their diet and foraging strategies. Raptors have a sharp-edged hooked beak for tearing meat; seedeaters have a thick beak that acts as a forceps and crushes; woodpeckers have a heavy, blunt beak that acts as a chisel to bore holes; and shorebirds have a long, delicate beak to probe for food in sandy areas. Beaks enable birds to find, grab, and sometimes kill food items and to tear food into smaller pieces to begin the digestion process.

Mouth

A bird's mouth consists of a hard upper palate, a soft lower palate, a distinctive tongue, salivary glands, and scattered taste buds. In some species of finches and pelicans, the soft palate enlarges to become a pouch for temporarily storing food. The **tongue** aids in manipulating food and moving it to the back of the mouth for easy swallowing. In parrots, it is highly muscular, but in many other species, it has few muscles and is moved by muscles of the jaw apparatus. Most birds have **salivary glands** located in the back of the mouth (pharynx), but seedeaters also have them in the soft palate. In these birds, the saliva moistens and lubricates dry seeds, and the glands secrete a starch-digesting enzyme. Some species, such as swifts and swallows, use dried saliva to build

Box 17-1 Avian Endocrine Glands and Their Function

Adrenal Gland
Secretes a stress hormone (corticosterone), sex hormones (androgens in males and estrogens and progesterone in females), and hormones that control concentrations of minerals in the body.

Bursa of Fabricius
Stimulates production of antibodies and lymphocytes.

Gonads
Testes in the male produce testosterone, ovaries in the female produces estrogens and testosterone. These regulate the secondary sex characteristics and control behavioral responses to the opposite sex.

Pancreas
Synthesizes hormones that regulate blood sugar and sugar metabolism in the liver (insulin, glucagon, and somatostatin). Also produces pancreatic polypeptide that inhibits gastrointestinal motility and secretion and induces a sense of satiety.

Parathyroid Gland
Produces parathormone that regulates calcium and phosphorus levels in the body.

Pituitary Gland
Anterior lobe secretes hormones that regulate other glands: thyroid-stimulating hormone (thyroid), adrenocorticotropic hormone (adrenal glands), follicle-stimulating hormone, luteinizing hormone, prolactin (female reproductive system). Posterior lobe secretes antidiuretic hormone to conserve water in the kidney and oxytocin to stimulate uterine contractions for egg laying.

Thymus Gland
Stimulates production of antibodies and lymphocytes.

Thyroid Gland
Secretes thyroxin to regulate growth of the body and feathers and may stimulate the migration urge.

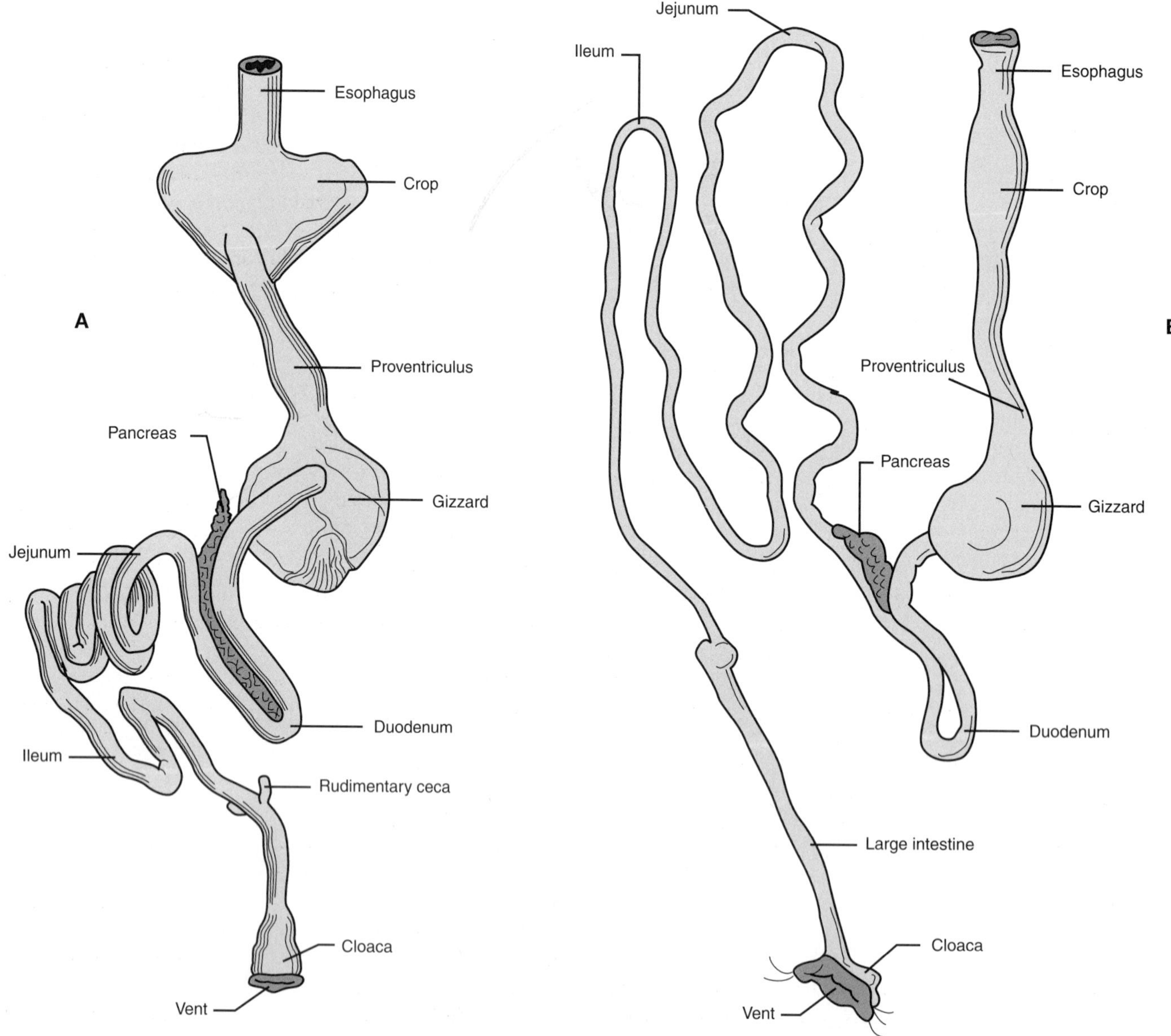

FIGURE **17-22** **General Diagram of Avian Digestive System. A,** Rock dove. **B,** Hawk.

nests, and woodpeckers use their sticky saliva to hold onto insects.

Esophagus

The esophagus is a somewhat muscular tube that extends from the pharynx to the stomach along the right side of the neck. The lining contains mucous glands that lubricate food to facilitate its passage into the stomach. In several species, the esophagus expands over the furcula to create a **crop,** which is a storage pouch for food. This crop can be a dilation of the esophagus, as seen in some fish eaters; a single pouch, as seen in hawks, seedeaters, grain eaters, and parrots; or a double pouch, as seen in pigeons. Birds that have well-developed crops generally eat a few larger meals per day instead of foraging and "nibbling" all day long.

Little digestion if any occurs in the crop. Its main function is to store, lubricate, and regulate the passage of food. In some species, it is modified for additional purposes. For example, in pigeons and doves, the mucosal lining of the crop thickens at breeding time and is broken down, forming "pigeon milk" that is fed to recently hatched chicks. Also, the crop lining in insect-eating birds consists of a heavy epithelium for protection from insects that are swallowed alive.

Stomach

The stomach of birds consists of two separated components: the glandular stomach and the muscular stomach. The anterior glandular stomach is called the **proventriculus.** This structure is unique to birds and is the organ in which chemical digestion begins. Its mucosa consists of columnar epithelial cells and mucosal glands that produce mucus to moisten food. The submucosal layer possesses digestive glands. These glands secrete pepsin, which begins the breakdown of proteins, and hydrochloric acid, which increases the acidity of the stomach to enhance the action of digestive enzymes. In birds the gastric juices can have a pH between 0.7 and 2.5.

The muscular stomach is called the **gizzard.** It consists of distinct bands of striated muscles that work to grind food components, such as bones, scales, and nuts. Also, many seedeaters and grain-eating birds actively seek and ingest small pieces of grit to aid in grinding food. In chickens, this grit enhances the digestibility of grain by about 10% (Welty, 1982).

Some characteristics of the gizzard are species specific. For example, the thickness of its walls varies with diet. Grain eaters (turkeys) have the thickest gizzard walls and can pulverize hard objects, such as steel needles and walnuts. The gizzard walls in carnivores are relatively thin, and those in omnivores are quite variable. In addition, the gizzards of owls, hawks, swifts, grouse, and herons grind indigestible food components into a **pellet** that is then regurgitated. Egestion of pellets in these species can be used as a clinical indicator of normal gastrointestinal motility.

Liver

The liver in birds is bilobed, and the right lobe is usually larger than the left. It stores excess fats and sugars, makes certain proteins, produces bile to neutralize the stomach acid and emulsify fats, and excretes waste products from the blood.

Pancreas

The pancreas is a relatively large gland in birds and rests in the loop of the duodenum. It is larger in fish and grain eaters and smaller in carnivores. It serves both an exocrine and endocrine function (see Chapter 14). In birds the endocrine portion of the pancreas occupies more tissue mass than in mammals, and the distribution of endocrine cells within the pancreas is more random.

Duodenum

The duodenum is the major organ responsible for the digestion and absorption of nutrients. In meat and fruit eaters, it is relatively short and thin walled. In seedeaters, it is long with several loops. In fish eaters, the duodenum is also relatively long but small in diameter.

Ceca

Ceca are paired sacs located at the junction of the small and large intestines in some species. Although their function continues to be studied, they appear to be important for water reabsorption and the bacterial fermentation of cellulose. The output from these sacs is dark brown and moist and has a distinctive odor. It is excreted a few times per week independently of the intestinal fecal material. Ceca are present in owls, ducks, geese, and Galliformes but are absent in other species, such as hawks, parrots, woodpeckers, and passerines.

Large Intestine

The large intestine is the segment that extends from the end of the small intestine to the cloaca. Its major role is the reabsorption of water and minerals.

Cloaca

The cloaca is located at the end of the digestive tract and is divided into three sections. The anterior section is called the **coprodeum** and receives excrement from the intestine. The **urodeum** receives discharge from the kidneys and genital ducts. The posterior **proctodeum** is accessed by both other sections and stores the excrement (see Figure 17-30). It is closed by a muscular anus that has powerful ejection muscles for the elimination of waste products. The waste products are organized into a **mute** in which a dark fecal center is surrounded by a ring of urates.

FEEDING HABITS

In general, a bird's intake is regulated by hunger. When a bird is hungry, it will seek out food, and when it is not, it will not waste the energy foraging. What stimulates hunger and foraging behavior is believed to be regulated by the hypothalamus of the brain. Sensory information from the stomach (full vs. empty), eyes (sight of food), skin (temperature), and body tissues (hydration status) is sent to the hypothalamus for pro-

CLINICAL APPLICATION Mutes: A Diagnostic Tool

Evaluation of a bird's mutes is an important diagnostic tool in assessing overall health. In many species the mutes normally have a dark fecal center surrounded by a white ring of urates. However, the color and consistency of a bird's mutes can be altered by diet, parasites, or disease, and any change in an individual bird's normal excreta should be investigated to discover the cause. For example, hawks fed day-old cockerels will have gold fecal centers in their mutes instead of dark ones, and parrots fed a fruity, pelleted diet often have a variety of colors to their mutes. These are normal changes and can be explained by diet. Birds suffering from the actions of some intestinal parasites, such as Coccidia, often have a tinge of green (and sometimes blood) in their output. Obtaining a complete patient history is important in evaluating these clinical observations. For pet birds, this should be easy. However, for wild birds with unknown histories, extensive laboratory testing may be necessary to explain abnormal output from the digestive and urinary systems. Tests performed often include fecal analysis for parasites, fecal Gram stain for bacteria, a complete blood count, a chemistry profile to assess organ function, and blood lead levels in species highly vulnerable to lead poisoning, such as bald eagles *(Haliaeetus leucocephalus)* and golden eagles *(Aquila chrysaetos)*.

cessing. If the information indicates a need for nutrition, a bird begins foraging for high-energy foods.

What a bird eats is species specific. The choice is determined by many factors, including a bird's physical characteristics (type of bill, feet, plumage, development of senses), its daily activity cycle (diurnal vs. nocturnal), flight style and endurance, and habitat. Some species are highly specialized, whereas others are more generalized and opportunistic. Diet also can be varied within a species. Sex, age, time of year, and geographical location greatly influence the availability of certain food items and a bird's ability to find and seize it. For example, recently fledged American kestrels maintain themselves primarily on insects, whereas the adults feed on small rodents, which are more nutritious but require greater hunting skill. Ruffed grouse *(Bonasa umbellus)* feed primarily on fruits in the summer and switch to aspen buds in the winter.

TEST YOURSELF

1. Which endocrine gland secretes hormones that regulate molting and the migratory urge?
2. List the endocrine and exocrine functions of the pancreas.
3. On which side of the neck is the esophagus located in birds? Does this differ from mammals?
4. List the two separated components of the avian stomach and their functions.
5. What is a mute? What can it tell us about the health of a bird?

CIRCULATORY SYSTEM

"The way to a man's heart is through his stomach." Although this phrase does not directly refer to the physiological functions of the two organs, it can be used to explain an important connection they possess. The digestive system, as mentioned previously, functions to break down foodstuffs into nutrients that can be absorbed into the blood. From here, the circulatory system takes over to deliver nutrient-rich blood to the tissues and remove metabolic waste. The system also functions to carry oxygen, minerals, and hormones to cells and blood helps to control and prevent diseases, as well as maintain a bird's body temperature.

ANATOMY

Heart

In birds the driving force behind this delivery system is a four-chambered heart that consists of a right atrium, right ventricle, left atrium, and left ventricle (Figure 17-23). The right side of the heart is smaller and less muscular, pumping blood only to the lungs. The left side is larger with well-developed muscles, and it pumps blood to the rest of the body. The heart is located in the cranial portion of the thoracoabdominal space. It is enclosed by a thin, fibrous pericardial sac, which contains fluid that aids in the lubrication of the heart muscle. This sac is adhered to several internal surfaces to keep the heart anchored in place.

Vessels

The heart is supported by a group of vessels that provide channels for the passage of blood. **Arteries** carry oxygenated blood from the heart to the tissues, and **veins** carry blood containing metabolic waste products away from the tissues back to the heart (see Figure 17-24, *A*). **Capillaries** are small vessels in which the exchange of gases and nutrients occurs. To meet the specific demands of the avian body, some of these vessels are highly specialized in the following ways:

1. The pectoral and brachial arteries, which provide blood to the flight muscles and wings, respectively, are relatively large.
2. Birds possess a **renal portal system** (Figure 17-24, *B*). A portal system begins and ends in a network of capillaries. Blood returning from the extremities (via the iliac veins) travels to the kidneys. Valves at the junction of the iliac veins and kidney (renal) veins steer blood either to the kidneys so metabolic waste products can be removed or directly to the heart via the posterior vena cava.
3. Many aquatic and terrestrial species possess a countercurrent system of heat exchange in their lower extremities. This system consists of a network of arteries and veins that are placed close together. Heat from arterial blood traveling to the lower extremities is transferred to

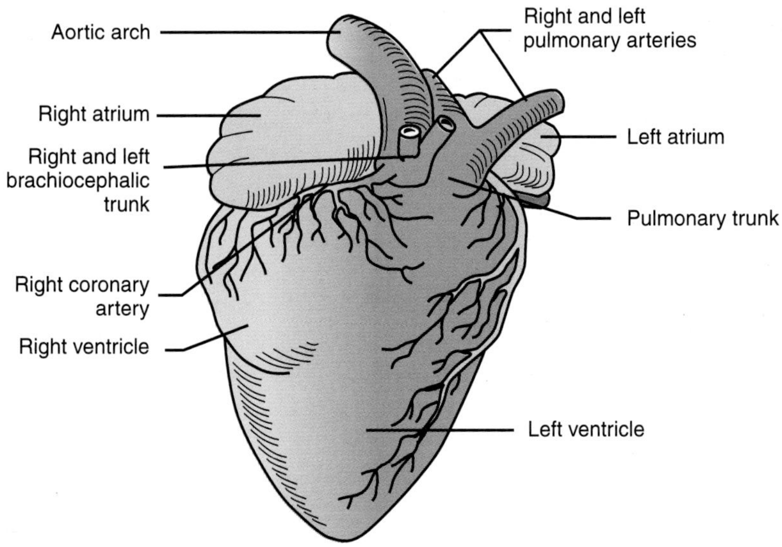

FIGURE **17-23** **Ventral Surface of the Avian Heart.**

the cooler venous blood returning to the heart. Thus blood reaching the lower extremities is cooler, and less of a temperature gradient exists with the environment. This feature reduces the amount of heat loss.

BLOOD FLOW

Birds are active creatures and have a relatively high body temperature between 37° to 42° C (Ritchie, Harrison, and Harrison, 1994). To maintain this temperature and generate body heat, they also have a relatively fast metabolism. This places high demands on the circulatory system to deliver oxygen and nutrients to the tissues quickly and efficiently. In "unstressed" chickens, it takes only 6 seconds for blood to make a complete circuit from the heart throughout the body and back (Welty, 1982).

Birds also have relatively fast heart rates (Table 17-1). The resting heart rate *(HR)* of a bird can be estimated by using the following formula (King and McLeeland, 1981):

$$\text{HR in beats/sec} = 12 \times (4 \times \text{weight in grams})^{-0.209}$$

ELECTROCARDIOGRAM

In birds, as the heart chambers contract and relax, the resulting changes in electrical voltage can be detected by placing electrodes in strategic locations on the wings and legs. The voltage changes are converted into visual peaks and valleys with the help of an electrocardiograph (ECG) machine. The ECG consists of a P, QRS, and T wave that correspond to the following muscular activities (Figure 17-25):

- P wave—contraction and relaxation of the atria
- QRS wave complex—contraction of the ventricles
- T wave—relaxation of the ventricles

In birds, the existence of the Q wave is in question. In many species, such as chickens and turkeys, it is believed to be completely absent, but in other species, such as some ducks, it appears to be prominent. The time intervals represented in the ECG are relatively fixed, with the exception of the T to P interval, which changes based on changes in the heart rate.

The ECG is an important tool to monitor a patient's stability during anesthesia and to diagnose malfunctions of the heart and major vessels.

BLOOD

We previously mentioned that the heart drives the circulatory system. The transport vehicle that it drives is the blood. Blood is made up of several components and functions to carry nutrients, oxygen, and hormones to cells; to carry metabolic wastes from cells to the lungs and kidneys; to control and prevent disease; and to regulate a bird's body temperature. Blood consists of red cells, white cells, platelets, and plasma (Figure 17-26).

Erythrocytes

Erythrocytes, or red blood cells, are oval, nucleated, and larger than those in mammals. In most species, they are formed in the bone marrow of adult birds, but in passerines (song birds), they are formed in the spleen and liver. The red cells possess hemoglobin for carrying oxygen to the tissues. The total number of red blood cells is dependent on several factors, including age, sex, diet, and time of year. In general, the percentage of red blood cells to total blood volume in a healthy adult bird should fall between 35% and 55% (Campbell, 1988).

Leukocytes

Leukocytes, or white blood cells, are important in helping a bird fight disease. In adults, they are primarily produced by the spleen, and in young birds, they are also formed by the liver, kidneys, pancreas, and the bursa of Fabricius (located on the dorsal wall of the proctodeum in the cloaca). There are several types of white cells, and each type has a different function.

A

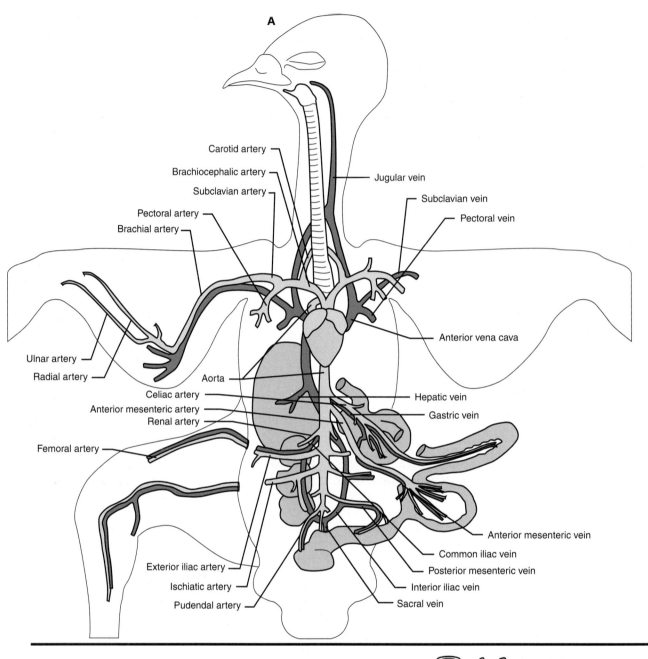

Carotid artery
Brachiocephalic artery
Subclavian artery
Pectoral artery
Brachial artery
Jugular vein
Subclavian vein
Pectoral vein
Anterior vena cava
Ulnar artery
Radial artery
Aorta
Celiac artery
Anterior mesenteric artery
Renal artery
Femoral artery
Hepatic vein
Gastric vein
Anterior mesenteric vein
Common iliac vein
Posterior mesenteric vein
Exterior iliac artery
Ischiatic artery
Pudendal artery
Interior iliac vein
Sacral vein

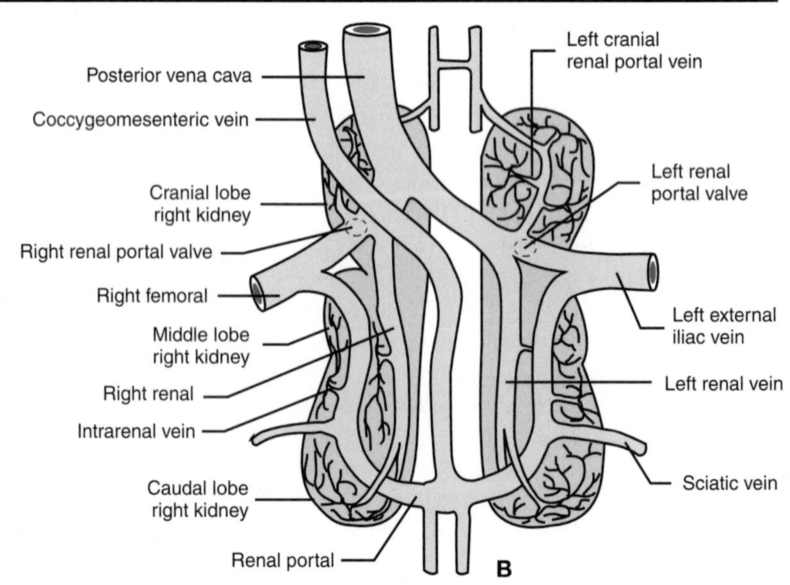

FIGURE **17-24 Vasculature of the Avian Circulatory System. A,** Blood vessels; **B,** renal portal system.

Heterophils. These cells are equivalent to the mammalian neutrophil. They are generally round, have a bilobed nucleus with clumped chromatin, and have rod-shaped red-orange granules in the cytoplasm. Heterophils are phagocytic cells that engulf foreign matter. A rise in the number of heterophils is usually seen with the onset of acute diseases.

Eosinophils. These cells are the same as the mammalian eosinophils. They are round cells with a lobed nucleus and large, red-orange, round granules in the cytoplasm. Their numbers increase in response to allergic reactions and heavy internal parasite loads.

Basophils. These cells are identified by a round, centrally placed nucleus and stain dark blue. The function of basophils is still being investigated.

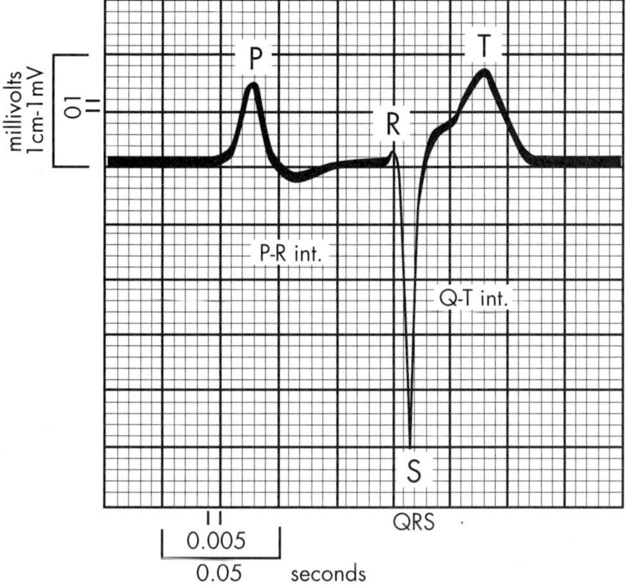

FIGURE **17-25** **Electrocardiogram of Healthy Racing Pigeon.**

Table 17-1 Heart Rates in Clinically Normal Birds

Bodyweight (g)	Heart Rate (beats/min) (Resting)	Heart Rate (beats/min) (Restrained)
25	274	400-600
100	206	500-600
200	178	300-500
500	147	160-300
1000	127	150-350
1500	117	120-200
2000	110	110-175
5000	91	105-160
10,000	79	100-150

From Ritchie B, Harrison G, Harrison L: *Avian medicine: principles and application,* Florida, 1994, Wingers Publishing.

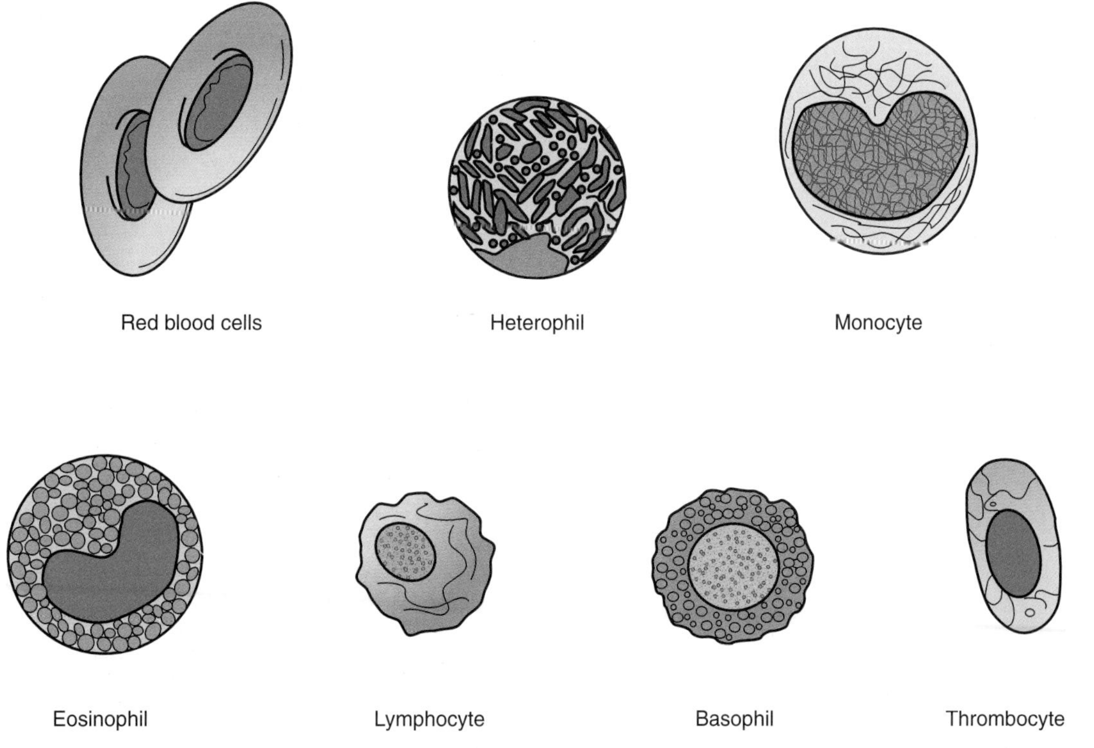

FIGURE **17-26** **Avian Blood Cells.**

CLINICAL APPLICATION — Sites of Venipuncture

Blood samples are taken for a variety of diagnostic purposes. In birds, blood can be drawn most easily from one of three vessels: a brachial vein, jugular vein, or medial metatarsal vein. The brachial vein is located on the ventral side of the wing, extending over the elbow and up the humerus. About halfway up the humerus, it joins the cutaneous ulnar vein and increases slightly in size. In raptors, the brachial vein is often used to take blood samples or insert temporary catheters for repeated intravenous treatments. The jugular veins are located ventrally, on each side of the trachea. The right jugular is larger than the left jugular and is most commonly used for venipuncture in psittacines. Lastly, the medial metatarsal vein is located on the ventral medial side of the leg, extending from the metatarsus dorsally over the heel joint. Blood samples are sometimes taken from this site for raptors but most commonly for waterfowl species.

Monocytes. These cells are phagocytic cells that act as a body's second line of cellular defense. The nucleus is often shaped like a kidney bean and can be located centrally or off to one side. An increase in monocyte production is often seen in cases of tuberculosis and aspergillosis.

Lymphocytes. These cells are the essential components of the immune system. Their centrally placed nucleus is round and contains densely clumped chromatin. They are produced by the thymus and bursa of Fabricius, with those originating from the latter producing humeral antibodies to help fight off infections.

Thrombocytes

Thrombocytes are nucleated cells that act as platelets. They are smaller than red blood cells and have a large, round to oval nucleus. They are important in blood clotting and are produced by bone marrow in adult birds.

Plasma

The plasma is about 80% water. The remaining 20% consists of a variety of substances, including salts, glucose, fats, amino acids, hormones, antibodies, vitamins, enzymes, waste products, and special blood proteins. These proteins are important for maintaining normal levels of water and blood in tissues by osmotic pressure.

TEST YOURSELF

1. What is the renal portal system?
2. What is the body temperature range of birds?
3. Describe the components of an avian ECG.
4. How do avian red blood cells differ from those in mammals?
5. List the three veins that are commonly used for venipuncture in birds. Where are they located?

RESPIRATORY SYSTEM

Because of the fast metabolism and high energy level of birds, the delivery of oxygen and removal of carbon dioxide from the body tissues must be quick and efficient. To accommodate this need, birds possess a respiratory system with highly specialized components (Figure 17-27).

ANATOMY

Oral Cavity

The oral cavity contains several structures involved in respiration. The **glottis** is the opening of the trachea located at the back of the tongue. Air is directed to the glottis via the mouth and nasal chambers. These two are linked via the **choanae,** which are two internal nares that open from the nasal chambers into the roof of the mouth. The **larynx** (a cartilaginous structure surrounding the glottis) has ligaments and muscle attachments that enable it to act as a valve to prevent solids and liquids from entering the trachea and lungs. It does not function in the production of sound as in mammals.

Trachea

The trachea consists of cartilaginous rings that are held together by bands of fibrous connective tissue. In a few species, such as swans and whooping cranes *(Grus americana),* the trachea is very long and coiled. For species that migrate at high altitudes, the long trachea helps provide moisture to the air inhaled and aids in the production of sound.

Syrinx

The enlargement of the trachea above the sternum is called the *syrinx*. It is essentially the voice box of birds and contains muscles, air sacs, and vibrating membranes (Figure 17-28). To create sound, air from the lungs and air sacs is forced over the membranes during expiration, causing changes in muscle tension and air pressure. These changes cause vibrations of the membranes. The complexity of a bird's vocalizations depends on the number of muscles present. Birds capable of complex vocalizations, such as many species of songbirds, have an average of seven pairs, whereas, on the other end of the spectrum, storks, vultures, and ostriches do not have any. Parrots fall in the middle, with three pairs of muscles in their syrinx (Welty, 1982).

Bronchi

At the level of the sternum, the trachea bifurcates into two branches called the *bronchi*. These branches pass through the ventral side of each lung and end in the posterior air sacs. Once they enter the lung, the bronchi lose their reinforcing cartilaginous rings and are called *mesobronchi*. The mesobronchi give rise to four to six ventrobronchi, which in turn divide into the parabronchi. The parabronchi are connected to air capillaries, where gas exchange occurs.

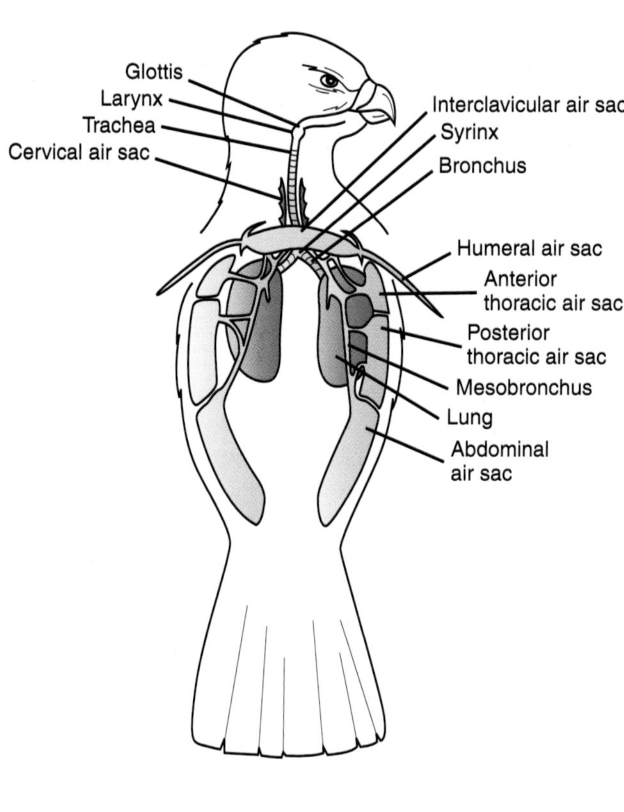

FIGURE **17-27 General Diagram of Avian Respiratory System.**

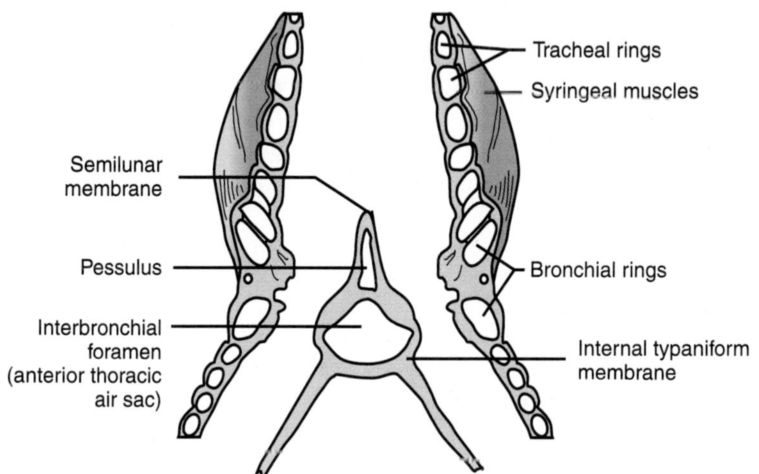

FIGURE **17-28 Cross Section of the Syrinx.**

Parabronchi

These small, parallel tubes originate from the ventrobronchi in the lungs and are connected to the tiny openings of air capillaries. The air capillaries, in turn, are surrounded by small blood capillaries. Gas exchange occurs between these two groups of capillaries.

Air Sacs

Air sacs are thin walled, lightly vascularized transparent membranes that make up about 80% of the total volume of the respiratory system. There are nine total, four of which are paired. The pairs include cranial thoracic, caudal thoracic, cervical, and abdominal air sacs. The unpaired sac is the interclavicular air sac, which is located in the thoracic inlet between the clavicles. Air sacs are connected to the primary bronchi (abdominal sacs) or secondary bronchi (cervical, cranial thoracic, caudal thoracic, and interclavicular sacs) and serve the following functions:

1. They act as reservoirs for air and provide warmth and moisture to facilitate its diffusion through the lung capillaries.
2. They help in thermoregulation to cool the body by the internal evaporation of water.
3. They help provide buoyancy to water birds. Many species of penguins and diving birds have large posterior and abdominal sacs, the volume of which can be adjusted during diving and floating.

Diverticula of some of the air sacs penetrate the skeleton. In many species, the interclavicular sac extends into the humerus bones, sternum, syrinx, and pectoral girdle. The abdominal sacs often extend into the legs and pelvic girdle.

Lungs

In the avian respiratory system, the lungs are relatively small, occupying only about 2% of the total body volume. They are attached to the thoracic vertebrae and ribs and are bright red, highly vascularized, and inelastic. They house the network of blood and air capillaries between which the exchange of gases occurs.

AIR FLOW

Two inhalations and two expirations are required to transport one pocket of air through the entire respiratory system (Figure 17-29). To begin the cycle, the *first inhalation* involves an expansion of the thoracoabdominal space (birds do not have a diaphragm, the major inspiratory muscle in mammals), creating a pressure gradient that brings air into the body. Most of the air flows into the posterior air sacs, where it is warmed and humidified. With the *first expiration,* this air is pushed into the lungs, where gas exchange occurs. The *second inspiration* results in the air moving out of the lungs and into the anterior pairs of air sacs, and the *second expiration* results in the air leaving the body through the trachea. The key factor in the flow of air through a bird's respiratory system is that air is pushed into the lungs, not pulled. More than any other group of animals, birds truly can get a "breath of fresh air." As previously mentioned, a bird's lungs are inelastic; they do not inflate and deflate as in mammals. Fresh air flows in a continuous unidirectional path in the lungs and does not get mixed with "dirty" air containing

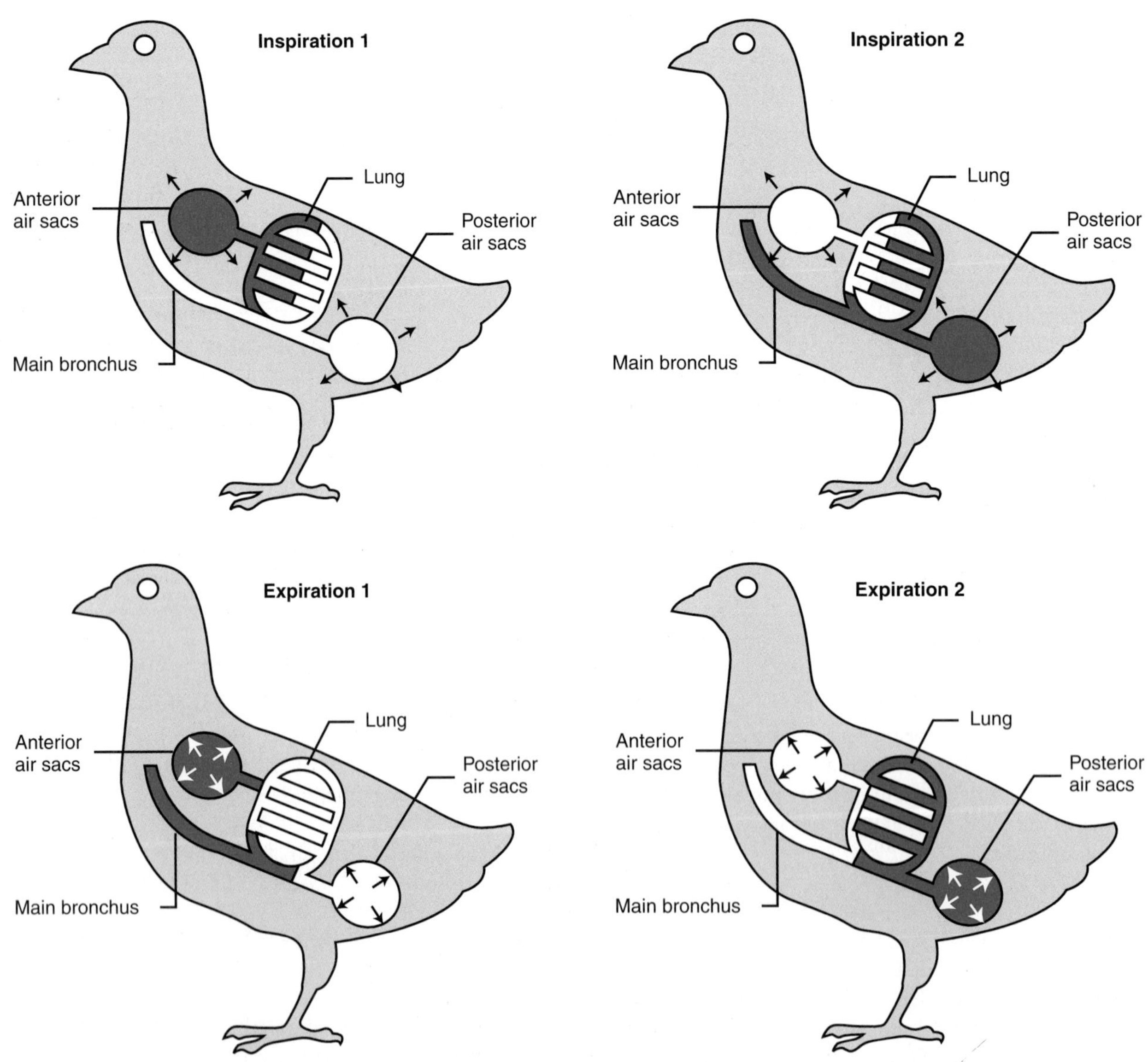

FIGURE **17-29** **Diagram of Air Flow Through a Bird's Respiratory System.**

waste products. This unique feature allows each breath of air to reach the lung capillaries with the maximum amount of oxygen possible (close to the 21% present in atmospheric air). In contrast, the lungs of mammals inflate and deflate, always leaving a quantity of residual air. When new air comes in, it mixes with the air remaining in the lungs, diluting the percentage of oxygen available for gas exchange.

Another unique feature of the avian respiratory system that contributes to its high efficiency is a countercurrent flow between the air and blood capillaries. The air capillaries are positioned at right angles to the blood capillaries so that carbon dioxide is continually removed from the blood and oxygen is continually added.

RESPIRATORY RATE

The breathing rate of birds varies with species, activity level, age, sex, time of day, and outdoor temperature. Smaller birds usually breathe faster than larger birds, and birds in flight have a higher respiratory rate than nonflying birds. In a thermoneutral environment at rest, chickens breathe 16 to 18 times per minute (Terres, 1980), whereas red-tailed hawks breathe about 40 times per minute (Chaplin, Mueller, and Degernes, 1989). A study by Odum (1943) found that at rest, house sparrows breathe 50 times per minute; when held in the hand, 102 times per minute; and when released and flying around a room, 212 times per minute. The variability in rate under different conditions can make it difficult to use respiratory rate as a diagnostic tool.

THERMOREGULATION

In addition to the exchange of gases, the respiratory system in birds also helps in thermoregulation. Air in the lungs picks up heat radiated by warm body tissues and blood and removes it from the body during the breathing process. The evaporation of water via the air sacs, lungs, and mouth cavity helps to cool the body to maintain a safe core temperature. This is most critical when outdoor air temperatures rise or when a bird participates in strenuous exercise, such as flight.

To increase the amount of cooling, a bird can increase the air flow over its mouth, pharynx, bronchi, and air sacs by increasing its breathing rate. This often results in panting or gular fluttering. The latter is often seen in owls, great blue herons *(Ardea herodias)*, quail, pigeons, and doves and involves rapid vibrations of their upper throat patch.

In addition to a bird's ability to use its respiratory system to remove excess heat, birds can control their body temperature in several other ways. To keep cool, birds bathe or reduce their activity level during the warmest parts of the day, and some species, such as turkey vultures and wood storks *(Mycteria americana)*, defecate on their legs for evaporative cooling. As mentioned previously, birds also can adjust the position of their body feathers to promote both heat loss and retention. To retain heat, many land and water species possess a special artery-vein arrangement in their lower extremities that limits heat loss through their bare legs. Birds also change their posture to conserve heat. This may include perching on one leg to reduce exposure of bare skin to the cold air or tucking their beak behind feathers in their back. Shivering to increase muscle heat production, moving to more protected locations (burrows, dense trees, etc.), and, in some smaller species (hummingbirds), short-term nocturnal torpor (body temperature is decreased several degrees and heart rate and oxygen consumption are reduced) also help to prevent loss of body heat during times of cold stress.

TEST YOURSELF

1. Where does gas exchange occur in the avian respiratory system?
2. List the nine air sacs and their main function in respiration.
3. Do birds have a diaphragm?
4. Describe the path of one breath of air through the respiratory system.

UROGENITAL SYSTEM

The urogenital system encompasses both the urinary and reproductive systems. Although these systems have very different functions, they are often studied together because of their close anatomical location in a bird's body (Figure 17-30).

URINARY SYSTEM

Like mammals, the urinary system consists of two main components: kidneys and ureters. Its major function is to remove nitrogenous waste products from the blood and eliminate them from the body. However, it also plays a role in maintaining the osmotic balance of electrolytes and salt in the blood and body tissues.

Anatomy

Kidneys. The **kidneys** in birds are located dorsally, in the slight depression formed at the level of the synsacrum. They are elongated and consist of three divisions, each of which is layered with an exterior **cortex** and an interior **medulla.** Within each layer, the divisions subdivide into lobules that possess nephrons, which are the "workhorses" of the urinary system. These nephrons radiate around a central vein (Figure 17-31). Unlike mammals, birds do not possess a renal pelvis, and thus the gross anatomy of the kidneys looks more homogenous.

Each nephron consists of a **glomerulus** and a **tubule.** The glomerulus is a filter that removes wastes, salt, glucose, gases, and water from the blood and passes them on to its tubule. The two types of tubules are looped and unlooped. The looped tubules (termed the **loops of Henle**) resemble those in mammalian nephrons and are located in large nephrons in the medulla of the kidney. The unlooped tubules are located in the smaller cortical nephrons and resemble those of reptiles. In both types, water, salt, and

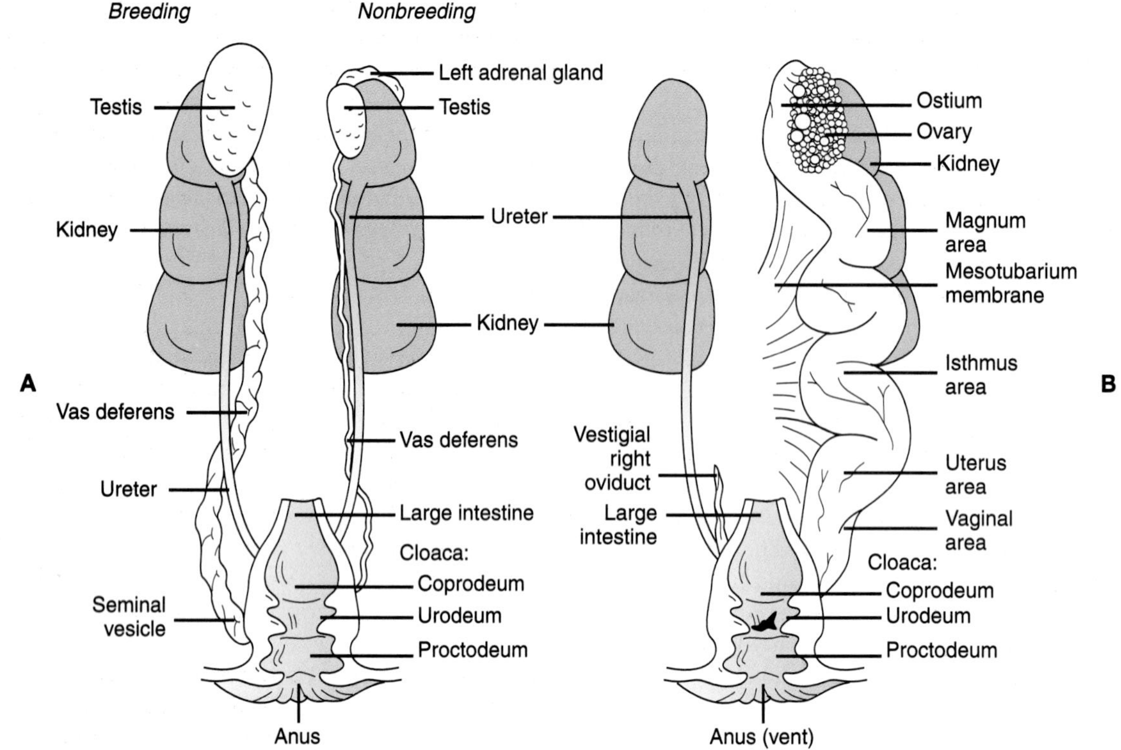

FIGURE 17-30 **Avian Urogenital System. A,** Male. **B,** Female.

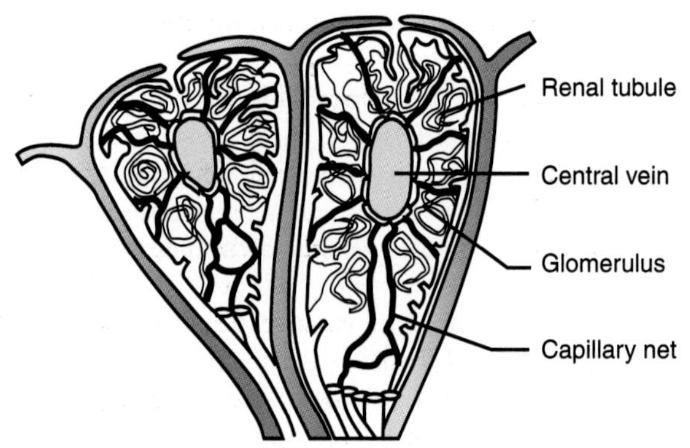

FIGURE 17-31 **Internal Anatomy of the Avian Nephron.**

glucose are selectively reabsorbed into the blood through capillaries, and the waste products are concentrated and passed into collecting ducts that empty into the ureters. About 66% to 99% of the water filtered into the kidney glomeruli is reabsorbed in the tubules.

Ureters. The ureters are an extension of the main collecting ducts. They are surrounded by smooth muscle and can "milk" urates from the kidney or inhibit their flow into the cloaca. Urine passing through the ureters ends in the urodeum of the cloaca and is either moved upward to the colon and ceca for further reabsorption of water or propelled outward through a bird's **vent** (sphincter separating the cloaca from the outside).

Renal Portal System. Birds, like reptiles, possess a special valve called the **renal portal valve** at the junction where the common iliac vein (carrying blood from the extremities) meets the renal portal vein entering the kidney (see Figure 17-24, *B*). This valve possesses a smooth muscle sphincter that opens and closes when receiving appropriate nervous stimulation. When the sphincter is closed, blood flows into the kidney; when it is open, blood bypasses the kidney and flows into the vena cava and heart.

Urine Composition

In chickens the composition of nitrogenous wastes eliminated by the kidneys consists of 75% uric acid, 10% to 15% ammonia, 2% to 10% urea, 1% to 5% creatine, and 2% amino acids (Welty, 1982). Clearly, the greatest component is uric acid and not urea, as in mammals. This finding is significant for several reasons. First, uric acid is more efficient in eliminating nitrogen; each molecule removes twice as much nitrogen as urea. Second, uric acid conserves water because it is relatively insoluble and can be eliminated with only a small volume of water. It takes 60 ml of water to excrete 1 g of urea, whereas it only takes 1.5 to 3 ml water to excrete the same amount of uric acid. Finally, the production of uric acid is critical to the survival of embryos within the egg. The only waste products that can be eliminated through an eggshell are gases. Other waste products must be stored in the egg throughout the embryo's development. Because urea requires a relatively large volume of water for excretion, the egg would not have enough room to house it. Also, high quantities of urea are toxic and would kill the embryo. The relatively small amount of nontoxic uric acid produced can be stored in the egg with no ill effects.

The final waste product is eliminated from the body as a paste. It is usually excreted in combination with a small quantity of fecal material from the digestive system. Collectively, the excreted product is called a *mute* and in a healthy bird is characterized by a dark fecal center (the color of which will vary with a bird's diet) surrounded by a ring of urates.

REPRODUCTIVE SYSTEM

Finally, we have reached the system responsible for creating the little package of genetic material that will develop into another amazing avian creature. Like most of the body systems in birds, the reproductive system is highly specialized and unique. The entire process of reproduction is periodic and under hormonal control. In temperate-zone birds, increasing daylight stimulates the hypothalamus to secrete substances that travel to the pituitary and cause the release of hormones that directly affect the reproductive process.

Anatomy

The major reproductive organs are called **gonads.** In males, these are the testes, and in females, these are the ovaries. In both sexes the organ on the left side of the body is larger, and in females the right ovary is rudimentary and not even functional. During the nonbreeding season, the gonads are relatively small. As breeding season approaches, hormones stimulate enlargement of the gonads, with up to a 300-fold increase in size of the testes in males. After the season ends, the gonads shrink. This is another adaptation that has allowed birds to reduce unnecessary weight for flight. Many species migrate long distances during the nonbreeding season and do not need to carry large, inactive gonads.

Male Reproductive System

The testes in birds are bean-shaped organs located ventral to the anterior part of the kidney (see Figure 17-30, *A*). Their anatomy and function are similar to those in mammals, as they produce the spermatozoa that are genetically ready to penetrate a developing ovum.

Spermatozoa of birds resemble tadpoles with relatively large heads and mobile tails. They swim out of the testes in seminal fluid produced by tubules in the testes, not by accessory glands as in mammals. They travel down a curvy ciliated tube, called the **vas deferens,** to a storage pouch called the **seminal vesicle.** The temperature in this pouch is about 4° C cooler than the core body temperature and can safely house the heat-sensitive spermatozoa.

Copulation. To pass sperm to the female, **copulation** must occur. This behavior is stimulated by androgens, which are male hormones produced in the testes by the **cells of Leydig.** The androgens travel to the hypothalamus in the brain and stimulate copulatory behavior. Copulation is achieved in one of two ways. In some species, such as ducks, geese, Galliformes, storks, and flamingos, a grooved erectile penis is attached to the wall of the cloaca to help transfer sperm into the female's vagina. However, in most species, sperm transfer occurs when the male and female bring their cloacae into close proximity. In pigeons, 200 million sperm are transferred during a single copulatory event. In the domestic chicken, 8 billion sperm are transferred (Welty, 1982).

Female Reproductive System

Eggs, or **ova,** are produced from follicles in the cortex of the ovary (see Figure 17-30, *B*) and are released in a manner similar to that of mammals. Several factors, including increasing day length, stimulate the anterior pituitary gland to secrete **follicle-stimulating hormone (FSH),** which increases the size of the follicles, and **luteinizing hormone (LH),** which stimulates both discharge of an egg from its follicle and development of the interstitial cells that produce sex hormones.

Anatomy. **Ovulation** is the process whereby the ovum leaves its follicle and enters the **oviduct.** This duct consists of three layers: an outer layer of connective tissue, a middle muscular layer that moves the egg down the oviduct by peristalsis, and an inner glandular layer that secretes various substances that are added to the egg during its passage. Lengthwise, the avian oviduct can be divided into the following five sections:

1. Infundibulum—Possesses folds that grab an ovum as it comes out of the ovary
2. Magnum—Secretes layers of albumin (egg white) around the egg
3. Isthmus—Deposits the keratin shell membrane
4. Uterus—Deposits watery albumin, a hard external shell, and pigmentation; large and muscular, it is also called the *shell gland*
5. Vagina—Secretes mucus to assist in egg laying; stores sperm for hours to several days

An egg spends the most time in the uterus when the shell and its pigments are being applied. Eggs come in different colors and may have speckles, blotches, or other irregular markings depending on how much they move when the tiny pigment glands apply color. During the egg production process, hormones alter a female's blood composition. Estrogen produced from the interstitial cells of the ovary stimulate a threefold to eighteenfold increase in fatty substances in the blood. Hormones from the thyroid, adrenals, and pancreas are responsible for doubling the blood sugar concentration, and the ovary and parathyroid glands stimulate an increase in blood calcium.

Clutch. The number of eggs that a female lays and incubates is called a **clutch.** This number varies among species but is fairly constant from year to year. Many species lay one egg per day.

CLINICAL APPLICATION Egg Binding

Eggs passing through the oviduct sometimes get lodged. This condition is called *egg binding* and is seen more often in small companion birds, such as parakeets, canaries, finches, and cockatiels. Birds suffering from this condition may be sluggish and reluctant to fly or perch, stand with a wide stance, droop their wings, have paralysis of the rear limbs, be anorexic, or have strained abdominal movements. Malformed eggs, excessive egg production, obesity, vitamin deficiencies, inactivity, environmental stress, or malfunction of the oviduct muscles can all result in egg binding. Removing the lodged egg may require drug therapy (oxytocin or prostaglandin to stimulate contraction of the uterus) or manual manipulation of the patient. The latter may include massaging the abdomen, administering an enema to lubricate the urodeum, or inserting a speculum into the urodeum to facilitate egg passage. If these techniques are unsuccessful, more intricate procedures may be necessary.

Others, such as ducks and geese, lay eggs every other day. Some larger species, such as eagles and condors, may lay at 4- to 5-day intervals.

The total number of eggs that a female can lay varies with the species. The two types of egg layers are determinate and indeterminate. **Determinate** layers have a specific number of follicles that develop in the ovary. Once these are laid, the clutch is complete, even if the eggs are removed. **Indeterminate** layers can produce more eggs than their normal clutch size and will continue to lay eggs if their eggs disappear. Visual, tactile, and hormonal influences cause them to stop laying when their clutch is complete. This concept has been used to remove and artificially incubate eggs of endangered species while still allowing a hen to lay and incubate her own clutch.

Incubation. Eggs must be kept warm and humidified during their development. An average incubation temperature for many species is 35° C. When a female bird is ready to lay her eggs, the pituitary acts again to secrete **prolactin,** which decreases the activity of the FSH and LH and promotes broodiness, or incubation behavior. Hormones also stimulate the development of a **brood patch,** which is an area of skin on the lower abdomen where heat is transferred to the egg. The hen plucks the feathers in this area because of the influence of prolactin, and estrogen stimulates thickening and wrinkling of the epidermis and an increase in the size and number of blood vessels.

The amount of time required for an egg to complete its development varies with the species. Generally, smaller birds have shorter incubation times (many passerines need 14 to 21 days) than larger birds (most hawk species need an average of 30 days).

The New Arrival

Hatching occurs with the help of powerful neck muscles and a specialized egg tooth on the outside of a chick's bill. The neck muscles atrophy greatly after hatching, and the egg tooth disappears.

The sex of the chick is determined by the genetic information passed on by the female. The female chromosome, Z, is dominant in eggs; the male chromosome, W, is recessive. Females can lay two types of eggs: those with a male chromosome (ZW), and those without (ZZ). Sperm all have the same sex chromosome (WW). Therefore only when the female contributes the W chromosome will a male result.

When hatched, chicks differ in the amount of feather cover they have, the status of their eyes (open or closed), and in their mobility. The four different classifications of newly hatched chicks are as follows:

1. Precocial—These chicks are covered with downy feathers, have their eyes open, and are quite mobile, leaving the nest quickly. Ducks and geese are good examples.
2. Semiprecocial—Some species, such as gulls and terns, are born with a downy covering and open eyes but are not mobile and cannot leave the nest.
3. Altricial—Songbirds are hatched with their eyes closed and their skin bare. They require a great deal of care before they can leave the nest.
4. Semialtricial—At hatching, these chicks are covered with down, are immobile, and may have their eyes open (hawks) or closed (owls).

TEST YOURSELF

1. What is the major component in the nitrogenous waste of birds? What are the advantages to producing this type of waste?
2. Explain how sperm are transferred from the male to the female in birds.
3. List the five sections of the avian oviduct and their functions.
4. What is the average incubation temperature?
5. What is a brood patch and how does it relate to incubation?
6. Describe the four classifications of newly hatched chicks.

CONCLUSION

With the general description of newly hatched chicks, we have come to the end of our brief study of the anatomy and physiology of birds. For most undomesticated species, a chick emerges from its shell and over the next few weeks to months develops physically and psychologically into a being destined to conquer the sky. Its body systems mature with all the specialized features mentioned, and its magnificent coat of feathers lifts it into the air. It may or may not travel great distances, but it will definitely experience the world as no other type of creature, even humans, ever can do.

APPENDIX 1

Bird Classification

Class: Aves
Orders: 29 with worldwide distribution (Gill, 1995)

Abbreviated List of Orders in the Class Aves

Order*	Species	Description
Anseriformes	Waterfowl—mallards, ducks, geese, swans	Aquatic birds with webbed feet and flattened bills with toothlike edges
Apodiformes	Swifts	Small aerial birds that eat insects on wing
Caprimulgiformes	Nighthawks, goatsuckers, frogmouths	Nocturnal species that eat insects on wing
Charadriiformes	Shorebirds, gulls, terns	Wading or swimming birds
Ciconiiformes	Herons, wood storks	Wading birds with long legs and bill; feed on aquatic life
Columbiformes	Pigeons, doves	Birds that eat grain, small seeds, corn.
Cuculiformes	Cuckoos	Slender birds with rounded wings, curved upper mandible; live in forest and eat caterpillars
Falconiformes	Hawks, eagles, falcons, vultures, osprey	Diurnal flesh eaters; with the exception of vultures, have sharp, hooked bills and strong feet for capturing live prey; some scavenge
Galliformes	Game birds—chickens, turkeys, quail, grouse, pheasant	Heavy bodied land birds with short, round wings and with curved upper bill; capable of short flights
Gaviiformes	Loons	Birds specialized for swimming and diving; live primarily on water
Gruiformes	Cranes, rails, coots	Wading birds with long legs; feed on variety of insect, aquatic, and rodent species
Passeriformes	Perching birds—starlings, crows, swallows, ravens, finches, songbirds	Vary in size, have three toes in front and one behind, and have well-developed syrinx
Piciformes	Woodpeckers—common flickers	Strong, sharp bill for boring holes into tree trunks for insects; stiff tail used as prop
Procellariiformes	Albatrosses	Birds of oceans, found mostly in the Antarctic, South America, Africa, Australia; have pronounced hook at end of their bill and external nostrils modified into tubes
Psittaformes	Psittacines—parakeets, parrots, budgerigars, cockatiels, cockatoos	Brightly colored tropical birds with strong, heavily curved beaks and short legs
Sphenisciformes	Penguins	Flightless birds on southern hemisphere adapted for living in cold water
Strigiformes	Owls	Mostly nocturnal, large headed, short-necked birds of prey with large eyes and facial disc
Struthioniformes	Ostriches	Large flightless birds of Africa; also bred in captivity in Australia, Europe, and United States

*Orders not described: *Casuariiformes* (emus, cassowaries), *Coliiformes* (mousebirds), *Coraciiformes* (kingfishers, bee-eaters, hoopes), *Dinornithiformes* (kiwis), *Musophagiformes* (turacos and plaintain eaters), *Pelecaniformes* (pelicans, gannets, cormorants), *Phoenicopteriformes* (flamingos), *Podicipediformes* (grebes), *Rheiformes* (rheas), *Tinamiformes* (tinamous), *Trogoniformes* (trogans).

APPENDIX 2

Life Spans of Common Pet Species

Bird	Maximum (Years)	Average (Years)	Bird	Maximum (Years)	Average (Years)
African Grey parrot	50	15	Macaw	50	15
Amazon parrot	80	15	Mynah	8	3
Budgerigar	18	6	Pionus parrot	15	5
Canary	20	8	Rainbow lorikeet	15	3
Cockatiel	32	5	Rosella	15	3
Conure	25	10	Sulphur-crested cockatoo	40	15
Domestic pigeon	26	15	Superb parrot	36	6
Eclectus parrot	20	8	Toucan	Unknown	4
Gouldian finch	Unknown	4	Zebra finch	17	5
Grey-cheeked parakeet	15	8			

From Ritchie B, Harrison G, Harrison L: *Avian medicine: principles and application,* Florida, 1994, Wingers Publishing.

SUGGESTED READINGS

Altman R, Clubb S, Dorrestein G, et al: *Avian medicine and surgery,* Philadelphia, 1997, WB Saunders.

Calder WA: Respiratory and heart rates of birds at rest, *Condor* 70:358-365, 1968.

Campbell T: *Avian hematology and cytology,* Ames, Iowa, 1988, Iowa State University Press.

Chaplin S, Mueller L, Degernes L: *Physiological assessment of rehabilitated raptors prior to release, Wildlife Journal* 12(1):7-8, 17-18, 1989.

Dorst J: *The life of birds,* vol 1, New York, 1974, Columbia University Press.

Faaborg J: *Ornithology: an ecological approach,* Englewood Cliffs, New Jersey, 1988, Prentice-Hall.

Freethy R: *How birds work,* United Kingdom, 1982, Blandford Books.

Gill F: *Ornithology,* ed 2, New York, 1995, WH Freeman.

King AS, McLeeland J: *Form and function in birds,* vol 2, London, 1981, Academic Press.

Korbel R: Klinischer untersuchungsgang. In Koenig H, Liebich H-G, eds: *Anatomie und propaedeutik des gefluegels,* Stuttgart, New York, 2001, Schattauer Verlag, pp 233-250.

Lucas A, Jamroz C: *Atlas of avian hematology,* Washington, 1961, Agriculture Monograph 25, United Stated Department of Agriculture.

Odum EP: Some physiological variations in the black-capped chick-adee, *Wilson Bull* 55:178-181, 1943.

Pettingill OS Jr, ed: Seminars in ornithology, Ithaca, NY, 1972, Cornell Laboratory of Ornithology.

Ritchie B, Harrison G, Harrison L: *Avian medicine: principles and application,* Florida, 1994, Wingers Publishing.

Stettenheim P: The integument of birds. In Farner DS, King JR, eds: *Avian biology,* vol 2, New York, 1972, Academic Press.

Terres JK: *The Audubon Society encyclopedia of North American birds,* New York, 1980, Alfred A. Knopf.

Welty JC: *The life of birds,* ed 3, Philadelphia, 1982, CBS College Publishing.

Whittow GC: *Sturkie's avian physiology,* ed 5, San Diego, Calif, 2000, Academic Press.

GLOSSARY

A

A bands Large, dark bands in a skeletal muscle fiber that alternate with lighter I bands to give a striped appearance to skeletal muscle fibers under a microscope. The A bands are composed of thick filaments of the contractile protein myosin.

abduction The joint movement whereby an extremity is moved away from the median plane.

abomasum The "true stomach" of the ruminant; secretes acids, mixes and contracts ingesta, and moves liquid chyme into the small intestine.

aboral direction Away from the mouth.

absorptive cell A cell commonly found in the small intestine that can absorb nutrients from the luminal surface via phagocytosis and pinocytosis. Absorptive cells have large surface areas as a result of the presence of microvilli. The expanded surface area increases the absorptive capability of the cell.

accommodation The focusing of the lens of the eye to allow close-up and faraway vision. It is accomplished by the muscles of the ciliary body that apply or relieve tension on the suspensory ligaments that attach it to the lens.

acetabulum The socket portion of the ball-and-socket hip joint. It is formed at the junction of the ilium, ischium, and pubis bones of the pelvis.

acetylcholine Neurotransmitter; associated with parasympathetic nervous system effects even though it is the neurotransmitter used in the preganglionic neuron in both the sympathetic and parasympathetic nervous systems; has a stimulatory effect on the gastrointestinal tract; increases secretions and muscle contractions in the esophagus, stomach, ruminant forestomachs, intestine, and colon.

acetylcholinesterase The enzyme that breaks down acetylcholine.

acinar gland The secretory units of exocrine glands that contain one or more saclike structures.

acromegaly A form of giantism that results from an excess of growth hormone (GH).

acrosome The caplike structure that partially covers the heads of spermatozoa. It contains digestive enzymes that are activated when the cells enter the female reproductive tract. They help the cell penetrate through the layers around the ovum to fertilize it.

ACTH *See* Adrenocorticotropic hormone.

actin A protein that composes microfilaments. It is found in the cytoskeleton, in myofibrils of muscle fibers, and in spindle fibers during cell division.

actin filaments One of the two contractile proteins of muscle (myosin is the other one) that slide over each other to produce the shortening of the muscle cell that we refer to as muscle contraction.

action potential The change in electrical charges that occurs during nerve depolarization; also called the nerve impulse; the changes in cellular polarity that define the electrical activity of cardiac tissue.

active immunity Activation of the immune system by either administration of a vaccine that contains a modified antigen or exposure to the antigen (e.g., by disease).

active site The specific area on an enzyme that connects with a substrate to cause a chemical reaction.

active transport The process that moves ions or molecules across the cell membrane and against the concentration gradient, requiring energy or ATP to be accomplished.

adduction The joint movement whereby an extremity is moved toward the median plane.

adenine (A) One of the nucleotides present in both DNA and RNA. It is a purine base that corresponds to RNA's uracil and DNA's thymine.

adenosine diphosphate (ADP) Adenosine diphosphate is the "discharged" form of adenosine triphosphate (ATP). It is a nucleotide that contains two phosphoric acid groups. When a phosphate group is split off an ATP molecule to produce ADP, energy is released that, in muscle, powers the sliding of the actin and myosin filaments over each other. When the phosphate group is reattached (which requires another energy source), ADP is converted back to ATP and the molecule is ready to provide energy again.

adenosine triphosphate (ATP) Adenosine triphosphate is a high-energy molecule produced in the mitochondria of cells. It is a nucleotide that contains three phosphoric acid groups. When a phosphate group is split off an ATP molecule to produce ADP, energy is released that, in muscle, powers the sliding of the actin and myosin filaments over each other. When the phosphate group is reattached (which requires another energy source), ADP is converted back to ATP and the molecule is ready to provide energy again. The more active a cell or body part is, the more ATP it will have produced and stored. For instance, muscles have a great deal of stored ATP, whereas fat has fairly little.

ADH *See* Antidiuretic hormone.

adipocyte A type of fixed cell in the connective tissue that stores fat (lipids) in its cytoplasm. The nucleus and other organelles are pushed to the periphery of the cell.

adipose cells *See* Adipocyte.

adipose connective tissue A subclass of connective tissue proper, adipose connective tissue is a vascularized type of connective tissue whose general functions are to protect, insulate, and provide a major source of energy to the body. Adipose connective tissue can occur as either brown or white adipose tissue. White adipose tissue, found commonly throughout the body, is a storage area for lipids. These lipids may be used for the production of energy or ATP. Brown adipose tissue, found in neonate and hibernating species, has its lipids converted to heat.

adipose Fat.

ADP *See* Adenosine diphosphate.

adrenal cortex The outer portion of the adrenal gland that produces glucocorticoid, mineralocorticoid, and sex hormones

adrenal glands Two endocrine glands located near the cranial poles of the kidneys. Each consists of an outer cortex and an inner medulla.

adrenal medulla The inner portion of the adrenal gland that produces the hormones epinephrine and norepinephrine.

adrenergic neurons Neurons that secrete catecholamines (e.g., norepinephrine) as their neurotransmitter.

adrenocorticotropic hormone (ACTH) A hormone secreted by the anterior portion of the pituitary gland, which in turn activates the adrenal gland. The adrenal gland then releases its own hormones. ACTH is vital to the normal function and development of the adrenal gland.

adult hemoglobin The primary type of hemoglobin found in the red blood cells of animals beginning a couple of weeks to a couple of months after birth.

aerobic metabolism Oxygen-consuming metabolism. The type of metabolism in muscle in which the supply of available oxygen is sufficient to keep up with the energy needs of the muscle fibers. Aerobic metabolism extracts the maximum amount of energy from glucose molecules.

aerobic respiration The cell function that produces chemical energy with the use of oxygen.

afferent glomerular arterioles The smallest arteriole branches that carry blood into the glomerulus for filtration.

afferent nerve Nerve that carries impulses toward the central nervous system.

afterbirth The name given to the placenta at parturition because it is delivered *after* the newborn.

afterload The sum of the forces that the heart must overcome during ventricular contraction

agglutination Precipitation or clumping of antigen-antibody complexes; one of the methods by which the immune system neutralizes antigens.

agranulocytes White blood cells without cytoplasmic granules. The agranulocytes are the monocytes and the lymphocytes; also known as nongranulocytes.

air sacs Nine thin, transparent membranes that are connected to the primary and secondary bronchi and act as reservoirs for air entering and leaving the lungs.

albumin Protein manufactured by the liver that plays an important role in maintaining the osmotic fluid balance between capillaries (blood) and tissues; a lack of albumin results in movement of fluid from the capillaries into the tissues, producing edema and fluid accumulation in body cavities.

aldosterone A mineralocorticoid hormone secreted by the cortex of the adrenal gland. It stimulates the kidney to conserve sodium ions and water and to eliminate potassium and hydrogen ions.

alimentary canal Also called the digestive tract, this encompasses all of the parts of the digestive system that transport food from the mouth to the anus: mouth, esophagus, stomach, small and large intestines, and anus.

alkaline The adjective that describes substances with a pH above 7 (basic). Basic or alkaline solutions have fewer hydrogen ions or more hydroxide ions than pure water.

allantoic sac Part of the placenta. It is a fluid-filled sac formed by the allantois that surrounds the amniotic sac.

allantois Part of the placenta. It is the membrane that forms the allantoic sac.

all-or-none principle Refers to the way in which a neuron depolarizes completely or not at all in response to stimulation.

all-or-nothing principle The principle that an individual muscle fiber either contracts completely or does not contract at all.

alopecia Loss of hair.

alpha$_1$-adrenergic receptors Receptors associated with the sympathetic nervous system response; these receptors, when stimulated by catecholamines, tend to cause vasoconstriction (constriction of blood vessels).

alpha cells Cells in the pancreas that produce glucagon.

alpha helix The coiled structure in a complex protein composed of hydrogen bonds and amino acids.

altricial Chicks that are hatched with their eyes closed and their skins bare and that are immobile.

alula Bone in birds that originates from the wrist and is comparable with a first finger; carries feathers that aid in steering.

alveolar ducts The smallest air passageways in the lungs. The alveolar ducts carry air to the alveolar sacs.

alveolar gland Secretory units of exocrine glands that are saclike in form; also called acinar gland.

alveolar sacs Clusters of alveoli at the ends of the alveolar ducts. The alveoli are arranged like bunches of grapes.

alveoli (*singular,* alveolus) Microscopic, thin-walled sacs surrounded by networks of capillaries. The interface between the wall of the alveoli and the wall of the capillary is where the actual exchange of gases takes place in the lungs.

amino acid The basic building block of peptides and proteins; those organic compounds, numbering around 80, that are made up of an amino group (NH_2) and a carboxyl group (COOH). Amino acids make up proteins when joined together in peptide bonds. They are naturally occurring in all plants and animals.

aminopeptidase Protease secreted in an inactive form from the pancreas and activated by trypsin.

amnion Part of the placenta. It is the membrane that forms the fluid-filled amniotic sac.

amniotic sac Part of the placenta. It is the fluid-filled sac that immediately surrounds the developing fetus.

amoeboid motion Amoeba-like movement accomplished by the extension of pseudopodia to create a streaming movement of cytoplasm.

amorphous Having no defined shape.

amphiarthrosis A slightly movable cartilaginous joint, such as the pelvic symphysis.

ampulla An enlargement in each semicircular canal that contains the receptor structure (the crista).

ampulla of the vas deferens An enlargement of the vas deferens just before it enters the urethra. It is present in some species and absent in others.

amylase Enzyme produced by the pancreas and, in some species, the saliva; attacks starch and breaks it into disaccharides (two sugar molecules).

amyloid An excessive amount of a waxlike, proteinaceous substance in the body's tissue.

anabolism The form of metabolism by which cells build complex compounds from simpler ones; the opposite of catabolism. The process by which the cell uses energy to manufacture large molecules from smaller ones; these molecules are used to maintain the cell and carry out metabolic processes.

anaerobic A biochemical pathway that can function without oxygen. The term also may be used to describe microbes that can live in the absence of oxygen.

anaerobic glycolysis An alternative expression for glycolysis referring to the fact that the reaction does not require oxygen.

anaerobic metabolism Nonoxygen-dependent metabolism. The type of metabolism in muscle that occurs when the need for energy to produce muscular activity exceeds the available oxygen supply. Anaerobic metabolism is not as efficient as aerobic metabolism and results in the formation of lactic acid as a byproduct. Lactic acid can cause discomfort in muscle tissue and requires oxygen to be converted back to glucose.

anaerobic respiration The cell function that produces energy chemically with the use of free oxygen.

anagen phase The active phase of hair growth.

anal sacs Perianal sacs, containing apocrine and sebaceous glands, that are located at the 5 o'clock and 7 o'clock positions relative to the anus. The sacs reside between the internal and external sphincter of carnivores and produce a strong smelling fluid when expressed. They are important for fecal territorial marking and are expressed during fearful episodes.

analgesia Decreased perception of pain.

anaphase The phase of mitosis when the daughter chromosomes begin to migrate to their respective centrioles, away from the center of the dividing cell.

anaphylaxis A severe, potentially life-threatening, allergic response.

anatomy The study of the form and structure of an animal body and its parts. Through anatomy we can describe where things are located in or on the animal body and what they look like.

anconeal process A beak-shaped process at the proximal end of the trochlear notch of the ulna. When it fails to unite with the ulna, an ununited anconeal process can cause the elbow joint to become unstable, leading to lameness.

androgens Hormones that promote the development of male characteristics; male sex hormones. The principal androgen is testosterone.

anemia Decreased oxygen-carrying capacity of the blood caused by insufficient numbers of red blood cells, decreased hemoglobin concentration, or a combination of both of these conditions.

anesthesia Complete loss of sensation.

anestrus The period when the ovary "shuts down" between the estrous cycles or breeding seasons of some animal species.

angle The angle of the hoof wall as viewed from a lateral aspect when the foot is flat on the ground.

anions A negatively charged atom or molecule; a negatively charged ion.

anisodactyly Toe position in which three toes face forward and once faces the rear.

antagonist Something that opposes the action of something else. An antagonist muscle or muscle group directly opposes the action of a "prime mover" muscle or muscle group that is directly producing a desired movement.

antebrachium The "forearm" region of the thoracic limb.

anterior chamber The portion of the aqueous compartment of the eye in front of (rostral to) the iris.

anterior pituitary gland The adenohypophysis; the rostral portion of the pituitary gland that produces seven hormones, many of which influence other endocrine glands.

antibodies Proteins produced by plasma cells (transformed B lymphocytes) in response to the presence of an antigen. A specific serum antibody is generated for a specific antigen.

anticlinal vertebra The thoracic vertebra whose spinous process projects straight up dorsally in contrast to the caudally inclined spinous processes cranial to it and the cranially inclined spinous processes caudal to it. It acts as a landmark on radiographs of the thoracolumbar region, particularly in dogs, in which it is the eleventh thoracic vertebra.

anticoagulant A substance that prevents blood from clotting when it is added to the blood.

anticodon The triplet pair of nucleotides in tRNA that correspond to the triplet bases or codons of mRNA.

antidiuretic hormone (ADH) A hormone released by the posterior pituitary. It facilitates water conservation in the body by promoting water reabsorption from urine in the collecting ducts. Low levels of ADH cause diabetes insipidus, a condition that results in excessive water loss from the body through increased urine volume.

antigens Cells or organisms that are "not self." An antigen also can be a structure on a cell membrane that the body recognizes as foreign. The presence of an antigen initiates an immune response in a healthy animal.

antineoplasticic drugs Drugs that inhibit the growth and spread of malignant cells and tumors; also known as chemotherapeutic drugs.

antiport system When two separate materials are moved across the plasma membrane in opposite directions at the same time.

antrum (1) The fluid-filled space within an ovarian follicle. (2) The muscular part of the stomach that is responsible for grinding of food; located between the body of the stomach and the pylorus.

anucleated Having no nuclei.

anuria Condition in which no urine is being passed from the body.

aorta Major artery of the systemic circulation that receives blood from the left ventricle.

aortic valve A semilunar valve; it separates the left ventricle and the aorta during diastole.

apex (tooth) The tip of the tooth root where the blood and nerve supply enter the tooth; the uppermost point of a structure.

apical surface The side of an epithelial cell that faces in toward the body cavity.

apocrine gland A gland whose secretions contain some of its cellular material. Part of the secretory cell is destroyed and must regenerate before the cell can secrete again. Examples of these glands are mammary glands and some sweat glands.

apocrine sweat glands Exocrine glands that secrete substances into the hair follicle rather than directly to the skin surface.

aponeurosis A broad sheet of fibrous connective tissue that attaches certain muscles to bones or to other muscles.

appendicular skeleton The bones of the limbs (appendages).

apteryla Bare areas of skin of birds where feathers do not originate.

aqueous compartment The compartment of the eye in front of (rostral to) the lens and ciliary body. It contains a watery fluid, called aqueous humor, and is subdivided by the iris into the anterior chamber and the posterior chamber.

aqueous humor The watery fluid that fills the aqueous compartment of the eye. It is produced in the posterior chamber and drained from the anterior chamber by the canal of Schlemm.

arachnoid The delicate, weblike layer of the meninges between the dura mater and the pia mater.

areolar connective tissue A soft, spongy connective tissue, also known as loose connective tissue. It is located throughout the body and is composed of a soft ground substance, numerous cell types (white blood cells, fibroblasts, macrophages), and all three types of fibers (elastic, reticular, and collagenous).

arrector pili muscles Smooth muscle that is attached to the base of the hair follicle. It is responsible for the involuntary "hair raising" response to cold and fear or aggression.

arthrodial joint A gliding joint in which two flat articular surfaces rock on each other. This type of joint usually allows only the movements of flexion and extension.

articular cartilage The thin layer of hyaline cartilage that covers the articular surfaces of long bones in synovial joints. It forms a smooth layer over the joint surfaces of the bones, which decreases friction and allows free joint movement.

articular process The process of a vertebra that forms a synovial joint with an adjacent vertebra.

articular surface The smooth joint surface of a bone that contacts another bone in a synovial joint.

arytenoid cartilages Two of the cartilages of the larynx. The vocal cords attach to the arytenoid cartilages. The arytenoid cartilages and the vocal cords form the boundaries of the glottis (the opening into the larynx).

ascites An abnormal condition in which an excessive amount of fluid accumulation is present in the abdominal cavity. Abdominal distention or a potbellied appearance can be clinically evident.

asternal rib A rib whose costal cartilage joins the costal cartilage of the rib ahead of it instead of directly joining the sternum.

ataxia Incoordination. An ataxic animal makes jerky, spastic movements.

atlas The first cervical vertebra. It forms the atlantooccipital joint with the occipital bone of the skull and the atlantoaxial joint with the axis (the second cervical vertebra).

atopy A type I hypersensitivity or allergic reaction to antigens that are inhaled, such as pollen and dust; often associated with a genetic predisposition.

ATP *See* Adenosine triphosphate.

ATP synthase The enzyme in the mitochondria of body cells that functions as a tiny "molecular machine" to regenerate ATP from ADP and detached phosphate groups. It is powered by the proton gradient present across interior mitochondrial membranes.

atrial septal defect Abnormal formation of the interatrial septum resulting in a communication (a hole) between the left and right atria.

atrophy Shrinkage.

auriculars Small contour feathers located around the external ear openings in birds.

autoimmune disease An abnormal condition in which the body starts recognizing some of its own cells as "not self" and initiates an immune response to destroy the cells.

autolysis The self-digestion of tissues or cells by enzymes that are released by their own lysosomes.

autonomic nervous system The part of the nervous system that controls smooth muscle, cardiac muscle, and endocrine glands automatically without conscious control; has motor and sensory branches.

autonomic reflex A reflex that results in stimulation or inhibition of smooth or cardiac muscle or endocrine gland function; mechanisms of homeostasis are autonomic reflexes.

avascular Without a vascular or blood supply.

axial skeleton The bones along the central axis of the body; made up of the skull, the hyoid bone, the spinal column, the ribs, and the sternum.

axis The second cervical vertebra. It forms the atlantoaxial joint with the first cervical vertebra (the atlas).

axon Extension of the neuron that conducts the nerve impulse away from the cell body to the terminal bouton (synaptic bulb) at the end of the neuron.

B

B lymphocyte The type of lymphocyte that is responsible for humoral immunity through its transformation into a plasma cell and production of antibody.

ball-and-socket joint Also called a spheroidal joint. It consists of a spherical joint surface (the ball) that fits into a closely matching concave joint surface (the socket). The shoulder and hip joints are ball-and-socket joints. Ball-and-socket joints allow the greatest range of joint movements.

barbs Slender projections off the main feather shaft that comprise a vane on each side of the shaft.

barbules Microscopic projections off feather barbs that help maintain a contour feather's structure.

basal bodies Refers to a pair of tubular structures. Each one is composed of nine microtubules surrounding another pair of microtubules. Basal bodies act as the base of cilia and flagella.

basal cell tumors Tumors of the stratum germinativum or basal layer of the epithelium. They tend not to metastasize and are most common in cats.

basal cells Cells located in the deepest layer of the epidermis that eventually mature to become keratinocytes.

basal surface The side of an epithelial cell that faces a lower level of connective tissue.

basement membrane A noncellular, collagen-based structure that supports epithelial tissue.

basopenia Theoretically, a decrease in the total number of basophils in peripheral blood. This condition is difficult to describe because basophils normally are rarely found in peripheral blood.

basophilia An increase in the total number of basophils in peripheral blood.

basophils One of the granulocytic white blood cells characterized by the presence of numerous, dark blue–staining granules in its cytoplasm.

belly The thick, central portion of a muscle.

benign A nonrecurrent, nonharmful growth.

beta$_1$-adrenergic receptors Receptors associated with the sympathetic nervous system response; these receptors, when stimulated by catecholamines, tend to cause an increase in rate and force of contraction of the heart.

beta$_2$-adrenergic receptors Receptors associated with the sympathetic nervous system response; these receptors, when stimulated by catecholamines, tend to cause dilation of the bronchioles (airways) and vasodilation of some blood vessels.

beta cells Cells in the pancreas that produce insulin.

beta-oxidation The breakdown of fatty acid chains into two carbon fragments in the mitochondria. These two carbon fragments can be broken down further into ketone bodies and acetyl-coA.

beta pleat The formation of a complex protein that is composed of hydrogen bonds corresponding with the spines of polypeptide chains.

bicarbonate Often referred to as sodium bicarbonate, it acts as a buffer in the secretions (pancreas, saliva) to reduce the acidity of the stomach or rumen; also helps to buffer the pH in the blood.

bifurcation of the trachea The division of the trachea at its caudal end into the left and right main bronchi, which enter the lungs.

bilateral symmetry The concept that the left and right halves of an animal's body are mirror images of each other. Paired structures, such as the kidneys, are located one on each side of the body, and single structures, such as the heart, are located near the median plane.

bile acids Hydrophilic (water-loving) molecules with a hydrophobic (water-hating) end secreted by the liver into the duodenum; combine with fat droplets to make them more water soluble.

bilirubin The yellow breakdown product of hemoglobin.

biopsy The removal of a small sample of tissue for microscopic examination. This procedure is often but not exclusively used to determine whether a tumor is benign or malignant.

biosynthetic Refers to a compound manufactured within a living thing.

blast A cell in the production stage of a particular substance.

blastic transformation Through this process, B lymphocytes become plasma cells that produce antibodies.

blastocyst The stage of development of a zygote that is ready for implantation in the uterus. It is shaped like a tiny, hollow ball of cells with a "bump" on one side that eventually develops into the embryo.

bloat The accumulation of gas within the rumen or monogastric stomach causing severe distention.

blood feather A developing feather that contains blood in its shaft for growth and nourishment.

blood-brain barrier The functional barrier between the capillaries in the brain and the nervous tissue itself; anatomically composed of capillary walls without the openings found in other capillaries and glial cells.

body of the penis The largest portion of the penis. It contains the majority of the erectile tissue of the organ.

body of the stomach The central part of the stomach between the fundus and the antrum.

bolus (of food) Amount of food swallowed at one time.

bone cortex The outer layer of a bone that is composed of compact bone.

bone marrow The soft material that fills the spaces inside bones. Two types of bone marrow are red bone marrow, which forms blood cells, and yellow bone marrow, which consists primarily of adipose connective tissue (fat).

bones of the cranium The bones of the skull that surround the brain. The externally visible bones of the cranium are the occipital bone, the interparietal bones, the parietal bones, the temporal bones, and the frontal bones. The internal (hidden) bones of the cranium are the sphenoid bone and the ethmoid bone.

bones of the face The skull bones that do not surround the brain. The externally visible bones of the face are the incisive bones, the nasal bones, the maxillary bones, the lacrimal bones, the zygomatic bones, and the mandible. The internal (hidden) bones of the face are the palatine bones, the pterygoid bones, the vomer bone, and the turbinates.

bovine spongiform encephalopathy (BSE) Also known as mad cow disease. This disease was first contracted by cows in Great Britain that had consumed the flesh of sheep thought to carry infectious prions.

Bowman's capsule Part of the renal corpuscle. It consists of two layers: an inner visceral layer that lies directly on the glomerular capillaries and an outer parietal layer. It functions as a plasma filter in the process of urine formation.

brachium The "upper arm." The area of the thoracic limb between the elbow and the shoulder.

brachycephalic Short-faced. Brachycephalic breeds of dogs include Boston terriers, pugs, English bulldogs, and Pekinese.

bradycardia Abnormally slow heart rate.

brain stem The connection between the brain and the spinal cord; composed of the medulla oblongata, the pons, and the midbrain; heavily involved in autonomic control functions related to the heart, respiration, blood vessel diameter, swallowing, and vomiting.

broad ligaments Paired sheets of connective tissue that suspend the uterus from the dorsal part of the abdominal cavity and attach it to the abdominal wall. They are often subdivided into the mesovarium, which supports the ovary; the mesosalpinx, which supports the oviduct; and the mesometrium, which supports the uterus.

bronchi The largest air passageways in the lungs. The left and right main bronchi are formed by the bifurcation of the trachea. The main bronchi divide into smaller and smaller branches within the lungs. The branching arrangement of the bronchi is referred to as the bronchial tree.

bronchial tree The air passageways in the lungs between the main bronchi and the alveoli. The branching nature of the bronchi as they form smaller and smaller air passageways resembles the branching of a tree.

bronchioles Some of the smallest branches of the bronchial tree. The bronchioles subdivide down to the alveolar ducts (the smallest air passageways that lead directly to the alveolar sacs).

bronchitis A lower respiratory tract infection affecting the lining of the larger air passageways in the lungs. Bronchitis can be a serious disease because the inflammatory fluids and excess mucus resulting from the irritation are difficult for the animal to cough up from down deep in the lungs.

bronchoconstriction Contraction of the smooth muscle that surrounds the air passageways in the lungs. Bronchoconstriction narrows the air passageways. It can be physiological, as when a mild degree of bronchoconstriction reduces the work of moving air in and out of the lungs at rest. Bronchoconstriction also can be pathological, as when inhaled irritants cause severe bronchoconstriction that makes breathing very difficult.

bronchodilation Relaxation of the smooth muscle that surrounds the air passageways in the lungs. Full bronchodilation causes the air passageways to dilate to their full, large diameters. Physiological bronchodilation occurs during intense physical activity when maximum air must be moved into and out of the lungs. A class of drugs called bronchodilators can be used to help relax severe bronchoconstriction, such as might occur in an asthmalike condition.

brood patch Area of thickened skin on the lower abdomen of birds where feathers are plucked to transfer heat to eggs during incubation.

brown adipose tissue "Brown fat" found commonly throughout the body of hibernating species and neonates. It is a specialized form of adipose tissue that releases its stored lipid reserves in the form of heat. This is accomplished because of the high degree of vascularization and concentration of mitochondria found in brown adipose tissue.

brush border The area on the free surface of an epithelial cell that is covered with microvilli.

buccal cavity Although this translates literally to "cheek cavity," the buccal cavity usually refers to the mouth or oral cavity; pronounced "BHU-kal."

buccal surface The surface of the caudal part of the upper and lower arcade teeth that face the cheeks; *bucco* is Latin for "cheeks."

bulb of the glans An enlargement in the penis of the dog and related species. It is made up of erectile tissue that slowly engorges with blood during copulation. When muscles surrounding the vagina and vulva of the female clamp down on the enlarged bulb, the male cannot withdraw the penis. He typically dismounts and turns so that the two animals are tail to tail. This position is known as the "tie" and usually lasts 15 to 20 minutes, after which the animals can separate.

bulbar conjunctiva The transparent membrane that covers the front (rostral) portion of the eyeball.

bulbourethral glands Male accessory reproductive glands that secrete a mucus-containing fluid just before ejaculation that lubricates the urethra for the passage of semen and clears it of urine. Bulbourethral glands are present in all common domestic animals except the dog.

C

calcaneal tuberosity Large process of the fibular tarsal bone that projects upward and backward; commonly referred to as the point of the hock; site of attachment of the gastrocnemius (calf) muscle; equivalent to the human heel.

calcified Hardening of organic tissue by the deposit of lime and calcium salts.

calcitonin The hormone secreted by the thyroid gland that prevents the level of calcium in the blood from getting too high.

callus The healing tissue between the ends of a fractured bone that is eventually replaced by true bone as the fracture heals.

calorigenic Heat producing.

CAM *See* Cell adhesion molecules.

canal of Schlemm The structure that drains aqueous humor from the anterior chamber of the eye. It is located out at the edge of the anterior chamber where the iris and the cornea meet.

canaliculi Tiny channels through the matrix of bone. Threadlike projections from osteocytes communicate with each other and with blood vessels through the canaliculi.

cancellous bone "Spongy" bone. A form of bone composed of seemingly randomly arranged "spicules" of bone separated by spaces filled with bone marrow. Appears spongelike to the naked eye. Found in the ends (epiphyses) of long bones and the interiors of short bones, flat bones, and irregular bones.

cancer The progressive, uncontrolled growth of abnormal cells or neoplasms that turn normal somatic cells into malignant ones. Ultimately, if left untreated, the cancer will metastasize, causing the disease to spread to other systems or areas of the body, leading to an eventual death.

canine parvoviral enteritis Caused by the canine parvovirus, this infectious disease has an extremely high mortality rate in puppies. Infections occurring in utero are known to cause acute myocarditis and overall poor health in the litter. Because it tends to attack cells in the mitotic phase, rapidly dividing epithelial tissue is particularly affected by parvoviral infections. Vomiting, diarrhea, bloody stool, and dehydration are clinical signs of disease. An immunization is available.

canine tooth Sharp, pointed tooth between the most caudal incisor and the most rostral premolar.

cannon bone The large metacarpal and metatarsal bones of the horse.

canthus The corner of the eyelids where they come together. Each eye has a medial and a lateral canthus.

capacitation The process spermatozoa undergo in the female reproductive tract before contact with the ovum that increases their fertility. Part of the process exposes the digestive enzymes in the acrosome. This helps the cell penetrate through the layers surrounding the ovum.

capillary refill time (CRT) The time it takes for mucous membranes to return to their normal pink color after being pressed to a white color. If the return to normal color is too slow or fast, it can indicate a diseased state.

capsular space The space between the visceral and parietal layers of Bowman's capsule.

carbohydrate metabolism Metabolic processes that store and release energy contained within carbohydrates for the purposes of growth, repair, and normal function of the body.

carbohydrates One of the essential nutrients necessary for all life functions. They are a quick source of energy and may be stored in the body as glycogen; sugars

carboxypeptidase Protease secreted in an inactive form from the pancreas and activated by trypsin.

carcinogenic Having those properties that cause cancer.

cardia The part of the stomach where the esophagus enters.

cardiac muscle Striated, involuntary muscle that is found exclusively in the heart. Cardiac muscle is controlled by the autonomic nervous system. It has one centrally located nucleus and intercalated disks that form special connections between the muscle branches.

cardiomyopathy Disease of the myocardium (heart muscle).

carnassial teeth Large rostral molar and last premolar in the dog that have deep roots.

carnivore An animal whose diet is primarily meat.

carpal bones The bones of the carpus. Consist of two parallel rows of short bones located between the distal ends of the radius and ulna and the proximal ends of the metacarpal bones.

carpus The joint composed of the carpal bones. Referred to as the "knee" of the horse and the "wrist" of humans.

carrier proteins Any protein that facilitates diffusion of a specific molecule through the cell membrane.

cartilage An opaque, dense connective tissue composed of a relatively small number of cells that are contained within a nonliving matrix. Cartilage absorbs shock and protects the epiphysial ends of bones. Cartilage is not innervated or vascularized, which makes it resistant to pain but also to healing. It is found in joints, body structures such as the ears and nose, the costal cartilage of the ribcage, and the fetal skeleton.

cartilaginous joint A joint in which the bones are united by cartilage; also called an amphiarthrosis. Only a slight rocking motion is permitted between the bones.

caruncle Numerous mushroomlike structures in the lining of the uterus of ruminant animals. They join with the cotyledons of the placenta to form placental attachment sites called placentomes.

catabolism The breaking down of nutrients into smaller and simpler materials for use by the cell to release energy; the opposite of anabolism.

catagen phase The transitional phase between anagen and telogen phases of the hair growth cycle.

catalase An enzyme found in almost all cells that breaks down hydrogen peroxide into water and oxygen.

catalysts Substances that induce chemical reactions by lowering the activation energy needed.

catecholamines The group of neurotransmitters that includes norepinephrine, epinephrine, dopamine, and other neurotransmitters with similar chemical properties.

cations Positively charged ions.

caudal A directional term meaning toward the tail end of an animal.

cecocolic orifice The opening between the cecum and the colon; most developed in the horse and other nonruminant herbivores.

cecum The blind pouch leading off from where the ileum meets the colon; in nonruminant herbivores the cecum can be very developed into a base, body, and apex (tip).

cell The most basic structural unit of all animals and plants. Cells make up all tissues of an organism and perform all of the functions by which life is defined, including growth, reproduction, and metabolism.

cell adhesion molecules (CAMs) Glycoproteins that aid not only in the bonding of cells but also in lubricating the movement of one cell past another. They also help to transport specialized cells to areas of need.

cell-mediated immune responses Response of the body's cells to regulate the destruction of infectious bacteria and viruses during specific immune responses.

cell-mediated immunity The portion of the immune system that produces "killer" cells that directly attack foreign invaders.

cell membrane The selectively permeable outer membrane of the cell that is composed of a phospholipid bilayer, protein, and cholesterol; also called plasma membrane or plasmalemma.

cell metabolism Functions that break down nutrients, produce ATP, use ATP, and create complex molecules from simple ones.

cellular respiration The oxidation of organic material to yield energy, carbon dioxide, and water.

cellulase An enzyme that breaks down the sugar cellulose.

cellulose Ruminant animals must convert this matter into volatile fatty acids to derive sustenance from it. This is accomplished through microbial fermentation. Cellulose is not digested by carnivores and most omnivores.

central nervous system (CNS) The brain and spinal cord

central sulcus The central depression of the frog in the equine hoof.

centriole A tubular organelle composed of nine triplets of microtubules that aids in the process of cell division. Centrioles split in two and migrate to opposite poles of a dividing cell to organize the spindle fibers, enabling the cell to divide in two.

centromere Also called a kinetochore; the protein disk that holds a pair of chromatids together as a chromosome and then holds that chromosome to a spindle fiber during cell division.

centrosome An area of condensed cytoplasm located near the nucleus that contains the centriole(s) of the cell.

cerebellar dysfunction Caused by inflammation, underdevelopment, or degeneration of the cerebellum, the disease is characterized by an exaggerated and awkward gait usually resulting from hyperextension of the legs. Cerebellar dysfunction does not exhibit any degree of paralysis, partial or complete.

cerebellum Second largest component of the brain; allows the body to have coordinated movement, balance, posture, and complex reflexes.

cerebral cortex Gray matter that makes up the outer layer of the cerebrum.

cerebral hemispheres The two halves of the cerebrum.

cerebrospinal fluid (CSF) Fluid that bathes and protects the brain and spinal cord from the hard surface of the skull and spinal vertebrae.

cerebrum That portion of the brain responsible for functions most commonly associated with "higher-order" behaviors (learning, intelligence, awareness); receives and interprets sensory information, initiates conscious (voluntary) nerve impulses to skeletal muscles, and integrates neuron activity that is normally associated with communication, expression of emotional responses, learning, memory and recall, and other behaviors associated with conscious activity.

cervical vertebrae The bones of the neck portion of the spinal column.

cervix The sphincter muscle "valve" between the uterus and the vagina; controls access to the lumen of the uterus from the vagina. It is normally closed except during breeding and parturition.

chemical control system The respiratory control system that monitors the pH of the blood and its content of O_2 and CO_2. If any of the measured values varies outside preset limits, the chemical control system initiates changes in the breathing pattern to bring them back into balance.

chemical digestion The breakdown of food by action of chemicals or enzymes.

chemical signaling The specific interaction of hormones and neurotransmitters to cell surfaces for the purpose of changing cell activity.

chemotaxis The movement of white blood cells into an area of inflammation in response to chemical mediators released at the site by injured tissue or other white blood cells.

chestnut Believed to be the vestigial remnants of the carpal and tarsal bones, they are horny, keratinized growths located on the medial forearm and hock of horses.

chief cells Cells in the stomach that produce the enzyme precursor pepsinogen.

choanae Two internal nares that open from the nasal chambers into the roof of the mouth.

cholecystokinin (CCK) A hormone released by the duodenum when chyme enters from the stomach. It slows gastric emptying and motility while increasing intestinal motility. It also stimulates the pancreas to release digestive enzymes into the duodenum.

cholesterol A steroid alcohol that is found in many fat-based tissues throughout the body. Cholesterol can be synthesized in the body or obtained through diet.

cholinergic neurons Neurons that secrete acetylcholine as their neurotransmitter.

cholinergic receptors Receptors for acetylcholine; may be muscarinic or nicotinic receptors.

chondroblasts Fixed cells that form cartilage.

chondrocyte Mature cartilage cell.

chondroitin sulfate A glycosaminoglycan found in cartilage.

chondronectin An adhesive glycosaminoglycan found in cartilage.

chordae tendineae Fine, threadlike cords that connect two atrioventricular valves to the appropriate papillary muscles in the ventricles.

chorion Part of the placenta; the outermost layer that attaches to the uterine lining. The chorion is linked to the fetus by the umbilical cord.

chorionic gonadotropin A hormone produced by the placenta of a pregnant animal.

choroid A portion of the uvea, or middle vascular layer, of the eye. The choroid consists mainly of pigment and blood vessels and is located between the sclera and the retina.

chromatids Strands of genetic material that, when joined together with another chromatid by a centromere, form a chromosome.

chromatin A material that is composed of DNA and proteins and makes up chromosomes.

chromosomes Threadlike accumulations of DNA in the nuclei of cells that are particularly visible during mitosis. The DNA of the chromosomes contains the genetic material of the cell. The number of chromosomes is constant within a given species.

chyle The "milky" appearing lymph from the intestines consisting of primarily small molecules of absorbed fats.

chylomicrons Microscopic particles of fat found in chyle and blood. Their numbers are highest after a meal.

chyme The semifluid, partially digested food that leaves the stomach and enters the duodenum.

chymotrypsin Protease secreted in an inactive form from the pancreas and activated by trypsin.

cilia Hairlike processes of the luminal surface of cells that assist in the movement of mucus, fluid, and solid material across the cell surface.

ciliary body A portion of the uvea, or middle vascular layer, of the eye. The ciliary body is a ring-shaped structure located immediately behind the iris. It contains the ciliary muscles that adjust the shape of the lens and the cells that produce aqueous humor.

ciliary muscle Multiunit smooth muscles of the ciliary body that adjust the shape of the eye's lens.

circular muscle The smooth muscle in the muscle layer of the gastrointestinal tract that encircles the organ and causes mixing or segmental contractions; plays a role in peristalsis; concentrated circular muscle compose the sphincters.

circulating pool of neutrophils Neutrophils found in the peripheral blood flowing through the center of blood vessels.

circumduction A joint motion whereby the distal end of an extremity moves in a circle.

cisternae A reservoir that stores fluid.

citric acid cycle A complicated metabolic pathway that is included in the metabolism of fats, proteins, and carbohydrates and that involves the oxidation of pyruvic acid and the release of energy. Other terms used are the Krebs cycle and the tricarboxylic acid cycle.

claws Accessory appendages of the integumentary system present mainly in carnivores for the purpose of grasping prey and self-defense.

cleavage The process of very rapid cell division after an ovum has been fertilized. The cells divide so rapidly that they do not have time to grow appreciably between divisions. The number of cells increases rapidly, but the overall size of the cell mass does not increase much.

clitoris One of the structures of the vulva of the female. Homologous to the penis of the male, the clitoris contains erectile tissue and is richly supplied with sensory nerve endings.

clutch The total number of eggs laid for a single nesting period.

CNS *See* Central nervous system.

coated pit Parts of the cell membrane that have a hairlike coating necessary for endocytic functions. These portions of the cell membrane pinch off to form vesicles that aid in the intracellular transport of materials.

coccygeal vertebrae The bones of the tail portion of the spinal column.

coccyx The human "tailbone." It consists of four to five coccygeal vertebrae fused into a solid structure.

cochlea The snail shell–shaped cavity in the temporal bone of the skull that contains the hearing portion of the inner ear.

cochlear duct A long, fluid-filled tube that runs the length of the cochlea. It contains the receptor organ of hearing (the organ of Corti).

codon The genetic code of an amino acid expressed in DNA or messenger RNA as three bases.

coenzymes An organic molecule that is required by an enzyme to carry out a metabolic reaction. Coenzymes, such as nicotinamide adenine dinucleotide (NAD), are often derived from vitamins.

cofactors Elements, such as coenzymes, that act concurrently with another element to carry out a chemical reaction.

coffin bone The distal phalanx bone, which is the entire third phalanx of the skeletal foot of the horse.

collagenous fiber A structural protein that is commonly located in tendons and ligaments.

collateral sulcus Deep ridge on either side of the frog that separates it from the bars in the equine hoof.

collecting ducts The tubule system that collects tubular filtrate from the distal convoluted tubules and carries it to the renal pelvis. They are not considered part of the nephron.

colloidal Referring to a gelatinous and viscous fluid.

colon The last large component of the intestinal tract; is responsible for absorption of water and electrolytes; is extensively developed in the nonruminant herbivores, like horses.

colostrum The initial secretion of the mammary gland before milk is produced. Colostrum is rich in nutrients, has a laxative effect on the newborn, and contains antibodies to the diseases the dam has been exposed to or vaccinated against. If the newborn drinks the colostrum within the first few hours of birth, the large antibody molecules will be absorbed intact by the intestine and impart passive immunity to the young animal.

columnar epithelial cells Tall, thin epithelial cells having nuclei located at their basal end; often ciliated.

columnar epithelium Epithelium composed of columnar cells.

comedones Pores clogged with an excessive amount of black sebum.

common bile duct The duct leading from the gallbladder to the duodenum; may be formed by the merging of the cystic duct from the gallbladder and the hepatic duct from the liver.

common vaginal tunic The outer connective tissue sac that surrounds the testis. It is derived from the layer of parietal peritoneum that was pushed ahead of the testis as it descended through the inguinal ring.

compact bone Heavy, dense bone made up of tiny, tightly compacted, laminated cylinders of bone called haversian systems; makes up the shafts (diaphyses) of long bones and the outer surfaces of all bones.

complement A group of inactive enzymes (proteins) in plasma that can be activated to rupture the cell membrane of a foreign cell. Complement can also act as an opsonin.

compound follicles Follicles through which more than one hair emerges.

compound gland An exocrine gland with branched ducts.

concentration gradient The spectrum between the area of highest concentration and the area of lowest concentration.

condyle A large, rounded articular (joint) surface. Examples are found on the distal ends of the humerus and femur.

congenital Present at birth.

cones Photoreceptors in the retina of the eye that perceive color and detail.

connective tissue Tissue made up of cells and extracellular substances that connects and supports cells and other tissues.

connexon Proteinaceous channel that aids in the intercellular transport of nutrients.

congestive heart failure Failure of the heart to maintain circulatory equilibrium with resulting congestion of the venous system. It is characterized by edema of the lungs, enlargement of the heart, increase in heart rate, and dilation of blood vessels.

conjunctiva The thin, transparent membrane that covers the front portion of the eyeball and lines the interior surfaces of the eyelids.

conjunctival sac The space between the bulbar and palpebral portions of the conjunctiva; the space between the eyelid and the eyeball.

connective tissue papilla The base of the hair follicle that ultimately provides the material necessary to create hair.

connective tissue proper Includes all types of connective tissue except for bone, blood, and cartilage. Connective tissue proper is divided into two subclasses: loose connective tissue and dense connective tissue.

contact inhibition That property that inhibits cells from dividing when in proximity to other cells.

contact signaling Cell-to-cell recognition, which is important in immune responses to infection.

contractile proteins Proteins that are essential to muscle contractions, such as myosin and actin.

contractility The inherent ability of the heart to develop a force by contracting, which increases chamber pressures.

contralateral reflex Reflexes that are initiated on one side of the body and travel to the opposite side to produce their effect.

contrast radiography Myelography; the injecting of dye into the epidural space to better visualize the spinal cord on radiographs.

coping The process of trimming and shaping a bird's beak.

coprodeum Anterior section of the cloaca that receives excrement from the intestine.

copulation The act of breeding; consists of intromission of the penis into the vagina, thrusting, and ejaculation.

corium The dermis of the skin.

cornea The clear "window" on the front of the eye that admits light to the interior of the eye; part of the outer fibrous layer of the eyeball.

corneal reflex Reflex closure of the eyelids when the surface of the cornea is touched; used in anesthesia monitoring to assess depth of anesthesia.

cornual process The "horn core" of horned animals; a process of the frontal bone. The hollow cavity within the cornual process is continuous with the frontal sinus (the paranasal sinus of the frontal bone).

corona radiata A thin layer of granulosa cells that surrounds the ovum as it develops in the ovarian follicle and after it is released by ovulation.

coronary band The part of the hoof that articulates with the skin.

coronary corium The part of the corium that has differentiated to provide nourishment to the hoof at the site of the coronary band.

corpus callosum White fibers that connect and provide communication pathways between the two cerebral hemispheres.

corpus cavernosum penis The larger of the two erectile tissue structures in the body of the penis. It is located dorsal to the smaller corpus cavernosum urethrae.

corpus cavernosum urethrae The smaller of the two erectile tissue structures in the body of the penis. It forms a "sleeve" around the urethra and is located ventral to the larger corpus cavernosum penis.

corpus hemorrhagicum The blood-filled remnant of the ovarian follicle immediately after ovulation.

corpus luteum Literally "yellow body." The solid endocrine structure that forms from the empty ovarian follicle after ovulation. Under stimulation from luteinizing hormone from the anterior pituitary gland, the granulosa cells left in the empty follicle multiply to form the solid corpus luteum. It produces progestin hormones, principally progesterone, that are necessary for the maintenance of pregnancy.

cortex The outer, superficial layer of an organ or structure. The outer portion of the kidney. It contains the renal corpuscles, proximal convoluted tubules, distal convoluted tubules, collecting ducts, and peritubular capillaries. In hair, it is the layer surrounding the medulla composed of hard keratin.

costal cartilage The cartilaginous, ventral portion of a rib.

costochondral junction The junction between the bony and cartilaginous portions of a rib.

cotyledon Numerous areas on the surface of the placenta of ruminant animals that join with the caruncles in the lining of the uterus to form placental attachment sites called placentomes.

cotyledonary placental attachment The type of placental attachment found in common ruminant animals. It consists of numerous cotyledons on the surface of the placenta joining with caruncles in the lining of the uterus to form attachment sites called placentomes.

cough A protective response to irritation or foreign material in the trachea or bronchi. The sudden, forceful expiration of air is intended to force the irritant or foreign material up and out of the respiratory tract. Productive coughs are moist and generally help an animal clear mucus and other matter from the air passageways. Nonproductive coughs are dry and generally not beneficial to the animal.

covalent Chemical bonds in which electrons are shared.

cranial A directional term meaning toward the head end of an animal.

cranial nerves Set of 12 pairs of nerves originating from the brain; may be sensory or motor or may contain both sensory and motor nerves.

cranial sacral system Another term that defines the parasympathetic nervous system based on the fact that the parasympathetic nervous system nerves emerge from the CNS cranial nerves and nerves from the sacral spinal cord segment.

cranium The cranial portion of the dorsal body cavity formed from several skull bones. It houses and protects the brain. It is the reference point for the directional term *cranial*.

creatine phosphate (CP) The molecule in muscle cells that splits to release the energy necessary to reattach the detached phosphate group to an adenosine diphosphate (ADP) molecule to convert it back to the high-energy molecule adenosine triphosphate (ATP).

cremaster muscle The bandlike muscle that raises and lowers the testes in the scrotum to help control their temperature. The testes must be maintained at a temperature slightly cooler than body temperature to produce spermatozoa.

Creutzfeldt-Jakob disease A disease in humans that was discovered by Hans Gerhard Creutzfeldt and Alfons Maria Jakob. The disease has no known cure and causes a fatal spongiform encephalopathy. Prions are known to be the infectious agent.

cribriform plate The sievelike area of the ethmoid bone through which the many branches of the olfactory nerve pass from the upper portion of the nasal cavity to the olfactory bulbs of the brain.

cricoid cartilage One of the cartilages of the larynx. The cricoid cartilage is ring shaped. It helps form and support the caudal portion of the larynx.

crista The short name for the receptor structure of the semicircular canals.

crista ampullaris The full name of the receptor structure of the semicircular canals.

cristae The folds within the mitochondria that increase ATP output by increasing the number of surface area reaction sites.

crop Dilation of the esophagus in some species of birds that acts as a storage pouch for food.

cross bridges Tiny "levers" on the myosin filaments of muscle. A muscle cell contracts by ratcheting the cross bridges back and forth to pull the thinner actin filaments toward the center of the myosin filaments.

cross extensor reflex Reflex initiated by a stimulation of a limb that result in extension of the limb on the other side of the body.

CRT *See* Capillary refill time.

crura A portion of the roots of the penis. The connective tissue bands that attach the penis to the brim of the pelvis.

cryptorchidism The condition of one or both testes failing to descend into the scrotum. Cryptorchid animals may be unilateral (one side only) or bilateral (both sides).

crypts Invaginations in the intestinal mucosa that produce the cells that form the villi.

cuboidal cells Cube-shaped cells having centrally located nuclei.

cuboidal epithelium Epithelium composed of cuboidal cells.

cumulus oophorus The small mound of granulosa cells on which the oocyte sits as it develops in the ovarian follicle.

cupula The gelatinous structure that sits on top of the receptor hairs in the crista ampullaris of the semicircular canals.

cutaneous membrane Also known as the integument. The outer layer (epidermis) is composed of keratinized stratified squamous epithelium. This helps to waterproof and prevent dehydration of the body. The inner layer or "dermis" is composed of dense irregular connective tissue, as well as collagenous and elastic fibers. This also helps the cutaneous membrane by giving it reinforcement and flexibility.

cutaneous muscles "Skin muscles"; thin muscles in the connective tissue beneath the skin. When a cutaneous muscle contracts, it causes the skin to twitch.

cuticle The single layer of cells that make up the outermost layer of the hair shaft.

-cyte Suffix meaning "cell."

cytochromes Essential to the final stage of the electron transport system, this copper-containing complex of enzymes transfers electrons to oxygen. The oxygen in turn can bond with hydrogen, thus producing water.

cytokinesis The separation of the cytoplasm into two separate daughter cells during the mitotic stage of cell division called telophase.

cytologist One who studies cells.

cytoplasm The part of the cell's protoplasm that is located outside of the nuclear envelope.

cytosine (C) One of the nucleotides present in both RNA and DNA. It is a pyrimidine base that corresponds to RNA and DNA's guanine.

cytosis The active transport of materials into or out of the cell. The transported material is bound by a membrane.

cytoskeleton The internal structure of the cell that maintains the cell's shape and aids in some functions. The cytoskeleton is composed of three types of filaments: microfilaments, microtubules, and intermediate filaments.

cytosol The fluid component of protoplasm that acts as its base.

cytotoxic T cells Also known as killer cells or killer T lymphocytes. They attach to antigenic cells and destroy them, but they are not themselves damaged.

D

DCT *See* Distal convoluted tubule.

deamination The process during catabolism in which the amino group NH_2 is removed.

deep A directional term meaning toward the center of the body or a body part; *see* Internal.

defecation The expelling of feces.

dehydration synthesis The combination of two or more simple materials to form one or more complex ones by removing water. For example, two monosaccharides can combine to form a disaccharide. Glucose + Galactose = Lactose + Water.

deltoid crest Thin, widened area on the proximal humerus where the wing muscles of a bird attach.

dendrite The receptive site of the nerve cell; extends from the cell body, giving the cell a starlike shape; receives stimuli and conveys them as nerve impulses to the soma.

dens Process on the cranial end of the second cervical vertebra (axis) that fits into the caudal end of the first cervical vertebra (atlas).

dense bodies Structures in smooth muscle cells to which the small contractile units of actin and myosin attach. The dense bodies of smooth muscle correspond to the Z lines of skeletal muscle to which the actin filaments attach.

dense connective tissue A highly fibrous connective tissue with little vascularization. It functions to reinforce and bind body structures. Dense connective tissue occurs as dense regular and dense irregular.

dense irregular connective tissue A collagen-based fibrous connective tissue that is found in the dermis, spleen, and liver. It has thicker bundles of fiber than dense regular connective tissue and is designed to withstand tension from multiple directions.

dense regular connective tissue Tightly bound, minimally vascularized fibrous connective tissue found in ligaments, tendons, and fascia. In ligaments, it binds joints; whereas in tendons, it binds muscle to bone. In fascia, it helps support surrounding tissues.

dental formula The shorthand abbreviation that shows the number of incisors (I), canines (C), premolars (P), and molars (M) that a species has; the first number of the pair indicates the number of teeth in half of the upper arcade, and the second number indicates the number of teeth in half of the lower arcade; lowercase letters indicate deciduous teeth; for example: I3/3 C1/1 P2/2 M3/3.

dental pad The hard, thick connective tissue pad that ruminants have in the space occupied by upper incisor teeth in other species.

dental prophylaxis The cleaning of teeth; slang is "dental prophy."

dentin The layer surrounding the tooth pulp; is more dense than bone but not as dense as the overlying enamel.

deoxyhemoglobin Hemoglobin that is not carrying any oxygen; also known as "empty hemoglobin."

deoxyribonucleic acid *See* DNA

depolarization The state of the neuron occurring immediately after sufficiently strong stimulation; the influx of sodium ions after stimulation.

dermal papillae Upward projections of the corium or dermis that insert into the epidermis. The projections are vascularized for the purpose of thermoregulation and waste removal. They are also innervated.

dermis The deep, connective tissue portion of the skin that contains blood vessels, glands, and hair follicles.

desmosome A type of intercellular attachment found in epithelial tissue. The bond is formed from the interlocking of filaments that connect the plasma membranes of adjacent cells.

determinate layer Species that can lay only the number of eggs in a normal clutch size.

development The growth of an organism to full size or maturity.

dewclaw A toe that does not reach the ground, such as the first digit of dogs and cats and the rudimentary medial and lateral toes of cattle.

diabetes insipidus A disease resulting from a deficiency of antidiuretic hormone from the posterior pituitary gland. It results in polyuria and polydipsia.

diabetes mellitus A disease resulting from a deficiency of the hormone insulin from the pancreatic islets. The lack of insulin prevents glucose from entering cells and being used as an energy source. This results in signs that include hyperglycemia, glycosuria, polyuria, polydipsia, polyphagia, weight loss, and weakness.

diapedesis The process by which white blood cells leave the blood vessel and enter tissue by squeezing through the tiny spaces between the cells lining the blood vessel walls.

diaphragm The thin, dome-shaped sheet of muscle that forms the boundary between the thoracic and abdominal cavities. A muscle that helps produce inspiration when it contracts. The diaphragm is dome shaped at rest with its convex surface directed cranially. When it contracts, the dome of the diaphragm flattens out, which increases the volume of the thoracic cavity and causes air to be drawn into the lungs.

diaphragmatic flexure Where the left dorsal colon of the horse bends back on itself to form the right dorsal colon.

diaphysis The shaft portion of a long bone.

diarthrosis A freely movable synovial joint.

diastole The part of the cardiac cycle associated with relaxation of the ventricles and the filling of the ventricles with blood in the atria.

diencephalon Serves as a nervous system passageway between the primitive brain stem and the cerebrum; three major structures of the diencephalon include the thalamus, the hypothalamus, and the pituitary.

diestrous Animals that have two estrous cycles per year.

diestrus The active luteal stage of the estrous cycle. During this period the corpus luteum has reached maximum size and is producing maximum amounts of progestin hormones.

differentiation The progressive acquisition of individual characteristics by cells to enable them to perform different functions.

diffuse placental attachment A "loose" form of placental attachment to the uterine wall; attachment sites are spread diffusely over the whole surface of the placenta and the whole lining of the uterus; found in horses and swine.

diffusion The tendency for molecules to move from an area of high concentration to an area of low concentration.

digestive system The collection of organs that take in and digest food for use by the body to maintain health and normal function. This system includes all structures of the mouth, esophagus, stomach, and the small and large intestines. Accessory organs such as the gallbladder and pancreas, although not directly involved in the mechanical functions of digestion, provide secretions that aid in the chemical part of the process.

digit A toe made up of two or three bones called phalanges.

dilated cardiomyopathy The enlargement of the heart resulting from dilation of the heart's chambers and thinning of the ventricular walls. If left untreated, the condition will ultimately lead to heart failure.

dimers Complex proteins containing two polypeptide chains.

diploid chromosome number The chromosome number in all of an animal's cells, except for the reproductive cells. It is always an even number.

disaccharides "Two sugars"; includes sucrose, maltose, isomaltose, and lactose.

discoid placental attachment Attachment of the placenta to the uterus in a single disk-shaped area; found in primates, rabbits, and many rodents.

distal A directional term used only for extremities of the body. It implies a position or direction *away from* the body proper.

distal convoluted tubule (DCT) The last tubular part of the nephron before it enters the collecting duct. DCTs are found in the kidney's cortex.

distal phalanx bone The bone of the phalanx (P-3) that is located most distally from the body; the tip of the digit.
distal sesamoid bone The "navicular bone" of horses. It is located in the digital flexor tendon deep in the hoof behind the joint between the middle and distal phalanges.
disulfide bonds Strong covalent bonds that unite amino acids in globular protein formations.
diuresis Producing and passing large amounts of urine.
DNA Deoxyribonucleic acid; the genetic material of a living thing found in strands called chromatin within the nucleus of the cell.
DNA polymerase An enzyme that reestablishes the double helix of DNA by uniting the nucleotide bases with their corresponding base pair. This creates a new strand for each original DNA strand.
dolichocephalic Long faced. The collie is a dolichocephalic dog breed.
dopamine A catecholamine neurotransmitter.
dorsal A directional term meaning toward the top surface of an animal when it is standing on all four legs; toward the backbone.
dorsal body cavity The space in the skull and spinal column that contains the brain and spinal cord. The portion in the skull is called the cranium, and the portion in the spinal column is called the spinal canal.
dorsal plane An anatomical reference plane that divides the body into dorsal (upper) and ventral (lower) parts that are not necessarily equal.
double helix Also called the Watson-Crick helix; the double coils as seen in DNA that have the specific nucleotides whereby one set determines the corresponding set.
dressing forceps A tweezerlike surgical instrument with serrated tips used to grasp gauze sponges and other surgical materials. It is not intended for use on tissue.
duct A tubelike channel that provides a route of exit for secretory or excretory products.
duodenum The first segment of the small intestine after the stomach. Chyme enters the duodenum from the stomach.
dura mater The outermost layer of the meninges that covers the brain and spinal cord; it is considered to be the toughest of the meninges.
dysfunction Abnormal functioning of an organ or body part.
dystocia A difficult birth. Dystocias usually result from a fetus that is too large for the birth canal or one that is oriented inappropriately for delivery.

E

eardrum Common name for the tympanic membrane. The paper-thin connective tissue membrane that is tightly stretched across the opening of the external ear canal into the middle ear.
eccrine glands Exocrine glands that secrete substances directly onto the skin without the loss of cellular material. They contain simple, coiled tube structures for excretory purposes.
eccrine sweat glands Sweat glands that cover the entire surface of the body for the purpose of thermoregulation.
eclampsia A condition seen in lactating dogs and cats that results from hypocalcemia. Early signs of eclampsia include muscle tremors and spasms.
edema An abnormal accumulation of fluid, either localized or generalized, within the tissues or cavities of the body.
efferent ducts of the testes The passageways that allow spermatozoa to move from the rete testis to the head of the epididymis.
efferent glomerular arterioles Arterioles that leave the glomerulus. They are carrying blood that has been filtered by the glomerulus; so it contains less plasma. Blood in the efferent glomerular arterioles has a relatively higher blood cell and plasma protein concentration than blood in the afferent glomerular capillaries.
efferent nerve Nerve that carries impulses away from the central nervous system.
effusion Excess fluid that has escaped into a body cavity to the detriment of normal body function.
ejaculation The reflex expulsion of semen from the penis.
elastase Protease secreted in an inactive form from the pancreas and activated by trypsin.
elastic cartilage Also called yellow cartilage; this cartilage is very similar to hyaline cartilage, except that it is more opaque and contains many elastic fibers. It is found in the external ear and the epiglottis.
elastic connective tissue Connective tissues composed of large numbers of elastic fibers and found in tissues that expand and contract, such as in the lungs and vocal cords.
elastic fibers Fibers composed of elastin. Elastic fibers form a delicate mesh in tissues.
electrocardiogram A recording of the electrical activity of the heart.
electrocardiograph An instrument that records and monitors the electrical activity of the heart.
electrolyte A substance that conducts an electric current in solution.
electron microscope A powerful microscope that magnifies a sample by using an electron beam for illumination.
electron transport system The final and most productive stage of cellular respiration, which takes place inside of the mitochondria.
embolus A blood clot that travels through a blood vessel and may obstruct a blood vessel at a location other than where the clot originated.
embryo The name generally given to the developing offspring during the first trimester of pregnancy. During this the period, the newly implanted zygote and its placenta are getting themselves organized and the body tissues, organs, and systems begin to form.

embryonic hemoglobin Hemoglobin found in red blood cells during early fetal life.

emulsification The mixing of fat or oil and water by agitation or shaking.

enamel Outer coating layer of the tooth; toughest substance in the body.

endocardium Innermost layer of the heart.

endochondral bone formation The type of bone formation whereby bone grows into and replaces a cartilage model. This is the method by which bones form in a developing fetus, starting with cartilage "prototypes" that are gradually replaced by bone. It is also the means by which long bones increase in length at the epiphyseal (growth) plates. New cartilage is created on the outside surfaces of the plates, and bone replaces old cartilage on the inside surfaces. This allows the bones to increase in length as the animal grows.

endocrine glands Glands or cells that release their regulatory products (hormones) directly into the bloodstream. Endocrine glands control most metabolic functions. Examples of endocrine glands include the pituitary, parathyroid, and pancreas.

endocrine system The system of glands that controls and regulates body functions through the internal secretion of hormones. The hormones are placed directly into the bloodstream, where they may act throughout the body.

endocrinology The study of the endocrine system.

endocytosis The taking in of a material from the outside of the cell by creating a "mouth" with the plasma membrane. The membrane engulfs the material and pinches off at the ends to form a vesicle. Endocytosis includes both the processes of pinocytosis and phagocytosis.

endolymph The fluid in the receptor structures of the inner ear.

endomysium The thin, delicate layer of connective tissue that surrounds each individual skeletal muscle fiber.

endoplasmic reticulum (ER) A system of channels within the cell that run from the nucleus to the exterior cell membrane. The two forms of ER have their own functions. Rough ER is the site for protein synthesis, and smooth ER is the site for lipid synthesis.

endosteum The fibrous membrane that lines the hollow interiors of bones.

endothelium Derived from mesothelium, the endothelium is composed of simple squamous epithelium. It lines the heart, blood vessels, and serous cavities of the body.

endotracheal (ET) intubation The placement of a soft rubber or plastic ET tube through the larynx and into the trachea to establish an open airway.

endotracheal tube A soft rubber or plastic tube that is passed through the larynx and into the trachea to establish an open airway; often used to administer inhalational anesthetics.

energy of activation The amount of energy necessary to initiate a reaction.

enteritis Inflammation of the intestines.

enterogastric reflex The reflex in which the presence of food in the stomach stimulates motility and digestive secretions on in the intestine.

enzyme A protein that speeds up chemical reactions in the body by acting as a catalyst and lowering the temperature as necessary for the reaction to take place. Specific enzymes are exclusive to specific reactions, and although they may change the rate of reaction, they are never changed themselves.

eosinopenia A decrease in the total number of eosinophils in peripheral blood.

eosinophil The granulocytic white blood cell characterized by the presence of numerous red-staining granules in its cytoplasm.

eosinophilia An increase in the total number of eosinophils in peripheral blood.

epicardium Outermost layer of the heart.

epidermal Referring to the epidermis.

epidermal orifice The actual opening of the hair follicle through which the hair emerges.

epidermis Composed of keratinized stratified squamous epithelium, it is the outermost layer of the skin.

epididymis The ribbonlike structure that lies along the surface of the testis. It is actually one long, convoluted tube that links the efferent ducts with the vas deferens. Spermatozoa are stored in the epididymis as they await ejaculation.

epidural anesthesia The administration of anesthetic agents into the space between the dura mater and the surrounding bone of the vertebrae.

epiglottis One of the cartilages of the larynx. The epiglottis is the most rostral cartilage. It projects forward from the ventral portion of the larynx. Its bluntly pointed tip usually tucks up behind the caudal rim of the soft palate when the animal is breathing. When the animal swallows, the epiglottis is pulled back to cover the opening of the larynx like a trapdoor.

epimysium The tough, connective tissue layer that covers and delineates individual muscles. It surrounds groups of skeletal muscle fascicles.

epinephrine A hormone secreted by the medulla of the adrenal gland under stimulation by the sympathetic portion of the autonomic nervous system. It produces part of the "fight or flight" response that results when an animal feels threatened; old name is adrenaline.

epiphyseal plate The growth plate of a long bone. Epiphyseal plates are located at the junction of the proximal and distal epiphyses with the diaphysis. They are areas where long bones increase in length by the process of endochondral bone formation. When an animal reaches its full size, the epiphyseal plates of its bones completely ossify and the bones cease their growth.

epiphysis The end of a long bone. Each long bone has a proximal and a distal epiphysis.

epithelial tissue A collection of tissues that are made up of layers of cells that line and cover body surfaces. These cells may be single layered or multilayered and can regenerate quickly.

epithelialization The rapid division of epithelial cells around a wound edge. Epithelialization attempts to cover the opening of a wound. This process is assisted by the contraction of collagen fibers, which bring the edges of the epithelial layer into close opposition.

equator The center of the spindle apparatus where the chromosomes line up during metaphase in cell division; also known as the equatorial plate.

equilibrium The balance of solutes and solution between the inside and outside of the cell. For example, in the case of salts and water, the concentrations on either side of the cell membrane will be equal in a state of equilibrium; the sense that helps an animal maintain its balance by keeping track of the position and movements of its head.

erectile tissue A spongy network of fibrous connective tissue and blood sinuses. When more blood flows into erectile tissue than leaves it, the sinuses engorge with blood and create hydraulic pressure that enlarges and stiffens the organ in which the erectile tissue is located.

erection Enlargement and stiffening of an organ that contains erectile tissue, such as the penis, clitoris, or nipple.

ergots Believed to be the vestigial remnant of metacarpal and metatarsal pads, they are the horny, keratinized growths located on the fetlocks of all equids.

eructation The expelling of gases orally; burping or belching.

erythrocytes Also called red blood cells or corpuscles, these cells are anucleated and biconcave in shape. They are responsible for carrying oxygen from the lungs to tissue. Erythrocytes are formed in the red bone marrow of adults and in the liver, spleen, and marrow of a fetus. They are also manufactured in the spleen of anemic and ill adults.

erythropoiesis Production of erythrocytes.

erythropoietin The hormone produced by the kidney that stimulates the red bone marrow to increase its production of red blood cells.

esophageal groove *See* Reticular groove.

essential amino acid An amino acid that cannot be produced in a sufficient amounts; therefore it must be obtained through diet. Different species have different essential amino acid needs.

essential fatty acids Unsaturated fatty acids such as linolenic, arachidonic, and linoleic fatty acids that are necessary for normal body functions yet are not synthesized by the body in sufficient amounts; therefore they must be supplemented by diet.

estrogens Hormones that promote the development of female characteristics; female sex hormones.

estrous cycle The period from the beginning of one heat period to the beginning of the next. It includes the stages of proestrus, estrus, metestrus, and diestrus.

estrus The heat period; the stage of the estrous cycle when the female is sexually receptive to the male and will allow breeding to take place.

ethmoid bone A skull bone; an internal bone of the cranium. The single ethmoid bone is located just rostral (ahead of) the sphenoid bone. It contains the cribriform plate, which transmits the many branches of the olfactory nerve to the olfactory bulb of the brain.

ethmoidal sinus The paranasal sinus in the ethmoid bone of horses and humans.

eukaryotes This classification of cells is found in all living things, such as plants and mammals, except for prokaryotes. Eukaryotes have a true nucleus that contains chromosomes and has a nuclear envelope. They also have membrane-bound organelles.

eustachian tube The tube that connects the middle ear cavity with the pharynx. It allows equalization of the air pressure on the two sides of the tympanic membrane.

euthanize To humanely put an animal to death.

excising Removing a sample of tissue or organ by cutting it out surgically.

excitatory neurotransmitters Chemicals released by neurons at the synapse that tend to cause excitation or depolarization of other neurons or target tissues.

excretion The elimination of waste materials from the cell or body.

excretory ducts Ducts that transport waste products or secretions out of an organ or gland.

exocrine glands Glands that release their secretions internally through ducts that lead directly to the location intended to be controlled. Some examples include sweat glands and salivary glands.

exocytosis The passage of materials too large to diffuse though the cell membrane by packaging them in vesicles, transporting them to the cell membrane, and then pressing them out of the cell.

exons Spaces of a gene's DNA sequence that are coded. Exons are separated by noncoded portions, called introns, which are spliced out to join exons together to form messenger RNA.

expiration Exhalation; the process of pushing air out of the lungs.

expiratory muscle A muscle whose action is to decrease the size of the thoracic cavity; this squeezes air out of the lungs, thereby producing expiration (exhalation).

extension The joint movement that increases the angle between two bones.

external acoustic meatus The bony canal in the temporal bone that leads into the middle and inner ear cavities of the bone. In the living animal, it contains the external ear canal.

external An alternative directional term for *superficial*. External also means toward the surface of the body or a body part.

external auditory canal The tube that begins at the base of the pinna and carries sound waves to the tympanic membrane. In most domestic animal species, it is L shaped, with a vertical portion leading down to a horizontal portion.

external ear The outer portion of the ear. It consists of the structures that collect and transmit sound waves to the middle ear: the pinna, the external auditory canal, and the tympanic membrane.

external respiration The process of respiration that occurs in the lungs. Oxygen and carbon dioxide are exchanged between the air inhaled into the alveoli of the lungs and the blood in the capillaries that surround them.

extracellular fibers The fibers of connective tissue located outside of the cells that perform a variety of functions depending on the degree of their elasticity or concentration.

extracellular fluid The fluid located outside of the cell.

extracellular matrix The nonliving substance found between cells that provides support and nourishment.

extraocular eye muscles The small skeletal muscles that move and position the eyeballs.

extravascular hemolysis Destruction of red blood cells outside of a blood vessel.

exudate The accumulation of fluid, pus, or serum in a cavity or tissue. Fluid or serum has often leaked through vessel walls or capillaries into the adjoining space.

eyelids The conjunctiva-lined folds of skin that protect and cover the eyeball.

F

fabella One of two small sesamoid bones located in the proximal gastrocnemius (calf) muscle tendon just above and behind the femoral condyles of dogs and cats.

facet A flat articular surface, such as between carpal bones and between the radius and ulna.

facilitated diffusion The diffusion of molecules across the cell membrane with the aid of carrier proteins. This reaction is otherwise unable to be performed as simple diffusion, and it requires no energy or ATP.

FAD *See* Flavin adenine dinucleotide.

false vocal cords The vestibular folds; connective tissue bands in the larynx of nonruminant animals in addition to the vocal cords. The false vocal cords are not involved in voice production.

fascia An arrangement of dense regular connective tissue that lies over muscle. This layer helps to support, separate, and connect muscle to other structures.

fascicle A group of skeletal muscle fibers bound together by a layer of fibrous connective tissue called the perimysium.

fatty acids The organic compounds of hydrogen, oxygen, and carbon that, when mixed with glycerol, form fat. There are several types of fatty acids. *Saturated fatty acids* are solid at room temperature and have no double bonds in their carbon chain. *Unsaturated fatty acids,* like the kinds in olive oil, are liquid at room temperature and have one or more double bonds. *Polyunsaturated fatty acids* contain two or more double bonds. *Volatile fatty acids* are created in the rumen and reticulum of ruminant animals, such as cows, through the process of cellulose fermentation and are essential for energy production. All fatty acids are insoluble in water.

fault bar Area on feather vane that lacks barbules. Also called a stress bar and is caused by an interruption of the feather's blood supply during development.

feak The act of rubbing the beak on a rough surface to clean it and maintain its shape.

feline panleukopenia Caused by the feline parvovirus, this infectious disease has an extremely high mortality rate in kittens. Infections in intrauterine cases are known to cause miscarriages, as well as fetal and newborn deaths. Because it tends to attack cells in their mitotic phases, epithelial tissue is at high risk for attack as a result of its constant cell division. Therefore characteristics of feline panleukopenia include vomiting, diarrhea, and dehydration. Vaccines are available.

femur The long bone of the "thigh" region. It forms the hip joint with the pelvis at its proximal end and the stifle joint with the tibia at its distal end.

fenestrations Small openings or holes in the walls of the glomerular capillaries. They allow certain molecules to leave the glomerular capillaries that would normally be too large to leave.

fermentation Anaerobic oxidative decomposition of cellulose into simpler compounds, such as volatile fatty acids. The enzymes that break down the cellulose are produced by microorganisms, which are contained in the rumen or cecum of herbivores.

fermentative digestion Digestive process in which food is broken down by enzymes produced by microbes.

fetal hemoglobin The predominant hemoglobin in red blood cells during the later part of gestation. It is gradually replaced by adult hemoglobin during the first few weeks to months after birth.

fetlock joint The lay term for the most proximal joint of the equine digit (the joint between the large metacarpal or metatarsal and the proximal phalanx). The proximal sesamoid bones are located on the caudal surface of this joint.

fetus The name given to the developing offspring beginning about the second trimester of pregnancy. The body tissues, organs, and systems develop in the early fetal period, and then the offspring grows to its full birth size.

fibrin A protein created when thrombin acts on fibrinogen. Fibrin is essential to the coagulation of blood. It forms a lattice of interwoven fibers around blood cells and platelets that solidify to form a blood clot.

fibrinogen A protein formed in the liver and released into the bloodstream, especially in the presence of inflammatory processes. Fibrinogen, when acted on by thrombin, forms fibrin, which creates the meshwork of a blood clot.

fibrinolysis Destruction of the fibrin strands that make up the matrix of a clot; part of the process of the breakdown of a clot.

fibroblast Fixed cell involved in the development of connective tissue. Fibroblasts can differentiate into chondroblasts and osteoblasts to create substances specific to their cell type.

fibrocartilage Found between the vertebrae of the spine, fibrocartilage is different from other types of cartilage in that it has no perichondrium. In addition, it possesses few chondrocytes and dense bundles of collagenous fibers. It is usually found intermingled with hyaline cartilage and has an excellent ability to resist compression.

fibrocyte Mature, fiber-forming cell.

fibrous adhesions Fibrous connections that are generated during the healing process; often seen in the abdominal and thoracic cavities after surgical procedures.

fibrous joint An immovable joint; also known as a synarthrosis. The bones of a fibrous joint are firmly united by fibrous tissue. The sutures that unite most of the skull bones are fibrous joints.

fibula A thin bone located beside the tibia in the lower leg region of the pelvic limb. It is a complete bone in the dog and cat, but only the proximal and distal ends are present in horses and cattle. The fibula does not support any appreciable weight. It mainly acts as a muscle attachment site.

"fight or flight" response A whole-body response resulting from an animal feeling threatened that prepares the body for intense physical activity. It results from a combination of direct sympathetic nerve stimulation and the release of epinephrine and norepinephrine into the bloodstream from the medulla of the adrenal gland. Effects in the body include increased heart rate and output, increased blood pressure, dilated air passageways in the lungs, and decreased gastrointestinal function.

filtration The passage of a solution by pressure through a semipermeable membrane that allows the liquid portion to pass through but not the solute.

fimbriae The muscular, fingerlike projections that form the fringe of the infundibulum of the oviduct. The fimbriae feel their way across the surface of the ovary to where follicles are developing. They help position the infundibulum so that the ovum or ova will be guided into the oviduct when ovulation occurs.

first-intention healing Healing that occurs in tissues in which the wound edges are held in close apposition to one another as in the case of a sutured wound. Little to no granulation tissue is formed. There is generally minimal scarring.

fission The asexual division of an organism or cell into two individual "daughter" cells.

fissures Deep grooves found in the cerebral cortex.

fixator A muscle that stabilizes a joint so that other muscles can produce effective movements of other joints.

fixed cells One of the two subdivisions of connective tissue cells. Fixed cells are stationary within the connective tissue and perform functions such as matrix production and regulation.

flagellum (*plural,* flagella)—The primary means of motility for spermatozoa and unicellular organisms. This threadlike tail propels the organism by means of a whiplike movement.

flat bone Bones that are relatively thin and flat. They consist of two thin plates of compact bone separated by a thin layer of cancellous bone. Many of the skull bones are flat bones.

flavin adenine dinucleotide (FAD) A coenzyme necessary for electron transport within the mitochondria.

flexion The joint movement that decreases the angle between two bones.

floating rib The most caudal rib or two in the rib cage. A rib whose costal cartilage does not unite with anything but just ends in the muscle of the thoracic wall.

fluid mosaic The constantly changing pattern of proteins and fluid between the two sides of the liquid bilayer.

follicle A fluid-filled structure or cavity. An ovarian follicle consists of an oocyte surrounded by fluid and the follicular cells that produced it. Thyroid follicles are microscopic and consist of small globules of thyroid hormone precursor surrounded by simple cuboidal cells.

follicle-stimulating hormone (FSH) The anterior pituitary hormone that stimulates the growth and development of follicles in the ovaries of the female. In the male, it stimulates spermatogenesis in the seminiferous tubules of the testes.

follicular atresia The shrinkage of ovarian follicles that began developing but stopped at some point in their development.

follicular cells The cells that surround oocytes in ovarian follicles. Also known as granulosa cells. They produce estrogen hormones in developing follicles.

foramen A hole in a bone.

foramen magnum The large hole in the occipital bone through which the spinal cord exits the skull.

fossa A depressed or sunken area on the surface of a bone. Fossae are usually occupied by muscles or tendons in living animals.

free radicals Molecules that contain an odd number of electrons, making them highly reactive with other molecules. They bond to other molecules in the body, creating a new free radical that often causes a chain reaction of free radical formation.

freely permeable Those structures that allow the passage of fluids.

frog The thick triangular pad located on both the plantar and palmar surfaces of the horse's hoof. It is one of the important structures of the "circulatory pump" in the equine foot.

frontal bones Skull bones; external bones of the cranium. The two frontal bones make up the "forehead" region of the skull. They contain the large frontal sinuses. The cornual process (horn core) in horned animals is an extension of the frontal bone.

frontal sinus The large paranasal sinus in the frontal bone of the skull.

fundus The blind pouch of the stomach that relaxes and distends with food.

G

G cells Cells in the antrum of the stomach that produce gastrin.

GABA (gamma-aminobutyric acid) Inhibitory neurotransmitter.

GAGs *See* Glycosaminoglycans.

gallbladder The muscular blind sac underneath the liver that stores bile until it is needed; cholecystokinin stimulates the gallbladder to contract, forcing the bile into the cystic duct and common bile duct and then into the duodenum.

ganglion (*plural, ganglia*) Cluster of neurons outside of the CNS.

gap junction Proteinaceous pores that exist in the intestinal epithelial cells of most animals. These pores allow for the passage of nutrients, as well as providing a channel for intercellular communication.

gastric atony The state in which the stomach is very relaxed, or has little or no muscle tone.

gastric Referring to or pertaining to the stomach.

gastrin A hormone produced in the lining of the stomach when food arrives. It stimulates the gastric glands to secrete hydrochloric acid and digestive enzymes to start the digestive process and cause the fundus to relax.

gastritis Inflammation of the stomach.

general anesthesia Complete loss of sensory perception accompanied by loss of consciousness.

general senses The senses that are distributed throughout the body. Their receptors are fairly simple, and they keep the central nervous system informed about general conditions inside and outside the body.

genes Specific sites on chromosomes that dictate heredity. Genes may control one specific phenotypic trait, whereas other traits require many genes for proper expression. Pairs of genes that control the same trait and are located on the same part of the chromosome are called alleles.

genetic code The unique order of pyrimidine and purine-based nucleotides that govern the arrangement and transmission of genetic information in all living things, with the exception of RNA-based viruses.

genetic material Materials, such as DNA, that perpetuate the genetic code through the function of reproduction.

gestation period The period of pregnancy.

GFR *See* Glomerular filtration rate.

gingiva The epithelial tissue that composes the "gums."

ginglymus joint A hinge joint in which one articular surface swivels around another. The only movements possible are flexion and extension.

gizzard Muscular stomach in birds that grinds food into a digestible form.

gland sinus The large space in the mammary gland into which the large milk ducts empty. It is located just dorsal to the teat.

glandular epithelia Epithelial tissue composed of one cell (goblet cell) or groups of cells that produce and secrete substances into the lumen.

glans of the penis The distal free end of the penis. It is richly supplied with sensory nerve endings.

glenoid cavity The concave articular surface of the scapula; the socket portion of the ball-and-socket shoulder joint. In birds, the wing is attached to the body by forming a joint in the depression.

glial cells Cells in the nervous system that support and protect the nervous system.

gliding joint An arthrodial joint in which two flat, articular surfaces rock on each other. The carpus is an example of a gliding joint.

globular proteins Complex proteins bearing a spherical shape.

glomerular capillaries Part of the renal corpuscle. Urine production begins here when plasma is filtered out of the glomerular capillaries and into the capsular space of Bowman's capsule.

glomerular filtrate The plasma that has been filtered out of the glomerular capillaries and into the capsular space.

glomerular filtration rate (GFR) The rate at which plasma is filtered into the capsular space. It is expressed in milliliters per minute.

glomerulus The tuft of capillaries found in the renal corpuscle; also called glomerular capillaries.

glottis The opening into the larynx. The arytenoid cartilages and the vocal cords form the boundaries of the glottis.

glucagon A hormone produced by the pancreas that raises blood glucose.

glucocorticoid hormones A group of hormones with similar actions secreted by the cortex of the adrenal glands. The most prominent effect of these hormones is to raise the level of glucose in the bloodstream.

gluconeogenesis The production of glucose from amino acids; occurs in the liver.

glucose Monosaccharide (simple sugar) that is used by the body for energy.

glycerol The main components of triglycerides present in all fats. Triglycerides are soluble in water and alcohol.

glycine Inhibitory neurotransmitter.

glycocalyx The outer covering of the cell, composed of glycoproteins, that not only aids in cell adhesion but also serves to identify the cell by other cells.

glycogenesis The creation of glycogen from glucose in the liver.

glycogenolysis The breaking apart of glycogen into glucose molecules.

glycolipid A compound composed of a carbohydrate, usually in the form of sugar, and a fatty acid together in a compound.

glycolysis The first step of cellular respiration that converts glucose into lactate or pyruvate and releases a small amount of ATP.

glycoprotein A compound composed of a carbohydrate, usually in the form of sugar, and a protein together in a compound.

glycosaminoglycans (GAGs) Carbohydrates composed of amino sugars, which are found in proteoglycans.
glycosuria The presence of glucose in the urine.
goblet cell A type of cell, located in the respiratory and intestinal tracts, that secretes mucus.
Golgi apparatus An organelle located near the nucleus that is shaped like flattened sacs that are stacked and flattened at the ends. It is believed to be involved in the synthesis of glycoproteins, lipoproteins, and enzymes.
gonad The organ that produces the reproductive cells; the testis in the male and the ovary in the female.
gonadotropin A hormone that stimulates the growth and development of the gonads (ovaries and testes). Usually refers to follicle-stimulating hormone (FSH) and luteinizing hormone (LH).
granulation tissue The new vascular and cellular tissue formed during the restoration of wounded tissue. It mostly consists of connective tissue and new blood vessels.
granulocytes White blood cells that are characterized by the presence of granules in their cytoplasm. The granulocytes are neutrophils, eosinophils, and basophils.
granulopoiesis A general term for the production of any or all of the granulocytes.
granulosa cells The follicular cells of the developing follicle. They produce estrogen hormones.
gray matter That part of the CNS made up of unmyelinated neurons.
greater curvature of the stomach The larger, outer curve of the stomach.
gristle Lay term for cartilage.
gross anatomy The study of body structures that are visible without additional aid to the naked eye.
ground substance The shapeless, viscous matrix present in connective tissue in which the cells receive nutrients and void waste products. It also helps to protect the body from infectious agents by acting as a barrier.
growth 1 phase (G1) Part of interphase. The cell enlarges and organelles replicate over a period, which varies between cell types.
growth 2 phase (G2) Part of interphase. During this phase, enzymes and proteins are synthesized and the centrioles complete their replication.
growth hormone (GH) The anterior pituitary hormone that promotes body growth in young animals and helps regulate the metabolism of proteins, carbohydrates, and lipids in all of the body's cells.
growth plate The epiphyseal plate of a long bone. Located at the junction of the proximal and distal epiphyses with the diaphysis. Growth plates are areas where long bones increase in length by the process of endochondral bone formation. When an animal reaches its full size, the growth plates of its bones completely ossify and the bones cease their growth.
guanine (G) One of the nucleotides present in both RNA and DNA. It is a purine base that corresponds to DNA and RNA's cytosine.
gubernaculum The short, inelastic band of connective tissue that attaches the testes into the scrotum. Growth of the embryo while the gubernaculum stays the same length results in movement of the testes caudally and ventrally. Eventually, they descend through the inguinal rings into the scrotum.
gular fluttering Rapid vibrations of the upper throat patch in many species of owls, herons, quail, pigeons, and doves. Used to increase cooling by the evaporative loss of heat from air passed over the oral cavity.
gustatory sense The sense of taste.
gut-associated lymph tissue (GALT) Lymphoid tissue scattered throughout the lining of the intestine. It is often compared with the bursa of Fabricius in birds, where B lymphocytes are processed.
gyrus (*plural,* gyri) The folds that provide the wrinkled appearance of the surface of the cerebral hemispheres.

H

hair bulb The bulbous portion of the hair follicle, located within the dermis, that provides the basis of material for hair production.
hair follicle Tubelike invaginations of the epidermis that traverse through the dermis into the connective tissue where the hair is rooted. The arrector pili and sebaceous glands are located within proximity of the hair follicle.
hair follicle matrix The layer of material that lies superficially over the connective tissue papilla. The matrix generates material for hair production.
hamuli Microscopic hooks that link barbules together.
haploid chromosome number The chromosome number in the reproductive cells. It is half of the diploid chromosome number.
haptoglobin A transport plasma protein that carries free hemoglobin from intravascular hemolysis to the macrophages of the mononuclear phagocyte system in the liver for further breakdown.
hard palate The bony roof of the mouth; the division between the mouth and the nasal cavity. The soft palate is immediately caudal to the hard palate. The hard palate is made up of portions of the maxillary and palatine bones.
hardware disease A disease process in ruminant animals caused by irritation of the lining of the reticulum by swallowed metal objects.
haustra Sacculations of the colon and cecum.
haversian canal The central canal that runs the length of a haversian system. The haversian canal contains the blood vessels, lymph vessels, and nerves that supply and nourish the osteocytes.
haversian system The microscopic, laminated cylinders of bone that make up compact bone. Oriented lengthwise in a long bone, haversian systems consist of a central haversian canal surrounded by concentric layers of bone. Osteocytes

in their lacunae are present at the junctions of the bony layers of the haversian system.

head A spheroidal articular surface on the proximal end of a long bone; present on the proximal ends of the humerus, femur, and rib. The head of a bone is joined to the shaft by an area that is often narrowed, called the neck.

health A state of normal anatomy and physiology that allows the body to function normally.

hearing The auditory sense; the mechanical sense that converts the sound wave vibrations of air molecules to nerve impulses that are interpreted by the brain as sounds.

heatstroke A dangerous body reaction to prolonged heat exposure. As the animal's core temperature rapidly rises, it becomes weak and confused and may lapse into unconsciousness that can lead to convulsions and death. Heatstroke often occurs in animals that are locked in automobiles in the hot summer sun or confined in sunny areas without water or access to shade. Heatstroke victims must be cooled rapidly to prevent brain damage or death.

heel The most posterior region of the hoof.

helper T cells The most numerous of the T lymphocytes. They help the immune response by secreting substances known as lymphokines into the surrounding tissue; this in turn increases activation of B lymphocytes and cytotoxic T cells.

hematocrit The percent of a total blood sample volume made up of red blood cells; the laboratory test performed to determine percent of red blood cells in a blood sample; also known as the packed cell volume (PCV).

hematopoiesis Blood cell production.

hematopoietic tissue Tissue that produces blood cells. Red bone marrow is hematopoietic tissue.

hemidesmosomes The half-units of desmosomes.

hemoconcentration A condition resulting from a loss of plasma from blood into tissue. The cells become more concentrated in the plasma. This condition is commonly seen in a dehydrated animal.

hemodilution A condition resulting from excess fluid entering blood from tissue or from intravenous injection of fluids. The cells become more diluted in the plasma. This condition can result from overhydration of an animal with intravenous or subcutaneous fluids.

hemoglobin The protein molecules found inside red blood cells that are responsible for carrying oxygen molecules.

hemoglobinemia Hemoglobin in plasma. The red blood cell membrane has ruptured, resulting in the release of hemoglobin. Hemoglobinemia is the result of intravascular hemolysis.

hemoglobinuria Free hemoglobin found in urine. The degree of intravascular hemolysis was great enough to release large amounts of hemoglobin. The excess hemoglobin over what could be bound to haptoglobin and carried to the liver is eliminated in urine.

hemolytic anemia An anemia caused by the hemolysis (rupture) of red blood cells; may be caused by an autoimmune disorder or from the toxic effects of certain chemicals or may be congenital.

hemorrhaging The abnormal bursting forth of blood from damaged blood vessels. It can be severe and may occur in arteries, veins, and capillaries.

hemostasis Controlling bleeding; stopping the flow of blood out of a blood vessel.

hemothorax An excess amount of bloody serous fluid present in the pleural cavity as a result of conditions such as pneumonia, cancerous tumors, or trauma.

heparin A polysaccharide manufactured by mast cells that acts as an anticoagulant to help continue the increased blood flow during the inflammatory response.

hepatic duct The duct that carries bile from the liver to the gallbladder (in those species that have gallbladders).

hepatic lobes The large divisions of the liver seen grossly during surgery or dissection.

hepatic lobules The small microscopic divisions of the liver.

hepatic portal system The blood vessels that carry blood from the capillaries of the intestine directly to the sinusoids of the liver.

hepatic Referring to the liver.

herbivore An animal whose diet is primarily plants.

hibernate To arrive at deep state of sleep, nearly to the degree of a comatose state. During hibernation, an organism's metabolism and body temperature are in a significantly lowered state.

hibernating gland An alternate nomenclature for brown adipose tissue owing to its glandular appearance and its vital role in providing body heat to an animal during hibernation.

hiccups Spasmodic contractions of the diaphragm accompanied by sudden closure of the glottis causing the characteristic "hiccup" sound. They are usually harmless and temporary.

hilus The isolated area of some organs where blood vessels and other structures, such as nerves, enter and leave. For example, the hilus of the kidney is the indented area on the medial side where blood or lymph vessels and nerves enter and leave and where the ureters leave the organ. The hilus of the lung is where air passageways, blood, and lymph vessels, and nerves enter and leave.

hinge joint A joint whereby one surface swivels around another like a door hinge; also called a ginglymus joint. The only movements possible in a hinge joint are flexion and extension. The elbow joint is an example of a hinge joint.

hip dysplasia A disorder of the hip joint in which the normally tight-fitting ball-and-socket hip joint is abnormally loose. The looseness (laxity) of the dysplastic joint allows the head of the femur to "rattle around" in the acetabulum, resulting in damage to the joint surfaces and osteoarthritis development. Movement of the damaged hip causes pain.

histamine Produced by mast cells from histidine during tissue injury, this biochemical increases blood flow and heart rate during the inflammatory response.

histiocytes Macrophages located in loose connective tissue.

histology The microscopic study of the structure of tissues and organs; microanatomy.

histones A globular protein found in the cellular nucleus that connects with nucleic acid to form nucleoproteins. Histones form a complex with DNA in chromatin and act as regulators of gene activity.

hock Ankle joint, or tarsus; joins the tibiotarsus and the tarsometatarsus.

holocrine gland A gland whose granular secretions contain not only the secretory product but also the cells themselves. Holocrine gland cells are destroyed in the process of secretion. The sebaceous gland is an example of a holocrine gland.

homeostasis A state of chemical equilibrium maintained in the body by feedback and regulation processes in response to internal and external changes; the maintenance of balance in the body. The concept of homeostasis includes the many mechanisms that monitor critical levels and functions in the body and stimulate corrective actions when things stray from normal. By keeping important activities within relatively narrow ranges, the process of homeostasis helps maintain normal body structure and function and therefore health.

homogeneous Having a uniform composition.

homologous Similar in basic structure and from the same embryological origin. The penis of the male and the clitoris of the female are homologous structures.

hoof wall The external, cornified portion of the hoof. It grows constantly downward from the coronet to the sole. The deepest layer articulates with the corium by way of the laminae.

Hooke Robert Hooke, in 1665, was the first person to identify the structure of the cell under a microscope.

hormones Chemical messengers of the body that are produced and excreted by specific cells for the purpose of regulating specific organs or cells.

horn A horny, keratinized extension of the frontal lobe in ruminate ungulates. At its root, it arises from the corium, being epidermal in origin. Horns vary in shape and size depending on age, sex, and species.

horn tubes Minute lines that traverse the hoof wall vertically from the germinating layer of the coronary band to the sole.

humerus The long bone of the brachium or "upper arm."

humoral immunity A type of defense immune response regulated by B lymphocytes. When B lymphocytes are activated by the presence of an antigen, they transform into plasma cells that produce antibodies against the antigen.

hyaline cartilage A bluish, semitransparent cartilage present in the costal cartilage, trachea, and embryonic skeleton. Hyaline cartilage is composed of densely packed collagen fibers and is covered by the perichondrium, except when present as articular cartilage in joints.

hyaluronic acid A small protein, containing no sulfate, that acts as an intercellular material present in the zonula adherens. It is important in the formation of tight junctions.

hyaluronidase An enzyme contained within white blood cells or infectious bacteria that hydrolyzes hyaluronic acid.

hydraulic pressure Pressure exerted by confined fluids. During erection of the penis, more blood enters the erectile tissue of the penis than leaves it. The resulting hydraulic pressure produces enlargement and stiffening of the penis.

hydrogen bonds Weak bonds that unite hydrogen with nitrogen or oxygen.

hydrolysis One of the most basic and prevalent life processes. Hydrolysis breaks down more complex materials into simpler ones by adding water. Water breaks down or dissociates into a hydrogen atom (H) and a hydroxyl group (OH), which cling to individual parts of the material, thus separating it into two simpler materials.

hydrophilic The tendency of a tissue to absorb or be attracted to water.

hydrophobic The tendency of a tissue to be repelled by water or to be insoluble.

hydrostatic pressure The force that propels a liquid.

hyoid apparatus The hyoid bone.

hyoid bone The bone in the neck region that supports the base of the tongue, the pharynx, and the larynx and aids the process of swallowing. It is usually referred to as a single bone, but it is composed of several portions. The hyoid bone is attached to the temporal bone by two small rods of cartilage.

hyperadrenocorticism Excessive secretion of hormones from the cortex of the adrenal gland; also called Cushing's syndrome.

hyperbilirubinemia An excess amount of bilirubin in plasma.

hypercalcemia An excess level of calcium in the blood.

hyperemia The reddish tinge of mucous membranes caused by an excessive flow of blood to the extremities.

hyperglycemia Too high a level of glucose in the blood.

hyperpigmented Referring to an abnormal degree of pigmentation.

hyperplasia Excessive development of a body part as a result of an abnormal proliferation of cells.

hyperreflexive Reflex response is more pronounced than normal.

hypersegmented neutrophil A neutrophil that has more than five nuclear lobes when seen in peripheral blood.

hypertension An abnormal elevation of blood pressure

hypertonic When the concentration of particles in solution is higher outside of the cell. This may cause water to move from the inside to the outside of the cell to attain equilibrium. In this way, the cell shrivels and becomes crenated.

hypoadrenocorticism Deficient secretion of hormones from the cortex of the adrenal gland; also called Addison's syndrome.

hypocalcemia Too low a level of calcium in the blood.

hypodermis *See* Subcutaneous layer.

hypoglycemia Too low a level of glucose in the blood.

hypophysis Pituitary gland.

hypoplastic Referring to an organ or tissue that is underdeveloped.

hyporeflexive Reflex response is less than normal.

hypotensive Having an abnormal decrease in blood pressure.

hypothalamus A portion of the brain stem that has extensive links to the brain and to the pituitary gland. It functions as an important bridge between the nervous and the endocrine systems.

hypothermia An abnormally low body temperature that slows down all metabolic processes. Hypothermia can result from prolonged exposure to cold environmental temperatures, or it may be drug-induced, such as with many general anesthetic drugs. Efforts should always be made to keep anesthetized animals and animals recovering from general anesthesia warm.

hypotonic When the concentration of a solution outside the cell is lower than it is on the inside of the cell. Water will tend to flow into the cell toward the higher concentration. This causes swelling and possible rupture of the cell.

hypoxia Oxygen deficiency; causes bluish tinge of mucous membrane. There are many causes for hypoxia, ranging from anemia to respiratory blockage.

I

I bands Large light bands in a skeletal muscle fiber that alternate with darker A bands to give a striped appearance to skeletal muscle fibers under a microscope. The I bands are composed of thin filaments of the contractile protein actin.

iatrogenic A condition caused by medical treatment given to an animal.

icterus The yellowish color given to tissues, membranes, and secretions by the presence of bile pigments; may indicate elevated levels of bilirubin, possibly resulting from liver failure; also known as jaundice.

IgA Immunoglobulin A. It can leave blood and enter tissue, where it plays an important role in preventing diseases caused by antigens that enter the body through mucosal surfaces.

IgD Immunoglobulin D; its function is unknown.

IgE Immunoglobulin E; it is associated with allergies.

IgG Immunoglobulin G; it is produced during the first exposure to an antigen; it is also made by newborn animals.

IgM Immunoglobulin M; It is produced after an animal has been exposed to an antigen for an extended time or when an animal is exposed to an antigen for the second time.

ileocecal sphincter The circular smooth muscle that regulates the movement of intestinal contents from the ileum to the cecum.

ileum The last of three segments of the small intestine; it empties into the colon or cecum.

ileus Intestinal obstruction; may be due to lack of movement of the bowel.

ilium The cranial-most of the three pairs of bones that make up the pelvis. It forms the sacroiliac joint with the sacrum.

immunization The process of creating immunity within an animal, usually by introducing the body to a killed or modified culture of the infectious agent to allow it to create antibodies; also called vaccination.

immunoglobulins Created by B-lymphocytes, these protein-based molecules (also called antibodies) are produced by exposure to an infectious agent's antigen. In future encounters with the same antigen, the antibodies will identify and fight it.

immunosuppressed Referring to an immune system that cannot elicit an immune response.

impermeable Referring to structures that do not allow the passage of fluid.

implantation angle The degree of angle with regard to a shaft of hair.

implantation Embedding of a developing blastocyst in the lining of the uterus.

incisive bones Skull bones that are part of the external bones of the face. The two incisive bones are the most rostral of the skull bones. In all common domestic animals, except ruminants, the incisive bones house the upper incisor teeth.

incisor The teeth in the front of the mouth that are narrowed into a sharp ridge at their tip.

inclusions The temporary component of the cell that is lifeless, having been brought into the cell via phagocytosis.

incus One of the three ossicles (the tiny bones that transmit sound wave vibrations across the middle ear). The incus, or anvil, is the middle of the three ossicles.

indeterminate layer Species that can produce more eggs than their normal clutch size.

infection Invasion and replication of microorganisms causing detrimental activity in the body.

inflammation The first step in the healing process when the body is injured. Its purpose is to "clean up" the damaged area through various inflammatory processes so healing can begin.

inflammatory process the series of cellular and metabolic events that take place primarily in connective tissue as the result of injury or loss of tissue. The inflammatory process acts to isolate and destroy infectious agents, as well as prepare the tissue for healing.

infraorbital pouch A pouch of cutaneous tissue found cranial to the medial canthus of the eye in sheep and other ungulates; also called lacrimal pouch.

infundibulum The cup-shaped ovarian end of the oviduct. Cilia lining the infundibulum beat rhythmically to ensure passage of the ovum into the oviduct.

inguinal pouch Also known as mammary pouch; a pouch of cutaneous tissue found within the inguinal area of sheep.

inguinal rings Slitlike openings in the abdominal muscles located in the groin (inguinal) region. The spermatic cords of the male pass through the inguinal rings from the scrotum to the interior of the abdominal cavity.

inhibitory neurotransmitters Chemicals released by neurons at the synapse that tend to depress or decrease depolarization of other neurons or target tissues.

inner ear The most internal portion of the ear. It is contained in the temporal bone and contains both hearing and equilibrium structures.

innervated Having a nerve supply.

insertion of a muscle The more movable of the attachment sites of a muscle. When a muscle contracts, it exerts traction on its insertion site, usually producing movement of a bone or other structure.

inspiration The process of drawing air into the lungs; inhalation.

inspiratory muscle A muscle whose action is to increase the size of the thoracic cavity; this causes air to be drawn into the lungs, thereby producing inspiration (inhalation).

insulin A hormone produced by the beta cells of the pancreatic islets. Its main action is to allow glucose to be absorbed into body cells and used for energy; this decreases the level of glucose in the blood.

integral proteins The proteins located within the lipid bilayer that create channels that aid in the selective permeability of the cell membrane.

integument The skin of the body, consisting of dermis and epidermis.

integumentary system The skin and all of its related components, such as nails, hair, hooves, and horns.

intercalated disks End-to-end attachment sites between adjacent cardiac muscle cells. The intercalated disks securely fasten the cells together and also transmit impulses from cell to cell. This allows large groups of cardiac muscle cells to function as a large single unit.

intercostal space The space between two ribs.

interdigital pouch A pouch of cutaneous tissue that exudes a waxy substance; found between the toes of sheep and other cloven-hoofed animals.

interferon A substance produced by a cell after a virus has invaded it. Interferon prevents further development or spread of the virus.

intermediate fibers Fibers that are specialized to the cell in which they are contained. They are composed of tough protein fibers that help to reinforce the cell in which they are contained.

intermediate filaments *See* Tonofilaments.

internal An alternative directional term for *deep.* Internal also means toward the center of the body or a body part.

internal respiration The exchange of oxygen and carbon dioxide between the blood in the capillaries all over the body and all the cells and tissues of the body.

interneuron Typically a short neuron that connects two other neurons; usually mentioned in context of the reflex arc.

interparietal bones Skull bones that are part of the external bones of the cranium. The two interparietal bones are located on the dorsal midline just rostral to the occipital bone. The interparietal bones are usually distinct in young animals, but in older animals, they may fuse into one bone and may even fuse to the parietal bones and become indistinguishable.

interphase The period between cell divisions during which all normal growth and functions occur.

interstitial cell–stimulating hormone (ICSH) The anterior pituitary hormone that stimulates the interstitial cells of the testes to produce androgens (the male sex hormones); also known as luteinizing hormone (LH).

interstitial cells Endocrine cells located between the seminiferous tubules of the testes. They produce androgens (the male sex hormones).

interstitial fluid All fluid contained within the tissue except for the fluid found within lymph and blood vessels.

intervertebral disk The cartilaginous disk located between the bodies of adjacent vertebrae. It acts as a "shock absorber" for the vertebrae.

intracellular fluid The fluid that is contained within the cell.

intramembranous bone formation "Membrane" bone formation. The type of bone formation that only occurs in certain skull bones when bone forms in the fibrous tissue membranes that cover the brain in a developing fetus.

intramuscular injection A route of drug administration that involves injecting a drug through a hypodermic needle that has been inserted into the belly of a muscle. The large blood supply of the muscle leads to rapid absorption of the drug into the bloodstream for distribution to the rest of the body.

intravascular hemolysis Destruction of red blood cells within a blood vessel.

intrinsic factor A protein produced by the stomach and required for absorption of vitamin B_{12}.

intromission Insertion of the penis into the vagina.

introns Spaces between coded exons of a gene's DNA sequence that do not contain codes.

involuntary muscle An old name for *smooth muscle.*

involuntary striated muscle An old name for *cardiac muscle.*

involution of the mammary gland "Drying up" of the mammary gland when the stimuli necessary to stimulate lactation cease; the cessation of milk production with shrinkage of the mammary gland back to near its prelactating size.

involution of the uterus Shrinkage of the uterus after parturition back to near its prepregnant size.

ions An electrically charged atom or molecule. Cations are positively charged ions, and anions are negatively charged ions.

ipsilateral reflexes The reflex stimulus and response are on the same side of the body.

iris A portion of the uvea, or middle vascular layer, of the eye. The iris is a pigmented, muscular diaphragm that controls the amount of light that enters the posterior part of the eyeball.

irregular bone A bone whose shape does not fit into the long bone, short bone, or flat bone categories. Irregular bones either have characteristics of more than one of the other three shape categories or have a truly irregular shape. Examples include vertebrae, some strangely shaped skull bones (such as the sphenoid bone), and sesamoid bones.

ischium The caudal-most of the three pairs of bones that make up the pelvis.

islets of Langerhans Clusters of cells in the pancreas that produce insulin and glucagon, as well as other endocrine products of the pancreas.

isotonic Equal tension present on either side of the cell membrane.

J

jaundice An abnormal condition characterized by the yellowing of the mucous membranes, skin, and sclerae as a result of an excess of bilirubin in the blood. It results from the movement of excess bilirubin in blood into tissues. This may be caused by liver failure, excessive destruction of red blood cells, or blockage of the bile ducts. Also known as icterus.

jejunum The second of three segments of the small intestine; usually the longest segment of the small intestine.

joint The junction between two bones. Joints can be completely immovable (fibrous joints), slightly movable (cartilaginous joints), or freely movable (synovial joints).

joint capsule The membrane that encloses the ends of the bones in a synovial joint; consists of an outer fibrous membrane and an inner synovial membrane that produces viscous synovial fluid that lubricates the joint surfaces.

joint cavity The fluid-filled potential space between the joint surfaces of a synovial joint; the joint cavity is normally filled by synovial fluid (the viscous, lubricating fluid produced by the synovial membrane lining of the joint capsule); also known as the joint space.

joint space Alternate name for the *joint cavity.*

junctional complex The point at which epithelial cells join to one another in very close proximity.

K

keel Bony ridge on the sternum of birds to which the flight muscles attach.

keratin A tough, waterproof protein that composes scales, the outer sheaths of beaks and claws, and feathers; a main component of the epidermis, nails, hair, horns and hooves.

keratin fibers The strong strands of the fibrous protein keratin that are insoluble in water.

keratinization The normal formation of keratin (a tough, waterproof protein) inside epithelial cells of the skin. As the epithelial cells mature, they fill with granules filled with keratin and at the same time give up vital organelles.

keratinized stratified squamous epithelium The epithelial classification of the epidermis. It is highly regenerative and waterproof, thereby helping the body to retain moisture and thermoregulate.

keratinocytes Cells that synthesize keratin. They have three distinct stages visible in the epidermis: the basal, prickle, and granular cell stage. As keratinocytes travel progressively away from the basement membrane toward the superficial epithelium, they lose their organelles to make way for more keratin. As a result of this process, the cells die by the time they reach the surface.

ketone bodies Products of lipid metabolism (lipolysis), including beta-hydroxybutyric acid, acetoacetic acid, and acetone. They are usually produced from acetyl-coA from fatty acids within the liver.

kinetochore *See* Centromere.

Krebs cycle The metabolism of sugars, fatty acids, and amino acids through oxidation to produce carbon dioxide, water, and energy.

Kupffer cells Macrophages present in the liver. Fifty percent of macrophages are Kupffer cells.

L

labia Literally means "lips." The external boundary of the vulva of the female.

labial Liplike or pertaining to the lips.

labial surface The surface of the rostral part of the upper and lower arcade of teeth that face the lips.

lacrimal apparatus The tear-producing and draining structures of the eyes.

lacrimal bones Skull bones; external bones of the face. The two small lacrimal bones form part of the medial portion of the orbit of the eye. In the living animal the lacrimal bones house the lacrimal sacs (part of the tear drainage system of the eye).

lacrimal gland The main tear-producing gland. It is located dorsal and lateral to the eyeball inside the bony orbit.

lacrimal puncta Openings in the upper and lower eyelid margins located near the medial canthus of each eye. They drain tears away from the surface of eyes.

lacrimal sac A small sac that receives tears from the lacrimal puncta and sends them down into the nasolacrimal duct.

lactation Milk production by the mammary gland.

lactic acid A waste product of anaerobic metabolism in skeletal muscle. The buildup of lactic acid in a muscle that has been forced into anaerobic mode by overstrenuous activity can cause discomfort; an end product of the metabolism of carbohydrates. It is created by the conversion of pyruvate into lactic acid after the fermentation of cellulose.

lactic acidosis In the ruminant, this is the same as grain overload and rumen acidosis; a condition in which too much carbohydrate is available to the rumen microbes, resulting in production of large amounts of lactic acid and subsequently causing severe changes in the rumen microflora and systemic acidosis.

lacunae Small cavities within the matrix of calcified tissues, such as cartilage and bone, within which cells (chondrocytes and osteocytes) are contained.

lamina propria The areolar connective tissue located in the mucous membrane.

laminae The interdigitations between the corium and hoof that serve as the attachment sites between the hoof and coffin bone.

laminitis Manifests itself as extreme pain and heat in the coronets because of swelling and inflammation of the sensitive laminae. It most often affects equids in their front feet, but in severe cases, it may involve all four feet. There are many causes, such as ingesting large quantities of grains and carbohydrates, drug reactions, retained placentas, and trauma. In severe cases, the coffin bone may penetrate the sole of the hoof; also called founder.

Langerhans' cells The macrophages of the epidermis that phagocytize invading microorganisms and produce antigens.

lanolin Fat-based secretion of the sheep's sebaceous glands; a byproduct of the wool industry and is used for lotions and ointments.

laryngeal hemiplegia The medical name for what is commonly called "roaring," a condition often seen in horses. It is produced by paralysis of the muscles that tighten the arytenoid cartilages and vocal cord on one side (usually the left) of the larynx. The result is that the paralyzed vocal cord partially obstructs the glottis and causes difficulty breathing, particularly when the animal tries to breathe heavily when exercising. Vibrations of the paralyzed vocal cord produce a characteristic roaring sound as the animal breathes.

laryngoscope An instrument used to aid the passage of an endotracheal tube through the glottis and down into the trachea. The laryngoscope consists of a handle that contains batteries and a long, narrow blade with a small light source near the end of it. The blade is used to gently press the tip of the epiglottis ventrally, exposing the opening of the glottis.

laryngospasm A spasmodic closure of the opening of the glottis; often occurs in cats during endotracheal intubation because of the sensitivity of a cat's larynx.

larynx The "voice box"; a short, irregular tube of cartilage and muscle that connects the pharynx with the trachea. Its functions are voice production, preventing foreign material from being inhaled, and controlling airflow to and from the lungs.

lateral A directional term meaning away from the median plane (center line) of the body.

lateral cartilages Two large bands of cartilage contained within the equid hoof that, in conjunction with the frog and digital cushion, aid in venous return.

lateral ventricles Blind pouches that project laterally between the vocal cords and the vestibular folds in the larynxes of nonruminant animals.

lesser curvature of the stomach The smaller, inner curve of the stomach.

leukemia "White blood"; a cancer or malignancy of one of the white blood cells. Production of that white blood cell is abnormal and uncontrolled.

leukocytes Also called white blood cells, leukocytes come in many different varieties, including basophils, eosinophils, neutrophils, lymphocytes, and monocytes. They may be granulated or nongranulated and are capable of amoeboid motion. The main function of leukocytes is body defense.

Leukocytopenia A decrease in the total number of white blood cells in peripheral blood.

leukocytosis An increase in the total number of white blood cells in peripheral blood.

leukopoiesis A general term for production of white blood cells.

ligament A band of fibrous connective tissue that is present in and around many synovial joints. When present, ligaments connect the bones of the joint to each other.

ligamentum arteriosum The normal remnant of the ductus arteriosus after it has constricted and fibrosed.

ligands Small molecules that bond to larger chemical groups or molecules.

ligation Surgically tying off blood vessels; usually done with suture material.

light microscopy The viewing of a sample by using natural light and magnifying the sample through the objective lenses of a microscope.

limbus The junction of the cornea and sclera of the eye.

linea alba The sheet of fibrous connective tissue (aponeurosis) that connects the abdominal muscles from each side on the ventral midline.

lingual surface The surface of the lower arcade of teeth that faces the tongue; *lingua* is Latin for "tongue."

lipase Enzyme produced by the pancreas and, in some species, the saliva; breaks apart fats into their components.

lipid bilayer A double-layered membrane made of phospholipids, such as the cell membrane and nuclear envelope.

lipids The group of fatty or fatlike substances that are insoluble in water. Alcohol, ether, chloroform, and other nonpolar substances can, however, dissolve them.

lipolysis The breakdown of fats.

lobe Each cerebral hemisphere is divided by sulci into lobes; different lobes of the cerebral hemispheres specialize in certain functions.

lobes (of the lung) Subdivisions of the lungs. Lung lobes are defined by major branches of bronchi entering them rather than grossly visible grooves and clefts.

local anesthesia Loss of sensation from a localized area of the body.

long bone Bones that are longer than they are wide. Most of the limb bones, such as the humerus, femur, and radius, are long bones.

longitudinal fissure Prominent groove that divides the cerebrum into right and left cerebral hemispheres.

longitudinal muscle The muscle in the intestinal tract layer that is responsible for shortening segments of the intestine when it contracts; is involved with peristaltic movement.

loop of Henle The middle part of the tubular portion of a nephron. It has a descending part that travels from the cortex to the medulla and an ascending part that travels back to the cortex. The loop of Henle is located between the proximal convoluted tubule and the distal convoluted tubule.

loose connective tissue A subclass of connective tissue proper, loose connective tissue is a vascularized type of connective tissue whose general function is to support the structures it surrounds. Loose connective tissue includes areolar, adipose, and reticular connective tissues.

lower arcade In reference to teeth, it means the teeth in the mandible, or the lower set of teeth in the mouth.

lower respiratory tract All of the respiratory structures within the lungs; includes all the respiratory passages from the bronchi down to the alveoli.

lumbar vertebrae The group of vertebrae located dorsal to the abdominal region.

lumen The opening in the middle of the intestinal tract (or any hollow organ).

luteinizing hormone (LH) The anterior pituitary hormone that stimulates ovulation in most species and then causes the empty follicle to develop into the corpus luteum.

luteolysis Destruction of the corpus luteum.

lymph Excess tissue fluid that is picked up by lymph vessels and returned to peripheral blood.

lymphocytes Nongranulocytic white blood cells that are involved in the immune response. The two types of lymphocytes are T lymphocytes, which are involved with cell-mediated immunity, and B lymphocytes, which are involved with humoral immunity.

lymphocytosis An increase in the number of lymphocytes in peripheral blood.

lymphokines Proteins that develop on the surface of helper T lymphocytes. The lymphokines activate killer T lymphocytes, which are responsible for cell-mediated immunity.

lymphopenia A decrease in the number of lymphocytes in peripheral blood.

lysosome An organelle that fights pathogens, repairs damaged tissues, and aids in intracellular digestion by engulfing materials with its membrane-bound vesicle bodies. It contains the digestive enzymes that help destroy microorganisms that have been phagocytized by the neutrophil.

M

macrophages Phagocytic cells that can engulf relatively large cells or bits of debris. They may be fixed in place or they may travel around in the tissues. Mature macrophages may become more mobile during times of infection and inflammation.

macroscopic anatomy Also called gross anatomy; the study of body parts large enough to be seen without magnification, such as a lung, leg, or brain.

macula A patch of sensory epithelium in the vestibule. It consists of hair cells covered by a gelatinous mass containing otoliths. The macula senses the position of the head.

malignant Any growth that is recurring and resistant to treatment and therefore considered to be harmful.

malignant melanoma A melanoma, composed of epithelial cells, that grows rapidly and often metastasizes. They are most common in horses, dogs, cats, and sometimes goats and sheep. In these cases the prognosis is poor. Melanomas in cattle and pigs are usually benign.

malleus One of the three ossicles (the tiny bones that transmit sound wave vibrations across the middle ear). The malleus, or hammer, is the outermost of the three ossicles and is attached to the tympanic membrane.

mandible A skull bone; one of the external bones of the face. The mandible is the lower jaw, the only movable skull bone. The mandible houses all of the lower teeth. It is usually referred to as a single bone, but in dogs, cats, and cattle, the two halves of the mandible are separate bones joined by a cartilaginous mandibular symphysis at the rostral end.

mandibular symphysis The cartilaginous joint (amphiarthrosis) that unites the two sides of the mandible at the rostral (front) end.

manubrium The first, most cranial sternebra. Its full name is manubrium sterni.

marbling The common name for fat deposits in the connective tissue layers of meat (skeletal muscle).

marginal pool of neutrophils Neutrophils found lining the walls of small blood vessels mainly in the spleen, lungs, and abdominal organs. These neutrophils are not circulating but are moving slowly along the walls of the vessels.

mast cell A transient cell of connective tissue containing heparin and histamine used in the inflammatory response. Mast cells recognize foreign invaders and release granules of histamine and heparin to increase blood flow. They resemble basophils, but they do not circulate in blood.

mastication Chewing.

mastitis Infection of a mammary gland.

matrix The intercellular material of connective tissue.

mature follicle An ovarian follicle that is fully developed and ready for ovulation; also known as a vesicular follicle or a Graafian follicle.

maxilla The bone of the upper jaw.

maxillary bones Skull bones; external bones of the face. The two maxillary bones make up most of the upper jaw and house the upper canine teeth, if present, and all of the cheek teeth (premolars and molars).

maxillary sinus The paranasal sinus in the maxillary bones.

mechanical control system The respiratory control system that sets inspiration and expiration limits for normal resting breathing; operates on the basis of stretch receptors in the lungs that communicate with the respiratory center in the brain stem.

mechanical digestion The physical breakdown of food into small particles.

meconium Dark, tarry material in the intestine of a newborn animal. The first feces passed by the newborn.

medial A directional term meaning toward the median plane (center line) of the body.

median plane An anatomical reference plane. A median plane is a sagittal plane that runs down the center of the body and divides it into equal left and right halves. It is also called a midsagittal plane.

mediastinum The area of the thorax between the lungs. It contains the heart and most of the other thoracic structures, such as the trachea, esophagus, blood vessels, nerves, and lymphatic structures.

medulla (1) The inner, deep layer of an organ or structure. (2) The inner part of the kidney. It contains the loop of Henle, peritubular capillaries, and collecting ducts. (3) The innermost layer of a hair strand made of two or three layers of flexible, soft keratin.

medulla oblongata The part of the brain stem just above (cranial to) the spinal cord.

megaesophagus A condition in which the esophagus loses muscle tones and dilates into a flaccid, saclike structure.

megakaryocytes Large, multinucleated cells in red bone marrow that are the parent cells of platelets. Platelets are formed when chunks of cytoplasm break off a megakaryocyte and enter circulation.

meibomian glands The tarsal glands of the eyelid margins. They produce a waxy substance that helps prevent tears from overflowing onto the animal's face.

meiosis The "reduction division" that reproductive cells undergo during their development. It results in a reduction of the chromosome number from the normal diploid number to the haploid number (half of the diploid number).

Meissner's corpuscles The oval, tactile nerve endings, both myelinated and unmyelinated, found within the dermal papillae of the epidermis. Sensitive to light touch, they are especially common in body parts with no hair follicles, such as the soles of the feet.

melanin That sulfurous pigment produced by melanocytes, especially when stimulated by sunlight. Melanin is present in the skin, hair, and choroid of the eye, and abnormally in melanomas.

melanocyte-stimulating hormone (MSH) The anterior pituitary hormone that apparently influences the pigment cells of the skin (the melanocytes). Its precise role in the body is not well understood.

melanocytes Cells located within the lower epidermis that process tyrosinase and melanin. Melanin, contained within melanosomes, is transferred to keratinocytes by way of the melanocyte's long projections.

melanosomes Granules filled with melanin that are transferred from the melanocytes to the keratinocytes.

melatonin A hormonelike substance produced by the pineal body. It apparently affects moods and wake-sleep cycles and may affect the timing of seasonal estrous cycles in some species.

membrane potential The difference in voltage that exists on either side of the cell membrane caused by the different concentrations of positive and negative charges.

membrane proteins Proteins imbedded in the cell's membrane, performing such functions as cell receptors and membrane transport molecules.

membrane receptors The integral proteins and glycoproteins that form binding sites and may aid in contact signaling.

memory cells After an initial immune response, some lymphocytes, called memory cells, are programmed to remember the antigen that caused the immune response and produce a more rapid immune response to that antigen the second time the body is exposed to it.

meninges Set of connective tissues that surround the brain and spinal cord; the three layers of the meninges, from outside to innermost layer, are the dura mater, the arachnoid, and the pia mater.

meniscus One of two concave, half moon–shaped cartilaginous structures on the proximal surface of the tibia that help support the condyles of the femur.

Merkel's cells Thought to aid in tactile sensory function, these cells are located in small numbers within the epidermal-dermal junction.

Merkel's disk The junction formed by Merkel's cells and sensory nerves.

merocrine gland A gland whose secretions contain none of its cells, thus leaving the gland cells intact. Examples include salivary and sweat glands.

mesoderm The middle layer of the fetal body's tissue. Located between the outer layer (ectoderm) and the inner layer (endoderm), the mesoderm gives rise to all connective and muscle tissues.

mesothelium A layer of cells that lines the body cavities of the fetus and that covers the serous membranes in adult animals.

messenger RNA (mRNA) One of the main components of protein synthesis; mRNA transfers the specific amino acid sequence of the genetic code of DNA to the cytoplasm, where protein is synthesized.

metabolic turnover The continuous breakdown of old cells and body matter to be replaced with new cells and body matter.

metabolism All of the complex, interrelated chemical processes that make life possible. Its two fundamental components are anabolism and catabolism.

metabolites Substances that are produced during metabolism.

metacarpal bones Bones of the forelimb that lie between the carpals and phalanges of quadrupeds.

metaphase The phase of mitosis when the newly formed chromosomes align on a medial plane or "equator" between the two centrioles located at either end of the dividing cell.

metaphase plate During metaphase, it is the site where chromosomes line up and are evenly distributed.

metastasis The progression of a disease from one organ or system to another organ or system, thus spreading the disease from the original neoplasm to secondary tumors.

metastatic masses The secondary tumors formed from the spread of malignant cells shed by the original malignant neoplasm during the process of metastasis.

metatarsal bones The bones of the pelvic limbs located between the tarsus and the phalanges.

metestrus The stage of the estrous cycle after ovulation when the corpus luteum develops. It occurs between estrus and diestrus.

micelle A very small droplet of fat surrounded by hydrophilic (water-loving) molecules that allows it to readily move in the liquid environment of the small intestine.

microanatomy *See* Histology.

microbe A microscopic organism that may or may not cause disease.

microfilament Closely associated with microtubules, these submicroscopic structures are found in most cells and are composed mostly of actin.

microglial cells Macrophages located in brain tissue.

microscopic anatomy The study of anatomical parts too small to be seen with the unaided eye, such as cells and tissues.

microtome A cutting instrument used to make extremely thin slices of tissue for microscopic study.

microtrabeculae A component of the cytoskeleton thought to add form, support, and substance to the cell's inner anatomy.

microtubules Tiny, hollow, tubelike structures that aid certain cells with rigidity and transportation. They also form the spindle fibers in the process of mitosis.

microvilli Fingerlike protrusions of the luminal surface of some epithelial cell membranes that increase the cell's exposed surface area.

micturition The process of expelling urine from the body; also called urination or uresis.

midbrain Mesencephalon.

middle ear The middle portion of the ear; an air-filled cavity in the temporal bone of the skull. It contains the ossicles and the opening of the eustachian tube. The middle ear amplifies and transmits sound wave vibrations from the tympanic membrane to the cochlea of the inner ear.

milk fever A disease seen in lactating cattle that results from hypocalcemia. The signs of milk fever include muscle weakness and an inability to stand.

milk letdown The immediate effect of nursing or milking. The movement of milk from the alveoli and small ducts down into the larger ducts and sinuses, where it is accessible for nursing or milking. It results from the release of oxytocin from the posterior pituitary gland. The oxytocin causes myoepithelial cells surrounding the alveoli and small ducts of the mammary gland to contract, squeezing the milk into the lower parts of the gland.

mineralocorticoid hormones A group of hormones secreted by the cortex of the adrenal glands that regulate the levels of some important electrolytes in the body. The principal mineralocorticoid hormone is aldosterone.

minute volume The volume of air that an animal breathes in and out during one minute. It is calculated by multiplying the animal's tidal volume by its respiratory rate (number of breaths taken per minute).

mitochondria The primary source of ATP formation for aerobic cell respiration. This organelle also contains DNA and RNA, making the mitochondria capable of its own protein synthesis and replication.

mitochondrial matrix The enzyme-rich liquid in the mitochondria that surrounds the cristae and provides them with the enzymes necessary for the proper function of the Krebs cycle.

mitosis Cell division of somatic cells for growth and to replace old or dead cells; the type of cell division that occurs in all body cells except the reproductive cells. When cells divide by mitosis, the chromosomes first duplicate themselves and then pull apart into two daughter cells. This preserves the diploid chromosome number.

mitotic phase The period during which cell division occurs. It is divided into the main phases of interphase, metaphase, anaphase, and telophase.

mitral valve Also called the left atrioventricular valve; separates the left atrium and ventricle and protects the pulmonary venous system from the high pressures in the left ventricle during systole.

mixed exocrine glands Exocrine glands, such as salivary glands, that can produce both mucous and serous secretions.

molar The grinding teeth located at the back of the mouth.

molting Process of feather replacement; occurs one to several times a year, depending on the species.

monocyte A large, phagocytic white blood cell. It is the largest white blood cell normally found in peripheral blood. It is an agranulocyte.

monocytopenia A decrease in the number of monocytes in peripheral blood.

monocytosis An increase in the number of monocytes in peripheral blood.

monoestrous An animal that has only one estrous cycle each year.

monogastric Having one stomach; usually refers to nonruminant animals that do not rely on fermentative processes to any great extent.

monoglyceride A product of triglyceride breakdown; made from one fatty acid plus a glycerol molecule.

mononuclear phagocyte system A collective term for monocytes and tissue macrophages found throughout the body.

monosaccharides Simple sugars; single sugar molecules, including glucose, galactose, and fructose.

morphological The unique structures and forms of each individual organ, tissue, cell, or organism as a whole.

morula The solid mass of cells into which the zygote has developed a few days after fertilization of the ovum. It resembles a tiny raspberry.

motor nerve Nerve that carries efferent impulses to muscles, although motor function may be used to describe any nerve that carries an efferent impulse, including those that supply endocrine glands and tissues that are not muscle.

motor neuron A neuron carrying impulses from the CNS to a peripheral effector organ such as a muscle or gland.

motor unit One nerve fiber and all the skeletal muscle fibers it innervates. Motor units with small numbers of muscle fibers per nerve fiber are capable of fine, delicate movements. Motor units with large numbers of muscle fibers per nerve fiber are capable of large, powerful movements.

mRNA *See* Messenger RNA.

mucin The main constituent of mucus, produced by goblet cells in the respiratory and intestinal tracts. It is composed of proteoglycans.

mucosa The inner layer of the intestinal tract; this layer usually contains glands that secrete into the lumen of the gastrointestinal tract.

mucous An adjective to describe something pertaining to mucus or structures that either secrete or are covered by mucus.

mucous cells Cells in the lining of the stomach that produce mucus which helps prevent the stomach lining from being digested along with the food.

mucous membrane The mucus-producing layer of stratified squamous or columnar epithelium found over the lamina propria. It is present in organs that have contact with the outside of the body. Mucus production in mucous membranes is commonly found in the digestive, respiratory, and reproductive tracts, with the exception only of the urinary tract. The mucus secreted in them helps to fight infection because it is loaded with antibodies. Mucus also helps to absorb nutrients and lubricate surfaces.

mucous secretions Thick viscous secretions composed mostly of glycoproteins.

mucus Complex, gel-like substance that is secreted by goblet cells or other mucous glands; acts as a lubricant and protective barrier.

multicellular Composed of many cells.

multimeric Complex proteins containing more than one polypeptide chain.

multinucleated Having more than one nucleus.

multiparous An animal that normally gives birth to more than one offspring at parturition.

multiunit smooth muscle The type of smooth muscle composed of individual smooth muscle cells or small groups of cells. Found where small, delicate involuntary contractions are needed. Multiunit smooth muscle requires nerve impulses to stimulate its contractions.

murmur An abnormal heart sound created by blood that is flowing in a turbulent fashion. Can be associated with physiological causes, leaky valves, or stenotic valves.

muscarinic receptor A type of cholinergic receptor that is stimulated by acetylcholine

muscle spindle A sensory organ located within muscle that detects stretch of the muscle.

muscle tissue A collection of tissues that support the body and enable it to move, thermoregulate, and transport materials. Some muscles may be controlled voluntarily, whereas others act involuntarily. Examples of involuntary muscle include cardiac and smooth muscle; voluntary muscle includes all of the skeletal muscles.

mutagen An agent that can create a transmissible genetic change in an organism's DNA.

mutation The sudden and irreversible genetic change that causes a difference between offspring and their parents.

mute Organized waste product of birds that is ejected from the cloaca by the muscular anus; normally consists of a dark fecal center surrounded by a ring of white urates.

myelin Fatty substance that covers some axons When fixed for microscopic examination, it appears white; hence myelinated neurons make up the "white matter" of the brain and spinal cord.

myelin sheath Cell membrane of glial cells (oligodendrocytes, Schwann cells) wrapped around an axon; increases speed of impulse conduction along the axon.

myelography The diagnostic procedure of injecting radiographic contrast dye into the epidural space to better visual the outline of the spinal cord.

myocardium The middle layer of the heart and the main muscle layer responsible for contraction during systole.

myoepithelial cells Cells in the mammary glands that have characteristics of both muscle cells and epithelial cells. They surround the alveoli and small ducts of the glands. When stimulated by the hormone oxytocin, they contract, squeezing milk down into the large ducts and sinuses; *see* Milk letdown.

myofibrils Microscopic, fiberlike structures that occupy most of the cytoplasm (sarcoplasm) in skeletal muscle cells. Myofibrils are composed of filaments of the contractile proteins actin and myosin and are packed together longitudinally in the muscle cells.

myoglobin A protein in muscle cells that has properties similar to hemoglobin. It can store and release large quantities of oxygen to fuel aerobic metabolic processes in the muscle cells.

myometrium The muscle layer of the uterus.

myosin A protein present in muscle fibers that aids in contraction and makes up the majority of muscle protein.

myosin filaments One of the two contractile proteins of muscle (actin is the other one) that slide over each other to produce the shortening of the muscle cell that we refer to as muscle contraction.

N

NAD *See* Nicotinamide adenine dinucleotide.

NADH *See* Nicotinamide adenine dinucleotide.

nares The nostrils.

nasal bones Skull bones that are part of the external bones of the face. The nasal bones form the "bridge" of the nose (the dorsal part of the nasal cavity).

nasal conchae Skull bones that are part of the internal bones of the face; also known as the turbinates. The nasal conchae are four thin, scroll-like bones that fill most of the space in the nasal cavity. In the living animal the turbinates are covered by the moist, vascular lining of the nasal passages.

Their scroll-like shape helps the nasal lining warm and humidify the inhaled air and trap tiny particles of inhaled foreign material.

nasal meatus Any of the main passageways in the nasal cavity. The nasal cavity is subdivided by the dorsal and ventral nasal turbinates into three main passageways: the dorsal, middle, and ventral nasal meatuses. A small fourth passageway, the common nasal meatus, is continuous with the three main passageways.

nasal passages The convoluted air passageways in the nose that conduct air between the nostrils and the pharynx.

nasal septum The midline barrier that separates the left and right nasal passages.

nasolacrimal duct The tube that carries tears from the lacrimal sac to the nasal cavity.

natural killer (NK) lymphocytes Lymphocytes that are neither T lymphocytes nor B lymphocytes and have the ability to kill some types of tumor cells and cells infected with various viruses.

navicular bone The distal sesamoid bone of the horse. The navicular bone is located deep in the hoof behind the joint between the middle and distal phalanges.

neck The area of a bone that joins the head with the main portion of the bone.

necrotic Referring to the death of a particular portion of tissue.

neonatal period The first few weeks and months after birth.

neonate A newborn organism.

neoplasia An abnormal growth of tissue or tumor.

neoplasms Also called tumors, neoplasms are growths that serve no purpose in an organism and continue to grow to the detriment of surrounding healthy tissue.

nephron The basic functional unit of the kidney. It is composed of the renal corpuscle and the tubule system, which is made up of the proximal convoluted tubule, loop of Henle, and distal convoluted tubule.

nephrosis An abnormal condition of the kidney involving degenerative changes, particularly in the renal tubules; may be associated with protein loss in the urine, which leads to a systemic hypoproteinemia.

nervous tissue A collection of tissues that collects, processes, and conveys information. Nervous tissue includes the brain, spinal cord, and nerves. Sensory (afferent) nerves convey information about the body's surroundings to the brain, whereas motor (efferent) nerves send instructions from the brain to the body. Some nerve tissues, called mixed nerves, can perform both functions.

neuroglia Cells in the nervous system that support and protect the neurons.

neuroglial cells The auxiliary cells of the nervous system. Examples include oligodendrocytes, microglia, and astrocytes.

neurology The study of the nervous system.

neuromuscular junction The "connection" between the end bulb of a motor nerve fiber and a skeletal muscle cell. There is actually a very small space (the synaptic space) between the end of the nerve fiber and the sarcolemma of the muscle fiber.

neurons Cells of the nerves that are structurally composed of a cell body (perikaryon), dendrites, and an axon. They not only initiate nerve impulses but also conduct them.

neurotransmitter The chemical released by the presynaptic neuron that diffuses across the synaptic cleft, binds with the receptor on the postsynaptic membrane, and stimulates (excitatory neurotransmitter) or inhibits (inhibitory neurotransmitter) the postsynaptic neuron.

neutropenia A decrease in the number of neutrophils in peripheral blood.

neutrophil A granulocytic white blood cell. Neutrophils are phagocytes and are known as the first line of defense against invading microorganisms because of their fast response time to the invasion.

neutrophilia An increase in the number of neutrophils in peripheral blood.

nicotinamide adenine dinucleotide (NAD^+ or NADH) The coenzyme used in many oxidation-reduction functions. When oxidized, it is written as NAD^+. In its reduced form (having given up an electron), it is written as NADH.

nicotinic receptor A type of cholinergic receptor that binds with acetylcholine.

nictitating membrane Thin, transparent third eyelid that moves across the eye from the nasal corner laterally. A T-shaped plate of cartilage covered by conjunctiva. It has lymph nodules and a gland that contributes to the tear film on its ocular surface. No muscles attach to the third eyelid. Its movements are entirely passive.

nociceptors Pain receptors.

nodes of Ranvier Unmyelinated areas of the axon between two adjacent Schwann cells that are involved in rapid conduction of nerve impulses along the axon.

nonessential amino acid An amino acid that is produced in the body in sufficient abundance so that it does not have to be supplemented by diet. Different species produce different nonessential amino acids; therefore what may be nonessential in one species may be essential in another.

nonspecific immunity Processes that protect an animal against anything it recognizes as foreign. It involves the protective barrier of the skin and mucous membranes that prevent antigens from entering the body, inflammation, and phagocytosis. The immune system is not activated during nonspecific immunity.

nonsteroidal antiinflammatory drug A drug that relieves pain (analgesia) and reduces inflammation but that is not related to the glucocorticoid hormones from the adrenal cortex. Glucocorticoid-like drugs are commonly referred to clinically as corticosteroids. Aspirin and ibuprofen are examples of nonsteroidal antiinflammatory drugs.

nonstriated involuntary muscle An old name for *smooth muscle.*

norepinephrine A hormone secreted by the medulla of the adrenal gland under stimulation by the sympathetic portion of the autonomic nervous system. It produces part of the "fight or flight" response that results when an animal feels threatened.

nuclear envelope A double-layered membrane made of lipids that surrounds the nucleus and separates the inner nucleoplasm from the outer cytoplasm; also called nuclear membrane.

nuclear membrane *See* Nuclear envelope.

nuclear pores Pores that traverse through both layers of the nuclear envelope, allowing the passage of protein molecules in and RNA molecules out of the nucleus.

nuclei Cluster of neurons within the CNS.

nucleic acids The class of substances that include RNA and DNA and are located within the cells of all living things. They are extremely dense and are composed of complex patterns of pentose sugars, phosphoric acids, and the nitrogen bases purine and pyrimidine.

nucleolus The dark, spherical object contained within the nucleus that is the site of ribosomal RNA synthesis. Nucleoli are composed of DNA, RNA, and protein. Each cell's nucleus may have more than one nucleoli.

nucleoplasm The gelatinous substance that is the protoplasm of the nucleus.

nucleotides The combinations of phosphoric acid, pentose sugars, and pyrimidine or purine bases that make up nucleic acids.

nucleus The part of the cell that contains DNA and aids in several body functions, including reproduction, metabolism, and growth.

nutrient foramen A large channel through the cortex of a large bone through which large blood vessels pass carrying blood to and from the bone marrow.

O

obturator foramen One of a pair of large holes in the pelvis located on either side of the pelvic symphysis. The role of the obturator foramina seems to be to lighten the pelvis because no large nerves or vessels pass through them.

occipital bone A skull bone that is one of the external bones of the cranium. The occipital bone is the caudal-most bone of the skull. It forms the atlantooccipital joint with the first cervical vertebra through the occipital condyles. The large foramen magnum in the occipital bone is where the spinal cord exits the skull.

occipital condyle One of two articular surfaces on the occipital bone. The occipital condyles are located on either side of the foramen magnum and form the atlantooccipital joint with the first cervical vertebra (the atlas).

occlusal surface The surface of the tooth that meets the surface of another tooth in the opposite arcade (e.g., the surfaces between the upper and lower premolar).

olecranon process The large process on the proximal end of the ulna that forms the point of the elbow. The olecranon process is the site where the tendon of the powerful triceps brachii muscle attaches.

olfactory sense The sense of smell. The receptors for smell are located in the nasal passages.

oligodendrocytes Glial cells in the brain and spinal cord whose cellular membrane forms the myelin sheath for axons in the CNS.

oligopeptides Chains of amino acids; also called polypeptides.

oliguria Passing small amounts of urine.

omasum A component of the ruminant "forestomach" that absorbs nutrients and water.

omentum The supportive mesenteries, which arise from the greater and lesser curvatures of the stomach.

omnivore An animal whose diet is a mixture of plants and meat.

oncogene Tumor viruses containing a gene that causes malignancy in cells.

oncotic pressure The difference between the osmotic pressure of blood and the osmotic pressure of interstitial fluid or lymph.

oocyte The immature form of the female reproductive cell.

oogenesis The production of female reproductive cells (ova) in ovarian follicles.

operculum Fleshy flap of skin at the external ear openings of some species that aids in funneling sound into the ear.

opsonin Plasma protein, usually an immunoglobulin, that coats an antigen, usually a microorganism, making it more attractive to phagocytes.

opsonization The process by which opsonins coat an antigen and make it more susceptible to phagocytosis.

optic disc The area of the retina where nerve fibers on its surface converge to form the beginning of the optic nerve. It contains no photoreceptors. It is the blind spot of the eye.

oral direction Toward the mouth; opposite is aboral.

orchiectomy A surgical procedure by which the testes are removed from a male animal; castration.

organ A group of tissues that work together for common purposes.

organ of Corti The receptor organ of hearing located in the cochlea. It consists of hair cells with a gelatinous structure (the tectorial membrane) resting on the hairs surrounded by fluid. Vibrations of the fluid cause distortion of the hairs, which generates nerve impulses that are interpreted by the brain as sound.

organelles Specialized organs within a cell that carry out specific functions of that cell. Examples of organelles include mitochondria, Golgi apparatus, lysosomes, and ribosomes.

organism A living individual, animal, or plant, unicellular or multicellular, that is capable of independent existence.

origin of a muscle The more stable of the attachment sites of a muscle. When a muscle contracts, its origin attachment site(s) do(es) not move much. This provides stability so that the insertion of the muscle can move bones or other structures.

oropharynx The opening at the back of the throat through which food and air both pass.

os cordis The visceral bone in the heart of cattle that helps support the valves of the heart.

os penis The visceral bone in the penis of dogs that partially surrounds the penile portion of the urethra.

os rostri The visceral bone in the snout of swine that strengthens it for the rooting behavior of pigs.

osmoregulators Proteins that regulate and adjust the osmotic pressure between the cell and extracellular fluids. Examples include albumin and enzymes.

osmosis The passive movement of water through a semipermeable membrane into a solution where the water concentration is lower.

osmotic diuresis Diuresis produced by excess dissolved substances in the fluid circulating through the tubules of the nephrons. The excess glucose in the tubular fluid of animals with diabetes mellitus produces an osmotic diuresis that results in polyuria.

osmotic pressure The force of water moving from one side of a membrane to the other side.

ossicles Skull bones that are the bones of the ear. The ossicles are six tiny bones (three on each side) in the middle ear that transmit sound wave vibrations from the tympanic membrane to the inner ear. From outside in, they are the malleus, the incus, and the stapes.

ossification The mineralization or hardening of bone.

osteoarthritis Inflammation of a joint characterized by progressive deterioration of the articular cartilage.

osteoblasts The cells that produce bone. They develop from cartilage cells and mature into bone-producing cells.

osteoclasts Large, multinuclear cells of the bone that absorb and reshape to remodel damaged bones.

osteocyte Mature bone cell. The osteocytes are located in spaces in the ossified matrix called lacunae.

otoliths The literal meaning of otolith is "ear stone." The otoliths are tiny crystals of calcium carbonate that lie in the gelatinous matrix that covers the hair cells of the macula (the sensory epithelium of the vestibule). The otoliths help the macula keep track of the position of the head.

oval window The membrane-covered opening into the cochlea that the stapes lies against. Vibrations of the oval window membrane set the fluid in the cochlea in motion; this stimulates the sensory structures in the organ of Corti and produces the nerve impulses that are interpreted by the brain as sound.

ovarian follicle The fluid-filled structure in the ovary in which immature oocytes develop into mature ova. The lining cells of the follicle, the granulosa cells, produce estrogen hormones.

ovaries The female gonads; they produce the female reproductive cell, the ovum, as well as estrogen and progestin hormones; homologous to the testes of the male.

oviduct Also called the fallopian or uterine tubes; the oviduct, by way of ciliary movement, transports ova from the ovary (via the infundibulum) to the uterus; site of fertilization in many species; tubular extensions of the uterine horns.

ovulation The traumatic rupture of a mature ovarian follicle that releases the ovum.

ovum (*plural,* ova) The mature female reproductive cell. The ovum is released from the mature follicle into the oviduct for fertilization by spermatozoa.

oxidation When a substance is combined with oxygen or when an atom loses electrons, thereby becoming more positively charged.

oxidative phosphorylation A process that allows free energy within the mitochondria to be used in the form of ATP.

oxyhemoglobin Hemoglobin that is carrying oxygen attached to iron molecules.

oxyntic cells Slightly older term for *parietal cells;* gastric gland cells that produce hydrochloric acid.

oxytocin One of the posterior pituitary hormones. It is produced in the hypothalamus and then stored and released from the posterior pituitary gland. It stimulates contraction of the myometrium of the uterus at breeding and parturition and contraction of the myoepithelial cells of the lactating mammary gland.

P

pacinian corpuscle Tactile nerve endings located within the subcutaneous tissue of the skin. These nerves can sense deep and heavy pressure, as well as stretch.

packed cell volume (PCV) The percent of red blood cells in a blood sample; also known as the hematocrit.

pain An unpleasant sensory response caused by the stimulation of pain receptors in the body.

palatal surface The surface of the upper arcade of teeth that faces the inside of the mouth; palatal means the teeth are facing the hard or soft palates.

palatine bones Skull bones that are part of the internal bones of the face. The two palatine bones make up the caudal portion of the hard palate.

palpate To feel.

palpebral conjunctiva The transparent membrane that lines the inner portion of the eyelid.

pampiniform plexus The network of veins in the spermatic cord of the male. It is derived from the testicular vein and surrounds the testicular artery. It functions as a heat-exchange mechanism that helps keep the testes slightly cooler than the rest of the body without cooling the body as a whole. Warm blood coming down the testicular artery is cooled by the blood in the pampiniform plexus; at the same time, the blood in the plexus, which is returning to the systemic blood supply, is warmed by the blood in the artery.

pancreas Endocrine and exocrine gland that produces and secretes digestive enzymes into the intestine and produces hormones, like insulin and glucagon.

pancreatic islets The endocrine portion of the pancreas; composed of thousands of microscopic clumps of cells scattered throughout the organ; also called the islets of Langerhans.

papilla A nipplelike protuberance; in birds, depressions in the feather tracts that give rise to new feathers.

papillary layer Layer of loose connective tissue that is intimately adjoined with the epidermis.

papillary muscle Muscles in the ventricles that have the shape of a papilla. Papillary muscles anchor chordae tendineae.

paraffin A fine, purified hydrocarbon wax that is used to preserve tissue samples and support them so that they can be sliced into thin sections for microscopic examination.

paralyzed Referring to the condition of temporary or permanent loss of muscle power or sensation.

paramecium A single-celled, ciliated protozoan.

paranasal sinus A space within a skull bone that is an outpouching of the nasal cavity. Depending on the species, paranasal sinuses are found within the frontal bones, maxillary bones, sphenoid bones, and ethmoid bones.

parasympathetic nervous system Part of the autonomic nervous system that is responsible for the "rest and restore" response; also called the craniosacral system because of the location of the parasympathetic nerves emerging from the brain stem and sacral vertebral segments.

parathyroid glands Endocrine glands consisting of several small nodules located in, on, or near the thyroid gland. They produce parathyroid hormone.

parathyroid hormone (PTH) The hormone secreted by the parathyroid gland that prevents the level of calcium in the blood from getting too low; also called parathormone.

parenteral A route of treatment other than via the digestive tract, such as intramuscular, intravenous, and subcutaneous.

paresis Partial or incomplete paralysis.

paretic Referring to a part of the body that suffers from paresis.

parietal bones Skull bones that are among the external bones of the cranium. The two parietal bones form the dorsolateral walls of the cranium. They are large and well developed in the dog and cat but relatively small in horses and cattle.

parietal cells Cells in the gastric glands that secrete hydrogen and chloride ions to form the acid in the stomach.

parietal layer The layer of pleura or peritoneum that lines the thorax or abdomen, respectively.

partial pressure In a mixture of gases, the partial pressure is the portion of the overall pressure each gas exerts. It can be calculated for a particular gas by multiplying the total pressure of the gas mixture by the percentage content of that particular gas.

parturition The birth process.

parvovirus A virus of the family Parvoviridae that is highly contagious and often deadly.

passive immunity The transmission of intact, preformed antibodies from one animal to another. The antibody molecules can help protect the recipient animal from disease-causing agents. An important source of passive immunity is colostrum, the first secretion of the mammary gland after parturition. If it is drunk by the newborn within the first few hours after birth, the antibody molecules will be absorbed into the bloodstream intact and help protect it; however, after that time, the antibody molecules will be broken down by digestion and not absorbed intact.

patagium Lightly vascularized web of skin in birds extending from the shoulder to the wrist; provides elasticity to the wing during flight.

patella The kneecap; the largest sesamoid bone in the body. The patella is located on the front surface of the stifle joint in the tendon of the large quadriceps femoris muscle. It rides in the trochlea of the femur.

patent ductus arteriosus Persistent fetal connection between the aorta and the pulmonary artery that can result in congestive heart failure if not corrected.

pathogen A microorganism or substance that can cause a disease.

PCT *See* Proximal convoluted tubule.

PCV *See* Packed cell volume.

pectin (1) Dark, ribbonlike structure attached to the retina and extending into the vitreous; thought to provide nourishment to the eye. (2) Sugar polymer commonly found in fruits.

pectoralis Large flight muscle originating from the keel and inserting on the humerus; contraction results in the downstroke.

pellet Tight bundle of indigestible food components (small bones, fur, feathers) that is eliminated by regurgitation.

pelvic flexure Where the left ventral colon of the horse bends back on itself to begin the left dorsal colon.

pelvic limb The hind limb.

pelvic symphysis The cartilaginous joint (amphiarthrosis) that unites the two halves of the pelvis ventrally.

pelvis The most proximal bony structure of the pelvic limb. Also known as the os coxae. The pelvis attaches to the sacrum dorsally at the sacroiliac joints and forms the hip joints with the heads of the femurs.

penis The male copulatory organ; homologous to the clitoris of the female.

pepsin A protease activated from pepsinogen in the stomach.

pepsinogen The enzyme precursor secreted by the chief cells in the stomach; pepsinogen is activated to pepsin.

peptidase Enzyme that breaks peptides into amino acids, dipeptides, and tripeptides.

peptide A molecule containing two or more amino acids joined together. Peptides combine to form proteins.

peptide bond Covalent joining of one amino acid to another to form peptides, which are the foundations of proteins.

pericardial fluid The transudate fluid secreted by the serous membrane around the heart. It helps to lubricate the beating of the heart.

pericardiocentesis The clinical technique of inserting a needle or catheter into the pericardial space with the intention of aspirating air or fluid.

pericardium Tissue that forms a sac around the heart to protect the heart and to control the movement of the heart within the thorax.

perichondrium The fibrous connective tissue surrounding the external surface of cartilage. The perichondrium is vascularized and provides a limited amount of nutrition to the cartilage.

periderm Epidermal covering of a new feather as it emerges from the skin.

perikaryon The cell body of the neuron; soma.

perilymph The fluid that surrounds the membranous portion of the inner ear, where the sensory receptors of the inner ear are found.

perimysium The fibrous connective tissue layer in skeletal muscle that surrounds groups of muscle fibers and binds them into groups called fascicles.

perinuclear cisterna The space between the internal and external layers of the nuclear envelope.

perioplic corium The narrow band between the coronary corium and the skin located beneath the periople.

periosteum The fibrous membrane that covers the outsides of bones except for their articular (joint) surfaces.

peripheral blood Blood outside of bone marrow that is carrying blood to and from the heart and lungs in blood vessels.

peripheral nervous system (PNS) Nerves outside of the central nervous system (brain and spinal cord).

peripheral proteins Proteins located on the inside of the cell's lipid bilayer that have enzymatic capabilities. These proteins are less mobile than integral proteins because they are attached directly to the cytoskeleton.

peristalsis A rhythmic, wavelike motion that progressively moves through a tube organ, such as the small intestine. Peristalsis assists in the movement of food through the alimentary canal. It is an involuntary movement that is stimulated when the tube is distended.

peritoneal fluid A fluid secreted by the peritoneum in the abdomen. It lubricates the movement of the internal organs over one another.

peritoneum The thin membrane in the abdominal cavity that covers the abdominal organs (the visceral layer of peritoneum) and lines the abdominal cavity (the parietal layer of peritoneum). A potential space between the two layers contains a small amount of lubricating fluid that allows abdominal structures to smoothly slide over each other.

peritonitis Inflammation of the peritoneum.

peritubular capillaries Capillaries that branch off from the efferent glomerular arterioles. They flow through the kidney closely associated with the tubules of the nephron and eventually converge and leave the kidney as the renal vein. Tubular secretion and reabsorption are associated with the peritubular capillaries.

peroxidase A catalyst enzyme that converts free radicals into hydrogen peroxide, a function that is essential for cellular respiration.

peroxisome Found in high numbers in kidney and liver cells of most vertebrate animals, this single-membraned vesicle detoxifies the body by releasing catalase and other enzymes.

petechiae A small hemorrhage found on the skin, mucous membranes, and serosal surfaces anywhere in the body.

pH A chemical concept defined as the negative logarithm of the hydrogen ion concentration. It is a number that indicates the relative acidity or alkalinity of something. The pH ranges from 0 to 14. The lower the pH number, the more acidic the environment, and the higher the pH number, the more alkaline the environment. A pH of 7 is neutral (neither acidic nor alkaline).

phagocytize The eating of a solid material by a cell.

phagocytosis Ingestion of microorganisms by phagocytic cells (neutrophils, monocytes, and macrophages).

phagosome The vesicle formed by phagocytosis, which contains material to be digested.

phalangeal bones The bones that compose the digits.

phalanx (*plural,* phalanges) A bone of a digit (toe or finger).

pharynx The throat; a common passageway for the respiratory and digestive systems.

pheomelanin A sulfur-based yellow-brown pigment that produces a reddish color in hair.

phonation Voice production.

phospholipid A molecule composed of three parts: phosphorus, fatty acids, and a nitrogenous base. Any lipid that contains phosphorus. Phospholipids are the main components of the cell membrane.

phosphorylation The addition of phosphorus into an organic compound.

photoreceptors The sensory receptors that convert photons of light energy to nerve impulses that are interpreted by the brain as vision; the rods and cones.

physiology The study of the functions of the animal body and its parts. Through physiology, we can describe how parts of the body work and what their functions are.

pia mater The innermost layer of the meninges.

pigmentation The degree of coloration dependent on the concentration of melanin. Higher concentrations of melanin (pigment) will create a darker color.

pillars (rumen) Muscular folds that divide the sacs of the rumen.

pineal body A structure in the brain located at the caudal end of the deep cleft that separates the two hemispheres of the cerebrum, just rostral to the cerebellum. It produces the hormonelike substance melatonin that appears to influence the body's biological clock.

pinna The externally visible part of the ear that collects sound waves and funnels them down into the external ear canal; the ear flap.

pinocytosis The engulfing of a liquid material through endocytosis ("cell drinking").

pitting edema The condition of "pitting" or dents left behind in edematous tissue when pressed firmly.

pituitary fossa A depression in the dorsal surface of the sphenoid bone that houses the pituitary gland in the living animal.

pituitary gland The "master endocrine gland." A pea-sized endocrine gland located at the base of the brain; made up of the anterior pituitary gland, which produces seven known hormones, and the posterior pituitary gland, which stores and releases two hormones from the hypothalamus; also called the hypophysis.

pivot joint A joint that allows only a rotary motion. The only true pivot joint in most animal bodies is the atlantoaxial joint between the first and second cervical vertebrae; also called a trochoid joint.

placenta A life-support system for a developing fetus; a multilayered, fluid-filled, membranous sac that surrounds the fetus and links it to the blood supply of the uterus. There is normally no direct mixing of fetal and maternal blood, but the blood vessels are close enough to each other that nutrients, wastes, and respiratory gases are easily exchanged between the fetal and maternal bloodstreams. It is also an important endocrine organ. At parturition, it is delivered last; so it is sometimes referred to as the afterbirth.

placentome The attachment site with the uterine lining for cotyledonary placentas. It is formed from the tight connection of a cotyledon on the surface of the placenta with a caruncle in the lining of the uterus. Normally, large numbers of placentomes link the placenta with the uterus.

plane of reference Any of four basic imaginary slices through an animal body oriented at right angles to each other. They provide points or areas of reference for descriptions of direction or location. The four anatomical planes of reference are the sagittal plane, median plane, transverse plane, and dorsal plane.

planum nasale The topmost plane of the muzzle in such species as cats, dogs, pigs, and sheep.

planum nasolabiale The topmost plane of the muzzle including the upper lip in such species as horses and cows.

plaque A flat, thickened site present in the desmosomes of the epithelial tissue.

plasma The liquid matrix of blood, which contains proteins and suspended cells. Plasma also contains diffused gasses, electrolytes, and a variety of biochemicals.

plasma membrane *See* Cell membrane.

plasmalemma *See* Cell membrane.

platelets Also known as thrombocytes. Platelets are small pieces of cytoplasm that break off cells (megakaryocytes) in the bone marrow and enter peripheral blood. They are involved in hemostasis by helping plug leaks in blood vessels and initiating the blood-clotting process. The majority (two thirds) of the body's platelets are found in the spleen; the rest are circulating through the blood.

pleomorphic Varying shapes; used to describe a monocyte nucleus that can take on many shapes without dividing into distinct segments.

pleura The thin membrane in the thoracic cavity that covers the thoracic organs (the visceral layer of pleura) and lines the thoracic cavity (the parietal layer of pleura). A potential space between the two layers contains a small amount of lubricating fluid that allows the thoracic structures to smoothly slide over each other as they and the thorax itself move.

pleural fluid The transudate fluid secreted by the serous membranes of the pleural cavity. It helps to lubricate the lungs during respiration.

pluripotent stem cell Primitive cell type found in red bone marrow. It is the cell type from which all blood cells are formed.

pneumonia A lower respiratory tract infection affecting the tiny bronchioles and alveoli in the lungs. Pneumonia can be a serious disease because the inflammatory fluids and excess mucus that is produced by the irritation are difficult for the animal to cough up from down deep in the lungs.

pneumothorax Air in the chest; an abnormal condition resulting from air leaking into the thoracic cavity from the lung or the outside world. It can result in collapse of the lung in that area because of loss of the normal partial vacuum in the thorax.

PNS *See* Peripheral nervous system.

point The portion of the frog that points to the cranial surface of the horse's hoof.

polar Having the quality of defined direction.

polar body A "garbage can" for excess chromosomes. The polar body is a byproduct of ovum development in the ovarian follicle; it will not develop into a mature ovum.

polled breeds Hornless animals from species that normally produce horns. The breeder achieves this by conscientiously selecting polled offspring in his breeding lines. An example of a common polled beef breed is the Hereford.

polychromasia "Many colors"; this term is used to describe immature red blood cell cytoplasm when it is still metabolically active and has started producing hemoglobin. This condition results in both acid (red) and basic (blue) stain being taken up by the cytoplasm, giving it a lavender color.

polycythemia An abnormal increase in the number of red blood cells in circulation.

polydipsia Excessive thirst.

polyestrous An animal that has continual estrous cycles if she is not pregnant. As soon as one cycle ends, another begins.

polymorphonuclear A term that describes a nucleus that can have many shapes.

polyphagia Excessive appetite.

polysaccharide "Many sugars"; a carbohydrate containing many monosaccharides that may be released in the process of hydrolysis. Polysaccharides are divided into the two groups: cellulose and starch.

polyuria Production of an excessive volume of urine.

pons A part of the brain stem located just rostral to the medulla oblongata.

pore A minute opening or space.

portal system An arrangement of blood vessels that carries blood from one organ or tissue directly to another organ or tissue before returning it to the heart.

posterior chamber The portion of the aqueous compartment of the eye behind (caudal to) the iris.

posterior pituitary gland The neurohypophysis; the caudal portion of the pituitary gland that stores and releases two hormones (antidiuretic hormone and oxytocin) that are produced in the hypothalamus.

postganglionic neuron In reference to the autonomic nervous system, it is the second of two neurons that typically comprise the nerves of the autonomic nervous system; so called because this neuron originates from a ganglion and carries the impulse from it to the target organ or tissue.

postprandial lipemia A condition of cloudy plasma that results from small fat particles found in blood soon after eating.

postsynaptic neuron The neuron that contains the receptors to which released neurotransmitter binds, causing depolarization or inhibition of depolarization of the neuron.

precocial Chicks that are hatched with downy feathers and their eyes open and that are mobile.

precursor Something that precedes or develops into something else.

preganglionic neuron In reference to the autonomic nervous system, it is the first of two neurons that typically comprise the nerves of the autonomic nervous system; so called because the first neuron is located "before" the ganglion.

prehend To grasp.

prehensile Capable of grasping.

preload Determined by venous return, it is the amount of blood in the heart at the end of diastole just before ventricular contraction.

premolar The teeth rostral to the molars.

prepuce The skin-covered sheath around the free end of the penis.

pressure The sense of something pressing on the body surface; often combined with the tactile sense (the sense of touch).

pressure gradient The spectrum between an area of highest pressure and an area of lowest pressure.

presynaptic neuron The neuron that is stimulated by the depolarization wave to release neurotransmitter into the synapse.

primary growth center The main growth area of a bone that is developing by the endochondral (cartilage) method. Primary growth centers are the areas of bone development that are located in the main portions of the cartilage rod bone templates in a developing fetus.

primary hairs The large, straight hairs predominant in complex hair follicles.

primary structure A long chain of amino acids held together with peptide bonds.

prime mover A muscle or muscle group that directly produces a desired movement.

prion A small, protein-based particle that is both infectious and resilient yet not a living pathogen.

process A general name for a lump, bump, or other projection on a bone. Processes can be either articular processes, which contribute to joint formation, or nonarticular processes, which are usually sites where tendons attach.

proctodeum Posterior section of the cloaca of birds that is accessed by the coprodeum and urodeum and stores the excrement until it is eliminated.

product The new substance created by the interaction of two or more chemical substances.

product molecules The product of an enzyme reaction caused by the enzyme's ability to weaken the bonds of the substrate molecule.

proestrus The stage of the estrous cycle when follicles are actively developing and growing in the ovary. As they grow, the follicles produce rising levels of estrogens, which gradually produce the physical and behavioral changes that prepare the animal for breeding.

progesterone The principal progestin hormone produced by the corpus luteum of the ovary. It helps prepare the uterus for implantation of the fertilized ovum and helps maintain pregnancy once it begins.

progestins Hormones produced by the corpus luteum of the ovary. They are necessary for the maintenance of pregnancy, particularly during the early gestational period. The principal progestin hormone is progesterone.

prokaryotes Included in the kingdom Monera, these unicellular organisms have no true nucleus, nuclear envelope, or membrane-bound organelles. Bacteria and Cyanobacteria are included in this classification.

prolactin The anterior pituitary hormone that helps trigger and maintain lactation.

promoters Codes within the DNA sequence that indicate where RNA synthesis should begin.

proper vaginal tunic The inner connective tissue "sac" that surrounds the testis. It is derived from the visceral peritoneum that covered the testis during its early development in the abdominal cavity.

prophase The phase during mitotic division when chromatin becomes visible and organizes into chromosomes by joining two strands by a centromere. The nuclear envelope and the nucleoli also disappear, and the centrioles divide and replicate, traveling to either "pole" of the cell.

propionic acid One of the key volatile fatty acids produced by anaerobic, fermentative metabolism in the rumen.

proprioception The sense of body position and movement. Stretch receptors in skeletal muscles, tendons, ligaments, and joint capsules send impulses to the nervous system to keep it informed of the positions and movements of the various body parts.

prostaglandins (PGs) Hormonelike substances that are produced and exert many effects locally in a variety of body tissues. Sometimes called "tissue hormones" because they regulate biochemical activities in the tissues where they are formed.

prostate gland The male accessory reproductive gland that generally surrounds the urethra just distal to the urinary bladder. The prostate gland is the only accessory reproductive gland in the dog; so it is quite large in that species.

proteases Enzymes that break down the basic structure of a protein by hydrolyzing the peptide bonds between the amino acids.

protective proteins Proteins that are a component of the immune response, such as antibodies.

protein Large organic compounds that are composed of amino acids held in peptide bonds to form polypeptides. They are synthesized by all living things and are essential for the basic maintenance of animal tissue.

protein synthesis *See* Translation.

proteoglycan The viscous intercellular material located in the gaps between the adjacent cells in the zonula adherens. It is composed of polysaccharide chains and small proteins.

proto-oncogene A weak gene predisposed to damage by carcinogens, thus making it the predecessor to an oncogene.

protoplasm The viscous fluid found within the cell.

proud flesh The condition occurring when large amounts of new tissue, also known as granulation tissue, develops in an otherwise nonhealing wound.

proventriculus Anterior glandular stomach of birds in which chemical digestion of proteins begins.

proximal A directional term used only for extremities of the body. It implies a position or direction *toward* the body proper.

proximal convoluted tubule (PCT) The first part of the tubular portion of a nephron. Its lumen is a continuation of the capsular space of Bowman's capsule in the renal corpuscle. A majority of tubular reabsorption takes place from the PCT.

proximal sesamoid bones Paired sesamoid bones in the legs of horses. They are located in the large digital flexor tendons behind the fetlock joints (the joints between the large metacarpal and metatarsal bones and the proximal phalanges).

pruritus Itching usually caused by parasitic infestations and allergic reactions. Pruritus is purely epidermal in origin.

Prusiner Dr. Stanley Prusiner was the winner of the 1997 Nobel Peace Prize for his work with prions. He proved that prions are proteinaceous units that lack nucleic bases yet are infectious. A prion's ability to change shape is what enables it to become pathogenic.

pseudocyesis Pseudopregnancy; an abnormally prolonged and exaggerated diestrus period that results in an animal acting and looking pregnant when it is not. Most cases resolve spontaneously.

pseudopodia "False foot"; the temporary extension of the cell's membrane and cytoplasm either for locomotion or engulfing nourishment.

pseudopods *See* Pseudopodia.

pseudopregnancy *See* Pseudocyesis.

pseudostratified columnar epithelium single-layered columnar cells that appear to be stratified because of the positioning of their nuclei. These epithelia are often ciliated and are good at moving material across their surface.

pterygoid bones Skull bones that are part of the internal bones of the face. The two pterygoid bones support part of the lateral walls of the pharynx (throat).

pterylae Seven tracts of skin where feathers originate.

pubis The smallest and most medial of the three pairs of bones that make up the pelvis. The pubis forms the cranial portion of the floor of the pelvis.

pulmonary An adjective referring to the lungs.

pulmonary artery Artery arising from the right ventricle that delivers blood into the pulmonary circulation.

pulmonary circulation The part of the circulatory system that delivers unoxygenated blood to the lungs and oxygenated blood to the left side of the heart.

pulmonic valve A semilunar valve; it separates the right ventricle and the pulmonary artery during diastole.

pulp (tooth) The latticelike material in the center of the tooth; contains the nerve and blood supply for the tooth.

pupil The opening in the center of the iris.

pupillary light reflex (PLR) Reflex in which light is shown in one eye, and the pupil constricts in both eyes.

pustules Small, pus-filled elevations of the skin that are easily expressed.

pygostyle Bony plate in birds formed by the fusion of several coccygeal vertebrae; supports the tail feathers.

pyknotic The term used to describe a nucleus that has died. The chromatin has become densely compacted; so no pattern is visible.

pylorus Ring of circular smooth muscle between the duodenum (small intestine) and the stomach; regulates the movement of liquid (chyme) from the stomach to the intestine.

pyridoxine Present in the water-soluble vitamin B_6, pyridoxine is necessary for the use of amino acids.

Q

quarters (1) The common name for the mammary glands that make up the udder of the cow. (2) The medial and lateral regions of the hoof.

quaternary structure A complex protein that contains two or more polypeptide chains held together by disulfide and hydrogen bonds.

queen A sexually mature, intact female cat.

R

radius One of the two bones (the ulna is the other) that form the antebrachium (forearm). The radius is usually the main weight-bearing bone.

ramus of the mandible The vertical portion of the mandible located at its caudal end. The ramus is where the powerful jaw muscles attach to the mandible.

reabsorption The process by which some constituents of plasma that were filtered out of the plasma by the glomerulus are returned to the bloodstream. Water, glucose, amino acids, and sodium are some of the substances that are reabsorbed.

receptor In the context of the nervous system, a specialized protein to which neurotransmitter binds.

receptor-mediated endocytosis A very specialized endocytosis that only allows the cell to incorporate those materials that have protein receptor sites specifically for that material on the cell.

red bone marrow The hematopoietic (blood cell–forming) type of bone marrow.

red pulp The area of the spleen that is filled with sinusoids and macrophages.

reflex arc The reflex arc is composed of the sensory receptor, sensory neuron, interneuron(s), motor neuron, and target tissue or organ involved with a stimulus and reflex response.

refractory period The period in the depolarization-repolarization cycle when the neuron cannot be stimulated to depolarize (absolute refractory period) or can only be depolarized with a greater than normal stimulation (relative refractory period).

regional anatomy A method of studying anatomy that examines all the component structures that make up each region of the body. For example, the regional approach to abdominal anatomy would examine all the cells, tissues, organs, muscles, blood vessels, and nerves that are present in the abdomen.

regulatory proteins Those proteins essential to maintaining normal body function with insulin and many other hormones.

regurgitation The movement of food back up the esophagus toward the mouth; is contrasted to vomiting in that regurgitation usually involves undigested food and is done without the violent abdominal contractions associated with vomiting.

remiges The primary and secondary flight feathers in the wing.

renal artery The major arterial blood supply to the kidney. It is a branch of the aorta and enters the kidney at the hilus. After entering the kidney, it begins branching into progressively smaller vessels that eventually become the glomeruli.

renal corpuscle The first part of the nephron. It is composed of the glomerular capillaries and Bowman's capsule. The capsular space of the renal corpuscle continues as the proximal convoluted tubule.

renal pelvis The collection point for tubular filtrate as it leaves the collecting ducts. When the fluid enters the renal pelvis, it is in the form of urine that must eliminated from the body. The renal pelvis continues as the ureter that carries urine to the urinary bladder.

renal portal system Network of veins that transport blood from the extremities to capillaries of the kidneys before returning it to the heart.

renal vein The major vein that drains the kidney. It is formed from venules that are formed from a convergence of the peritubular capillaries. It leaves the kidney at the hilus.

repolarization The process following depolarization wherein potassium ions diffuse rapidly out of the neuron.

reproductive cells Cells found in the ovary and testicle that carry the genetic code. Each cell (called an ovum and sperm for female and male, respectively) contains one half of the genetic code apiece, which are expressed as haploid numbers of chromosomes.

reproductive system The group of organs that function to produce offspring. The organs of the reproductive system includes not only those of the genital tract (such as the ovaries and testicles) but also all the organs of the endocrine system that regulate reproductive hormones.

residual volume The volume of air remaining in the lungs after the maximum amount of air has been forced out of the lungs by expiration.

respiratory center The area in the brain stem that controls the breathing process.

respiratory system the group of organs that function to fortify blood with oxygen and remove carbon dioxide. The respiratory system includes the lungs, trachea, and the respiratory center in the medulla oblongata. Supportive thoracic muscles and the diaphragm also play important roles in respiration.

resting membrane potential The electrical charge of some cells at rest caused by differing concentrations of ions inside and outside of the cell membrane.

resting state In reference to neurons, more sodium ions are outside of the cell membrane than inside, and more potassium ions are inside the cell; it is the state of the neuron before stimulation.

rete testis A complex of ducts in the testis that conduct spermatozoa from the seminiferous tubules to the efferent ducts.

reticular cell Phagocytic cells of reticular connective tissue. Reticular cells are particularly important in lymphatic and myeloid tissue.

reticular connective tissue A form of connective tissues composed of networks of reticular fibers and cells; found principally in bone marrow, lymph nodes, blood vessels, liver, and kidney.

reticular fibers Extremely fine fibers in reticular connective tissue.

reticular groove A muscular groove found in young ruminants that conveys milk and liquids from the cardia directly to the omasum; also called the esophageal groove.

reticular layer Layer of irregular connective tissue that composes the majority of the dermis. It is intimately associated with the papillary layer by collagen fibers.

reticulorumen Pertaining to both the reticulum and rumen; often describes the contractions of the rumen and reticulum together.

reticulum The most cranial part of the forestomach; it has a honeycomb appearance inside.

retina The inner nervous layer of the eye where the photoreceptors are located. The refractive structures of the eye form an image on the retina that is converted to nerve impulses by the photoreceptors (the rods and cones). The nerve impulses from the retina are transmitted by the optic nerve to the brain, where they are converted to visual images.

retinal degeneration The progressive degeneration of the rods and cones, eventually leading to blindness. It occurs because of an inherited disease in dogs and a taurine deficiency in cats.

retractor penis muscle An elastic, bandlike muscle that pulls the nonerect penis of animals with a sigmoid flexure back into its S-shaped configuration.

retrices Tail feathers.

retroperitoneal Behind the parietal layer of peritoneum that lines the abdominal cavity, outside the abdominal cavity proper.

ribonucleic acid *See* RNA.

ribosomal RNA (rRNA) One of the main components of ribosomes that aids in protein synthesis and the combination of amino acids to create protein molecules.

ribosome An organelle composed of ribonucleic acid located on the rough endoplasmic reticulum or suspended in the cytoplasm, where protein synthesis takes place.

ribs Long bones of the axial skeleton that form the lateral walls of the thorax. Their dorsal portions are made of bone and form synovial joints with the thoracic vertebrae. Their ventral portions are made of cartilage (the costal cartilages).

rigor mortis Literally the "stiffness of death." The stiffness of skeletal muscles that usually occurs shortly after death. It results from insufficient sources of energy in dead muscle fibers to allow them to relax.

RNA (ribonucleic acid) The nucleic acid used in protein synthesis. It differs from DNA because it uses ribose instead of deoxyribose and also because RNA's pyrimidine "uracil" replaces DNA's "thymidine." The three types of RNA are transfer RNA (tRNA), messenger RNA (mRNA), and ribosomal RNA (rRNA).

RNA polymerase An enzyme that aids in transcription by converting DNA base sequences into RNA base sequences.

roaring *See* Laryngeal hemiplegia.

rods Photoreceptors in the retina of the eye that perceive dim light images in shades of gray.

root hair plexus The arrangement of sensory nerves located at the root of the hair follicle, enabling it to sense touch.

root The anchor of the hair that attaches it to the connective tissue layer.

roots of the penis The structures that attach the penis to the brim of the pelvis. They consist primarily of the two connective tissue crura covered by the ischiocavernosus muscles.

rostral A directional term meaning toward the tip of the nose. Rostral is generally used to describe positions and directions only on the head, where the term *cranial* loses its meaning.

rotation A joint movement that consists of a twisting motion of a part on its own axis.

rough endoplasmic reticulum (rough ER) The portion of the ER that is studded with ribosomes and is involved in protein synthesis.

round window The membrane-covered opening into the cochlea that functions as a pressure-relief device. When the stapes pushes on the membrane covering the oval window, the fluid in the cochlea pushes on the membrane covering the round window, making it bulge outward. When the stapes pulls on the oval window membrane, the round window membrane bulges inward. This allows the fluid in the cochlea to freely vibrate with the movements of the ossicles and stimulate the hearing receptors in the cochlea.

rRNA *See* Ribosomal RNA.

rugae Folds of the inner lining of the stomach.

rumen A large, fermentative section of the forestomachs of ruminants; the rumen is responsible for production of volatile fatty acids, microbial protein, and other essential nutrients needed by the ruminant.

ruminants An herbivore that has a large fermentative section of forestomach called a rumen; cattle, sheep, and goats are examples of ruminants.

rumination The process of regurgitating food from the reticulorumen, rechewing the food, and swallowing it again; called "chewing the cud."

S

SA node *See* Sinoatrial node.

saccule One of two saclike spaces (the utricle is the other one) in the vestibule that contain sensory structures that monitor the position of the head.

sacral vertebrae The vertebrae of the pelvic region. The sacral vertebrae fuse into a solid structure called the sacrum. The sacrum forms a joint with the ilium of the pelvis on each side called the sacroiliac joint.

sacroiliac joint The joint between the pelvis and the sacrum that joins the pelvic limb to the axial skeleton.

sacrum The solid structure formed by the fusion of the sacral vertebrae.

sacs Blind pouches.

sagittal plane An anatomical reference plane; the sagittal plane runs lengthwise with the body, dividing it into left and right parts that are not necessarily equal halves; *see* Median plane.

saliva The liquid secretion of the salivary glands. Saliva is secreted into the mouth in response to food, stimulation of the mouth, or thinking about eating; in most species, it contains enzymes and buffers.

salivary glands Glands located in and around the mouth that produce saliva; includes the parotid, mandibular, and lingual salivary glands.

saltatory conduction The skipping of the depolarization wave (action potential) in a myelinated axon from one node of Ranvier to the next node of Ranvier; means "leaping" conduction.

sarcolemma The cell membrane of a muscle cell.

sarcomere The basic contracting unit of skeletal muscle. It consists of the actin and myosin filaments between Z lines in a muscle cell. Myofibrils are composed of many sarcomeres stacked up end to end.

sarcoplasm The cytoplasm of a muscle cell.

sarcoplasmic reticulum The organelle in a muscle cell that is equivalent to the endoplasmic reticulum of other cells. It stores calcium ions (Ca^{++}) necessary to initiate the muscle contraction process. Release of Ca^{++} from the sarcoplasmic reticulum is stimulated by a nerve impulse.

saturated fatty acids Such as those found in animal fats; have no double bonds in their carbon chains and are solid at room temperature.

scapula The shoulder blade; the most proximal bone of the thoracic limb. In domestic animals, no bony connection exists between the scapula and the axial skeleton.

Schleiden Mathias Schleiden's work with plant tissue helped him to develop the cell theory, which states that all living things are composed of cells.

Schwann cells Glial cells associated with the peripheral nerves whose cellular membrane forms the myelin sheath for axons in the PNS.

Schwann Theodor Schwann was a German anatomist whose work with animal tissue helped to develop the cell theory, which states that all living things are composed of cells.

sclera The white portion of the eye; part of the outer fibrous layer of the eyeball.

sclerotic ring Bony plates that act as a protective border of the eye sockets.

scrapie A contagious and fatal disease caused by prions, occurring in both sheep and goats; the incubation period is around 2 years before symptoms, such as a disabled gait, and eventually a long illness resulting in death.

scrotum The sac of skin that houses the testes and, by raising or lowering them, helps control their temperature.

seasonally polyestrous An animal that has continuous estrous cycles during (a) certain portion(s) of the year and no estrous cycles at other times.

sebaceous glands Simple holocrine glands that secrete a substance called sebum through the hair follicle.

sebum Secretion of the sebaceous gland containing oils and epithelial cells. It is released into the hair follicle to lubricate the skin.

second-intention healing Healing in wounds that are not sutured and that form granulation tissue. Epithelialization, fibrosis, and contraction of the wound are part of the healing process.

secondary growth center Secondary areas of growth in bones developing by the endochondral (cartilage) method. Secondary growth centers are areas of bone development located outside the main portions of the cartilaginous bone templates in a developing fetus.

secondary hair The smaller, yet most numerous hairs in an animal's undercoat.

secondary structure The coiled and crimped portions of a protein's primary structure.

secretin A hormone produced in the lining of the duodenum when chyme enters from the stomach. It stimulates the pancreas to release a fluid rich in sodium bicarbonate to help neutralize the acidic chyme. It inhibits gastric motility and delays gastric emptying.

secretion The process by which a cell or gland produces and expels some useful product; also used to refer to the product itself.

secretory granules Materials that have been brought into the cell and are separated from the cytoplasm by a single membranous boundary.

secretory unit The portion of a multicellular exocrine gland that is composed of secretory cells and produces a secretion.

segmental contractions Contractions of the circular muscles in the intestine; mixes intestinal contents and slows transit of liquid feces.

selectively permeable Structures that allow some things to pass through but not others.

semialtricial Chicks that are hatched with a downy feathers, are immobile, and may or may not have their eyes open.

semicircular canals Three semicircular canals in each inner ear that are part of the vestibular system. They sense rotary motion of the head.

seminal vesicles Accessory reproductive glands that contribute various materials to semen. Seminal vesicles are present in all common domestic animals except the dog and cat.

seminiferous tubule The site where spermatogenesis (spermatozoa production) takes place in the testis.

semiprecocial Chicks that are hatched with downy feathers and eyes open but are not mobile.

senescence The process of aging.

sensory nerve Nerves that carry afferent impulses from sensory receptors toward the central nervous system.

sensory neuron Neuron carrying impulses toward the CNS.

sensory receptor A modified nerve ending that converts mechanical, thermal, chemical, or electromagnetic stimuli into nerve impulses that travel to the CNS and are interpreted as the appropriate sensation.

septum (*plural,* septa)—A partition or dividing structure in an organ or area.

serosa The outermost layer of the intestinal tract.

serous membrane A membrane that lines a serous cavity, such as the thorax or abdomen. Serous fluid produced by serous membranes help to lubricate organs.

serous secretions Thin, watery secretions composed mostly of enzymes; a transudate.

Sertoli cells Large "nurse" cells to which spermatozoa are attached during their development. Sertoli cells normally produce small amounts of estrogen hormones. If they grow abnormally and form a Sertoli cell tumor, the abnormally high amount of estrogens produced by the tumor can cause feminization of the affected male animal.

serum The fluid portion of blood that has had the clotting factors removed. Serum is produced by letting a blood sample clot before the fluid is removed.

sesamoid bones Bones present in some tendons where they change direction markedly over joints. Sesamoid bones act as "bearings" over the joint surfaces, allowing powerful muscles to move the joints without the tendons wearing out as they move over the joints.

sex chromosomes Two of the normal diploid chromosome complements. The sex chromosomes determine the genetic sex of the individual. If there are two X sex chromosomes, the individual is genetically female. If there is an X and a Y sex chromosome, the individual is genetically male.

sex hormones Hormones that target the reproductive tissues. The male sex hormones are the androgens, and the female sex hormones are the estrogens.

shaft The keratinized, visible portion of hair that extends above the surface of the epithelium.

shaft of the mandible The horizontal portion of the mandible that houses all the lower teeth.

short bone A small bone shaped like a small cube or marshmallow. The bones of the carpus are examples of short bones.

short-chain fatty acids *See* Volatile fatty acids.

sigh A deeper than normal breath. A sigh may correct a minor oxygen or carbon dioxide imbalance in the blood, or it may expand the lungs a little more than the normal breaths do. In humans, sighs can have an emotional basis also.

sigmoid flexure The S-shaped bend in the nonerect penis of the bull, ram, and boar.

simple ciliated columnar epithelium Single-layered, columnar-shaped epithelium containing cilia; found in the respiratory tract and oviduct.

simple columnar epithelium Single-layered columnar epithelium found in the stomach and intestines because of its ability to absorb and secrete.

simple cuboidal epithelium Single-layered, cube-shaped epithelium found on the ovaries and in many of the ducts of the body because of its ability to aid in secretion.

simple diffusion The ability of some molecules, such as oxygen, water, and carbon dioxide, to pass through the cell membrane without the additional aid of carrier proteins.

simple epithelium Epithelium composed of a single layer of cells.

simple gland An exocrine gland with unbranched ducts.

simple squamous epithelium Delicate, single-layered, flat-celled epithelium found in the lungs and blood vessels.

simple sugars Monosaccharides, such as glucose and fructose.

sinoatrial (SA) node A group of specialized cardiac muscle cells in the wall of the right atrium of the heart that act as the heart's pacemaker. The impulse that starts each heartbeat is initiated in the SA node.

sinus hairs *See* Tactile hairs.

sinuses Also known as the paranasal sinuses; outpouchings of the nasal passages that are housed within spaces in areas of the skull bones.

sinusitis Inflammation and swelling of the lining of a paranasal sinus.

skeletal muscle fiber A skeletal muscle cell. Because of their long, thin fiberlike appearance, skeletal muscle cells are often called skeletal muscle fibers.

skeletal muscle Multinucleated, striated, voluntary muscle that enables conscious movement of an animal; the type of muscle that moves the bones of the skeleton and is under conscious control.

skull The collective name of the 37 or 38 bones of the head. The skull is the most complex part of the skeleton. It houses the brain and all the special sense organs.

small ribonucleoproteins RNA protein complexes that remove noncoded introns from messenger RNA and splice together the coded exons to create a complete and identical copy of the DNA gene.

smell The olfactory sense; a chemical sense that detects odor molecules in the inhaled air. The olfactory epithelium is located up high in the nasal passages.

smooth endoplasmic reticulum (smooth ER) The portion of the ER that is without ribosomes and is involved in the synthesis of lipids.

smooth muscle Nonstriated, involuntary muscle having only one nucleus; the type of muscle found in soft internal organs and structures. Smooth muscle gets its name because its cells do not have a striped appearance under the microscope like skeletal and cardiac muscle cells do. Smooth muscle is not under conscious control. Smooth muscle is found in the digestive tract, where it assists with the movement of food through the gut (peristalsis).

sneeze A protective reflex stimulated by irritation or foreign matter in the nasal passages. Consists of a sudden, forceful expiration of air that is directed through the nose and mouth in an effort to eliminate the irritant.

sodium cotransport The process by which glucose and amino acids are passively reabsorbed back into circulation in the proximal convoluted tubule. These two substances bind to the same transport protein to which sodium is attached. When the sodium is actively transported into the tubular epithelial cells, the glucose and amino acids follow.

sodium-potassium pump Active transport molecule that moves sodium molecules out of the neuron and potassium molecules into the neuron to maintain the resting state.

soft palate The soft mucosal flap that extends caudally from the hard palate on the roof of the mouth.

sole The concave plantar and palmar portion of the hoof. The sole is avascular and lacks innervation.

soma The cell body of the neuron; perikaryon.

somatic cells Nonreproductive cells found throughout the body containing a diploid number of chromosomes and replicating themselves through the cell division process of mitosis.

somatic nervous system Conscious or voluntary nervous system controlling skeletal muscles; somatic motor function is the efferent branch, and the somatic sensory function is the afferent branch.

somatic reflex A reflex resulting in the stimulation or inhibition of skeletal muscle contraction.

special senses Taste, smell, hearing, equilibrium, and vision. The organs of special sense are organized into complex organs and structures that are all located in the head.

specialization The ability of an organism to differentiate to acquire new characteristics.

specialized connective tissue Tissue including bone, blood, and cartilage. Specialized connective tissue may be subdivided into supportive connective tissue (including bone and cartilage) and vascular connective tissue (including blood).

specific immunity Reactions of the immune system aimed at destroying specific antigens.

spermatic cord Cordlike connective tissue structures that enclose blood vessels, nerves, lymphatic vessels, and the vas deferens as they pass between the testes and the abdominal cavity through the inguinal rings.

spermatogenesis The production of spermatozoa in the testis.

spermatozoon (*plural,* spermatozoa) The male reproductive cell.

sphenoid bone A skull bone that is one of the internal bones of the cranium. The sphenoid bone forms the floor of the cranium and contains a depression, the pituitary fossa, which houses the pituitary gland.

sphenoidal sinus The paranasal sinus in the sphenoid bone.

spheroidal joint A ball-and-socket joint, such as the shoulder or hip joint.

spinal canal The long, flexible caudal portion of the dorsal body cavity formed by the adjacent arches of the vertebrae of the spine. It houses and protects the spinal cord.

spinal column Also known as the vertebral column; the collective name for the cervical, thoracic, lumbar, sacral, and coccygeal vertebrae.

spinal nerves Nerves of the peripheral nervous system that originate from the spinal cord.

spindle apparatus The structure that during mitosis connects to the centromeres of the chromosomes for the purpose of division.

spindle fibers Visible during the metaphase stage of cell division, the fusiform structure is made up from the microtubules that extend from the centrosomes. These fibers aid in mitosis by connecting to the cell's chromosomes at their centromeres, creating the pull necessary to divide them.

spinous process The single, dorsally projecting process of a vertebra.

spliceosomes Specialized areas in the nucleus created by small ribonucleic proteins that remove noncoded introns from messenger RNA.

splint bones The vestigial metacarpal and metatarsal bones of a horse's leg. There are two splint bones in each leg: one on either side of the cannon bone (the large metacarpal or metatarsal bone).

squamous cell carcinoma Composed of squamous epithelium, these cancerous masses are locally invasive and also may metastasize. They occur in a variety of species, most commonly on the conjunctiva, skin surface, urogenital tissue, mouth, and stomach.

squamous cells Flat, hexagonal cells that compose squamous epithelia.

squamous epithelium Epithelium composed of squamous cells.

stapes One of the three ossicles (the tiny bones that transmit sound wave vibrations across the middle ear). The stapes, or stirrup, is attached to the membrane that covers the oval window of the cochlea. It is the innermost of the three ossicles.

steatorrhea Fatty, greasy stools.

stenosis The narrowing of an opening, such as a heart valve.

sternal flexure Where the right ventral colon of the horse bends into the left ventral colon on the ventral floor of the peritoneal cavity.

sternal rib Rib whose costal cartilage directly joins the sternum.

sternebra A bone of the sternum.

sternum The breastbone; The series of rodlike bones called sternebrae that form the floor of the thorax.

stifle joint The joint between the femur and the tibia. In humans it is called the knee joint.

storage proteins Proteins that are stored for later use, such as those found in egg whites.

stratified cuboidal epithelium Multilayered, cube-shaped epithelium found in excretory tracts of the body.

stratified epithelium Epithelium composed of layers of cells.

stratified squamous epithelium Epithelial tissue composed of multiple layers of flat squamous cells; found in the vagina, mouth, and anus; possesses the ability to regenerate rapidly.

stratum basale *See* Stratum germinativum.

stratum corneum The horny layer of the epidermis lying most superficially on the skin's surface. The cells of this layer are anucleated and keratinized, being the dead remnants of keratinocytes. This is the predominant layer of the epidermis.

stratum germinativum The base layer of the epidermis, composed of a single layer of cuboidal cells that divide to replenish the constantly eroding superficial layer of the epidermis.

stratum granulosum The granular layer of epidermis containing keratohyaline and lamellated granules, located between the stratum germinativum and the stratum lucidum. This layer of the epidermis aids in waterproofing the skin.

stratum lucidum The clear layer of epidermis present only in very thick skin, such as that of the paw pads, located beneath the stratum corneum.

stratum spinosum The prickle cell layer; the weblike layer of epidermis dense with intercellular attachments located between the stratum granulosum and the stratum basale.

streak canal The passageway at the tip of the teat of the cow that carries milk from the teat sinus outside the body.

stretch reflex Reflex initiated by stretch receptors within a muscle that results in contraction of the muscle to compensate for the stretching.

striated muscle Muscle that looks striped because of alternating light and dark bands. Examples of striated muscle are skeletal and cardiac muscle.

striated Striped.

stroma The foundation-supporting tissues of organs.

structural proteins Proteins that form body structures, such as hair and collagen.

subcutaneous layer The layer of adipose tissue located beneath the epidermis and dermis that insulates and protects the body.

submucosa The second innermost layer of the intestinal tract; lies between the mucosa and the muscle layer.

substrate Substance acted on by an enzyme.

sulcus (*plural,* sulci) Shallow grooves in the cerebral cortex.

superficial A directional term meaning toward the surface of the body or a body part; *see* External.

superovulation Production of an abnormally high number of ova in the ovaries by the administration of drugs with follicle-stimulating hormone-related activity. Usually done as the first step in transferring embryos to other animals.

suppressor T cells Lymphocytes that inhibit helper T cells and cytotoxic T cells by negative feedback. They also prevent B lymphocytes from transforming into plasma cells. These cells provide the means by which the immune response can be shut down.

supracoracoideus Small, deep flight muscle originating on the keel and inserting on the top of the humerus; contraction results in the upstroke.

surfactant A component of the fluid that lines the alveoli in the lungs. Surfactant helps reduce the surface tension of the fluid, which helps prevent the alveoli from collapsing shut as air moves in and out during breathing.

suspensory ligaments The tiny ligaments that attach to the periphery of the lens of the eye and connect it to the ciliary body. They are the means by which the ciliary muscles exert and relieve tension on the lens to adjust its shape for near and far vision.

suture The immovable fibrous joint that unites most of the skull bones; also known as synarthrosis.

sweat glands Coiled glands, being merocrine or apocrine, located in the corium of all the body's subcutaneous flesh with few exceptions. The ducts of these glands pass through the dermis to the surface of the epidermis, where the sweat evaporates, aiding in thermoregulation.

sympathetic ganglion chain Series of ganglia located outside the thoracolumbar area of the spinal column and associated with the sympathetic nervous system.

sympathetic nervous system Part of the autonomic nervous system that is responsible for the "fight or flight" response; also called the thoracolumbar system because of the location of the sympathetic nerves emerging from the thoracic and lumbar vertebral segments.

symport system A system in which all of the substances are moved in the same direction.

synapse The junction between two neurons or a neuron and another target cell.

synaptic cleft Physical gap between two communicating neurons or a neuron and its target cell.

synaptic end bulb Button at the end of the axon that releases neurotransmitter; also called synaptic knob or terminal bouton.

synaptic knob *See* Synaptic end bulb.

synaptic transmission The continuation of the nerve impulse across the synapse from one neuron to another or from one neuron to its target cell.

synarthrosis An immovable fibrous joint, such as the suture that unites most of the skull bones.

synergist Something that aids the action of something else. A synergist muscle contracts at the same time as a prime mover and assists it in carrying out its action.

synovial fluid Viscous fluid formed by the lining layer of the joint capsule of a synovial joint; lubricates the joint surfaces.

synovial joint A freely movable joint; also known as diarthrosis.

synovial membrane The membrane that lines joint capsules. It is composed of connective tissue and produces a synovial fluid, which helps reduce friction in the joint.

synsacrum Strong bony plate created by fusion of the distal lumbar vertebrae, the sacral vertebrae, and the first few coccygeal vertebrae. It fuses with the pelvis and provides a stiff framework to support the legs.

synthetic phase (S phase) The period spent in preparation by the cell before cell division. The cell begins to replicate and synthesize DNA in preparation for cellular division.

syrinx Enlargement of the trachea above the sternum. Contains muscles, air sacs, and vibrating membranes that collectively form the voice box of birds.

system Groups of organs that are involved in a common set of activities.

systematic anatomy A method of studying anatomy that examines each system of the body (e.g., skeletal system, reproductive system) as a separate topic.

systemic circulation The part of the circulatory system that provides blood flow to and away from the body tissues.

systole The part of the cardiac cycle associated with contraction of the ventricles and ejection of blood into the arterial systems.

T

T lymphocyte The type of lymphocyte that is responsible for cell-mediated immunity.

T tubules Transverse tubules; a system of tubules in a skeletal muscle cell that extend from the sarcolemma (cell membrane) into the depths of the cell. They help carry an impulse caused by nerve stimulation of the muscle cell into its interior.

T_3 Triiodothyronine; the main thyroid hormone.

T_4 Tetraiodothyronine or thyroxine; thyroid hormone that is largely converted to T_3 before exerting an effect on target cells.

tachycardia An abnormally high heart rate.

tactile elevations Small elevations located throughout the surface of the epidermis, usually containing a tactile hair; important in the perception of touch.

tactile hairs Hairs sensitive to touch.

tactile sense The sense of touch.

tail glands An oval region filled with many sebaceous and apocrine glands, located over the eighth coccygeal vertebrae. It aids in signaling heat and personal identification.

talons The claws of birds of prey.

tapetum (*full name,* tapetum lucidum); a highly reflective area of the choroid in the back of the eye of most domestic animals (except swine). It acts as a light amplifier to aid dim light vision by reflecting light back through the photoreceptors after it has passed through them once.

target (hormone target) An organ or tissue that responds to a particular hormone.

tarsal bones The bones of the tarsus, Consisting of two rows of short bones located between the distal ends of the tibia and fibula and the proximal ends of the metatarsal bones.

tarsal glands The meibomian glands of the eyelid margins. They produce a waxy substance that helps prevent tears from overflowing onto the animal's face.

tarsus The joint composed of the tarsal bones; referred to as the hock of most animals and the ankle of humans.

taste The gustatory sense; a chemical sense that detects taste molecules dissolved in the saliva in the mouth.

teat sinus The large space within the teat of the cow that fills with milk when milk letdown occurs.

tectorial membrane The gelatinous sheet that lies on the hair cells of the organ of Corti in the cochlea. Movements of the cochlear fluid produced by sound wave vibrations cause the tectorial membrane to distort the sensory hairs, producing nerve impulses that the brain interprets as sound.

telogen effluvium "Blowing the coat"; the overall hair loss that occurs from the hair follicles being in a synchronized telogenic phase. It may be brought on by many factors, such as stress, medication, malnutrition, and postpartum hormonal changes in dogs.

telogen phase The resting phase of hair growth.

telophase The phase of mitosis when the daughter chromosomes return to being long-fiber chromatids, the nuclear envelope and nucleoli reappear, and the cell has completed its formation into two completely independent daughter cells.

temperature sense The sense of hot and cold.

temporal bones Skull bones that are part of the external bones of the cranium. The two temporal bones form the lateral walls of the cranium, contain the middle and inner ear structures, and are the skull bones that form the temporomandibular joints with the mandible (lower jaw).

temporomandibular joint (TMJ) The hinge joint on each side of the lower jaw (mandible) that connects it with the rest of the skull. Each joint is formed by the convex condyle of the mandible articulating with the concave articular surface on the ventral portion of each temporal bone.

tendons Fibrous connective tissue bands that connect skeletal muscles to bones.

terminal bouton Button at the end of the axon that releases neurotransmitter; also called the synaptic end bulb or synaptic knob.

terminators Codes within the DNA sequence that indicate where RNA synthesis should end.

tertiary structure The spiral, three-dimensional coil of globular proteins caused by the individual charges of the hydrophobic and hydrophilic "R" groups.

testes The male gonads. They produce the male reproductive cells, spermatozoa, as well as androgen hormones.

testosterone The principal male sex hormone.

tetraiodothyronine T_4 or thyroxine; thyroid hormone that is largely converted to T_3 before exerting an effect on target cells.

tetramers Complex proteins containing four polypeptide chains.

thalamus Part of the diencephalon that acts as a relay station for regulating sensory impulses to the cerebrum.

thermolabile enzymes Enzymes that are affected by changes in temperature and are therefore changed in structure themselves.

third eyelid The nictitating membrane. A T-shaped plate of cartilage covered by conjunctiva. It has lymph nodules and a gland that contributes to the tear film on its ocular surface. No muscles attach to the third eyelid. Its movements are entirely passive.

third-intention healing The healing process that occurs in extensive, gaping wounds that cannot be sutured. It is similar to second-intention healing but more extensive. The formation of granulation tissue and the contraction of the wound (even if incomplete) are important parts of third-intention healing. Scaring and permanent hair loss may be significant after healing is completed.

thoracic cavity The chest cavity. It is separated from the abdominal cavity by the thin, sheetlike diaphragm.

thoracic duct A large lymph vessel found in the thorax. It empties its contents of lymph into large blood vessels in the thorax.

thoracic limb The front limb.

thoracic vertebrae The group of vertebrae located dorsal to the thoracic region.

thoracolumbar system Sympathetic nervous system; so named because most of the nerves of the sympathetic nervous system emerge from the thoracic and lumbar segments of the spinal cord.

thorax Another name for the thoracic, or chest, cavity.

threshold The required level of stimulation, or degree of change in cell's electrical potential, necessary to initiate an action potential.

thrombocytes Also known as platelets. Platelets are small pieces of cytoplasm that break off megakaryocytes in the bone marrow and enter peripheral blood. They are involved in hemostasis and the blood-clotting process.

thrombopoiesis The production of platelets.

thrombus A blood clot that obstructs a blood vessel at the site of the clot's formation.

thymine (T) One of the nucleotides present only in DNA. It is a pyrimidine base that corresponds only with adenine.

thymopoietin A hormonelike substance produced by the thymus. It influences the development of T cells, important components of an animal's cell-mediated immunity.

thymosin A hormonelike substance produced by the thymus. It influences the development of T cells, important components of an animal's cell-mediated immunity.

thymus An organ that is important in the development of a young animal's immune system. It produces hormonelike substances, such as thymopoietin and thymosin.

thyroid cartilage One of the cartilages of the larynx. It is shaped as a V that forms and supports the ventral portion of the larynx. The human thyroid cartilage is commonly referred to as the "Adam's apple."

thyroid gland An endocrine gland made up of two parts located on either side of the larynx in the neck region. It produces thyroid hormone and calcitonin.

thyroid hormone The collective name given to two hormones produced by the thyroid gland T_3 and T_4. It helps an animal generate body heat; influences the metabolism of proteins, carbohydrates, and lipids; and encourages the growth and development of young animals.

thyroid-stimulating hormone (TSH) The anterior pituitary hormone that stimulates the growth and development of the thyroid gland and causes it to produce its hormones.

thyroxin T_4 or tetraiodothyronine; thyroid hormone that is largely converted to T_3 before exerting an effect on target cells.

tibia The main weight-bearing bone of the lower leg. It forms the stifle joint with the femur proximal to it and the hock with the tarsus distal to it.

tibial crest A longitudinal ridge on the front of the proximal end of the tibia.

tidal volume The volume of air breathed in and out in one breath. It varies according to the body's needs. The tidal volume is lowest at rest and higher during physical activity.

tie The process by which male and female dogs become temporarily "attached" to each other as a part of the breeding process. Muscles in the female clamp down around the enlarged bulb of the glans of the penis, making it impossible for the male to withdraw the penis for awhile. The male dismounts and turns so that the two animals stand tail to tail. The tie lasts about 15 to 20 minutes and does not seem uncomfortable to either animal.

tight junction A type of intercellular connection that is impermeable to leaks. Passage of extracellular substances can occur only through the cell itself. Tight junctions are formed by the fusion of one cell's plasma membrane to another cell's plasma membrane.

tissue A group of cells that are similar in structure and perform the same function. The four basic tissues in the animal body are epithelial tissue, connective tissue, nervous tissue, and muscle tissue.

tissue forceps A tweezerlike surgical instrument with delicate tips; used for grasping and moving tissue. The delicate tip is designed to be gentle on the tissues it grasps.

toe The most anterior region of the hoof.

tonofilaments Thin filaments that provide the structural support for certain membrane junctions. Tonofilaments are especially important in tissue that needs to flex.

touch The tactile sense; the sensation of something being in contact with the surface of the body.

trachea The windpipe; the short, wide tube that extends from the larynx down into the thorax, where it divides into the left and right main bronchi that enter the lungs. The trachea is held open by incomplete hyaline cartilage rings that are spaced along its length.

transamination The process of amino group transfer to other amino acids or within the same compound.

transcription The process of transcribing the genetic code from DNA and RNA through protein synthesis using messenger RNA.

transfer RNA (tRNA) The type of RNA that transfers amino acids to the ribosome for protein synthesis. Each of the 20 amino acids has its own specific type of tRNA, which places it in the appropriate order for the specific type of protein being synthesized. tRNA's nucleotides or "anticodons" base-pair with mRNA's codon triplets to accomplish the process.

transient cells One of the two subdivisions of connective tissue cells, transient cells have a mobile existence, traveling in and out of the connective tissue as needed.

transitional epithelium Epithelium that can expand and contract, thus enabling it to hold a good deal of volume. Transitional epithelium is found in the urinary bladder and ureters. The appearance of the epithelial cells varies depending on the level of tension on the tissue. Transitional epithelium therefore may appear columnar, cuboidal, or squamous.

translation Referring to the process of protein synthesis using messenger RNA to transfer genetic information in the form of nucleotides into amino acid form. This process occurs in the cytoplasm on ribosomes.

transport proteins Proteins that transport substances such as hormones from their origin to where they are needed.
transudate The thin, fluid-containing little protein that has been passed through a membrane. Normal serous fluid is a transudate.
transverse plane An anatomical reference plane across the body that divides it into cranial (head-end) and caudal (tail-end) parts that are not necessarily equal.
transverse process A lateral-projecting process of a vertebra.
transverse tubules *See* T tubules.
tricuspid valve Also called the right atrioventricular valve; separates the right atrium and ventricle.
triglycerides A glycerol composed of three fatty acids, which are the main storage form of water-insoluble lipids.
triiodothyronine T_3; the main thyroid hormone.
trimers Complex proteins containing three polypeptide chains.
trimesters The three main divisions of pregnancy. They are not equal thirds but give a convenient way to describe the events occurring during pregnancy.
tRNA *See* Transfer RNA.
trochoid joint Also known as a pivot joint; one bone pivots on another in a rotary motion. The only true pivot joint in the bodies of most domestic animals is the joint between the first and second cervical vertebrae.
trypsin Protease secreted as an inactive form, trypsinogen, from the pancreas.
trypsinlike immunoreactivity (TLI) test Test that identifies the presence of pancreatic trypsin in the blood; a positive test result is suggestive of pancreatic disease.
trypsinogen Precursor for trypsin secreted from the pancreas.
tubular filtrate The glomerular filtrate after it has passed into the proximal convoluted tubule. It will be called the tubular filtrate throughout its entire journey through the nephron tubules even though its chemical composition will change many times before it enters the collecting duct.
tubular gland Secretory unit of exocrine glands either containing or composed of tubules.
tubular secretion The process by which substances that the body needs to eliminate but that are not filtered out of plasma in the glomerulus are moved into the tubular filtrate. Hydrogen ions and the breakdown products of many medications are actively secreted into the tubular filtrate to become part of the composition of urine.
tubulin A protein present in the microtubules that gives support to the microtubule and also aids in the motility of the cell.
tubuloacinar Referring to secretory units of exocrine glands that possess both tubular and acinar (or alveolar) parts.
tubuloalveolar *See* Tubuloacinar.
tunica albuginea The tough, fibrous connective tissue capsule of the testis.
turbinates Skull bones that are part of the internal bones of the face; also known as the nasal conchae. The turbinates are four thin, scroll-like bones that fill most of the space in the nasal cavity. In the living animal the turbinates are covered by the moist, vascular lining of the nasal passages. Their scroll-like shape helps the nasal lining warm and humidify the inhaled air and trap tiny particles of inhaled foreign material.
twitch contraction A single, skeletal muscle fiber contraction. It can be divided into three phases: a brief latent phase, a longer contracting phase, and an even longer relaxation phase.
tylotrich hairs Tactile hairs used to aid in the perception of touch. They are located in close association with tactile elevation or "tylotrich pads."
tympanic membrane The eardrum. The paper-thin, connective tissue membrane that is tightly stretched across the opening of the external ear canal into the middle ear.
tyrosine melanin The pigment that produces brown-black colors in hair.

U

ulna One of the two bones (the radius is the other) that form the antebrachium (forearm). The ulna forms a major portion of the elbow joint with the distal end of the humerus.
ultraviolet rays Electromagnetic radiation contained within normal sunlight. Although they have beneficial qualities, such as encouraging vitamin D production, they also can damage the skin in cases of prolonged exposure.
umbilical arteries Arteries that carry carbon dioxide–rich, waste-filled blood from the fetus to the placenta through the umbilical cord.
umbilical cord The link between the fetus and the placenta. It is a cordlike structure that contains blood vessels and a drainage tube from the urinary bladder (the urachus).
umbilical vein The vein in the umbilical cord that carries oxygen and nutrient-rich blood from the placenta to the fetus.
uncinate process Projection on the complete rib that overlaps the adjoining rear rib to strengthen the rib cage.
ungual process The process on the distal end of the distal phalanx of dogs and cats that is surrounded by the claw in the living animal.
ungula An alternate name for the *hoof.*
ungulate The taxonomic classification of animals that includes all hoofed animals, both wild and domestic.
unicellular exocrine gland The only known example is the goblet cell. It is a ductless exocrine gland that secretes mucus. Goblet cells are located in the respiratory and intestinal tracts.
uniparous An animal that normally gives birth to only one offspring at parturition.
unsaturated fatty acids Breakdown products of fat metabolism. Unsaturated refers to the fact that not all the chemical binding sites of the molecules are filled. Such as those found in plant oils; have one or more double bonds in their carbon

chains and are liquid at room temperature. Examples include arachidonic, linolenic, and oleic acids.

upper arcade In reference to teeth, it means the teeth in the maxilla, or the upper set of teeth in the mouth.

upper respiratory tract The respiratory structures outside the lungs. Includes the nose, pharynx, larynx, and trachea.

urachus A tube in the umbilical cord that drains urine from the fetus' urinary bladder into the allantoic sac of the placenta.

uracil (U) One of the nucleotides present only in RNA. It is a pyrimidine base that corresponds only with DNA's adenine.

urea A nonprotein source of nitrogen used by rumen microbes; a compound produced by the liver and excreted into the rumen. One of the final products of protein metabolism.

uremia Literally urine in the blood. Refers to a buildup of waste materials especially urea in the blood because of insufficient removal by the kidneys.

uresis Expelling urine from the body; also called micturition or urination.

ureters The muscular tubes that leave the kidney at the hilus and connect to the urinary bladder. They move urine to the bladder by peristaltic, smooth muscle contractions.

urethra The tube that connects the urinary bladder with the outside world. In the female it only conducts urine. In the male it conducts urine and semen.

urinary calculi (*singular,* calculus) Uroliths or urinary tract stones.

urinary stones *See* Uroliths.

urination *See* Uresis.

urodeum Section of the cloaca that receives waste products from the kidneys and genital ducts.

urolithiasis An abnormal condition characterized by the presence of urinary tract stones.

uroliths Urinary tract stones; precipitated aggregates of mineral crystals that form macroscopic stones or sand anywhere in the urinary tract.

uropygial gland Also called the preen gland; secretes an oily substance that cleans and waterproofs feathers.

uterus The womb; where the fertilized ovum implants and lives while it grows and develops into a new animal.

utricle One of two saclike spaces (the saccule is the other one) in the vestibule that contain sensory structures that monitor the position of the head.

uvea The middle vascular layer of the eye. It includes the choroid, the ciliary body, and the iris.

V

vacuole A clear space in the cytoplasm of a cell; it is surrounded by cell membrane. Phagocytized microorganisms are found in vacuoles.

vagina The tube that connects the cervix with the vulva. It receives the erect penis at breeding and serves as the birth canal at parturition.

vaginal tunics Two connective tissue layers that surround the testes in the scrotum. They are derived from layers of peritoneum that were pushed ahead of the testes when they descended through the inguinal rings into the scrotum.

vagus nerve The nerve of the parasympathetic nervous system that is involved in regulating gastrointestinal motility and secretion; acetylcholine is the neurotransmitter of the vagus nerve.

valvular regurgitation When a valve leaks.

valvular stenosis When the opening of the valve is smaller than it should be.

vas deferens The muscular tubes that carries spermatozoa and the fluid they are suspended in from the epididymis to the urethra for emission as a component of semen.

vascularized Region of the body supplied with a blood source via blood vessels.

vasoconstriction Constriction of blood vessels.

vasodilation Dilation of blood vessels.

velvet skin The soft skin on the antlers of deer that provide a vascular source necessary during the early seasonal growth of the antler. Later in the season, the buck will scrape the velvet off, allowing the antler to harden. These hardened antlers are used for sparing with competing males during the breeding season. The velvet is often eaten by the buck because of its high nutritive value.

vent Opening of the cloaca to the outside in birds.

ventral A directional term meaning toward the bottom surface of an animal when it is standing on all four legs; toward the belly.

ventral body cavity The large space in the body that is divided by the thin, sheetlike diaphragm muscle into the cranial thoracic cavity (chest) and caudal abdominal cavity (belly).

ventricular septal defect Abnormal formation of the interventricular septum, resulting in a communication (a hole) between the left and right ventricles.

vertebra One of the bones of the spinal column.

vertebral column Also known as the spinal column; the collective name for the cervical, thoracic, lumbar, sacral, and coccygeal vertebrae.

vesicle A small sac that contains fluid.

vestibular folds The false vocal cords; connective tissue bands in the larynx of nonruminant animals in addition to the vocal cords. The vestibular folds are not involved in voice production.

vestibule The portion of the inner ear that senses the position of the head. Its sensory epithelium is contained in two saclike spaces: the utricle and the saccule.

vestibule of the vulva The entrance into the vulva; the short space between the labia and the entrance into the vagina. The urethra of the female opens into the vestibule.

vestigial structure A small, primitive structure left over from a previous stage in a species' development. The splint bones of the horse are vestigial remnants of fully developed metacarpal and metatarsal bones that were present in ancestors of the modern horse.

VFAs *See* Volatile fatty acids.

villi Fingerlike projections on the surface of the small intestine that increase surface area for absorption; contain the microvilli brush border that digests nutrients.

vincristine A drug used in chemotherapy. It is derived from the periwinkle plant and halts malignant growth of a tumor in metaphase by destroying asparagine, which is the tumor's primary source of nourishment.

virulent Capable of causing disease.

virus The simplest organism, composed of DNA or RNA, is surrounded by a protein sheath and sometimes an additional envelope. Viruses cannot live or reproduce independently; therefore they must establish a parasitic relationship with another cell to perform these functions. Individual viruses are identifiable by their antigens.

viscera (*singular,* viscus) Refers to the soft, internal organs enclosed within a body cavity, such as the lungs, kidneys, and intestines. The term is particularly used to describe the organs of the abdominal cavity.

visceral layer The layer of pleura or peritoneum that lies directly on the surface of organs in the thorax or abdomen, respectively.

visceral sensations Miscellaneous interior body sensations. They include hunger and thirst and stretching sensations from hollow internal organs.

visceral skeleton Bones formed in soft organs (viscera). Examples include the os penis in the penises of dogs, the os cordis in the hearts of cattle, and the os rostri in the snouts of swine.

visceral smooth muscle The type of smooth muscle found in the walls of many soft internal organs, such as the intestine, urinary bladder, and uterus. Its cells are linked to form large sheets that show rhythmic waves of contraction without external nerve stimulation.

vitamin D A fat-soluble vitamin essential for life in most organisms. Vitamin D enables the body to use calcium and phosphorus and is necessary for the formation of healthy teeth and bones. Vitamin D may be found in many common food sources, as well as produced in the skin when exposed to ultraviolet rays in sunlight. An insufficient amount of vitamin D can cause rickets or osteomalacia.

vitreous compartment The compartment of the eye behind (caudal to) the lens and ciliary body. It contains a soft, gelatinous fluid called vitreous humor.

vitreous humor The soft, gelatinous fluid that fills the vitreous compartment of the eye.

vocal cords Two fibrous connective tissue bands attached to the arytenoid cartilages that stretch across the lumen of the larynx and vibrate as air passes over them; also known as the vocal folds.

vocal folds *See* Vocal cords.

volatile fatty acids (VFAs) Also called short-chain fatty acids, these are the main energy source of ruminants. They are created by the microbial fermentation of cellulose in the rumen and in the colon of nonruminant herbivores. Common VFAs include acetic acid and propionate.

Volkmann's canal One of countless tiny channels through the matrix of bone that brings blood in from the periosteum to the haversian canals in the centers of the haversian systems. The haversian systems run lengthwise in long bones. Volkmann's canals come in at right angles to the haversian systems and join with the haversian canals.

voltage The potential electrical energy created by separation of opposite electrical charges caused by the cell membrane.

voluntary muscle Also known as skeletal muscle; muscle involved in the conscious movements of the body.

voluntary striated muscle An old name for *skeletal muscle.*

vomer bone A skull bone that is one of the internal bones of the face. The vomer bone forms part of the nasal septum.

vulva The external portion of the female reproductive system. It consists of the vestibule, the clitoris, and the labia.

W

wave of depolarization The opening of sodium channels starting at the point of stimulus and continuing down the length of the neuron to the end of the axon; also called the nerve impulse and the propagation of the action potential along the neuron.

white adipose tissue "White fat"; found commonly throughout the body. It is used for thermoregulation, protection, and support of the body and its organs. It is also a storage compartment for lipids. White adipose tissue is highly vascularized so that the lipids contained within can be readily converted to energy via triglyceride metabolism.

white line The white or light-colored region that marks where the wall and sole of the hoof adjoin.

white matter Myelinated axons in the CNS.

white pulp The area of the spleen that contains lymphocytes.

whole blood Blood that contains plasma and all the formed elements (cells and platelets).

withdrawal reflex Reflex arc in which painful stimulus on skin causes contraction of the affected limb; also called the flexor reflex.

wool-type hairs Hair coats composed primarily of secondary hairs, as seen in sheep.

X

xiphoid The last, most caudal sternebra. Its full name is the xiphoid process.

Y

yawn A slow, deep breath taken through a wide-open mouth. It may be stimulated by a slight decrease in the blood oxygen level, or it may just be due to boredom, drowsiness, or fatigue.

yellow bone marrow The most common type of bone marrow in adult animals. Yellow bone marrow consists mainly of adipose connective tissue (fat). It does not produce blood cells, but it can revert to red bone marrow if the body needs greater than normal blood cell production.

Z

Z line The dark line in the center of the light band (I band) of skeletal muscle. Z lines are actually disks to which the actin filaments are attached. They look like lines because of the angle at which they are usually viewed.

zonary placental attachment The type of placental attachment to the uterus that is in a belt-shaped area that encircles the placenta; found in dogs and cats.

zygodactyly Toe position in some birds in which the fourth digit is opposable and can be positioned forward or to the rear.

zygomatic arches Bony arches below and behind the eyes of common domestic animals. In dogs and cats, they form the widest part of the skull. The zygomatic arches are made up of the rostral-facing zygomatic process of the temporal bone joined with the caudal-facing temporal process of the zygomatic bone.

zygomatic bones Skull bones that are part of the external bones of the face. The zygomatic bones form a portion of the orbit of the eye and the rostral portion of the zygomatic arch.

zygote The fertilized ovum.

INDEX

A

Page numbers followed by f indicate figures; t, tables; b, boxes.

B

C

D

E

F

G

H

I

J

K

L

M

N

O

P

Q

R

S

T

U

V

W

X

Y

Z